Severin's Veterinary Ophthalmology Notes

Glenn A. Severin, DVM, MS
Diplomate ACVO and ACVIM

Third Edition
1996

Manuscript editor: Helen Mawhiney
Digital Imaging & Layout: Dennis Giddings, MS, AMI
Printer: DesignPointe™ Communications Inc.

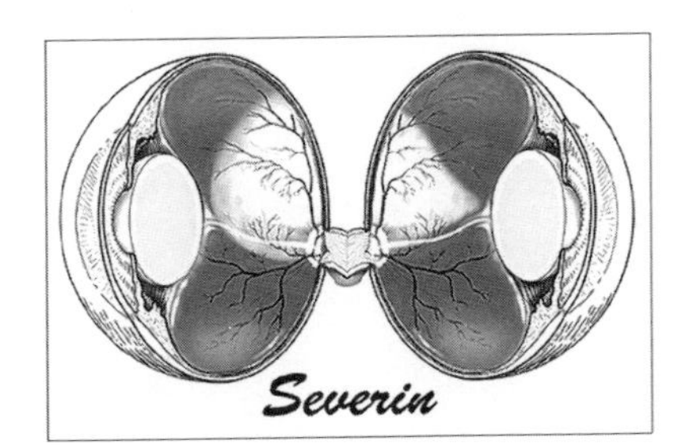

Second Printing, 1996
Third Printing, 1998
Fourth Printing, 2000

For information, address Veterinary Ophthalmology Notes, 1701 South Whitcomb, Fort Collins, Colorado 80526-1932

ISBN 0-9646143-0-8

Dedicated to my wife Joan,
without whose support this book would not have been possible.

TABLE OF CONTENTS

- CHAPTER 3 -
OPHTHALMIC INSTRUMENTS AND SUTURE

- CHAPTER 4 -
PRINCIPLES OF OCULAR SURGERY

- CHAPTER 5 -
EYELIDS

- CHAPTER 6 -
THIRD EYELID

- CHAPTER 7 -
LACRIMAL APPARATUS

- CHAPTER 8 -
CONJUNCTIVA

- CHAPTER 9 -
SCLERA

- CHAPTER 10 -
CORNEA

- CHAPTER 11 -
ANTERIOR CHAMBER

- CHAPTER 12 -
ANTERIOR UVEA

- CHAPTER 13 -
LENS

- CHAPTER 14 -
VITREOUS

- CHAPTER 15 -
RETINA AND OPTIC NERVE

- CHAPTER 16 -
GLAUCOMA

- CHAPTER 17 -
ORBIT AND GLOBE

- APPENDIX I -

- APPENDIX II -

- APPENDIX III -

- APPENDIX IV -

- INDEX -

CHAPTER 1 - EXAMINATION OF THE EYE

A routine ophthalmic examination consists of careful elucidation of the patient's ocular history, thorough examination of the adnexa and eyes in a well lighted room, followed by examination in a darkened room. Large animals should first be examined outside in bright light before bringing indoors.

BASIC INSTRUMENTATION AND DRUGS FOR A COMPLETE EYE EXAMINATION

INSTRUMENTS

Examining lights - round and slit beam
Magnifying lens - 20 diopter
Binocular loupe - Optivisor number 5 lens plate
Lacrimal cannula - 20, 22, 25, 27 gauge
Cytology spatula
Direct ophthalmoscope
Schiotz tonometer
Goniolens

DIAGNOSTIC AGENTS

Mydriatic - tropicamide 1%, and 2.5% phenylephrine
Fluorescein stain
Topical anesthetic
Irrigating solution
Goniolens solution
Schirmer tear strips
Culture swabs and transport media

HISTORY

The history should begin with determining the current changes that prompted the owner to present the patient for examination. Then, a more complete history should be taken to further assist in accurate diagnosis and management of the problem.

Presenting signs - The presenting manifestations of ocular disease fall in four categories.

1. Change in appearance of the orbit, lids or eye
2. Increased ocular discharge
3. Pain
4. Decreased vision

Additional questioning regarding presenting signs

1. Duration of lesion?
2. Are signs continuous or intermittent?
3. Are there circumstances when the signs are more severe?
4. Has any treatment been administered? If so, what was given and how did the patient respond?
5. Have there been any previous ocular problems?

General History - This is of special importance if the ocular problem is suspected to be secondary to a systemic disease.

1. Have there been previous health problems?
2. Have any medicines been given; if so, what and when?
3. Travel history

LIGHT ROOM EXAMINATION

Light room examination consists of evaluating the eye and surrounding structures in a systematic fashion. Overhead lighting from a surgery light is excellent. If this is not available, a transilluminator or penlight should be used.

GROSS APPEARANCE OF THE EYES AND FACE

Avoid contact with conjunctival surfaces to prevent contamination. Determine if the lesions are unilateral or bilateral. Check for:

Ocular discharge

1. Epiphora (tearing) - from irritation to the eye or obstruction of lacrimal drainage system
2. Inflammatory discharge - due to conjunctivitis, blepharitis or keratitis
3. Evaporative residue - mucous and cellular debris buildup from keratoconjunctivitis sicca
4. Reflux drainage - dacryocystitis

Size of the eye

1. Smaller than normal - microphthalmia or acquired phthisis bulbi
2. Normal
3. Larger than normal - macrophthalmia or chronic glaucoma (buphthalmos)

Position of the eye

1. Enophthalmos will occur:
    a. If the eye is smaller than normal
    b. From contraction of extrinsic muscles of the eye - ocular pain caused by corneal ulcer or injury, anterior uveitis, or posterior episcleritis
    c. From relaxation of sympathetic smooth muscles - Horner's syndrome
    d. From loss of tissue mass in the orbit (dehydration, absorption of postorbital fat)
2. Exophthalmos - space-occupying lesions of the orbit, extrinsic muscle degeneration, deformity of the orbit and shallow orbit because of breed predisposition. This can be evaluated by visual examination, palpation and digital retropulsion of the eye through the upper eyelid.
3. Strabismus - deviation of the eye that the patient cannot overcome
    a. Esotropia (crossed eyes) - seen most frequently in Siamese cats and occasionally in dogs
    b. Exotropia (lateral deviation) - dogs, most common in brachycephalic breeds (Boston terrier, Pekingese, pug). Cats, rare. Herbivore, common.
    c. Hypertropia - upward deviation of the eye
    d. Hypotropia - downward deviation of the eye

Periorbital swelling - Allergic reactions, orbital infections, neoplasia or trauma. The eye is in normal position, but swelling in the lids and adjacent tissues may make it appear similar to exophthalmos.

INITIAL PROCEDURES

Quickly evaluate the eyelids and globe to determine what diagnostic tests may be required.

Microbial cultures and tear formation measurement must be done at the beginning of the examination because other examination procedures may invalidate their results. Swabs for conjunctivitis can be taken from the inferior cul-de-sac. If ulcers are present, it is recommended to make the swab from the ulcer.

Bacterial cultures and sensitivity - Aerobic cultures are routinely indicated. Anaerobic cultures should also be considered in dacryocystitis. Commercial systems such as Culturette (Fig 1-1) can be refrigerated and will preserve organisms several hours. Unfortunately, ocular cultures frequently have small numbers, therefore culture plates should be inoculated ASAP.

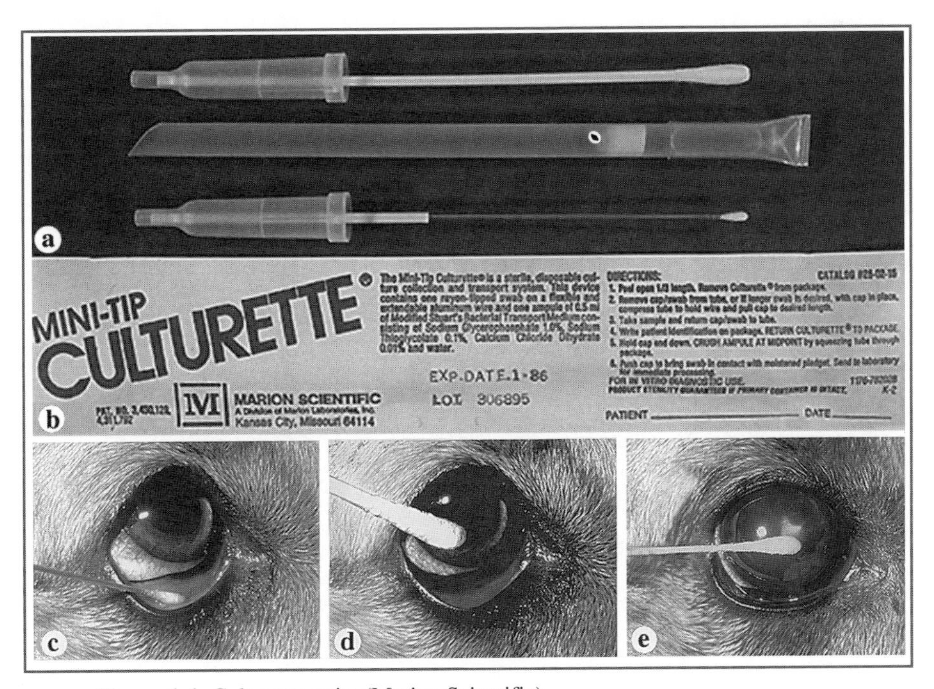

Figure 1-1. Culturette units (Marion Scientific).
- a. Standard and MINI-TIP culturette swabs
- b. MINI-TIP culturette packet
- c. Collecting culture from inferior cul-de-sac with MINI-TIP swab
- d. Collecting corneal culture with standard swab
- e. Collecting corneal culture with MINI-TIP swab

Fungal cultures - Most ocular pathogens are saprophytic fungi that require enriched medium such as Sabouraud's enriched media or blood agar. Separate swabs should be submitted.

Viral cultures - Swabs should be taken from the conjunctiva and/or cornea and placed in viral transport media. The diagnostic laboratory you are using should be contacted for the transport media they recommend (or provide). Transport media will keep virus viable at least 7 to 10 days. Swabs should be refrigerated (4°C) or kept on wet ice, viruses will remain viable for three to four days. Freeze-thaw cycles destroy virus (decrease numbers).

Schirmer tear test

1. Materials (Fig 1-2)
   - a. Commercial tear testing strips - standardized strips, Sno Strips (Akorn), Color Bar (Eagle Vision, Schering-Plough)
   - b. Strips can be made from #40 Whatman filter paper (5 x 40 mm strips with a notch 5 mm from the end)

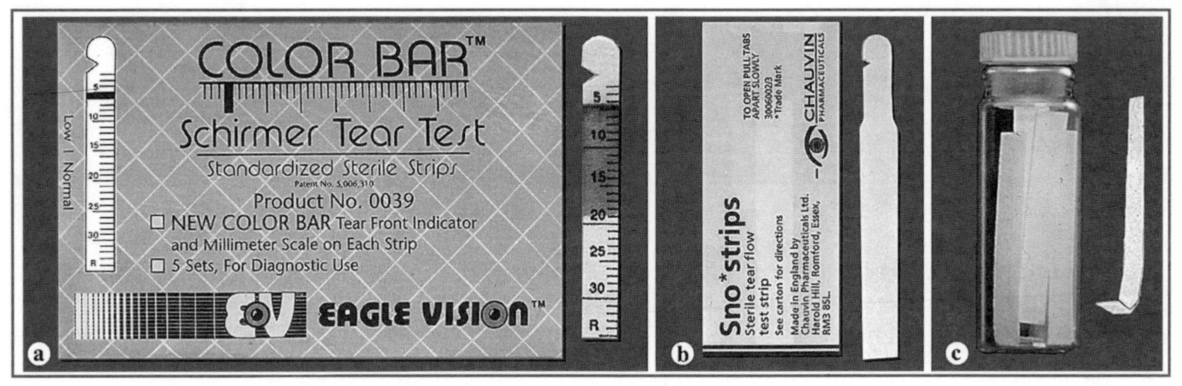

Figure 1-2. Schirmer tear test strips.

a. Color Bar™ standardized sterile strips (Eagle Vision) - envelope containing 5 sets and a strip turned blue with moisture.
b. Sno Strips (many sources e.g. MWI) - packet and individual strip
c. Tear test strips cut from #40 Whatman filter paper

2. Schirmer tear test without anesthetic (STT). This is the routine test done in animals. It measures basal tear production and the tear response from the Schirmer strip in the eye.
   a. Place 5 mm tip between lower eyelid and cornea. Hold the eyelids closed. Leave in place 1 minute (5 minutes in man).
   b. Immediately after removing the strip from the eye, measure the amount of moisture on the strip, excluding the 5 mm tip that touched the eye. The moistened area of the strip becomes transparent. If the strip is placed on the millimeter measuring scale with the notch at zero, the scale can be read through the transparent area.
3. Interpretation
   a. Small animals - cats are usually 2 to 3 mm less than dogs
      1) 9 or more: normal. Most dogs and cats exceed 17 mm.
      2) 5 to 9: probably decreased. Dogs and cats can have as little as 5 mm and appear healthy.
      3) Less than 5 mm is definitely decreased formation. Severely affected patients will not even moisten the 5 mm tip.
   b. Large animals - most have abundant tears, with as much as 20 mm in 30 seconds
      1) Normal: exceeds 15 mm/min
      2) Suspect: 10-15 mm/min
      3) Abnormal: less than 10 mm/min
4. Schirmer tear test with topical anesthetic (STTa).
   a. Seldom done in animals. Measures the basal tear production after topical anesthesia and drying the inferior cul de sac with a cotton swab. The normal value in dogs should be > 5 mm in 60 seconds.

SYSTEMATIC EXAMINATION OF ADNEXA AND ANTERIOR SEGMENT

A binocular loupe is recommended for this examination. The animals should be handled so that excitement is kept to a minimum. If only one eye is involved, always examine the normal eye first. The order of examination and signs to be considered are:

Eyelids

1. Blepharitis - discharge, discoloration, swelling, and loss of hair
2. Blepharospasm - blepharospasm results from pain (superficial or intraocular) or from constant facial nerve stimulation. It may lead to entropion.
3. Entropion - moderate to severe pain, lacrimal discharge, corneal changes
4. Ectropion - discharge and conjunctivitis
5. Eyelash diseases - lacrimation, pain, entropion and/or superficial corneal disease

6. Lagophthalmos - observed with protruding eyes and facial nerve paralysis. It predisposes to exposure keratitis.
7. Ptosis - seen with Horner's syndrome and oculomotor nerve paralysis
8. Lacrimal drainage - increased tear formation or failure of nasolacrimal system
9. Neoplasms

Third eyelid (nictitating membrane) - normally not prominent but may appear more prominent if nonpigmented or protruding.

1. Follicular conjunctivitis and folliculitis
2. Eversion of the cartilage
3. Prolapse of gland of third eyelid
4. Conjunctival hyperplasia
5. Neoplasms
6. Protrusion

Conjunctiva - examine for:

1. Vascularity
2. Edema (chemosis)
3. Surface moisture
4. Subconjunctival hemorrhage
5. New growths
6. Foreign bodies

Sclera - examine for degree of vascularity and new growths

1. Diffuse anterior episcleritis
2. Nodular scleritis
3. Necrotizing scleritis
4. Nodular fasciitis
5. Thinning from glaucoma
6. Erosion from intraocular tumors
7. Traumatic injury
8. Scleral melanosis and melanomas

Cornea - normally a clear avascular structure

1. Loss of transparency (leukoma)
    a. Edema
    b. Inflammatory cell invasion (corneal abscess)
    c. Scar tissue
2. Development of vascularity
    a. Superficial
    b. Deep
3. Cellular infiltration
    a. Pigment
    b. New growths
4. Ulceration
5. Change of contour (keratoconus, keratoglobus)

Anterior chamber - is altered when the tissues forming it are diseased (cornea, iris or lens)

1. Depth

   a. Deep - posterior lens luxation, small lens, chronic glaucoma. A deep anterior chamber occurs naturally in cats and some breeds of dogs.
   b. Shallow - iris bombé, anterior synechia, anterior lens displacement and anterior uveal tumors
2. Contents
   a. Blood (hyphema)
   b. Pus (hypopyon)
   c. Fibrin (plasmoid aqueous)
   d. Lipid aqueous
   e. Abnormal tissues (pigment epithelium cysts, tumors and granulomas)
   f. Foreign bodies
3. Filtration angle
   a. Width of angle (narrow or wide)
   b. Congenital abnormality (goniodysgenesis)
   c. Acquired obstruction (tumors, peripheral anterior synechia)

Iris - examine for:

1. Congenital conditions that affect the appearance but do not necessarily interfere with sight
   a. Polycoria - more than one pupil
   b. Coloboma - fissure in the iris
   c. Heterochromia - multicolored iris
   d. Thin iris - hypoplasia is seen in blue-eyed animals
2. Congenital conditions that may affect sight
   a. Persistent pupillary membrane
   b. Severe abnormal iris development (absence of pupil, aniridia)
3. Size of pupil - see pupillary light response
   a. Anisocoria (unequal pupils) - may result from unilateral constriction or dilation
   b. Mydriasis (dilated pupil)
      1) Unilateral - glaucoma, topical drug effects, efferent nerve dysfunction, or iris sphincter dysfunction (iris atrophy)
      2) Bilateral - bilateral retinal and optic nerve diseases, systemic drug effect, optic chiasm or brain lesions affecting pupillary reflex pathway
   c. Miosis (constricted pupil) - anterior uveitis, drugs, or Horner's syndrome
   d. Hippus (rhythmic contraction and dilation of pupil)
4. Reflectivity of light and change in color - inflammation results in a darkened iris
5. Synechia - anterior or posterior
6. Acquired atrophy

Lens - normally not seen until aging changes occur

1. Size
   a. No lens - aphakia
   b. Small lens - microphakia
   c. Large lens - intumescent cataracts
2. Position - displacement (luxation or subluxation)
   a. Anterior - may push the iris forward to cause shallow anterior chamber or luxate into anterior chamber
   b. Posterior - results in a deep anterior chamber
   c. Subluxation along equator - causes an uneven iris surface and a tremor of the iris may occur when the head is moved (iridodonesis)
3. Opacities (cataract)
   a. Acquired cataracts
   b. Developmental cataracts
4. Lenticular sclerosis - a natural aging change that is most prominent in the nucleus

Vitreous - normally not seen unless changes are present

1. Congenital abnormalities
   a. Persistent hyaloid artery
   b. Hyaloid remnants
2. Acquired opacities
   a. Vitreous floaters after uveal or retinal infections
   b. Transudates/exudates - acute pars planitis or posterior segment disease
   c. Asteroid hyalosis - small white opacities suspended in the vitreous
3. Liquefaction (syneresis)
   a. Syneresis is the process of the liquefaction of vitreous. Synchysis is the liquefied state after syneresis. Syneresis may result from lenticular displacement, as a degenerative change, or after hemorrhage into the vitreous. Syneresis predisposes to retinal detachment.
   b. Synchysis scintillans - the falling snow effect seen behind the lens after liquefaction of the vitreous. As the vitreous liquefies, opaque material may be present. If the eye is moved, this material will rise and then slowly settle.

BASIC NEUROLOGIC TESTS

Oculocephalic reflex (vestibulo-ocular reflex or VOR, doll's head reflex). This tests cerebellum, oculomotor n., and abducens n. Move the head gently from side to side. Note the slow and fast nystagmus. Slow will be away from the direction of the head movement and fast will be in the same direction as the head movement.

Blink reflex (tests trigeminal n. - afferent; facial n - efferent).

1. Tap the medial canthus, or
2. Touch the conjunctiva (conjunctival reflex), or
3. Touch the cornea with a wisp of cotton or Q-tip (corneal reflex)

The animal should blink and possibly move its head to avoid the stimulus. If the cornea or conjunctiva are sensitive (trigeminal n.) but the eyelids are paralyzed (facial nerve disease), the eye will be retracted by the extrinsic muscles of the eye but there will not be a blink.

Nystagmus - evaluate for resting or position changes.

Oculocardiac reflex - decrease in heart rate due to vagal inhibition when pressure is applied to the eye or the eye manipulated during surgery.

Anisocoria - Observe for symmetry of pupil sizes in room light. In a darkened room, observe for equal dilatation. This can be easily accomplished by standing at arm's length from the animal and looking through a direct ophthalmoscope set on 0.

Visual tests - **See Chapter 1, page 60**

1. Menace reflex
2. Moving object
3. Dazzle reflex
4. Maze testing

PUPILLARY LIGHT REFLEXES (PLR)

Pupillary motion is a dynamic process; the stronger parasympathetic sphincter is dominant and the weaker sympathetic dilator is subordinate.

PLR pathway. The neuronal pathway for the pupillary light reflex and vision has the same origin in the retina. See Fig 1-3 Optic pathway.

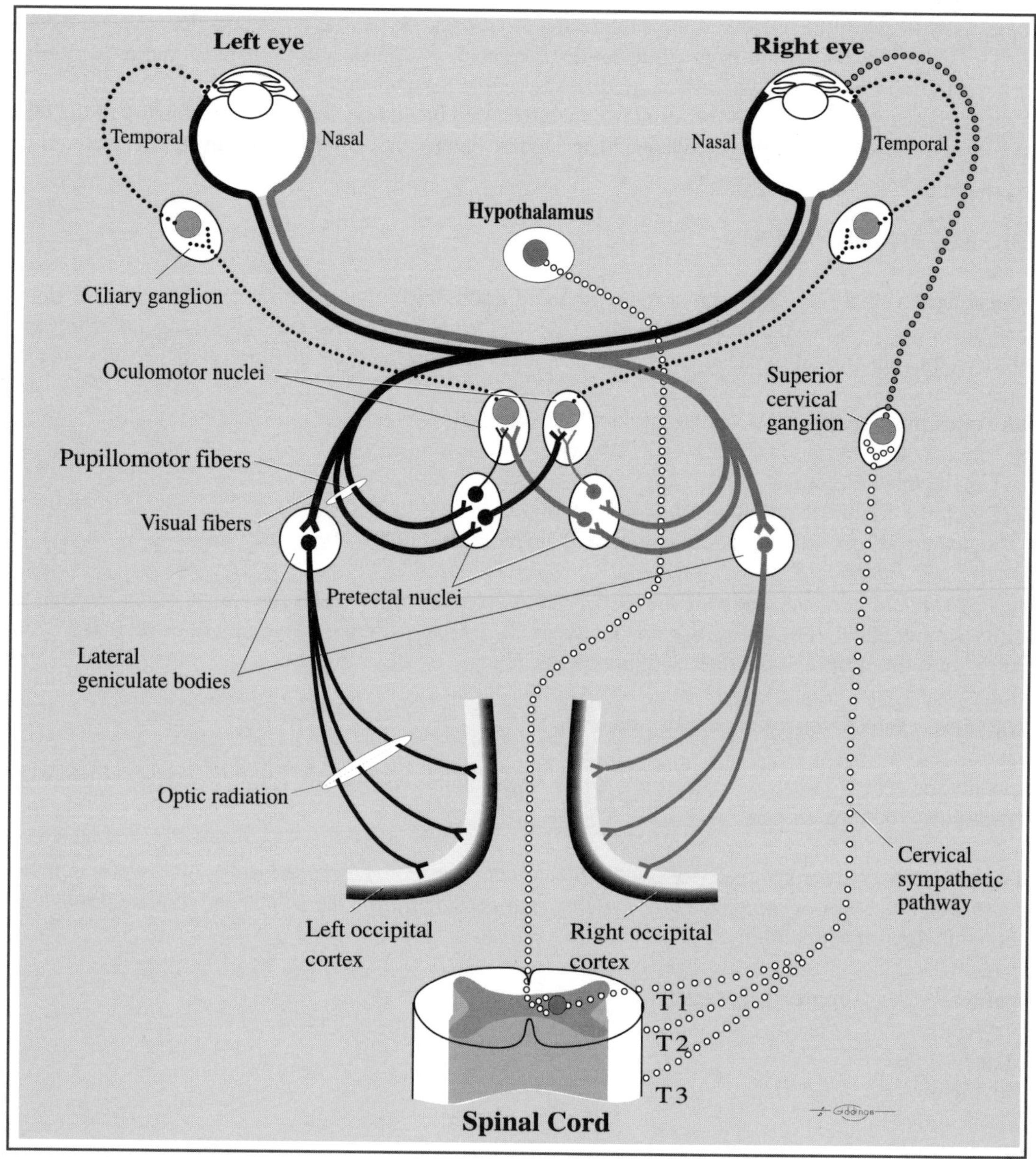

Figure 1-3. Optic pathway.

The pupillary light reflex is entirely subcortical. Approximately 20% of the fibers leave the optic tract before the visual fibers synapse at the lateral geniculate body. These fibers synapse at the pretectal nucleus. The majority go to the contralateral parasympathetic oculomotor nucleus and the remaining fibers go to the ipsilateral oculomotor nucleus. The efferent pupillary reflex pathway leaves via the oculomotor nerve (CN-III), going to the ciliary ganglion and from there to the iris sphincter by means of the short ciliary nerve.

The pupillary dilator muscle is supplied by the cervical sympathetic pathway and controlled by the hypothalamus. It does not play an active part in the pupillary light reflex.

1. The *afferent* pathway is a three-neuron system
   a. First order neurons are composed of photoreceptors and bipolar cells
   b. Second order neurons are the retinal ganglion cells that extend beyond the eye as the optic nerve. At the optic chiasm, decussation (crossover) of nerve fibers occurs. In man, decussation is 50%, cats 65%, dogs 75%, horses and cattle 83%, and in most nonmammalian species 100%. The pupillomotor fibers leave the optic tract near the lateral geniculate body and synapse in the pretectal nucleus.
   c. Third order neuron fibers from the pretectal nucleus again decussate; the majority go to the contralateral parasympathetic oculomotor nucleus (CN-III) and fewer go to the ipsilateral nucleus.
2. The *efferent* pathway is a two-neuron parasympathetic pathway
   a. Preganglionic fibers accompany CN-III until they leave to synapse at the ciliary ganglion
   b. Postganglionic fibers are the short ciliary nerves. In the dog there are five to eight and in the cat there are two, a medial and lateral ciliary nerve.

PLR technique (Fig 1-4)

This test can be performed in a light or dark room but is more sensitive in a dark room. A strong focal light should be used for best results. The animal should be calm and time should be allowed for it to adjust to the examination room.

1. Direct - The direct response of an eye to a light
   a. Carnivores have a brisk response to light that results in rapid miosis. The strongest response will occur when the light is directed at the area centralis. A normal dog will dilate to less than 5 mm with a bright light. Cats have the most rapid constriction but may take longer to dilate when light stimulation ceases.
   b. Herbivores have a slower PLR, especially horses. This should not be misinterpreted as a pathologic change.
2. Indirect (consensual) reflex - The response of the pupil of an eye when a light is directed in the other eye. In domestic animals, the indirect PLR is less prominent than the direct PLR because of the decussation, which results in more efferent pupillomotor fibers that return to the ipsilateral side of the brain. This is referred to as dynamic contraction anisocoria. The difference is most noticeable in horses and least noticeable in cats.
3. Swinging light test. Directing a light into an eye for two to four seconds and then redirecting it in the other eye for an equal time.
   a. Normal - When moving the light source from one eye to the next, the newly illuminated pupil should always be semiconstricted and then constrict down more when the light hits it.
   b. Abnormal - If the newly illuminated pupil dilates under direct illumination, the eye is abnormal (a positive swinging light test). This is diagnostic of a prechiasmal lesion in the affected eye.

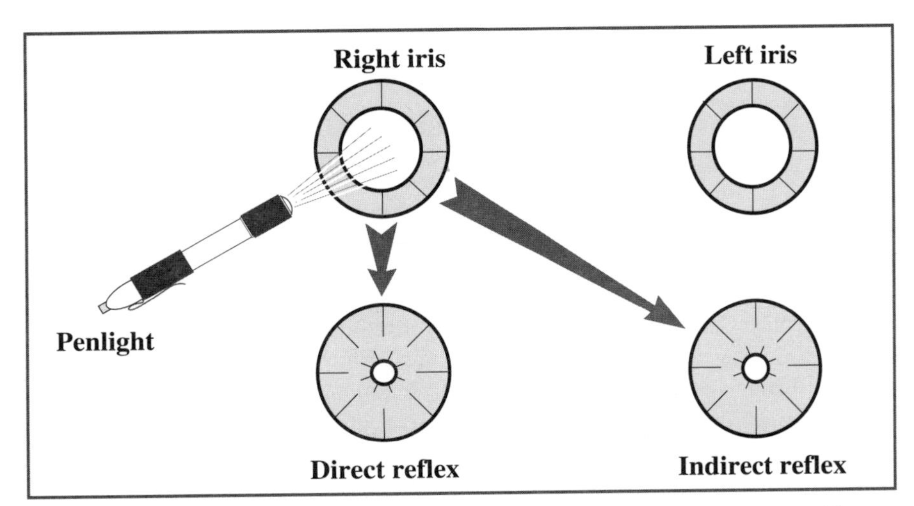

Figure 1-4. Pupillary light reflexes. Direct and indirect reflexes are demonstrated for a light beam directed into the right eye.

Interpretation of the pupillary reflexes

1. Positive direct reflex indicates:
   a. The afferent pupillary reflex pathway of the stimulated eye is intact. It requires that the retina and the optic nerve are functional to the level of the optic chiasm but does not discriminate if there is any unilateral dysfunction between the optic chiasm and the oculomotor nucleus.
   b. The efferent pathway and the pupillary constrictors to the eye are functional
   c. A positive direct reflex does not indicate the patient can see.
2. Positive indirect reflex indicates:
   a. The afferent pupillary reflex pathway of the stimulated eye is functional
   b. The efferent pathway and the pupillary constrictors of the consensual eye are functional
3. Differential diagnosis of a miotic pupil
   a. Pharmacologic - miotic agents (parasympathomimetics)
   b. Parasympathetic afferent nerve stimulation - ocular pain (anterior uveitis, ocular trauma)
   c. Sympathetic efferent nerve failure (Horner's syndrome)
4. Differential diagnosis of a dilated pupil - iridoplegia is dysfunction of the iris sphincter.
   a. Pharmacologic - mydriatic agents (parasympatholytics) that cause sphincter end-organ dysfunction or adrenergics stimulating the dilator muscle
   b. Efferent nerve dysfunction - damage to parasympathetic fibers or oculomotor nerve nucleus (blunt trauma, dysautonomia). Pharmacologic testing is beneficial when differentiating dysautonomia (Key-Gaskell syndrome) from other causes of a dilated pupil (Table 1-1).
   c. Bilateral afferent nerve dysfunction - retina, optic nerve, chiasm, optic tracts
   d. Iris disease - synechia, iris sphincter atrophy

Table 1-1. Pharmacologic testing for dysautonomia

Effect on pupil	**Normal**	**Dysautonomia**
Pilocarpine 1% (direct action)	None or slight	Immediate miosis
Echothiophate 0.06% (indirect action)	Miosis 10-15 min	No change
Effect on third eyelid		
Epinephrine 1:10,000*	No change	Immediate retraction
Cocaine 10%	Retraction	No change

*Epinephrine 1:10,000 does not affect the pupil of the normal or dysautonomic animal.

Re-examine anterior segment

Using a penlight or transilluminator, examine all structures previously examined in the light room examination. Give special attention to the cornea, anterior chamber and iris. Subtle changes may be seen that were not noticed in the lighted room.

Dilate the pupil

1. Normal eyes - Tropicamide 1% is preferred. Two applications 10 minutes apart should dilate the pupil in 20 to 30 minutes
2. Slow-to-dilate pupils - anticipated with anterior uveitis, puppies, color-dilute eyes with microphthalmia
   a. Phenylephrine 2.5%; administer 1 to 2 minutes after tropicamide
   b. Murocoll 2 (10% phenylephrine and 0.3% scopolamine, Muro Co). Administer at 10 minute intervals. The drop is irritating and may maintain mydriasis in a normal eye as long as four days.
   c. Horses with severe anterior uveitis - subconjunctival injection of 1 mg atropine and 5 mg phenylephrine is very effective

While waiting for mydriasis - Special examinations that would be deemed appropriate for this patient can be performed.

EXAMINATION AFTER MYDRIASIS

Transillumination - The cornea, anterior chamber, lens and vitreous can be examined with a penlight or transilluminator.

1. Purkinje-Sanson reflexes - The examining light will produce three reflections (images) (Fig 1-5).
   a. The larger and most superficial reflection is from the cornea
   b. The second originates from the anterior lens capsule
   c. The deepest originates from the posterior lens capsule
   d. *Comment* - If the light is moved, the images formed by the cornea and anterior lens capsule move with the direction of motion of the light. The image from the posterior capsule moves in the opposite direction. The images are valuable in determining the depth of the anterior chamber and the thickness of the lens.

      If a biomicroscope or similar magnifying instrument is used, two corneal reflexes instead of one are seen, one on the anterior lens surface and the other at the endothelium.

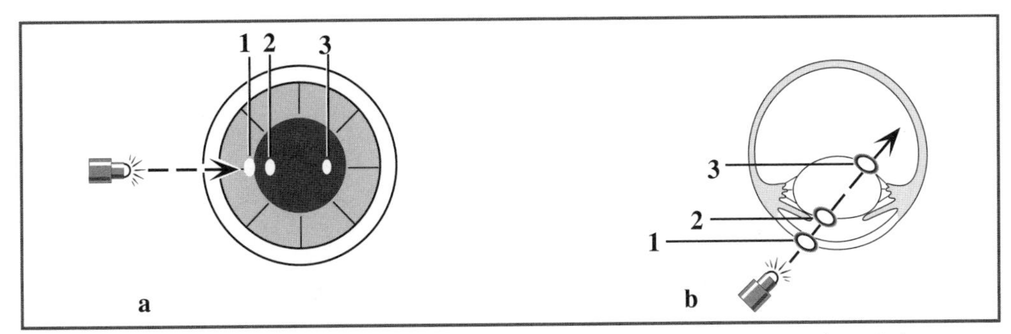

Figure 1-5. Purkinje-Sanson reflexes (images). When a focal beam of light passes through the eye, reflection will result from: 1) the cornea, 2) anterior lens capsule, and 3) posterior lens capsule.
a. Anterior view
b. Cross-sectional view

2. Corneal examination. With the observer located in front of the eye, light directed transversely from the temporal side will result in slight translucency of the cornea. If there are corneal opacities, they will be readily visible against the dark background of the dilated pupil.
3. Anterior chamber examination. With the observer located in front of the eye, a slit or small round beam of light directed at a 45° angle to the eye will not result in any internal reflection of light from the aqueous. Therefore, the anterior chamber will appear clear. If there are any solids (protein, cells) in the aqueous, there will be reflection of light from these particles (Tyndall effect) (Fig 1-6). This reflection is referred to as flare and may be graded + for slight to ++++ when severe.

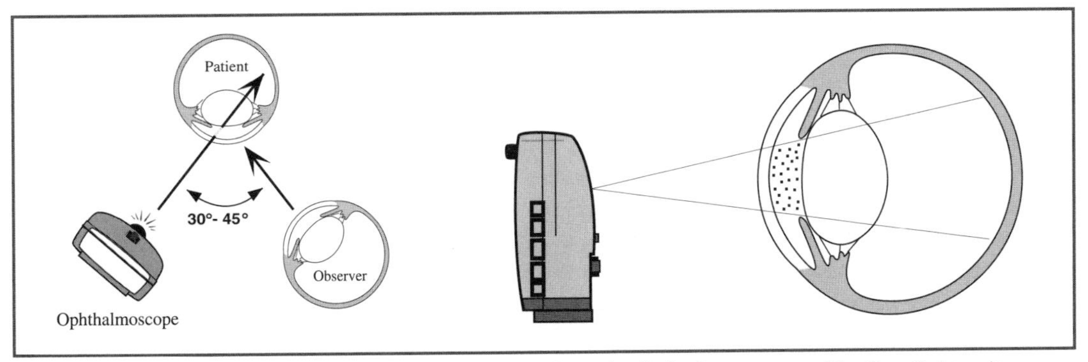

Figure 1-6. Aqueous flare. In an inflamed eye, protein and cells in the aqueous will reflect light as it passes through. This is referred to as aqueous flare.

4. Lens examination

Transillumination. The examiner is located in front of the eye and a beam of light directed at the lens with a 45 degree angle to transilluminate the lens (Fig 1-7a).

Retroillumination. The lens visualized through an ophthalmoscope with examiner in front of patient using round beam of light (Fig 1-7b).

a. *Normal "Y" suture visualization.* The normal "Y" sutures are easily seen in young dogs using transillumination. The anterior is upright and the posterior inverted (Fig 1-7a.1). The posterior Y sutures are more readily seen than the anterior. Normal Y sutures cannot be seen with an ophthalmoscope (Fig 1-7b.1).

b. *Nuclear sclerosis.* With transillumination of patients with nuclear sclerosis, the nucleus will have a gray translucence and the cortex will remain clear (Fig 1-7a.2, 1-7a.3). If the lens is viewed through an ophthalmoscope, the lens will appear clear with the pupil filled with tapetal reflex and a junction ring will be seen at the nuclear-cortical junction (Figs 1-7b.2, 1-7b.3).

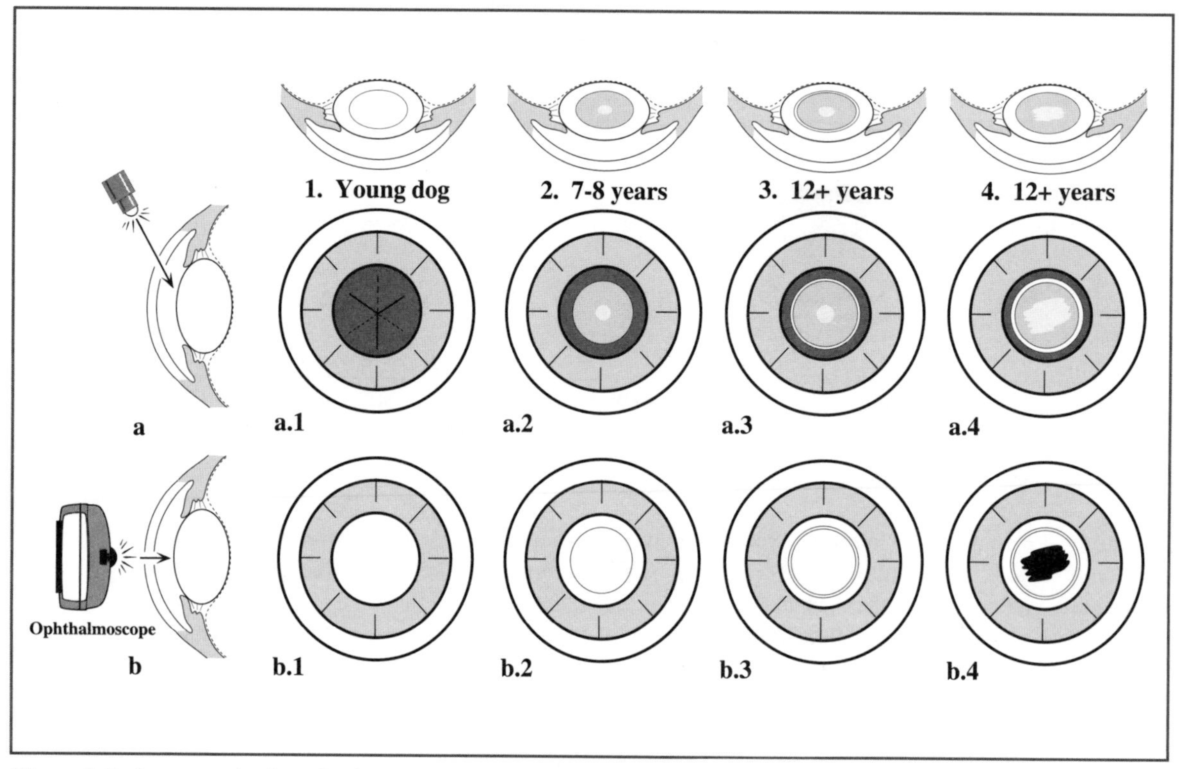

Figure 1-7. Lens examination of a dog: 1. young; 2. eight years with beginning nuclear sclerosis; 3. 12 years, with advanced nuclear sclerosis; 4. 12 years with early nuclear cataract and nuclear sclerosis.
a. Examination with transilluminator
b. Examination with an ophthalmoscope set at 5D and positioned 8 inches from the patient.

c. *Attachment of the suspensory ligaments to the lens equator* (Fig 1-8). The lens equator and zonular attachment can be visualized in an eye with a well dilated pupil. Aided with a focal light beam, the examiner should look across the eye from the limbus toward the opposite edge of the pupil. Immediately behind the edge of the pupil, indentations can be seen on the equatorial lens capsule where the zonules attach. They have a "picket fence" appearance where they attach to the lens equator.

d. If cataracts are present, they will appear white when transilluminated (Fig 1-7a.4) and black when observed on retroillumination with an ophthalmoscope (Fig 1-7b.4). The black outline results from the cataract absorbing light reflected from the tapetum.

5. Vitreous examination. Transillumination of the normal eye will often reveal:

a. Small posterior polar remnants of the hyaloid artery

b. Areas of light reflection between vitreous planes. These are similar to the jet trail left by an airplane.

c. *Comment.* Neither of the above can be seen with an ophthalmoscope

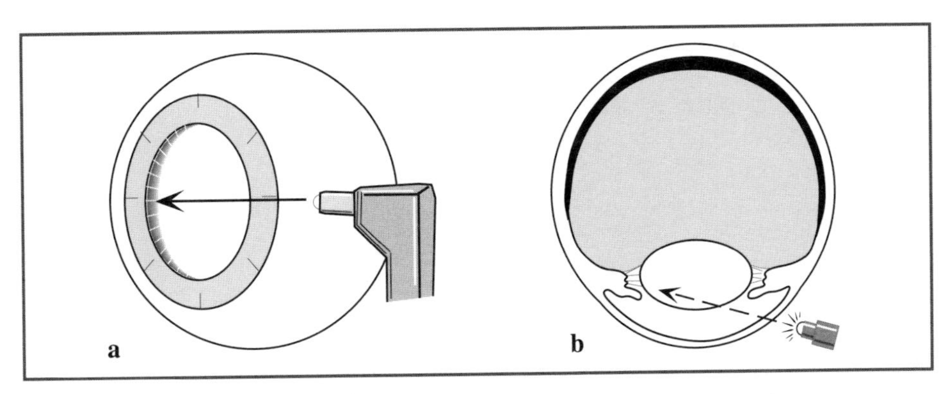

Figure 1-8. Transillumination to demonstrate zonular attachments at the lens equator.
- a. Observer's view
- b. Horizontal section

Slit-beam light examination

1. Examination with a slit lamp microscope, slit beam of an ophthalmoscope (Fig 1-9), or slit beam penlight
2. The slit-light beam will cut an optical section through the eye, making it possible to identify the cornea, depth and contents of the anterior chamber, irregular surface areas of the iris, layers of the lens, and anterior vitreous

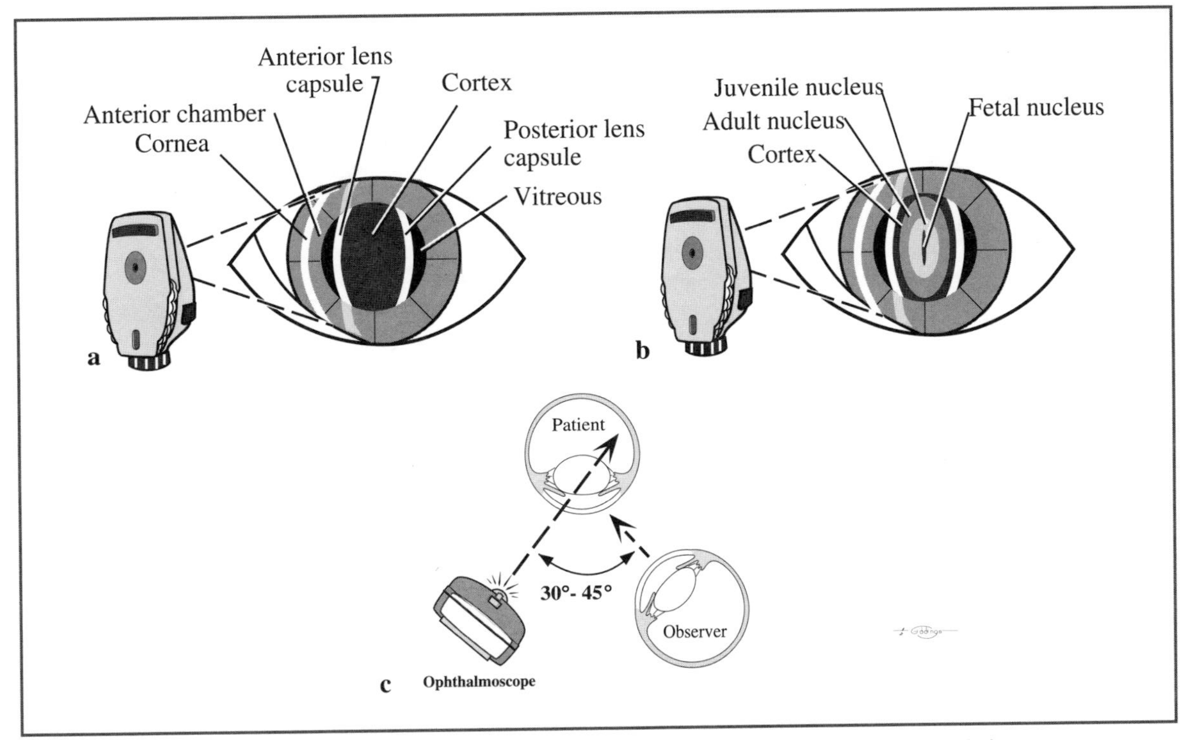

Figure 1-9. Transillumination with an ophthalmoscope slit-beam. The slit beam of an ophthalmoscope cuts an optical section through the normal eye, identifying the cornea, anterior chamber, lens and vitreous.
- a. Young dog lens - appears homogeneous
- b. Old dog lens - The layers of the lens seen from the surface inward are: anterior capsule, cortex, adult nucleus, and juvenile nucleus; central fetal nucleus (dark area); and posterior juvenile nucleus, adult nucleus, cortex and capsule.
- c. Dorsal view showing relationship between patient, ophthalmoscope and observer.

BASIC OPTICS AND REFRACTION

To better understand the fundamentals of ophthalmoscopy, it is necessary to review some basic principles of optics and refraction.

TERMS

Beam - a collection of parallel light rays
Concave lens - a divergent or negative lens
Convex lens - a convergent or positive lens
Diopter - the unit of measure of the refractive power of a prism or lens
Focal point - the point where parallel light rays are brought together by a lens
Focus - a convergent or divergent beam of light
Opaque - substances that do not transmit light
Reflection - light reflected from the surface of a medium
Refraction - bending of light when it passes from one medium to another
Refractive index - the light-bending capability of a transparent medium
Translucent - substances that transmit light poorly (frosted glass)
Transparent - substances that transmit light freely (glass, air, etc)

Principles of refraction and reflection

When light contacts a smooth surface or a transparent medium, some of it is reflected and the rest is refracted into it. This bending is the result of a change in velocity of the light entering the medium. Light travels slower in a denser medium.

The angle of reflection (i´) and the angle of refraction (r) depend on the angle of incidence (i) of the light. They are measured from the normal, which is perpendicular to the surface of the medium at the point of incidence (Fig 1-10).

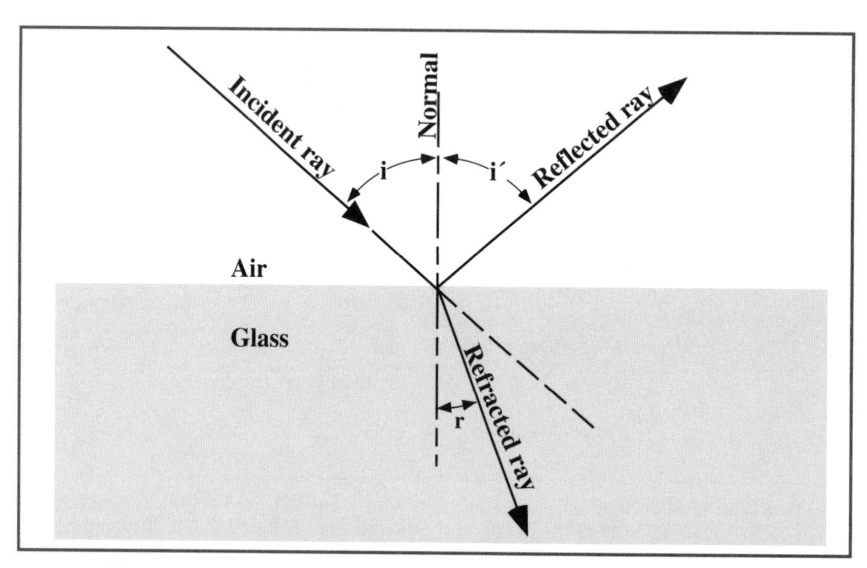

Figure 1-10. Refraction and reflection of light between air and glass.
i = angle of incidence
i´ = angle of reflection
r = angle of refraction

The angle of incidence = the angle of reflection. Symbolically this is:

$$\text{angle } i = \text{angle } i'$$

The angle of refraction = the angle of incidence times the refractive index for that material. The Greek letter mu (μ) is used for the refractive index. Symbolically this is:

$$r = i\mu$$

The refractive index (μ) is the ratio between the velocity of light in a vacuum (c) and the velocity in a medium (v).

$$\text{Refractive index} = \frac{\text{Velocity in vacuum}}{\text{Velocity in medium}} \quad \text{or} \quad \mu = \frac{c}{v}$$

Some refractive indices of importance in ophthalmology are:

air	=	1.00029 or 1.00
water	=	1.33
glass	=	1.50
cornea	=	1.34 (some authors give 1.33)
aqueous	=	1.33
lens	=	1.42
vitreous	=	1.33

Diopter determination of a prism

When light passes through a prism it is bent toward the base of the prism. The diopter strength of a prism is the number of centimeters a beam of light is deviated toward the base in a distance of one meter.

A 1 diopter prism deviates a beam of light 1 cm in one meter and likewise a 5 diopter prism results in a 5 cm deviation (Fig 1-11).

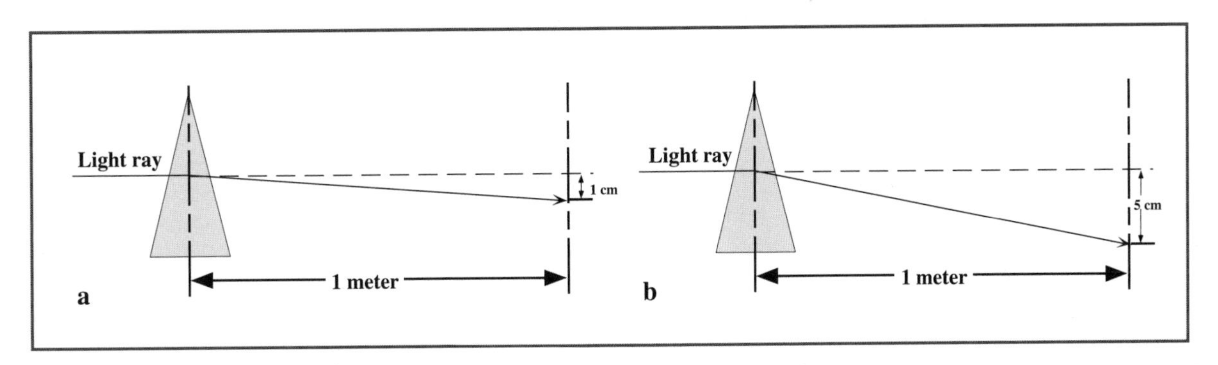

Figure 1-11. Refraction using a prism.
a. Effect of a 1 diopter prism on a light ray
b. Effect of a 5 diopter prism on a light ray

Diopter determination of lenses

Lenses may be convex or concave. The degree of curvature of the lens determines its specific refraction. A convex (convergent) lens is capable of producing an image of the light source at its focal point. A convex lens with a diopter rating of 1 has a focal length of one meter (Fig 1-12). Focal length (f) is the distance between the center of the lens and the focal point (fp).

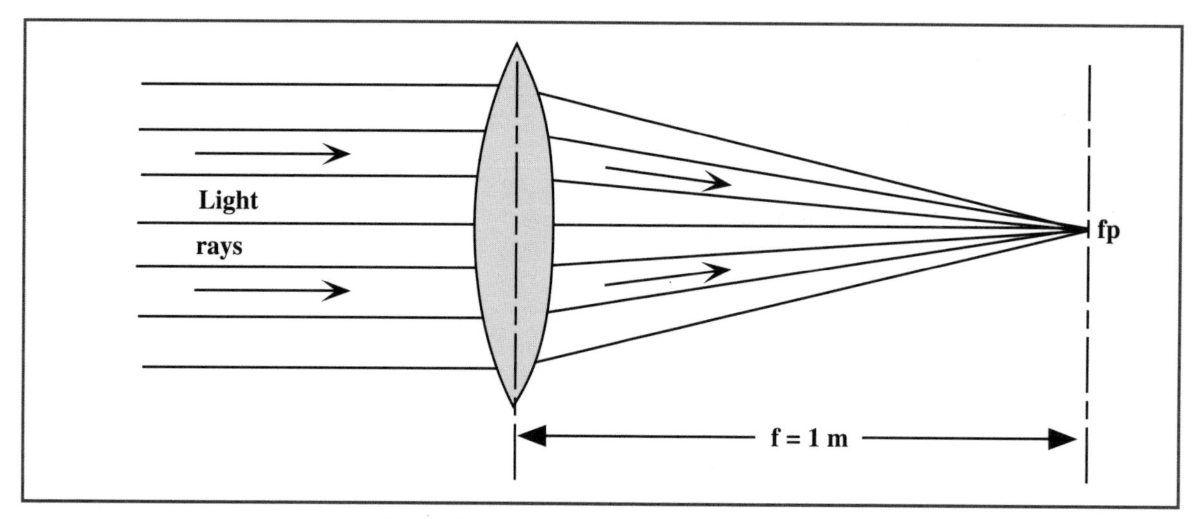

Figure 1-12. Focal length of a 1 diopter lens.
f = focal length
fp = focal point

Parallel light rays passing through the lens will all meet at the focal point. The focal point is the same as the point where a lens will project an image on a flat surface.

The diopter strength (D) of a convex lens is the reciprocal of the focal length in meters (f).

$$\text{Diopters} = \frac{1}{\text{focal length}} \quad \text{or} \quad d = \frac{1}{f}$$

The focal length of a convex lens (f) in meters is the reciprocal of the diopter strength (D) (Fig 1-13).

$$\text{Focal length} = \frac{1}{\text{diopters}} \quad \text{or} \quad f = \frac{1}{d}$$

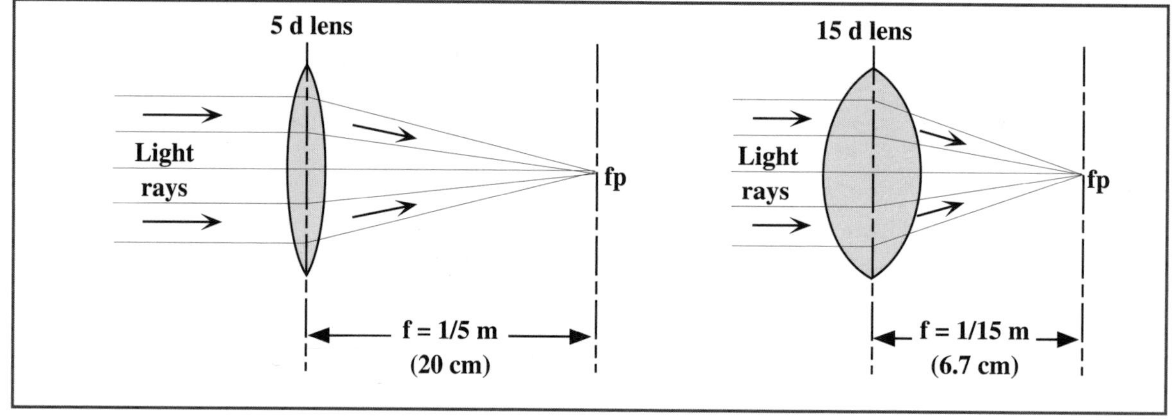

Figure 1-13. Focal length of 5 and 10 diopter convex lenses.

Although the diopter definition for a prism appears different from a convex lens, they are related. Consider a convex lens to be a series of prism segments with their bases located toward the center of the lens and each prism segment is progressively stronger toward the periphery (Fig 1-14).

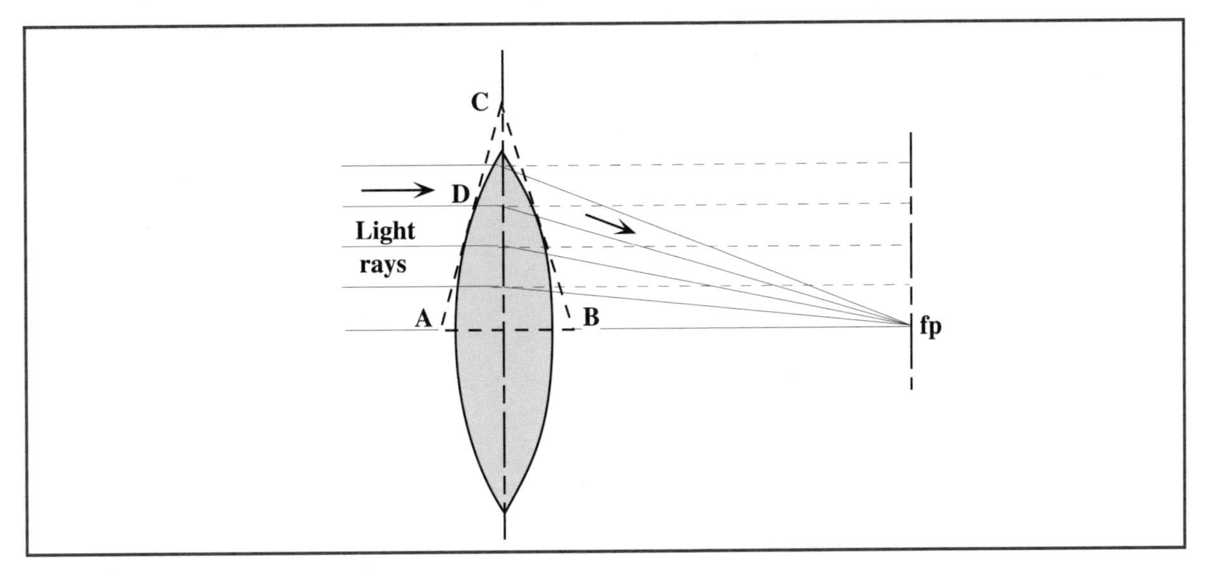

Figure 1-14. Comparison of a convex lens with a series of prisms. A-B-C represents a prism that has the same characteristics as point D on the lens.

Concave (divergent) lens spread light rays and do not produce a focused image. They have a virtual image at the focal point that is located between the light source and the lens. The focal point of a -1 diopter concave lens is 1 meter from the lens (Fig 1-15).

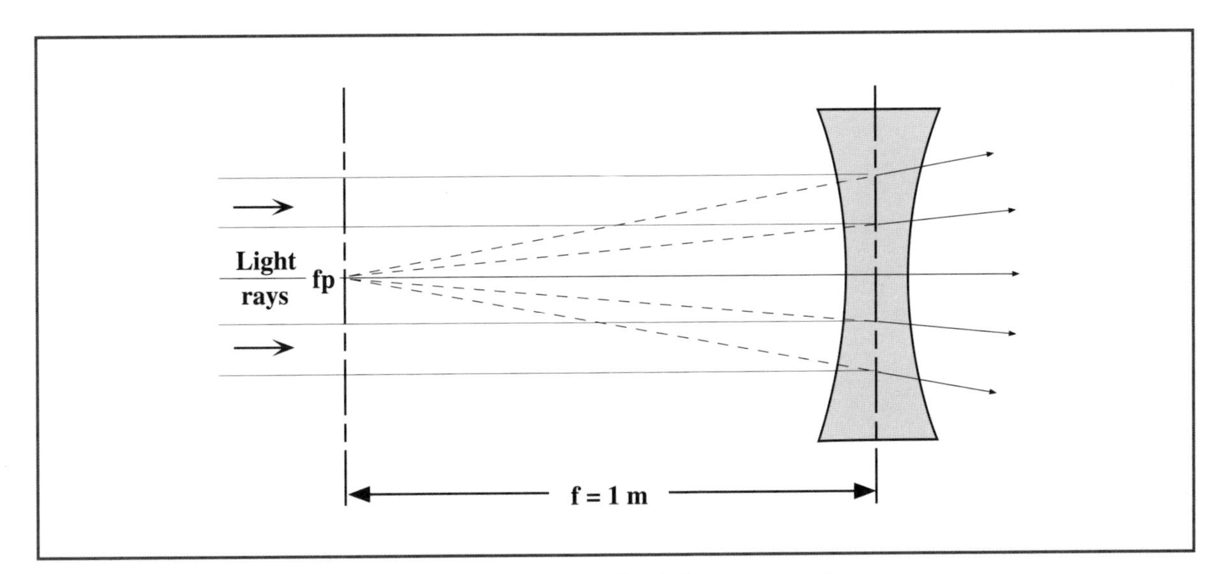

Figure 1-15. Focal point of a -1 diopter concave lens.

The same calculations as for convex lenses are used to determine the refractive strength of concave lenses.

$$d = \frac{1}{f} \quad \text{and} \quad f = \frac{1}{d}$$

The relative focal points for -5 and -15 diopter concave lenses are shown in Fig 1-16.

When using convex and concave lenses it is easier to refer to them as positive and negative. A convex lens is referred to as a positive lens and a concave lens as a negative lens. On the ophthalmoscope dial, black letters are used for the diopter strength of the convex lenses and red represents the concave lenses.

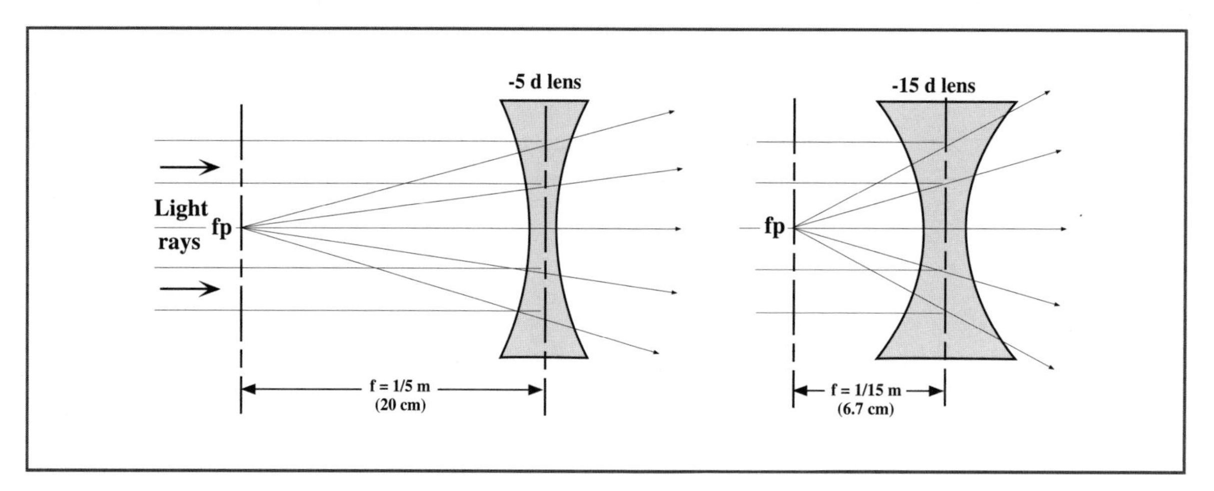

Figure 1-16. Focal lengths of -5 and -15 diopter concave lenses.

OPHTHALMOSCOPY

TERMS **(Fig 1-17)**

Ametropia - any form of abnormal refractive power of the eye
Axial myopia - myopia due to largeness of the eye, the common form of myopia
Emmetropia - normal sight
Hyperopia (farsighted) - focal point of the eye behind the retina
Myopia (nearsighted) - focal point of the eye is ahead of the retina
Presbyopia - the loss of accommodation in man occurring with hardening of the lens. This begins at about 45 years of age.
Refraction myopia - myopia due to excessive refraction strength of the eye

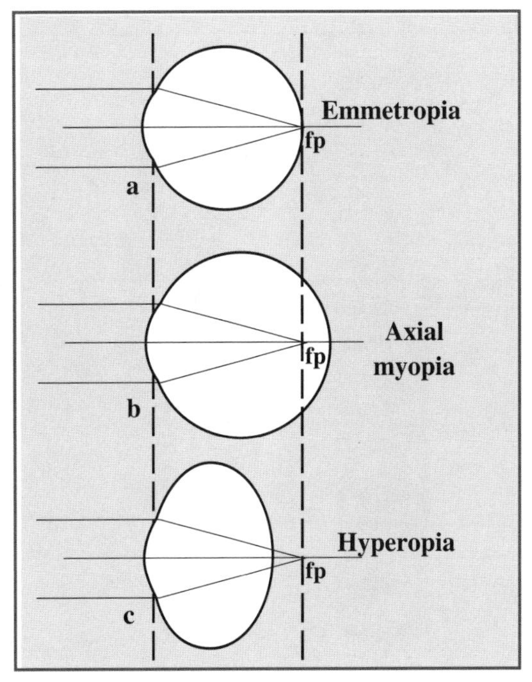

Figure 1-17. Diagrams of normal and abnormal refraction of the eye.
a. Emmetropia - normal vision
b. Myopia - nearsighted vision
c. Hyperopia - farsighted vision

Ophthalmoscopy is difficult to master and requires continuous use to maintain proficiency. It can be either direct (looking directly into the eye), or indirect (using a handheld lens and a light source to view a projected image of the fundus). Each technique has advantages and disadvantages, but the beginner can often master indirect techniques faster than the direct ophthalmoscope.

DIRECT OPHTHALMOSCOPY

Instrumentation

1. Ocular transilluminator (Fig 1-18) - the fastest and simplest way to do a screening examination of large animals, especially horses. A darkened room is sufficient to allow the horse's pupil to dilate to permit an examination. The light source is held against the examiner's face and below his pupil so that the light is easily directed through the horse's pupil. A large fundus area (5 or 6 times greater than can be seen with a direct ophthalmoscope) is visible. The entire fundus is not in clear focus, but can be seen adequately to screen the eye for pathology. Detail of pathologic areas can then be studied using the direct ophthalmoscope. This technique also works well for cattle and llamas.

   The reason for success of this examination in large animals is that their pupils remain more dilated during examination. This method is generally not successful in cats and dogs without dilating the pupil, then only animals with large eyes.

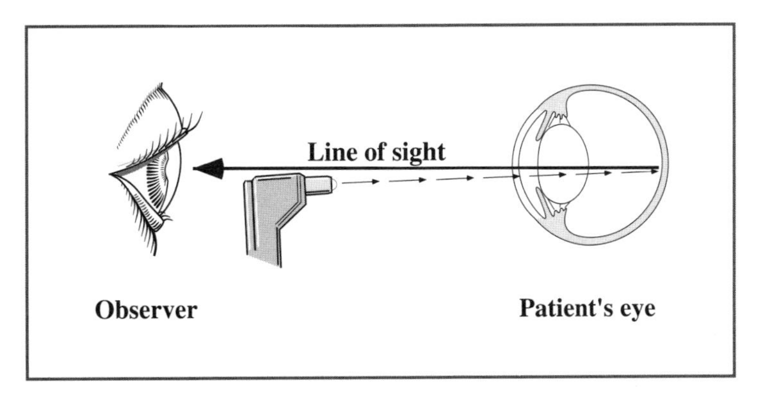

Figure 1-18. Transilluminator used as an ophthalmoscope.

2. Ophthalmoscope - The instrument has a light source directed into the patient's eye so the beam is nearly parallel with the examiner's line of sight (Fig 1-19).

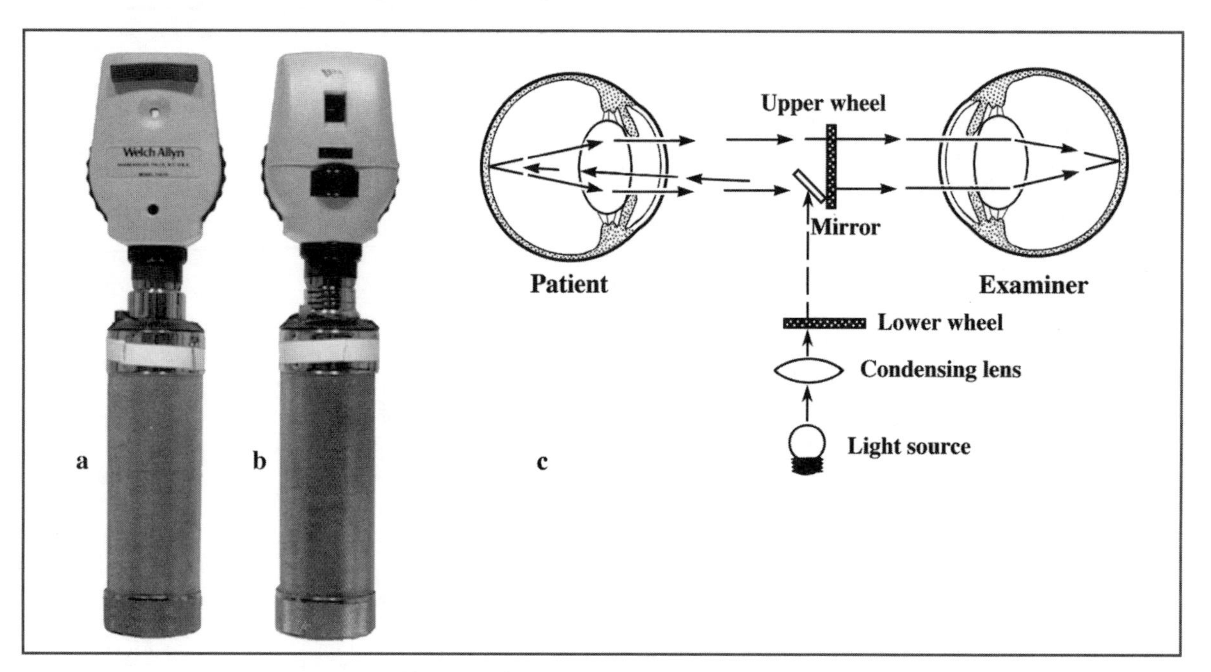

Figure 1-19. Direct ophthalmoscope.
a. Back of ophthalmoscope
b. Front of ophthalmoscope
c. Schematic drawing of direct ophthalmoscopic examination

The upper lens wheel gives the examiner a selection of lenses ranging from 40 D to -25 D (Fig 1-20). The lower wheel has five apertures (Fig 1-21): 1) a slit to help evaluate elevation of the lesions, 2) a small diameter opening, 3) a large diameter opening (this one is used most of the time), 4) a grid-marked aperture to evaluate relative size of lesions, and 5) a red-free green lens to differentiate red pigment from retinal hemorrhage or a cobalt blue lens to enhance fluorescein visualization. In a red fundus such as in man, hemorrhage will appear black when examined with a red-free light.

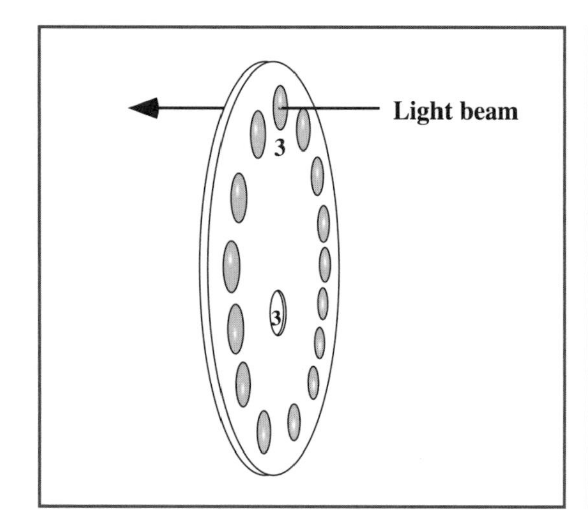

Figure 1-20. Upper lens wheel with variable diopter strength lenses.

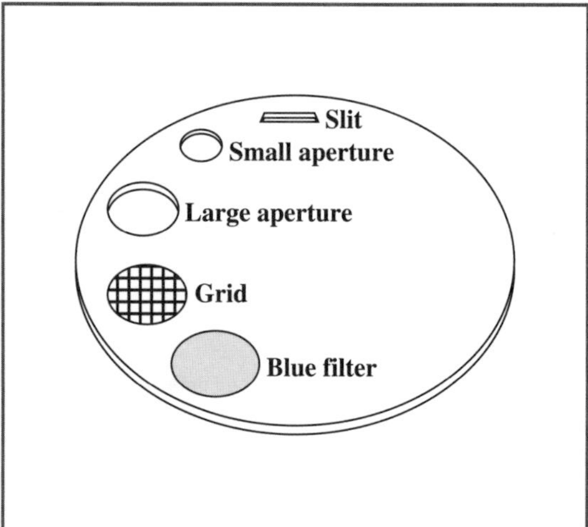

Figure 1-21. Lower lens wheel with slit opening, small aperture, large aperture, grid marker and blue filter.

Technique of ophthalmoscopy

An instruction booklet accompanies new ophthalmoscopes and should be studied thoroughly before use. To successfully examine the eye, it is desirable to have a semidarkened or completely darkened room and a well dilated pupil.

1. Set the ophthalmoscope at "0".
2. The small animal patient's right eye should be examined with the examiner's right eye and the left with the left. In large animals, the examiner can use his dominant eye for either patient eye.
3. To examine the right eye (Fig 1-22a):
   a. The ophthalmoscope is held vertically in the right hand, in front of the examiner's right eye, resting it against his eyebrow and the bridge of his nose. The ophthalmoscope is directed about 15° to the left of the examiner's forward line of sight. This will allow the examiner to avoid the patient's nose as he moves close to the patient. If the examiner wears glasses and wishes to keep them on, the ophthalmoscope is held in contact with the glasses.
   b. The examiner places his left hand on the patient so that the index finger controls the movement of the upper eyelid and the thumb controls the lower. Be sure that the pressure is placed only on bones of the face. Pressure placed directly on the eye causes enough increase in intraocular pressure to reduce the size of fundus blood vessels.
4. The left eye is examined by holding the ophthalmoscope in the left hand, using the examiner's left eye, and holding the lids open with the right hand (Fig 1-22b).

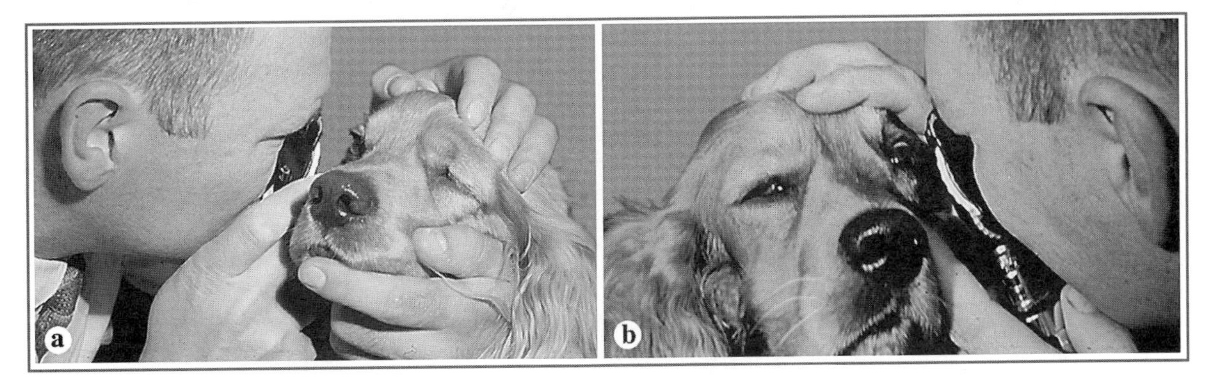

Figure 1-22. Direct ophthalmoscope examination technique.
a. The patient's right eye is examined with the examiner's right eye and the ophthalmoscope is held about 2 inches from the patient.
b. The patient's left eye is examined with the examiner's left eye.

Examination protocols

Two protocols are recommended.

1. *Variable distance examination.* The examiner sets the ophthalmoscope at 0 diopters, positions himself at 18-24 inches from the patient, and adjusts his position until the fundus light reflex is maximal. At this distance the scleral, iris and fundus reflex are clearly seen. If the transparent media (cornea, aqueous, lens and vitreous) are normal, they cannot be seen. The examiner then moves continuously toward the patient, allowing the optics of the patient's eye to bring internal structures into clear view. If there is opacity in the transparent media, a black image will be seen in the fundus light reflex as a result of the shadow from the opacity. Corneal opacity and blood vessels will appear black. Lens changes are clearly seen at about 14 inches and pathology immediately behind the lens at 10 to 12 inches. Vitreous changes are visible until about 6 inches away when fundus detail begins to appear.
2. *Fixed distance examination.* The examiner sets the ophthalmoscope at 20 diopters and positions himself 1.5 to 2 inches from the patient. This setting will allow examination of the adnexa, cornea, and sclera. Then, rotating the lens wheel toward "0" D, the ophthalmoscope brings deeper structures into clear view.

Ophthalmoscope settings for examining the normal eye at an examination distance of 1.5 to 2 inches (5 cm)	
Structure	**Ophthalmoscope setting in diopters**
Adnexa and sclera	20
Cornea	15 to 20
Iris	12 to 15
Anterior capsule of lens	12 to 15
Posterior capsule of lens	8 to 12
Vitreous	2 to 8
Optic disk and fundus	2 to -2

Fundus Examination

The fundus is best seen at 1.5 to 2 inches from the patient. The more dilated the pupil, the better the view. If there is a bright corneal reflection (specular reflex) from the center of the cornea, this can be reduced by looking through the cornea off center.

1. Starting with the ophthalmoscope set at "0" D, the upper lens wheel should be rotated toward negative (red) numbers until the fundus adjacent to the disk is clearly visible. This is generally -2D to -4D. If the fundus becomes indistinct, rotate the lens wheel toward the positive lenses. Note the lens that gives the clearest view. The fundus can now be examined. The normal sensory retina is transparent, allowing visualization of deeper structures.
2. To examine the optic disk, reset the ophthalmoscope to "0". Again, turn toward negative lenses. The setting that gives the clearest visualization of vessels near the center of the disk is determined. In normal patients, the setting should be within 1 D of the setting for the fundus. A more negative setting for the disk indicates disk depression (glaucoma, atrophy, congenital depression). A more positive setting indicates disk elevation (papillitis, papilledema, tumors, physiologic enlargement [pseudopapilledema]).
3. *Comment.* Domestic animals, especially the dog, have been reported to be myopic. The degree of myopia has been exaggerated because the inexperienced examiner accommodates 1 to 3 D without realizing it. This accommodation results in the eye appearing accordingly myopic. If you accommodate 2 D and the patient is 1 D myopic, the setting for the ophthalmoscope will be -3 D for clear visualization. If a retinoscope is used, most dogs are between $\pm$ 0.5 D. The retinoscope is an instrument used only for diopter determination of the eye. It eliminates accommodation and refractive error of the examiner.

Advantages of direct compared to indirect ophthalmoscopy

1. Simple instrumentation
2. Moderate equipment expense - $150 for a basic ophthalmoscope head
3. Upright image
4. Offers greatest magnification of fundus features, giving a more detailed examination. The natural magnification of the eye is approximately 17x in dogs, cats 19, horses 8 and cows 11. (Murphy CJ, Howland HC. Optics of comparative ophthalmoscopy. Vision Research 27:599-607, 1987.) Structures 30 to 90 microns can be examined.
5. Both depth and height of lesions can be determined with the diopter settings.

Disadvantages of direct compared to indirect ophthalmoscopy

1. Small field of vision (4-5 mm with regular ophthalmoscope). Transilluminators permit visualization of a much larger area.
2. Clear fundus visualization is limited to a shallow depth of field; 3 d = 1 mm depth for dogs and humans.

INDIRECT OPHTHALMOSCOPIC EXAMINATION

Examination of the eye with a lens held near the patient and a light source near the examiner's eye. A large area of the fundus can be seen. This facilitates rapid screening and evaluation of the fundus. The depth of field with indirect examination is greater than with direct ophthalmoscopy. Pupil dilation is necessary for thorough examination. The examination may be performed monocularly or binocularly.

Lenses (Fig 1-23)

Fourteen to 28 diopter lenses are used for routine examinations. A 20 D lens gives an excellent image. For laboratory and exotic animals with small eyes, 40 to 78 D lenses may be preferred.

The quality of the lens determines the ease and clarity of fundus visualization. A precision ground biconvex, aspheric, achromatic 20 D lens may cost $145 or more; a 5x (20 D) plastic magnifying lens costs less than $10. Therefore, lens quality is the choice of the examiner. Precise lens distance from the patient is more critical with a 14 D lens than a 28 D lens. Therefore, a 20 D or higher lens is recommended for the beginner. The smaller the diopter rating, the greater the magnification.

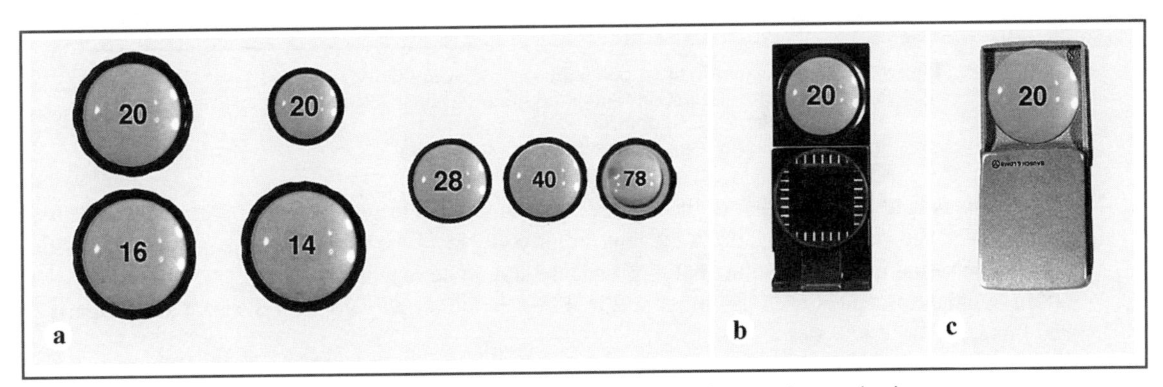

Figure 1-23. Examples of lenses used for indirect ophthalmoscopic examination.
- a. Optical lenses
- b. Thread counter, available in fabric stores
- c. 5x (approximately 20 diopter) Bausch & Lomb magnifying lens, available from Arista Surgical and many book stores

Monocular indirect ophthalmoscopy (Fig 1-24)

1. Light sources
   - a. Modified otoscope (author's preference)
   - b. Transilluminator
   - c. 3.5 volt ophthalmoscope (setting the ophthalmoscope at 2 to 5 D lens will reduce the working distance between the examiner and the patient).
2. Technique
   The examiner takes a position about 18 to 20 inches in front of the patient, holding the light source in front of his dominant eye and just below the pupil. The light is directed at the patient's eye until the tapetal reflex is obvious. The lens is held with the observer's thumb and forefinger. The other fingers can stabilize the upper lid and steady the lens. The greatest curvature of the lens should be toward the examiner. Then the lens is placed in the line of vision immediately in front of the patient's eye and slowly moved toward the examiner until an inverted image fills the lens. With a 20 D lens, this will occur when the lens is about two inches from the patient's eye. The image in the lens is upside down, and right and left are reversed. Until the examiner becomes experienced, this reversal makes it difficult to make correct movements to examine the entire fundus. To bring an area into better view, the observer's head and the hand holding the lens should be moved synchronously in the same direction as the area he wants to view.

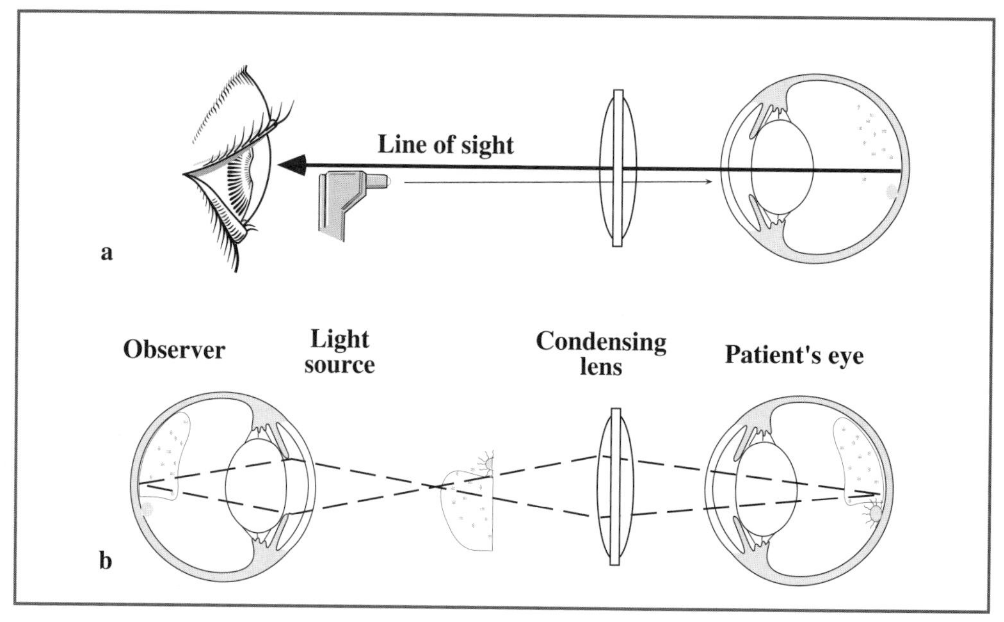

Figure 1-24. Monocular indirect ophthalmoscopic examination.
a. Indirect examination with a modified otoscope used as a light source and a 20 diopter lens
b. Optical schematics for monocular examination

If the lens is held perpendicular to the viewer's line of sight, a bright specular reflection will be seen in the center of the visual field. Tilting the lens slightly will send the reflexes to the sides. If the patient moves or the visual image is lost, the entire procedure should be repeated.

If an ophthalmoscope is used, setting it at 2 to 4 D will shorten the working distance and magnify the visual image.

A/O Reichert monocular indirect ophthalmoscope (Fig 1-25)

It is simple to use and works on the same principle as looking through a 3x telescope held backwards. It decreases magnification of the eye by one-third, increases visual field 3-fold, and has excellent depth of field. It is the easiest to use of all ophthalmoscopes and has all the advantages of indirect examination. It is an excellent ophthalmoscope for an examiner who has an ophthalmic problem that makes it difficult to see the patient's fundus clearly with a direct ophthalmoscope. It costs about $1,500.

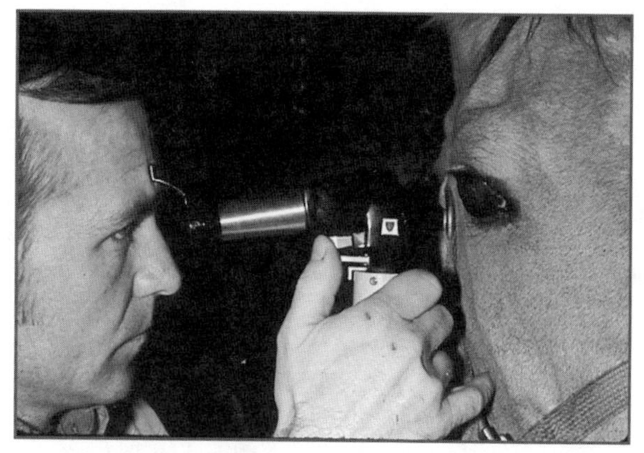

Figure 1-25. A-O Reichert monocular indirect ophthalmoscope. It provides an upright image of the fundus and permits examination without mydriasis.

Binocular indirect ophthalmoscopy (Fig 1-26)

Available from many sources. Cost varies - $1200 to $1800. These allow stereoscopic vision and give an intensified image. The technique is difficult to develop but when mastered it is the best method to use for screening the fundus. The examining light is built in and much brighter than the light in other ophthalmoscopes, therefore there is a greater chance to see fundus lesions when opacities are present in other tissues. Mirrors or prisms reduce the observer's interpupillary distance so that he can see through the patient's pupil with both eyes (Fig 1-27). Examination technique is the same as monocular indirect.

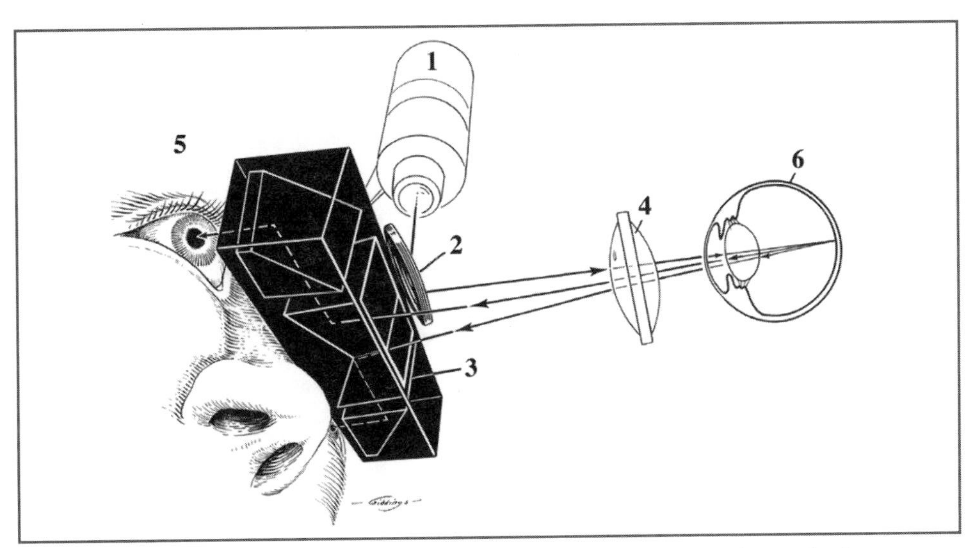

Figure 1-26. Schematic diagram of binocular indirect ophthalmoscopic examination.

1. Light source
2. Reflecting mirror for light source
3. Prisms to reduce interpupillary distance
4. 20 diopter lens
5. Examiner's eye
6. Patient's eye

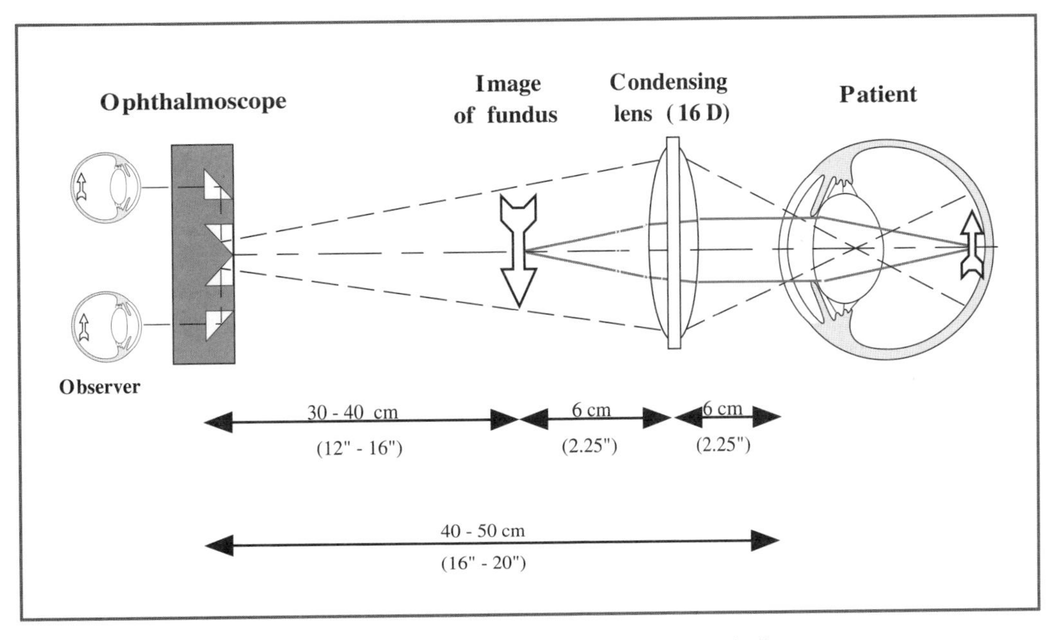

Figure 1-27. Optics and working distances for binocular indirect ophthalmoscopic examination using a 16 diopter lens.

Advantages of indirect when compared to direct ophthalmoscopy (A/O monocular not considered)

1. Large area of fundus visible; therefore, can quickly check eye for abnormalities
2. Great depth of field. Lesions in vitreous and fundus are clearly seen simultaneously.
3. Binocular gives stereoscopic image
4. More light; therefore, can see through diseased cornea and vitreous when direct examination is not possible

Disadvantages of indirect compared to direct ophthalmoscopy (A/O monocular not considered)

1. Technique difficult to master
2. Image inverted with right-left reversal
3. Visual image magnification is determined by the strength of the lens
   14 D = 5x magnification (about 1/3 of magnification)
   28 D = 3.5x magnification (about 1/4 of magnification)
4. Need dilated pupil
5. Need dark room
6. Bright light may be uncomfortable to the patient and potentially damage the retina

CLINICAL EXAMINATION WITH THE OPHTHALMOSCOPE

Cornea and iris (the direct ophthalmoscope can be used as a magnifying loupe when set at 15 or 20 D) - examine for:

1. Blood vessels
2. Pigment
3. Scarring

Lens - examine for:

1. Cataracts
2. Lenticonus
3. Persistent hyaloid remnants
4. Nuclear sclerosis

Vitreous - examine for:

1. Congenital remnants (persistent hyperplastic primary vitreous)
2. Exudates
3. Hemorrhage
4. Vitreous floaters
5. Retinal detachment displacing liquified vitreous

Fundus - the posterior portion of the eye seen with an ophthalmoscope includes optic nerve, retina, choroid (tapetum/nontapetal). The visual retina is transparent with only the blood vessels visible. The retinal pigment epithelium is nonpigmented in the area of the tapetum and pigmented in the nontapetal fundus.

1. Optic disk - examine for:
   a. Color
   b. Presence of physiologic cup
   c. Degree of vascularity
   d. Presence of hemorrhage
   e. Size
   f. Presence of pits, fissures or colobomas
   g. Abnormal masses

2. Retina - examine for:
   a. Size and number of blood vessels vary between species
      1) Holangiotic - the entire retina has blood vessels (dog, cat, pig, ruminants)
      2) Paurangiotic - blood vessels limited to peripapillary area (horse, guinea pig)
      3) Merangiotic - blood vessels localized to a region of the retina (rabbit)
      4) Anangiotic - no retinal blood vessels (birds)
   b. Hemorrhage
   c. Edema and exudates
   d. Detachment - results in loss of transparency
   e. Thinning - results in tapetal hyperreflectivity
   f. Retinal dysplasia
3. Tapetal fundus
   a. Tapetal hyperreflectivity (due to retinal thinning)
   b. Changes in tapetal color (inflammatory/dysplasia)
   c. Pigment changes (depigmentation/hyperpigmentation)
   d. Genetic lack of tapetal development (subalbinotic/collie eye syndrome)
   e. Blood vessel attenuation will be exaggerated by tapetal hyperreflectivity. Reduced light will result in better visualization.
4. Nontapetal fundus - pigment responsible for the color of nontapetal fundus is derived from retinal pigment epithelium and choroid pigment. Examine for:
   a. Congenital lack of pigmentation (seen with subalbinotic changes/choroidal hypoplasia)
   b. Acquired depigmentation (postinflammatory)
   c. Hyperpigmentation - a latent change after inflammatory depigmentation

CANINE

Ophthalmoscope settings for the fundus vary with the examiner.

Lens

The normal lens is not seen with the ophthalmoscope. It will become visible in cataracts and lenticular sclerosis. It can be best visualized with a direct ophthalmoscope with it set at 5 D and the examiner positioned about 20 cm from the eye.

Vitreous

The vitreous is usually clear. It may have slight opacities that can be seen with transillumination and the slit lamp, but are not visible during ophthalmoscopic examination. Asteroid hyalosis is the most common degenerative change seen.

Fundus (Fig 1-28)

The fundus is usually brightly colored in the area of the tapetum lucidum and dark brown in the nontapetal area.

1. Optic disk
   a. Size - approximately 1.5 mm in diameter
   b. Location - it is slightly nasal and inferior to the longitudinal axis of the eye and may be within the tapetum lucidum, the nontapetal fundus or at their junction
   c. Shape - round or irregular in outline depending on the amount of myelination extending from the optic nerve. Myelination of the retrobulbar optic nerve extends through the lamina cribrosa and terminates at the limits of the optic disk. The nerve ending is represented by a round area seen within the disk. In young animals, myelination is often limited to the nerve ending and the optic disk is round with a circumpapillary ring of pigment. As the dog matures, myelination may extend from the optic nerve, which gives an irregular appearance.

d. Color - Blood supply gives the disk a definite pink cast
e. Physiologic cup - a gray cleft is seen near the center of the optic disk, representing the termination of the hyaloid canal in the optic nerve
f. Blood vessels - the blood vessels are not bilaterally symmetrical. Three or four large venules return to the central disk area and may anastomose. The arteries are brighter red, more numerous, much smaller and emerge from the periphery of the disk. The blood vessels should be examined for size and relative number.

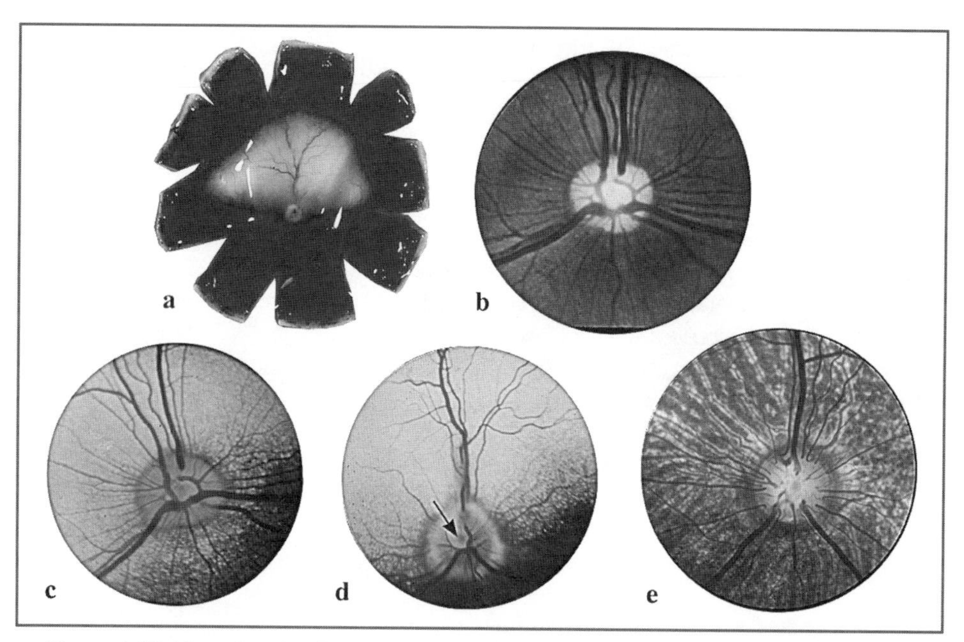

Figure 1-28. Normal canine fundus.

a. Dissected left eye. Tapetum is roughly triangular with the most acute angle nasally. Optic disk located along lower border of tapetum.
b. Fundus, six week old border collie. Tapetum has not developed.
c. Fundus, puppy in "b", now three months old. Tapetum has developed.
d. Fundus, normal dog. Myelination of optic nerve fibers extends beyond edge of optic nerve, giving optic disk roughly triangular appearance. Physiologic cup indicated by arrow.
e. Nontapetal fundus seen in Dalmatian. Note minimal pigment below optic disk. Retinal blood vessels can be seen crossing over much broader choroidal blood vessels.

2. Retinal blood vessels
   a. There are usually 3 to 4 major nerves exiting at the optic disk and 10 to 12 much smaller arteries coming from it. Arteries are bright red with the veins much darker. Normal blood vessels extend beyond the superior limits of the tapetum. Any decrease in size results in attenuation of how far the blood vessels can be seen peripherally.
   b. Healthy veins and larger arteries have a hollow appearance (essential reflex) extending away from the optic disk. This is more prominent in the nontapetal fundus. This reflex disappears with generalized retinal disease.
   c. Area centralis - a relative avascular area in the axial retina slightly temporal and superior to the optic disk. This region has the greatest cone density.
3. Tapetum lucidum
   a. Has a triangular appearance and is seen in the upper one-half of the fundus. It is located in the choroid beneath the choriocapillaris and is 9 to 15 cells thick. The retinal pigment epithelium is nonpigmented over the tapetum, allowing the tapetum to be seen.
   b. Color - varies a great deal: yellow, orange, green, blue or combinations
   c. The tapetum may have homogeneous appearance with slight flecking or appear to be composed of a mixture of color plaques

d. Lack of tapetum - may occur in subalbinotic dogs, especially with blue irides. If the retina is nonpigmented and the tapetum is missing, choroid blood vessels can be seen, resulting in red and white background. If the tapetum is missing and retinal pigment is present, the entire fundus is quite uniform in color.

4. Nontapetal fundus - This represents the greatest part of the fundus (usually 3/4 or more). The nontapetal area gets its color from retinal pigment epithelium and choroidal pigment.
   a. Color - may be gray, light or dark brown. In most animals these pigments are dense enough to obscure choroidal blood vessels.
   b. Variations in appearance - if retinal and choroidal pigment is deficient, the choroidal vasculature becomes visible. Tigroid stippling (stripes) is the mildest form of decreased pigment. The more marked the hypopigmentation, the clearer the choroidal features. Nearly total nonpigmentation occurs in severe color dilution animals.

FELINE (Fig 1-29)

Cats are often more difficult to examine than dogs because the third eyelid is more prone to protrude during examination. Cats are less myopic than dogs.

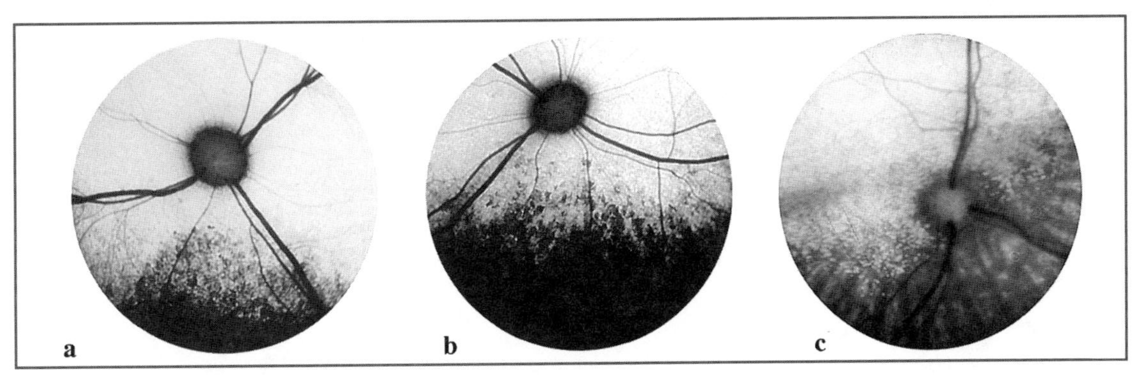

Figure 1-29. Normal feline fundus.
a & b. Normal fundus. Right and left eyes are shown. Optic disk is dark because of photographic technique. There are three major paired blood vessels.
c. Right eye, normal Siamese. Choroidal blood vessels can be seen because of lack of pigment.

Optic Disk

1. Size - about 1 mm in diameter; much smaller than the dog
2. Location - in the inferior tapetum
3. Color - white to gray. Myelination of the optic nerve ends as it perforates the lamina cribrosa, giving a slightly depressed appearance to the disk.
4. Physiologic cup - present in center, but not as easily seen as in the dog
5. Blood vessels - arteries and veins arise from the periphery. No central veins or anastomosis as seen in the dog.

Retina

1. Major arteries and veins are paired
2. Essential reflexes are not as prominent
3. Distinct area centralis that is nearly free of blood vessels

Tapetum

1. Shape - nearly circular, much larger than in the dog, and in a similar location
2. Color - yellow, green, red or mixed. More reflective than in the dog. In Siamese cats the area centralis may have thinning of the tapetum, resulting in the red color of the choroid showing through. This can be mistaken as hemorrhage.

3. Texture - usually quite even except in Siamese cats, where it may appear granular
4. Lack of tapetum - the tapetum may be poorly developed in subalbinotic animals and Siamese cats

Nontapetal area

1. Color - may be reddish, light or dark brown and in some cases a dark gray
2. Variations - usually well pigmented but in subalbinotic cats, especially Siamese, may show lack of pigment similar to dogs

BOVINE AND OVINE (Fig 1-30)

The bovine and ovine are so similar in appearance, they can be described together.

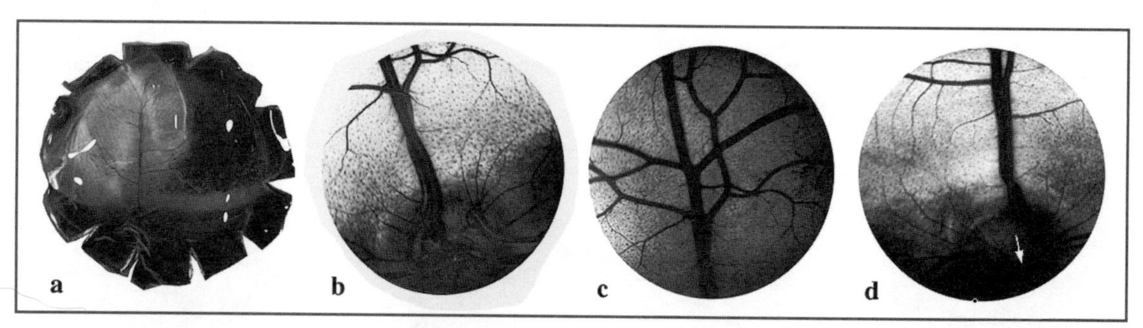

Figure 1-30. Normal bovine and ovine fundus.
- a. Dissected bovine right eye. Note incomplete tapetal development. Major blood vessels are paired. Optic disk is nonmyelinated.
- b. Normal bovine. Optic disk is nonmyelinated and pigmented. Dorsal artery and vein are entwined and tapetum has black flecking.
- c. Same eye, following dorsal artery and vein as they continue above the optic disk.
- d. Normal ovine. Fundus is indistinguishable from bovine. A hyaloid remnant is barely visible (arrow) at 6 o'clock near the rim of this disk.

Optic nerve

1. Size and shape - a horizontal oval and slightly smaller than the horse. The margins are indistinct.
2. Color - most of the myelination of the optic nerve stops at the lamina cribrosa, resulting in an optic nerve that is colored the same as surrounding fundus. Some myelination may occur, which results in white patches in the disk area and on occasion most of the optic disk is myelinated.
3. Location - the disk in the nontapetal fundus is below and temporal to the posterior pole of the eye.
4. Physiologic cup - an opaque hyaloid remnant is generally present located centrally on the disk.
5. Blood vessels - the blood vessels emerge from the central optic disk in the area of the hyaloid canal. Paired arteries and veins are usually present and consistent enough in distribution to be designated as dorsal, temporal and nasal pairs. The blood vessels are so large that they appear lying on the optic disk rather than being a part of it.

Retina

1. The veins and arteries are the largest retinal blood vessels in domestic animals. They appear to be lying on the retina and project into the vitreous.
2. Color - a very distinct color difference between the red arteries and blue veins.
3. The dorsal artery and vein is the largest pair and give off branches that go horizontally across the tapetum. The paired temporal and nasal vessels go horizontally in the nontapetal area and parallel the major branches of the dorsal artery and vein.
4. There is a relatively avascular horizontal area centralis on either side of the optic disk between these sets of parallel vessels.

Tapetal area

1. Not as extensive and varies in shape
2. Color - usually blue-green but may have a reddish cast. Has the same black flecked appearance and texture as horses.
3. Shape - irregular with the lower limit sometimes only a horizontal line above the optic disk.

Nontapetal area

It is usually heavily pigmented and may be brown, red or nearly black.

EQUINE (Fig 1-31)

The preferred instrument for ophthalmoscopic screening is a modified otoscope or transilluminator.

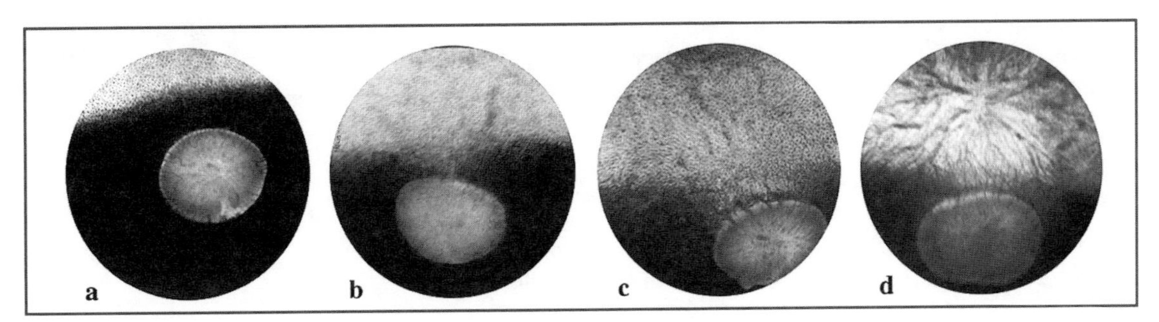

Figure 1-31. Normal equine fundus.
- a. Six month old colt. White border at 6 o'clock represents where optic fissure closed.
- b. Adult horse. Optic disk more oval. Blood vessels can be seen extending further horizontally than vertically. Note black flecking of tapetum.
- c. Adult horse. Several large choroidal blood vessels at dorsal rim of the optic disk. More variation in tapetal and nontapetal coloration.
- d. Adult horse. Color-dilute fundus with choroidal blood vessels visible above optic disk.

Optic disk

1. A large round to oval shaped disk. In adults, the horizontal diameter is 6 to 7 mm and vertical is 4 to 5 mm. The disk is large enough that the large beam from a standard ophthalmoscope barely illuminates the entire disk. The lower border has a white irregular edge that represents where the optic fissure closed and should not be confused with scarring.
2. Physiologic cup - a slight central cupping with a gray spot
3. Color - salmon pink. Myelination penetrates the lamina cribrosa but does not extend beyond the optic nerve.
4. Location - about 15 mm below and 3 to 4 mm lateral to the posterior pole of the eye in nontapetal fundus
5. Some small blood vessels can be seen on the optic nerve

Retina

1. Vascular pattern - paurangiotic. Blood vessels limited to a small area surrounding the optic disk. The nonvascular portion of the retina is nourished from the choriocapillaris of the choroid.
2. Thirty to 40 small blood vessels arise from the optic disk and extend 1 to 1.5 disk diameters horizontally and less than one vertically.
3. Venules and arterioles cannot be differentiated.

Tapetal area

1. Shape - semicircular in appearance with a nearly straight lower border running horizontally above the

optic disk. It extends nearly to the equator of the globe. If the retina is removed and the pigmented retinal epithelium is removed from the area around the optic disk, the tapetum will be seen to extend well beyond the lower border of the optic disk. This accounts for the tapetum that becomes exposed after chorioretinitis in the apparently nontapetal fundus near the optic disk. Repigmentation may follow the pattern of choroid blood vessels, which gives a cross-hatched appearance of pigment over hyperreflective tapetum. If the scars are beyond the tapetum, the depigmented scar will appear white.

2. Color - usually blue or blue green, less frequently yellow to rust. Color varies with haircoat genetics.
3. Texture - there is black flecking (stars of Winslow) that represents where choriocapillaris vessels alter the tapetum as they approach the retina. Purple streaks are sometimes present that represent large superficial choroidal blood vessels.
4. Variations - the tapetum may be partially or totally lacking in subalbinotic animals, allowing large choroidal blood vessels to be observed.

Nontapetal fundus

1. The nontapetal area is usually black or brown. Circumpapillary scarring is a common change observed in adult animals that have had subclinical attacks of equine recurrent uveitis.
2. Color dilute animals may show mild to severe chorioretinal hypoplasia; albino horses lack visible retinal or choroidal pigment.

PORCINE (Fig 1-32)

The porcine eye is nontapetal with a grey to reddish-grey fundus. White reflexes from the internal limiting membrane are often seen extending on either side of the optic disk.

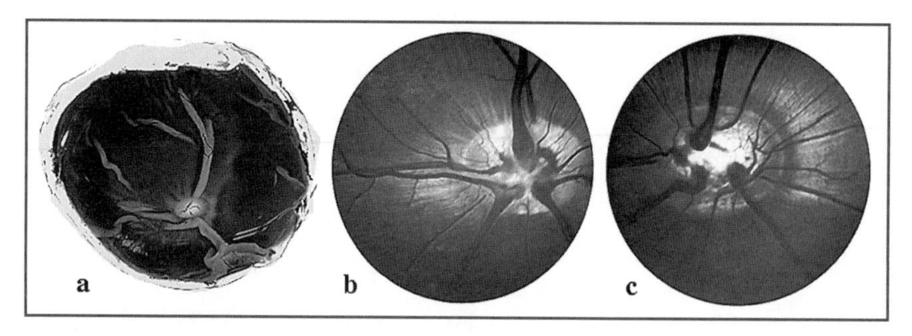

Figure 1-32. Normal porcine (Yucatan miniature pig).
- a. Dissected eye. Retinal folds occurred during dissection. Optic disk is myelinated and oval. The fundus is nontapetal. White pigs will have a pink fundus.
- b. Normal fundus. Vessels are paired with three or four major arteries. Note the medullary rays extending from the optic disk and central hyaloid remnant.
- c. Normal fundus. This eye has minimal myelination of the optic disk.

Optic disk

1. It is oval, large and partly myelinated to give a blotchy white appearance.
2. Location - similar to dogs. Located below and nasal to the posterior pole of the eye.
3. Large veins and smaller arteries that may be located central or peripheral

Retina

1. Blood vessels prominent similar to dog
2. Very definite area centralis temporal and superior to optic disk

Fundus

1. Color may be brown, reddish brown or purple
2. White striations can be seen leaving the optic disk, possibly representing reflections from the internal limiting membrane. These are extremely prominent in young pigs but are less noticeable as the animal ages.

GOATS (Fig 1-33)

Optic disk

1. Usually round and well myelinated
2. Hyaloid remnants may be seen but less common than sheep or cattle
3. Located centrally, below posterior pole of the eye

Fundus

1. Well developed tapetum - blue, green or may have yellow tones. Texture is more homogeneous than sheep and cattle.
2. Nontapetal fundus - dark brown or reddish
3. Blood vessels large but not obviously paired like sheep and cattle

LLAMA (Fig 1-33)

Optic disk

1. Round to oval
2. May or may not be myelinated. If myelinated, it is not unusual to see myelinated nerve fibers on either side of this disk.
3. Hyaloid remnants are common

Fundus

1. Nontapetal fundus
2. The color is usually red and brown or rust, or red with a blue cast. Small areas of yellow can sometimes be observed.
3. Blood vessels are large and usually paired.

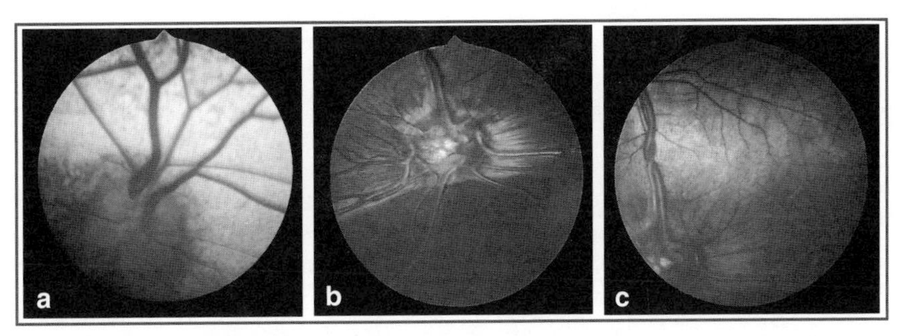

Figure 1-33. Normal goat and llama.

a. Normal goat. The optic disk is round and smaller than sheep and usually well myelinated. Blood vessels are large as is characteristic of sheep.

b & c. Normal llama. Optic disk is poorly myelinated with large paired blood vessels. Note some myelinated nerve fibers on the nasal side of the disk. The llama is considered to be nontapetal, but note the yellowish (light area) discoloration above the optic disk.

RABBIT (Fig 1-34)

Merangiotic vascular pattern with blood vessels confined to a horizontal zone on either side of the optic disk

Optic disk

1. Located 1 to 2 disk diameters above the posterior pole of the globe
2. Slightly oval in shape
3. Deep physiologic cup, especially in New Zealand white rabbits. ***Do not confuse this with a coloboma.***

Fundus

1. Retinal blood vessels with accompanying medullary fibers can be seen on both sides of the disk.
2. New Zealand white rabbit - nonpigmented fundus with choroidal blood vessels easily seen
3. Pigmented rabbits (e.g. Dutch belted) - fundus is brown in color and choroidal blood vessels are not visible. Medullary fibers are usually seen radiating below and on both sides of the optic disk.

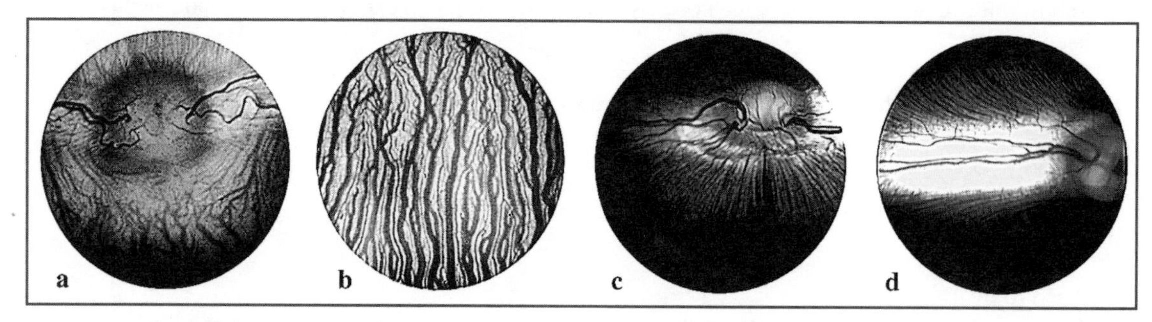

Figure 1-34. Normal rabbit.

a & b. Normal New Zealand white. Nonpigmented fundus with horizontal retinal blood vessels on both sides of the disk. There is a large physiologic cup. Choroidal blood vessels are visible.

c & d. Normal Dutch belted. The fundus is darkly pigmented. Medullated nerve fibers and the merangiotic vascular pattern are easily seen.

SPECIAL EXAMINATIONS

After the routine light room examination has been completed, a mydriatic (tropicamide 1%) should be administered and then repeated in 10 minutes. Within 20 to 30 minutes of the first drop, the pupil should be dilated. This waiting period is an opportunity to perform any additional examination procedures that would be deemed appropriate based on the findings of the initial light room examination.

EXAMINING LIGHTS (Fig 1-35)

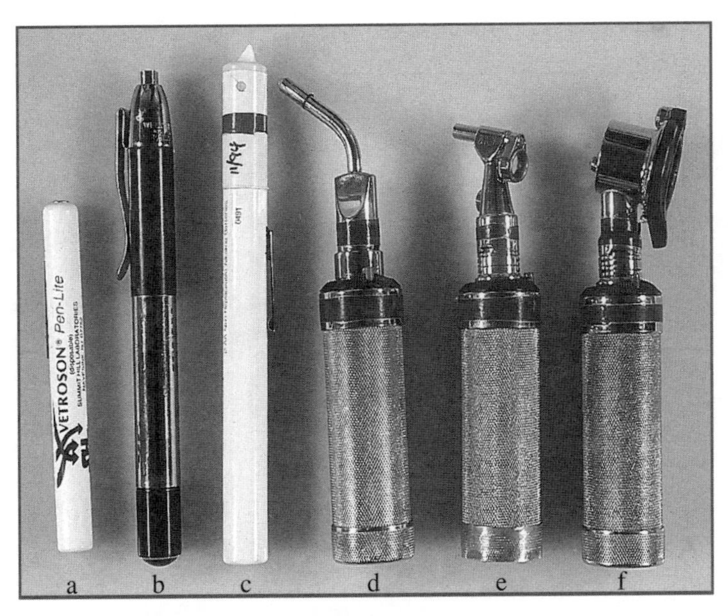

Figure 1-35. Examining lights.
a. Disposable penlight
b. Welch Allyn focusing penlight
c. Slit-beam penlight
d. Welch Allyn Finnoff transilluminator
e. Modified operating otoscope
f. Pneumonic otoscope

Penlights

Available from many sources

1. Round beam for general examination
2. Slit beam for examination of the cornea, anterior chamber and lens (Concept and Vetroson)

Transilluminators

Brighter than penlights, provide a more focused beam, and can be used as a light source for indirect ophthalmoscopy.

1. Welch Allyn Finnoff transilluminator - a cobalt blue filter is available for fluorescein intensification
2. Operating otoscope (can be modified by removing the speculum bracket). This is the author's preferred transilluminator.
3. Pneumonic otoscope can be used as a transilluminator or as a magnifying lens and light.

Ultraviolet (Wood's lamp)

Useful to visualize normal lens by turning it opaque and intensifies fluorescein fluorescence

BINOCULAR LOUPES (many available)

Optivisor (Donegan Optical) (Fig 1-36)

Available with several lens powers. The #5 lens plate has a focal length of 8 inches and 2.5 power magnification. This is satisfactory for most examinations and minor surgery.

Surgical binoculars (Fig 1-37)

Have compound lenses similar to opera glasses, thus allowing magnification and a comfortable working distance. These are much more expensive. Custom made loupes are available with variable magnification and focal distance.

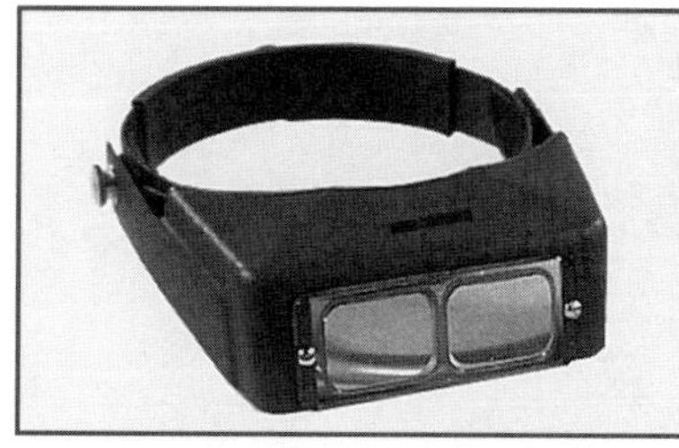

Figure 1-36. Optivisor binocular loupe with number 5 lens plate (2.5x magnification and 8 inches focal length).

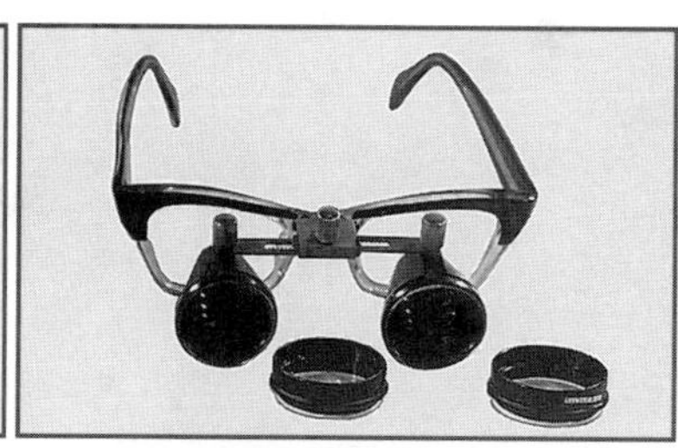

Figure 1-37a. Surgical binocular loupe. Magnification 1.8x and auxiliary lens give 2.5x.

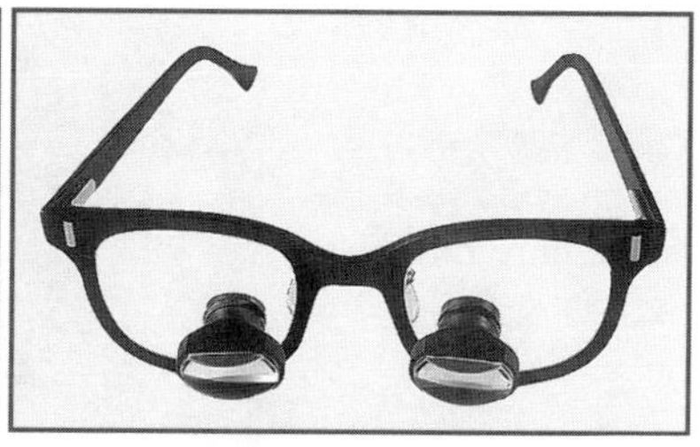

Figure 1-37b. Designs for Vision's custom-made surgical telescope (Deseret Health Medical).

CYTOLOGY - Scraping, impression smears, aspirates

Conjunctival scraping (Lavach JD et al. Cytology of normal and inflamed conjunctivitis in dogs and cats. J Am Vet Med Assoc 1977;170:722).

1. Spatula for ocular cytology (Fig 1-38) - the Kimura platinum tip spatula is designed specifically for exfoliative cytology but, unfortunately, is expensive. A satisfactory substitute can be an iris spatula or repositor, chemistry measuring spatula, lens cortex spatula, or the grooved tip of a #3 Bard Parker scalpel handle.
2. Topical anesthetic is instilled in the eye three to four times at 30-second intervals

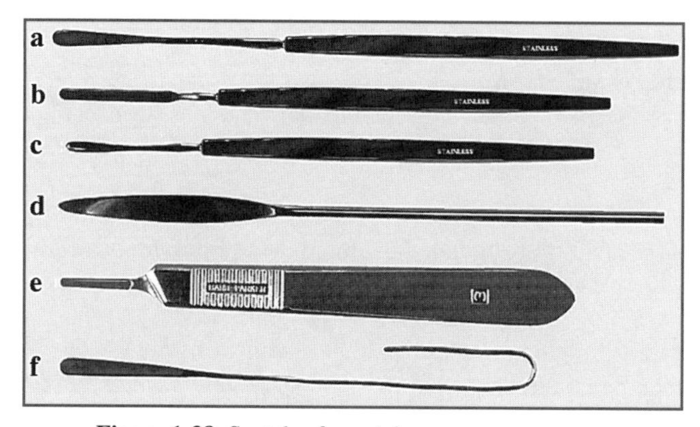

Figure 1-38. Spatulas for cytology.
a. Kimura platinum spatula
b. Iris repositioning spatula
c. Lens cortex spatula
d. Chemistry spatula
e. #3 Bard Parker handle
f. Stainless steel wire spatula

3. Generalized conjunctivitis - using a conjunctival or suitable spatula, a scraping is made from the palpebral or bulbar conjunctiva (Fig 1-39 a and b). The lower palpebral conjunctiva works very well in small animals and the upper palpebral conjunctiva is preferred in large animals. Scraping from the center of the lid will yield the most representative cells. Avoid scraping near the fornix. This will show an excess number of goblet cells. Scrapings made near the eyelid margin may have keratinized cells. Scraping from the dorsal globe will yield excellent cells but is more difficult because the bulbar conjunctiva is very mobile. If there is excess mucus or inflammatory discharge, clean the eye thoroughly with an eye wash before collecting the sample. Air-drying of the slide is satisfactory if staining will not be delayed. If staining of slides will be delayed, a spray slide fixative is generally recommended.
4. Focal lesions - scraping should be made directly from the lesion. This is very important with melting corneal ulcers (Fig 1-39.c).

Impression smears (Fig 1-39.d)

Impression smears are used less frequently than scrapings. They have their greatest value in corneal ulcers and growths suspected of being neoplastic. Corneal lesions with stromal involvement that are epithelialized will require rubbing off the overlying epithelium before making the impression smear. Biopsies can also be used for making impression smears before being placed in formalin.

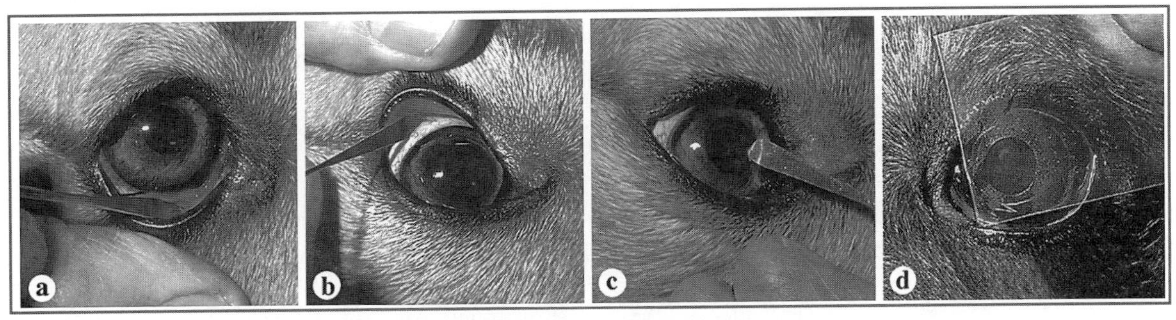

Figure 1-39. Collecting cytology specimens.
a. Scraping from lower eyelid conjunctiva
b. Scraping from dorsal bulbar conjunctiva
c. Scraping from corneal ulcer
d. Impression smear from corneal ulcer

Centesis anterior chamber and vitreous

Samples drawn from the anterior chamber or vitreous are useful for cytology, serologic examination, and/or culturing. From 0.2 to 0.5 ml can be safely withdrawn depending on the species.

Fine needle aspiration from suspected tumors involving the iris has a high risk of spreading the tumor. If the tumor is adherent to the cornea, aspiration can be performed with a corneal puncture without danger of releasing tumor cells into the aqueous.

1. Anterior chamber centesis
   a. Restraint
      1) Small animals - general anesthesia is recommended
      2) Equine - topical anesthesia and sedation are usually adequate. Short general anesthesia eliminates risks of injuring a visual eye.
   b. Technique (Fig 1-40)
      1) Small animals - Using a small forceps, the conjunctiva is elevated several millimeters from the limbus. A 25 to 27 gauge needle is introduced, bevel up, at this site and it is advanced beneath the conjunctiva to a scleral site 2 to 3 mm from the limbus. This will result in the conjunctival needle wound being further from the limbus than the scleral wound so that when the needle is withdrawn aqueous loss will form a conjunctival bleb. The needle is

directed against the sclera so that when it enters the anterior chamber it will be anterior and parallel with the iris. A drilling motion will facilitate traversing the sclera. The needle is passed far enough so that the entire bevel surface is in the anterior chamber. When the needle is withdrawn, the conjunctival wound is pinched with forceps. Anterior chamber volume is replaced within minutes with aqueous production.

2) Equine - The technique is the same as for small animals except the site for aspiration should be the dorsal limbus to take advantage of the scleral extension beyond the base of the iris.

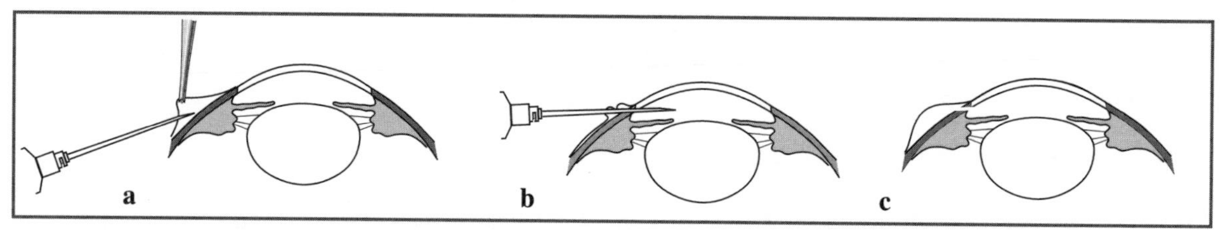

Figure 1-40. Anterior chamber centesis.

a. Pick up the conjunctiva several millimeters away from the dorsal or dorsolateral limbus. Introduce a 25 or 27 gauge needle at this spot and tunnel beneath the epithelium as the needle is advanced toward the limbus.
b. Traverse the limbus using a drilling motion with the needle and withdraw the desired amount of aqueous.
c. When the needle is withdrawn, a subconjunctival aqueous bleb will develop. This disappears in several hours.

2. Vitreous centesis
   a. Restraint
      1) Small animals - deep sedation or general anesthesia
      2) Equine - topical anesthesia and deep sedation is usually adequate
   b. Technique (Fig 1-41)
      1) Small animals - a 23 gauge needle is inserted through the conjunctiva and sclera about 8 mm posterior to the limbus (over the pars plana of the ciliary body). The needle is directed toward the optic nerve to avoid the lens. If the pupil is dilated, the needle may be directed visually to a specific location. A larger needle will allow easier aspiration but may result in greater vitreous loss or possible hemorrhage when the needle is withdrawn.
      2) Equine - same technique as small animals except the needle is introduced 10 to 15 mm posterior to the limbus. Because of the dorsal scleral overhang, a greater distance from the limbus is needed with a dorsal than a temporal site.

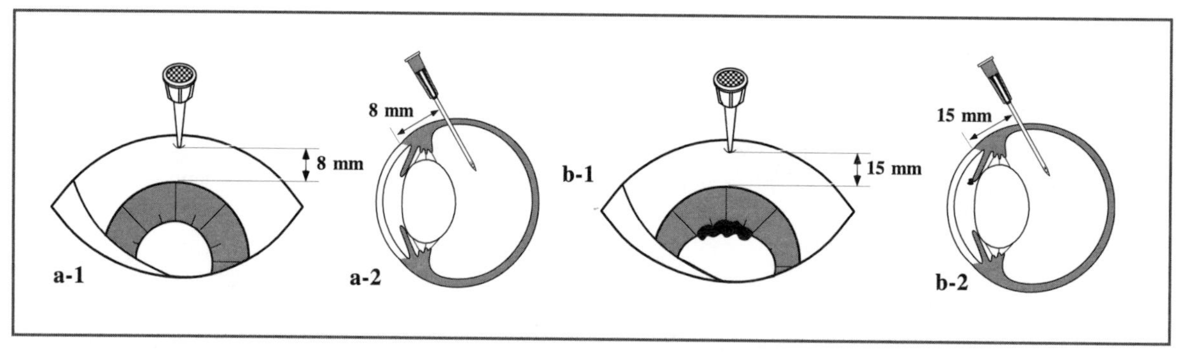

Figure 1-41. Vitreous centesis/injection. A 23 gauge needle is inserted through the conjunctiva and sclera with the needle directed toward the optic nerve to avoid the lens.

a. Small animals. Insertion 8 mm dorsal to limbus. 1) Anterior view 2) Sagittal view
b. Equine. Insertion 15 mm dorsal to the limbus. 1) Anterior view 2) Sagittal view
An alternate site would be 10 mm lateral to the limbus (not shown).

ASSESS PATENCY OF NASOLACRIMAL SYSTEM

Physiologic patency

Fluorescein placed in the conjunctival sac will usually appear in the nostril in small animals in 1 to 5 minutes; cats more rapidly than dogs. In horses it may take 20 minutes or more. Failure of fluorescein to appear in the nose is not proof of obstruction.

Flushing the nasolacrimal duct

This will determine anatomic patency. See Chapter 7, page 225, for anatomy.

1. Cats and dogs - the conjunctiva should be topically anesthetized
   a. Lacrimal cannulas (Fig 1-42)

Figure 1-42. Lacrimal cannulas.
- a. Human cannula with 23 gauge tip on 19 gauge needle
- b. Modified 20 gauge needle
- c. Modified 22 gauge needle
- d. Modified 25 gauge needle
- e. Modified 27 gauge needle
- f. 30 gauge air injection cannula

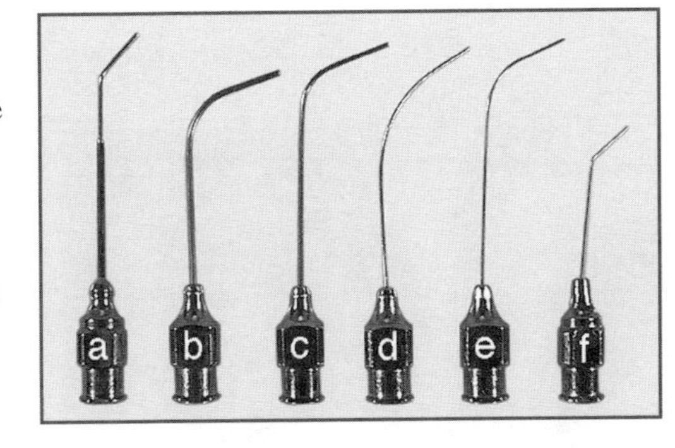

1) Lacrimal cannulas can be made from 20, 23, 25, or 27 gauge disposable hypodermic needles by cutting off the point with scissors. If a stylus is placed in the needle before cutting, it will prevent crushing the tip when the needle is cut.
2) Human lacrimal cannulas are satisfactory. Most have a 23 gauge tip on a 19 gauge needle. The tip may be straight or angled at 45°.
3) Curved lacrimal cannulas (20, 23, 25, 27, 30 gauge) are available from Sontec Instruments.

   b. Technique - topically anesthetize the eye. Place the largest cannula that will go into the punctum on a 3- or 6-cc syringe. Hold the syringe so that the plunger can be pushed without changing the grip on the syringe. Restrain the patient's head with the nose down at a minimum of a 20° angle. This will eliminate irrigating fluid from flowing toward the pharynx and stimulating coughing. The upper punctum (Fig 1-43) is generally the easiest to cannulate, but both are satisfactory. Cannulate about 5 mm and then irrigate with considerable force on the plunger. Irrigating solution will come out the opposite palpebral punctum and the nostril if the duct and canaliculi are patent. If there is duct obstruction, it may be necessary to occlude the opposite punctum and reflush. Retrograde flushing at the nasal punctum requires general anesthesia.

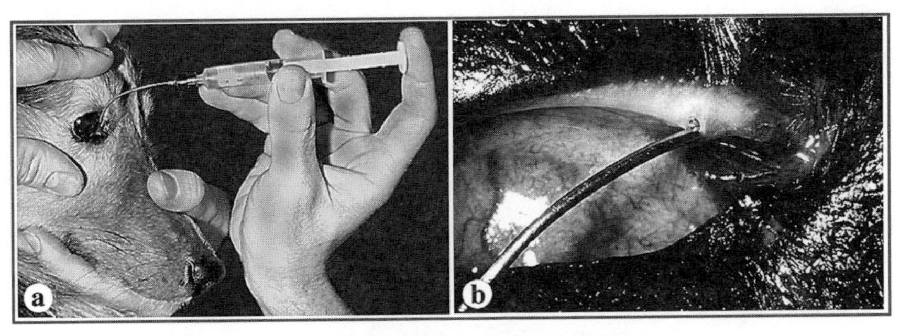

Figure 1-43. Flushing canine palpebral punctum.
- a. Head positioned with nose lowered
- b. Lacrimal cannula in upper eyelid punctum

2. Rabbits - have only a lower eyelid punctum located further from the nasal canthus and the edge of the eyelid.
3. Large animals - can be flushed from the palpebral or nasal punctum (Fig 1-44). Sedation is recommended.
   a. Palpebral punctum - topical anesthesia is recommended
      1) Cannulas - lacrimal cannulas, tomcat catheter, IV catheter, male urinary catheter (5-6 Fr), or polyethylene tubing
      2) Technique - the palpebral puncta can be difficult to visualize. A 12 cc syringe is preferred because of the large fluid capacity of the nasolacrimal duct. The lower punctum is larger than the upper.
   b. Nasal punctum - In horses and cattle, the nasal punctum is easily visualized on the floor of the nares and therefore is more frequently used. It is more difficult to visualize in llamas.
      1) Cannulas - 5 or 8 French feeding tube, teat cannula, 160 polyethylene tubing, large IV catheter, a curved tip irrigation syringe, or tomcat catheter
      2) Technique - Attach a 12 or 20 ml syringe to the cannula. Pass the cannula until it fits snugly in the punctum or has been passed 3 to 4 inches. To prevent backflow, it is advisable to apply pressure with a finger where the cannula enters the punctum. Eight to 15 ml of irrigating fluid may be needed before any fluid appears at the palpebral puncta.

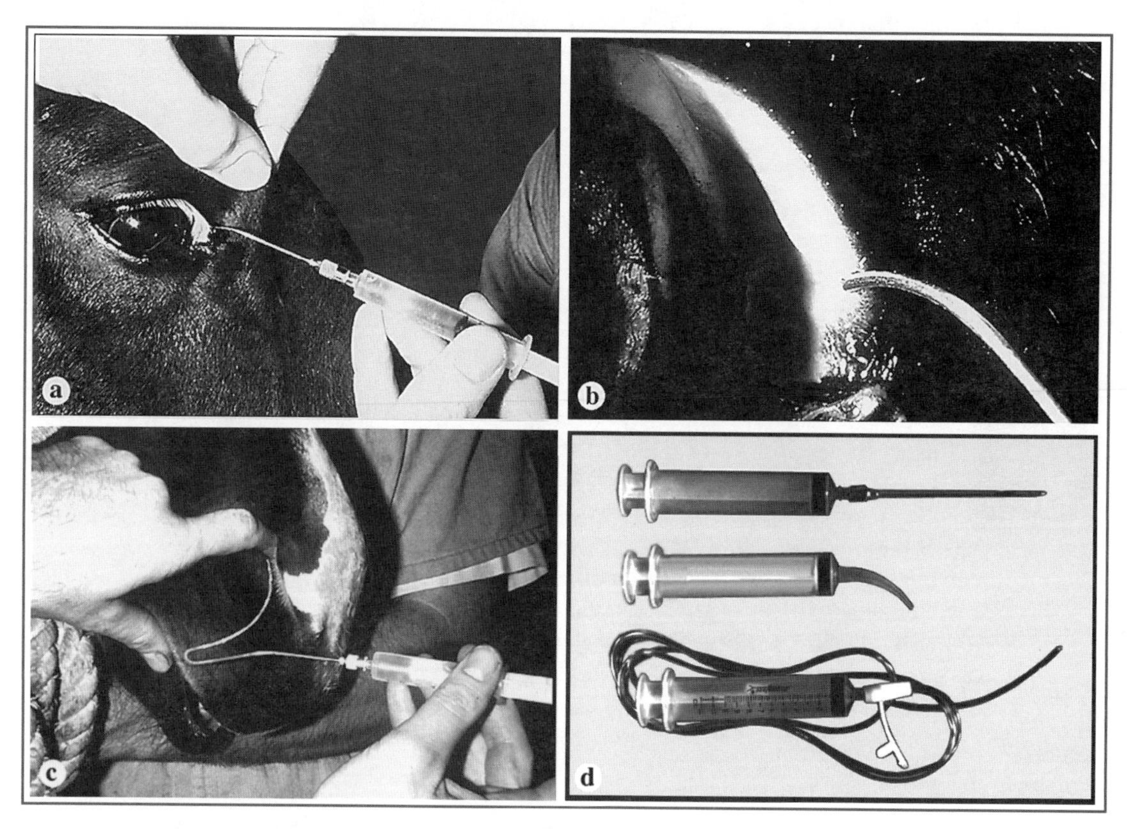

Figure 1-44. Flushing equine nasolacrimal system.
- a. Flushing upper punctum with 20 gauge lacrimal cannula
- b. Close-up showing superior punctum location
- c. Flushing nasal punctum with syringe and PE160 polyethylene tubing
- d. Other cannulas: teat tube, irrigation syringe, 8 French feeding tube

Catheterization

If flushing the duct is unsuccessful, then catheterization is indicated. See Chapter 7, page 239 for technique.

EXAMINATION OF THE THIRD EYELID

Animals with sudden onset unilateral ocular discharge and pain should always be examined for foreign bodies.

Fornix examination

A curved mosquito forceps or strabismus muscle hook is excellent to elevate the eyelid away from the globe. Start at the canthus, lift the eyelid up and work the muscle hook (or closed forceps) all the way around eyelid allowing visualization of the fornix dorsally and the palpebral cul-de-sac inferiorly.

Third eyelid examination

1. Anterior surface - retropulse the eye to protrude the third eyelid so that the palpebral surface can be visualized
2. Posterior surface - ***AVOID grasping the margin of the third eyelid with a 1 x 2 forceps and pulling the eyelid away from the globe!***
    a. Small animals (Fig 1-45) - The technique preferred by the author entails grasping the third eyelid along its border with a curved mosquito forceps so that the forceps lies parallel with the free margin of the eyelid and then "rolling" the third eyelid up on the forceps, which will allow visualization of the bulbar surface of the third eyelid and expose the inferior fornix. An alternate technique would be to grasp the free edge of the third eyelid with a Graefe fixation forceps (Chapter 3, page 131) and pull the third eyelid away from the globe.
    b. Large animals - Manipulating the third eyelid with a Graefe forceps, or perpendicular grasping with a mosquito forceps, is satisfactory.

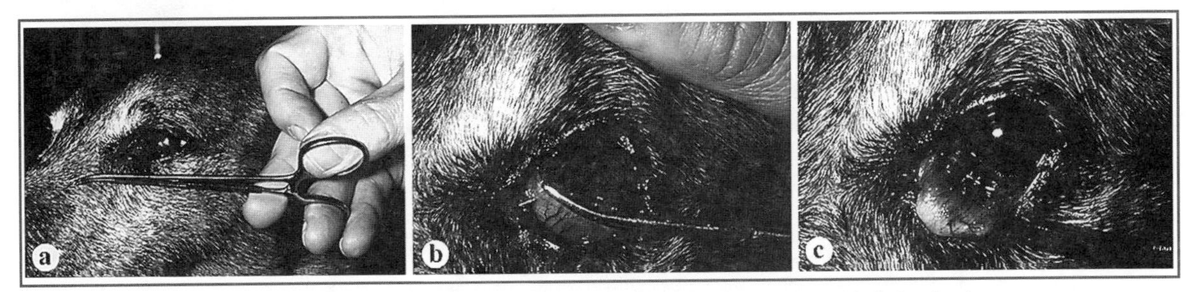

Figure 1-45. Examining the posterior surface of the third eyelid and inferior fornix.
a. Curved mosquito forceps in front of eye
b. Grasping third eyelid along its border with curved mosquito forceps
c. Third eyelid rolled up on forceps

CORNEAL STAINS

Corneal stains are used to determine the health and integrity of the corneal and conjunctival epithelium, and determine physiologic flow of the nasolacrimal system.

Sodium fluorescein

Sodium fluorescein is water soluble, appears yellow-orange in high concentration, and green when diluted. It will not penetrate intact epithelium of the cornea or conjunctiva. If the ocular epithelium is disrupted, it will produce a green stain in the corneal stroma and subconjunctival tissues. Staining is enhanced with an ultraviolet or blue light.

1. Sources
    a. Sterile strips with 1 mg fluorescein
    b. Ophthalmic solution 0.5 to 2.0%. Fluorescein neutralizes common preservatives, therefore solutions may become contaminated.
    c. Topical combination of fluorescein and proparacaine
    d. 10 to 25% fluorescein IV solution for fluorescein angiography
2. Corneal and conjunctival staining
    a. Sterile strips are most frequently used (no danger of contamination)
        1) Moisten the strip with an irrigating solution or topical anesthetic. A dry strip can scratch the eye or if the eye is dry, fail to transfer fluorescein.
        2) Touch the strip to the conjunctiva dorsal to the limbus. Only a minute amount is needed. Gently irrigate the eye. This will disperse the fluorescein and wash away the excess. Cotton or a gauze sponge placed below the eye will absorb the overflow. ***Do not touch the strip to the cornea because this will leave a fluorescein-positive imprint.***
        If the dorsal conjunctiva is not accessible, apply the strip to the palpebral surface of the third eyelid. Irrigation will still distribute the fluorescein over the eye.
    b. Solutions
        1) Commercial solution - one drop applied directly on the cornea, followed by irrigation
        2) Large animals - a solution can be made by placing the fluorescein-impregnated tip of a strip in a 3 cc syringe and then fill the syringe with irrigation solution. Place a 25 gauge needle on the syringe and break off the needle at the hub. The solution can be directed from the syringe gently across the cornea (Chapter 2, page 66). Rinsing is usually unnecessary.
    c. Interpretation
        1) Corneal ulcers - fluorescein will produce a bright green stain of the exposed corneal stroma that persists 15 to 30 minutes. If there is severe stromal involvement and endothelial damage, fluorescein will enter the aqueous through the damaged endothelium.
        2) Small corneal defects or epithelial toxicity - may require a darkened room, magnification, and the use of a blue or ultraviolet light to identify subtle changes.
        3) Conjunctival injuries - may appear yellow-orange with white light or fluoresce green with a blue light.
3. Other uses
    a. Testing for aqueous leakage from corneal wounds (Seidel's test). Fluorescein applied over the wound will develop a green rivulet where the aqueous escapes from the wound.
    b. Physiologic nasolacrimal patency, see page 39.
    c. Fluorescein angiography. Intravenous fluorescein is useful in detecting abnormalities in retinal vascular permeability, the intercellular barriers between the regional pigment cells (zonula occludens), and the flow pattern of retinal blood vessels.
    d. Fluorescein will result in a faint green staining of degenerate corneal and conjunctival epithelial cells that is visible only with a blue or ultraviolet light, thus acting as a vital stain.
4. *Comment* - False positive staining can occur where Schirmer tear strips touch the cornea and after the use of proparacaine topical anesthesia.

Rose bengal

Rose bengal (a fluorescein derivative) is a vital stain that stains dead or degenerating epithelial cells of the cornea and conjunctiva. Its main indication is demonstrating epithelial changes seen with dry eye, especially in early cases.

1. Sources
    a. Sterile ophthalmic strips with 1.3 mg rose bengal
    b. 1% ophthalmic solution. This may cause irritation that can be prevented with topical anesthesia.
2. Staining technique
    a. Same as fluorescein
    b. Excess mucus will stain intensely and require ocular irrigation before epithelial staining can be evaluated.

3. Interpretation - A red stain to affected conjunctiva and epithelium indicates devitalized cells. It is not unusual for the corneal epithelium protected by the third eyelid to be negative. Slight patchy epithelial staining is normal.
4. Epithelial toxicity has been observed

TONOMETRY

Measurement of tension or pressure. Direct tonometry is the measurement of intraocular pressure with a manometer and is not clinically practical. Indirect tonometry determines the intraocular pressure by measuring corneal tension.

Digital tonometry

Estimation of intraocular pressure by applying digital pressure to the eye. This is a crude estimate and does not replace the use of a tonometer. It is dependable when marked pressure difference exists. A painful eye will be enophthalmic and in turn feel softer than the normal eye. An exophthalmic eye that cannot be retroposed will feel harder than a normal eye even though the intraocular pressure may be normal.

1. Digital pressure on the globe through the upper eyelids. Acute glaucoma with enophthalmos and chemosis may not feel firmer than the normal eye when palpated through the lid. Chronic glaucoma with significantly high pressure can be detected quite easily.
2. Digital pressure directly on the cornea. After topical anesthesia, the eye can be touched with a moistened finger and the indentability of the cornea evaluated. The author has found this more dependable than palpation through the eyelid.

Indentation tonometry (Fig 1-46a)

There is a correlation between indentability of the cornea and intraocular pressure. The higher the pressure, the less the indentability. Topical anesthesia is necessary.

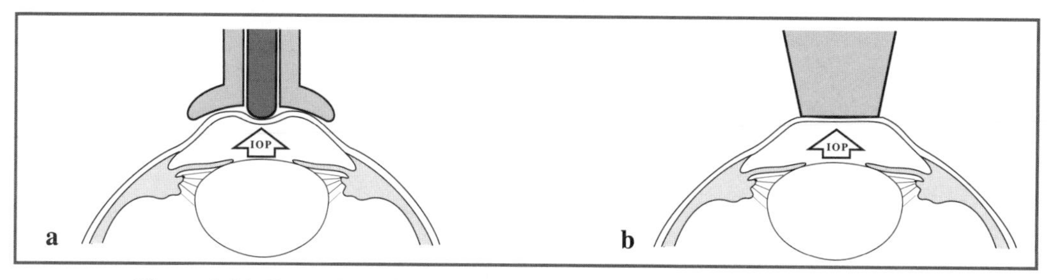

Figure 1-46. Comparison of indentation and applanation tonometry.
a. Indentation tonometry determines pressure by indenting the cornea
b. Applanation tonometry determines pressure by flattening the cornea

1. Touching cornea with a muscle hook, curved mosquito forceps or cotton swab. After the eye has been topically anesthetized, the cornea can be lightly touched with the tip of a muscle hook or curved hemostat. Gradually allow the weight of the instrument to rest on the cornea until indentation is noted. Hypotonic eyes will show obvious indentation before the examiner is aware the cornea is supporting any of the weight of the instrument. Normal eyes will indent slightly when the examiner is aware that the cornea is starting to support the weight of the instrument. Eyes with increased pressure will support the weight of the instrument without significant indentation or may actually require pressure from the examiner before indenting. This is superior to digital tonometry but is still a crude estimate and does not replace the use of a tonometer for evaluating intraocular pressure.
2. *Schiötz indentation tonometer* (Fig 1-47a) - The Schiötz tonometer is an accurate instrument to estimate intraocular pressure in the dog and cat. It cannot be used in large animals unless they are in lateral recumbency. It is the least expensive tonometer available. Cost varies from $150 (Arista) to $250. The less expensive instruments have a wider edge to the footplate, which makes it more difficult to slip the footplate between the third eyelid and cornea. The tonometer has a 5.5 gm plunger that sets on the cornea and will indent the cornea slightly when intraocular pressure is normal. The plunger movement controls a rocker arm with a pointer that moves over a millimeter scale. One millimeter of corneal

indentation results in a 20 mm displacement on the scale. If the pressure is elevated, the indentability of the cornea is reduced and the scale reading may be 0 to 3 mm. When this happens, weights are provided that can be added to make the plunger weigh 7.5 or 10 gm.

a. Restraint and positioning - The eye must be looking vertically so that the tonometer can rest on the center of the cornea. Sitting animals will usually roll their eye downward, eliminating proper positioning of the tonometer (Fig 1-47b). When this occurs, the patient must be placed in dorsal or dorsolateral recumbency (Fig 1-47c).

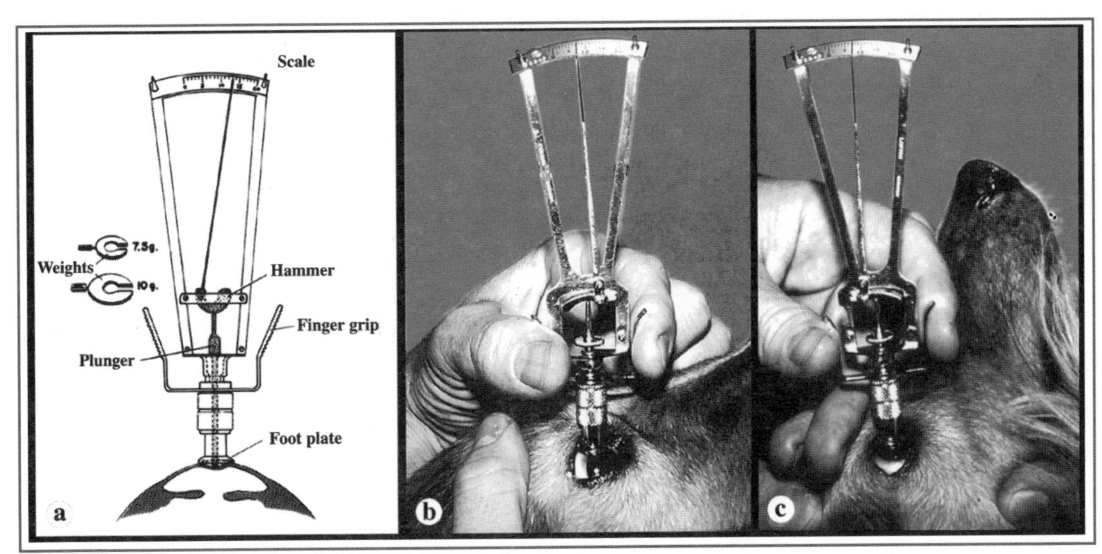

Figure 1-47. Restraint and positioning for Schiötz tonometry.
a. Schematic drawing of Schiötz tonometer
b. Dog in sitting position with nose turned up. Eye rolls down.
c. Dog in dorsal recumbency. Eye directed toward ceiling.

b. Techniques - After the eye has been topically anesthetized, the tonometer is held directly above the cornea so that when the tonometer footplate touches the cornea the tonometer will be vertical. Tilting the tonometer will result in an inaccurate reading. If the footplate extends over the sclera, the chance for error is increased. Allow the instrument to rest its entire weight on the cornea for one to two seconds. A scale reading the moment after the total weight of the tonometer is on the cornea is most accurate. Repeat placing the tonometer on the cornea until two to three repeatable readings are determined.

c. Interpretation of scale readings - The most accurate scale readings are between 4 and 8, therefore a scale reading less than 4 should be repeated using a 7.5 gm plunger load mass. Acute glaucoma may require using a 10 gm plunger load mass before the lever will leave zero. Always measure both eyes because the differential pressure may be more significant than the individual pressures.

1) Human conversion table. A conversion table for the human eye comes with the Schiötz tonometer. The corneoscleral rigidity of animals is less than man. Therefore, if this conversion table is used to estimate intraocular pressure in animals, the pressures determined will be less than the patient's actual intraocular pressures. Fortunately, the error is constant and the table can still be used. When the human table is used, the author has found normal values to be:

Canine: 12 to 24 mm Hg (most dogs are below 20)
Feline: 12 to 26 mm Hg (most adult cats are between 18 to 22; young patients slightly lower)
Equine: 14 to 22 mm Hg (requires lateral recumbency)
Bovine: 14 to 22 mm Hg (requires lateral recumbency)

2) Dog and cat calibration tables - Because of the error when using the human conversion table, calibration tables have been developed for the dog (Table 2) and the cat (Table 3). Normal pressures in dogs are about 15 to 28 and cats about 16 to 30 mm Hg.

Table 1-2. Calibration table for Schiötz tonometry in dogs*

Schiötz scale reading	IOP (mm Hg) 5.5 g wt	IOP (mm Hg) 7.5 g wt	IOP (mm Hg) 10.0 g wt
0.5	46	61	75
1.0	44	59	73
1.5	43	56	70
2.0	40	53	66
2.5	33	47	61
3.0	26	40	55
3.5	23	35	49
4.0	21	32	44
4.5	20	29	41
5.0	19	27	38
5.5	18	26	36
6.0	17	24	33
6.5	16	23	31
7.0	15	22	30
7.5		20	28
8.0	14	19	27
8.5	13		25
9.0		18	24
9.5	12	17	23
10.0		16	22
10.5	11	15	21
11.0			20
11.5	10	14	19
12.0		13	18
12.5			17
13.0		12	16
13.5	8	11	15
14.0			
14.5		10	14
15.0	7		13
15.5		9	12
16.0			
16.5	6	8	11
17.0			10
17.5		7	
18.0	5		9
18.5		6	
19.0			8
19.5			7
20.0		5	

*Pickett et al, ACVO Proceedings 1988

Table 1-3. Calibration table for Schiötz tonometry in cats*

Schiötz scale reading	IOP (mm Hg) 5.5 g wt	IOP (mm Hg) 7.5 g wt	IOP (mm Hg) 10.0 g wt
0.5	44	73	
1.0	42	71	
1.5	40	68	
2.0	37	65	80
2.5	33	61	76
3.0	30	56	71
3.5	27	48	66
4.0	25	42	61
4.5	24	37	56
5.0	22	34	51
5.5	21	31	47
6.0	20	29	44
6.5	18	27	40
7.0		25	37
7.5	17	24	35
8.0	16	22	33
8.5	15	21	31
9.0	14	20	29
9.5	13	19	27
10.0		18	25
10.5		17	23
11.0	12	16	22
11.5	11	15	20
12.0		14	19
12.5	10	13	18
13.0		12	17
13.5	9		15
14.0		11	14
14.5	8	10	13
15.0			12
15.5		9	11
16.0	7	8	10
16.5			9
17.0	6	7	8
17.5		6	7
18.0			6
18.5	5	5	5
19.0			
19.5			
20.0			

*Pickett et al, ACVO Proceedings 1988

3) Rule of 2 - This is an estimate of intraocular pressure without using a conversion table to record intraocular pressure in mm Hg. Dogs and cats with normal pressure usually have a scale value that is within 2 mm plus or minus the weight of the plunger. This is:

Plunger weight	Scale range for normal eyes
5.5 gm	3.5 to 7.5
7.5 gm	5.5 to 9.5
10.0 gm	8 to 12

Scale readings less than the above values would indicate increased pressure and higher readings would indicate decreased pressure.

Applanation tonometry (Fig 1-46b)

Applanation tonometers measure the amount of flattening (area of contact) of the cornea when a weight touches the cornea. The higher the pressure, the more weight it takes to flatten the cornea. This type of tonometer is the most frequently used in human ophthalmology. The most widely used human applanation tonometer is adapted to the slit lamp, thus making it impractical for use in animals. Several types of electronic tonometers are suitable for animal use.

1. Tono-Pen (Oculab) (Fig 1-48) - a small hand-held electronic applanation tonometer that is completely portable. It is accurate when the examiner becomes experienced in using it. It is less expensive than fixed-base electronic tonometers. In the dog and cat it overestimates pressure in the low range, accurate in the normal, and underestimates high pressure. In the horse, it underestimates at all pressures.

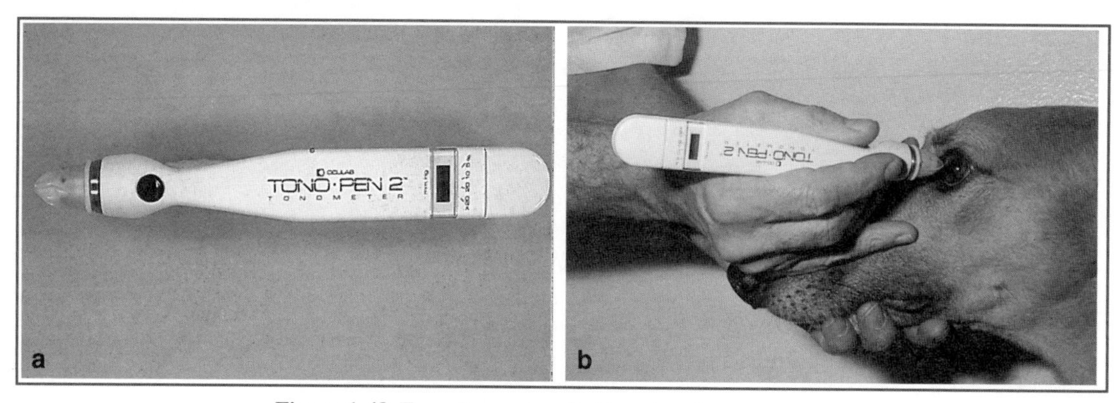

Figure 1-48. Tono-Pen - a handheld applanation tonometer.
a. Tono-Pen
b. Measuring pressure with Tono-Pen

2. Countertop electronic tonometers have been used for many years and several are available. Examples are:
   a. The McKay-Marg applanation tonometer (Biotronics) has been extensively used in veterinary ophthalmology and has been dependable. It is no longer manufactured but reconditioned units are available.
   b. Challenger tonometer (Mentor O & O)
   c. Mentor O & O makes several models of pneumotonometers. Mentor Model 30 Classic pneumotonometer is shown in Fig 1-49.

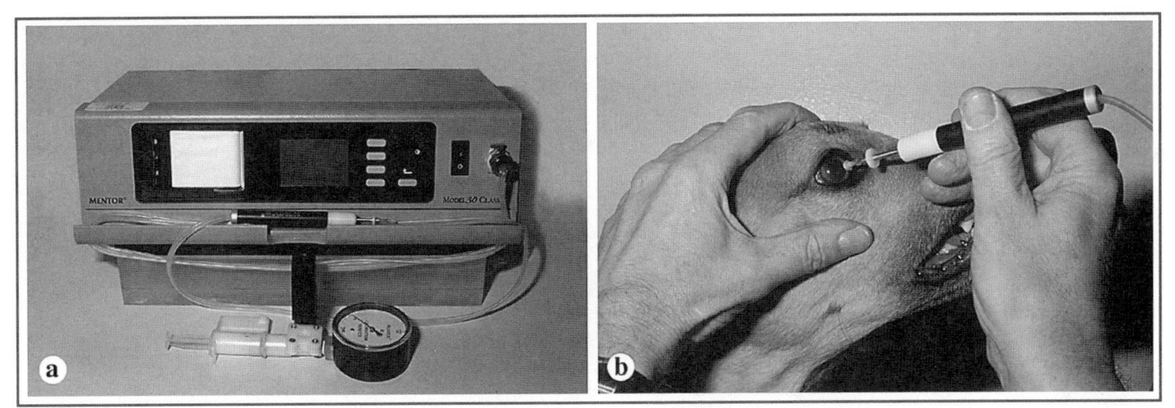

Figure 1-49. Mentor, Model 30 Classic pneumotonometer.
a. Instrument
b. Measuring intraocular pressure

Comment

1. Tonometry is useful in the differential diagnosis of the diseases that cause a red eye.
   a. Increased pressure - glaucoma
   b. Normal pressure - conjunctivitis, exophthalmos from space-occupying lesions of the orbit
   c. Decreased pressure - anterior uveitis, episcleritis, severe vascular hypotension (hemorrhagic shock, dehydration, Addison's disease)
2. Corneal diseases that will affect accuracy of readings:
   a. Corneal edema increases indentability and will result in reduced pressure readings
   b. Corneal lesions with an irregular surface - deep ulcers; tumors, granulation. Schiötz tonometer readings are more susceptible to irregularities than applanation tonometers.

GONIOSCOPY

Gonioscopy is the examination of the filtration (iridocorneal) angle.

Anatomy

1. Horses (Fig 1-50) - the filtration angle is visible through the cornea at the nasal and temporal limbus
2. Small animals (Fig 1-51) - the sclera overlaps the filtration angle and internal reflection from the cornea prevents adequate visualization of the filtration angle unless special contact lens (goniolens) is used

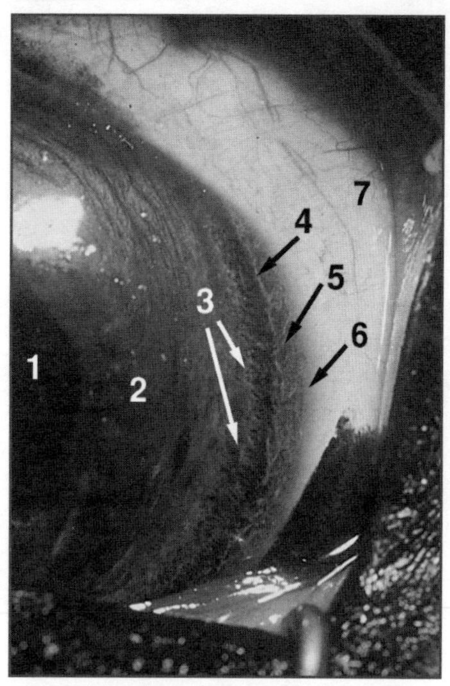

Figure 1-50. Normal equine filtration angle as seen at temporal limbus.
1. Pupil
2. Iris
3. Pectinate ligaments
4. Pectinate ligament insertion on cornea
5. Trabecular meshwork seen through cornea
6. Limbus
7. Conjunctiva

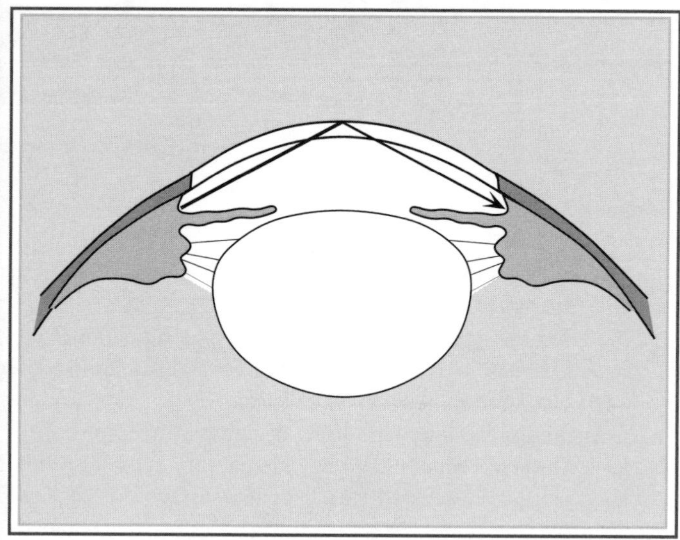

Figure 1-51. Internal reflection of light prevents visualization of filtration angle in small animals.

Indications for gonioscopy

1. Important in determining the cause for glaucoma
2. Examining for congenital abnormalities (goniodysgenesis) of the filtration angle
3. Evaluating peripheral iris tumors, cysts or injuries

Instrumentation

The minimal equipment needed is a goniolens, magnification loupe, light source and gonioscopic solution (Fig 1-52).

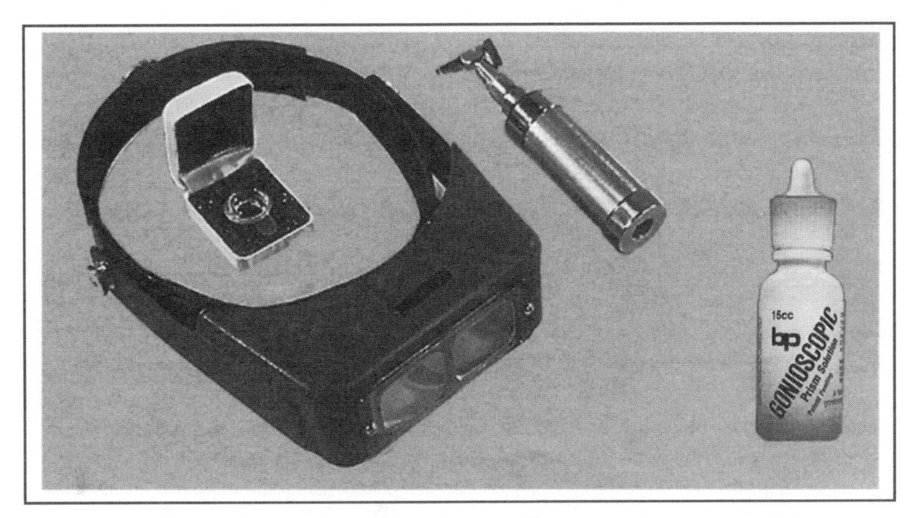

Figure 1-52. Minimal equipment for gonioscopy. Optivisor, transilluminator, Franklin goniolens, and gonioscopic lens solution.

1. Goniolenses - many styles are available (Fig 1-53)
   a. Franklin gonioscopic lens with latex cuff (no longer avsilable). Simple to use.
   b. Other goniolenses - Cordona, infant Koeppe, and Lovac Barkan (House of Vision)

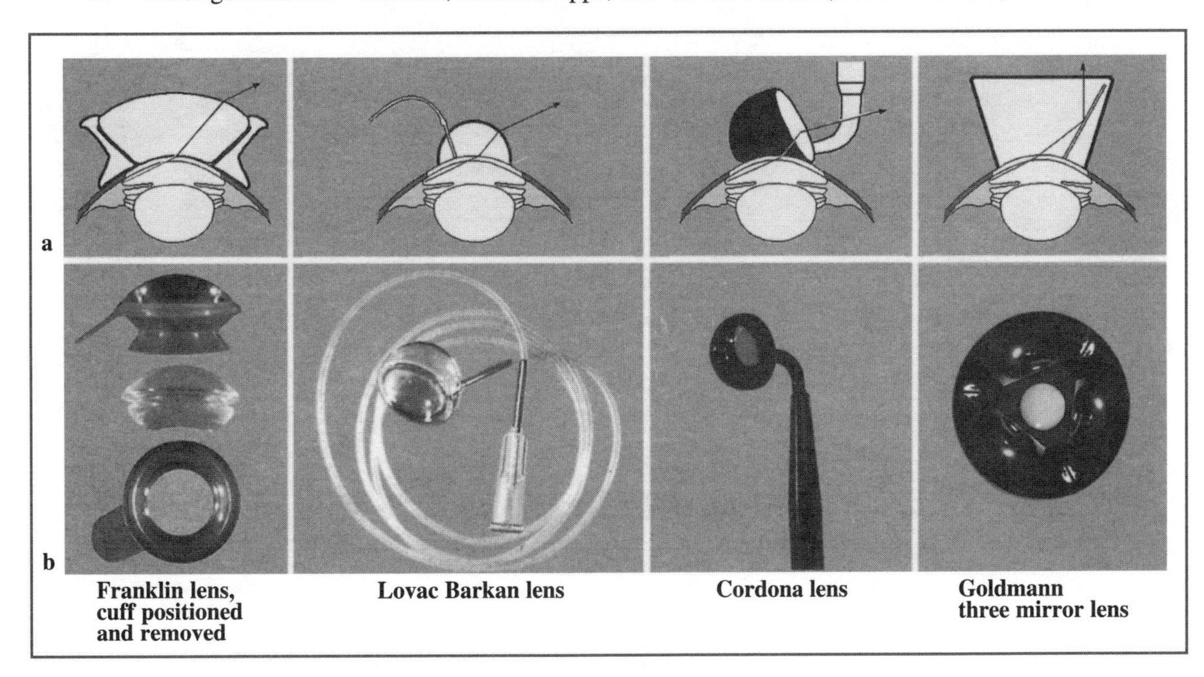

Figure 1-53. Goniolenses. Internal corneal reflection of light necessitates the use of a goniolens to visualize the canine filtration angle.
a. Schematics representing how respective goniolenses overcome internal reflection of light
b. Respective goniolenses

2. Magnification and light source
    a. Optivisor and a transilluminator are adequate
    b. Weck-Cordona fiberoptic goniolens - this combines a light source with a goniolens. It is an excellent instrument. It can be used on kittens and puppies but unfortunately is quite expensive. The examiner can still wear an Optivisor for additional magnification.
    c. Slit lamps (hand-held or stationary)
    d. Gonioscope - hand-held binocular microscope made specifically for gonioscopy
    e. Operating microscope
3. Gonioscopic lens solution

Technique using Franklin goniolens with latex cuff in small animals (Fig 1-54)

1. The lens cup is filled with gonioscopic solution and then placed on the eye. The gonioscopic coupling solution will fill in the space between the lens and the cornea to provide clear optics. If air bubbles appear in the space, the lens must be removed, refilled with gonioscopic fluid and then repositioned. The cuff is positioned beneath the eyelids and provides a degree of self-retention that facilitates keeping the lens securely on the eye.
2. The transilluminator light is placed near the goniolens with the beam directed across the iris as the examiner looks from behind the light toward the opposite side of the eye. The pectinate ligaments will be seen extending between the base of the iris and cornea. The examiner must rotate around the eye visualizing the entire circumference of the filtration angle.
3. Cats have a deep anterior chamber with enough doming of the cornea to allow partial visualization of the filtration angle when looking across the eye from the limbus using a transilluminator and Optivisor. A gonioscopic lens will provide better visualization and, if available, should be used (Fig 1-55d).

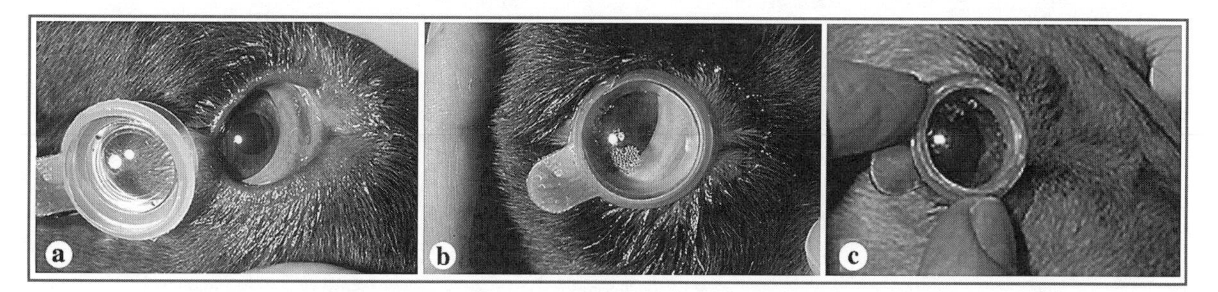

Figure 1-54. Technique of gonioscopy with Franklin goniolens.
    a. After the eye is topically anesthetized, the lens cup is filled with gonioscopic lens solution, the eyelids held open and the lens quickly placed.
    b. The lens is self-retaining when the eyelids are released.
    c. The third eyelid retracts, allowing filtration angle visualization.

Technique in horses

The filtration angle is visible in horses at the temporal and nasal limbus, therefore a goniolens is not needed.

An Optivisor and transilluminator are adequate. It can be assumed that the portion of the filtration angle visualized is representative of the rest of the filtration angle (Fig 1-50).

Interpretation (Fig 1-55)

The angle should be examined for width, the character of the pectinate ligaments, goniodysgenesis and the presence of peripheral anterior synechia, neoplasia, or injury.

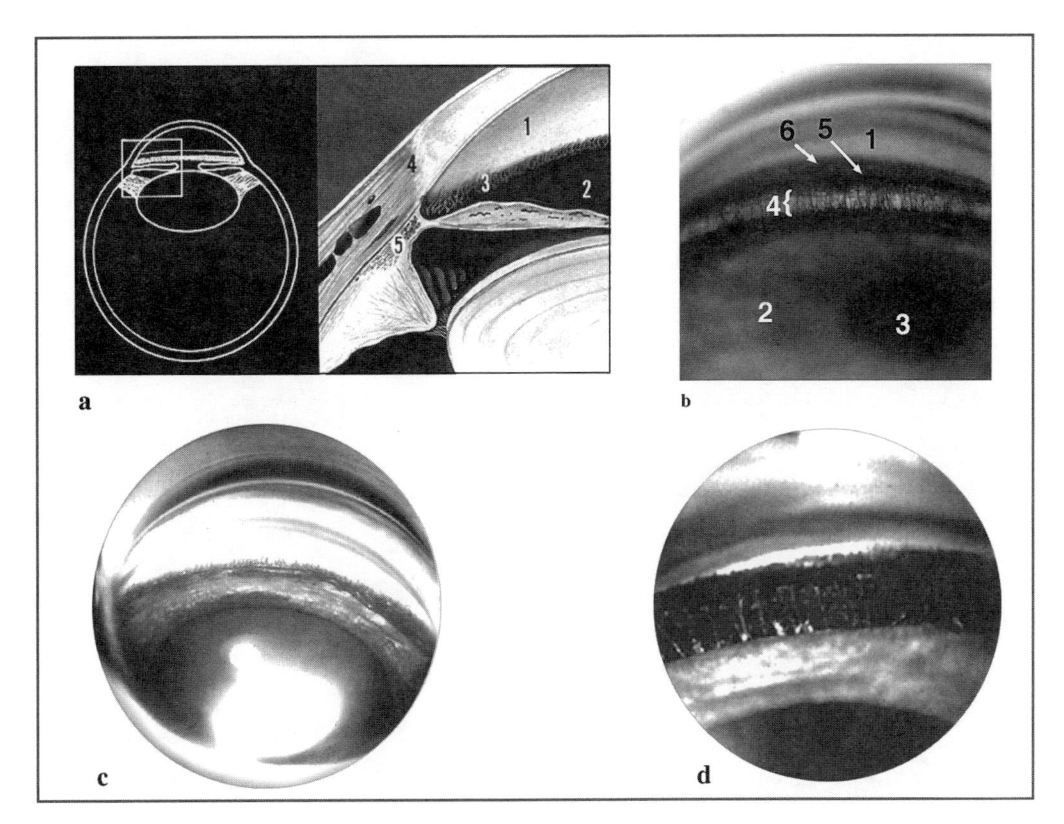

Figure 1-55. Normal canine and feline filtration angle.

a. Schematic cross-section iridocorneal angle (Courtesy Dr. Milt Wyman). 1) Cornea. 2) Iris. 3) Pectinate ligaments. 4) Limbus. 5) Trabecular meshwork.

b. Normal pigmented filtration angle. 1) Cornea. 2) Iris. 3) Pupil. 4) Pectinate ligaments. 5) Inner pigment. 6) Outer pigment.

c. Normal nonpigmented filtration angle.

d. Normal feline filtration angle. Note the wide angle with long sparse pectinate ligaments.

ELECTRORETINOGRAPHY

The electroretinogram (ERG) is the electrical response recorded when the retina is stimulated with light. It is not a measure of vision but it is a measure of the functional integrity of the entire outer portion of the retina and the pigmented epithelial layer.

Equipment requirements

1. Electroretinograph - Several years ago, electroretinographs were constructed by purchasing and assembling the primary component parts: a light source (photostimulator), high-gain amplifier, and a recorder. Now, commercial ERGs are available, many of which are computerized, thus making it possible to do screening ERGs without general anesthesia (Fig 1-56).

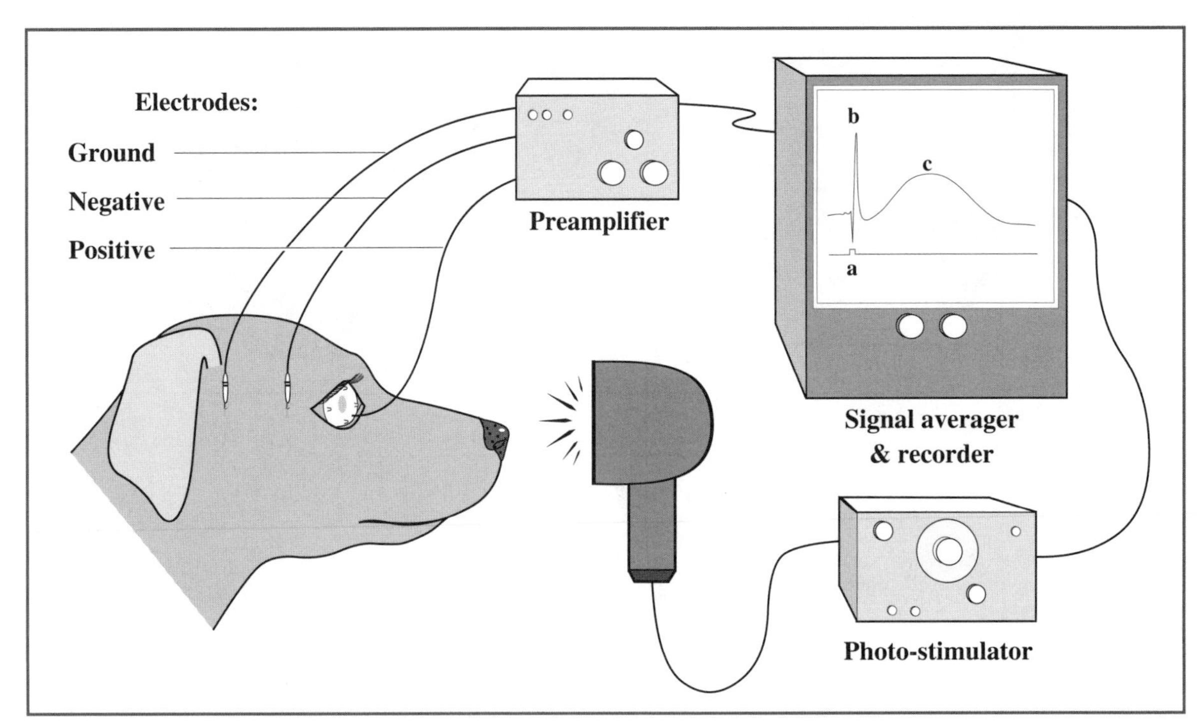

Figure 1-56. Components of a computerized electroretinograph (ERG). Electrodes, preamplifier, signal averager and recorder, and photostimulator.

2. Photostimulator
   a. Grass strobe photostimulator
   b. Projector bulb with electronic shutter
   c. Ganzfeld - a white shell that the head may be placed in so that light stimulation is evenly distributed over the entire retina. A Grass photostimulator is the light source (Fig 1-57).
      1) Not necessary for preoperative ERGs
      2) Provides a controlled environment for in-depth ERGs, but is not universally accepted by researchers
   d. Filters for photostimulators
      1) Rod response (scotopic)
         a) red
         b) dim blue
      2) Cone response (photopic)
         a) bright blue
         b) white light - variable intensities are used

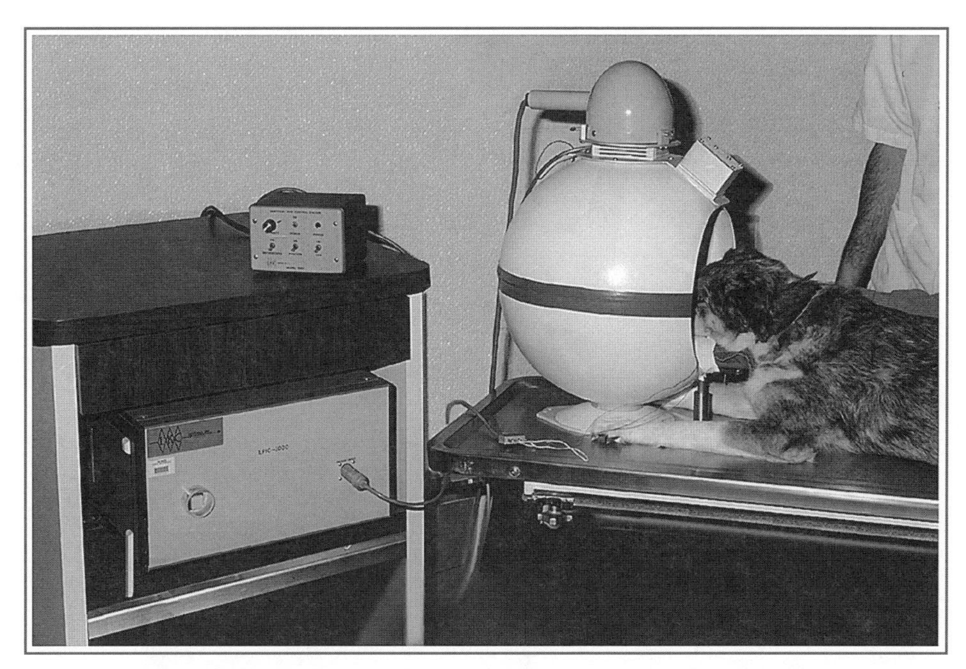

Figure 1-57. Computerized ERG with Ganzfeld shell for technical ERGs.

3. Electrodes - three electrodes are needed:
   a. Positive (active) corneal electrode - this can be a specifically designed corneal contact such as the ERG-jet gold contact (Life Tech Incorporation) or a saline agar wick.
   b. Negative (reference) electrode - this is a needle electrode placed in the skin "behind the eye". Actual placement is subcutaneously along the zygomatic arch, about one-half the distance between the lateral canthus and the base of the ear, behind the retina.
   c. Ground (indifferent) electrode - this is also a needle, usually placed subcutaneously over the temporal area or forehead
4. Coupling agent for corneal contact - gonioscopic lens solution works very well for this

Technique

1. Clinical retinal screening - indicated when the retina cannot be seen because of cataract, opaque cornea, hyphema, etc. If a computerized ERG is available, this type of ERG can be performed without general anesthetic. The pupil is dilated with Mydriacyl and the patient dark-adapted for a minimum of 20 minutes. Test each eye in the following order: red, blue and white light. A single flash can be attempted if the animal is quiet. If there is too much movement, 6 to 10 flashes averaged by the computer will produce an acceptable ERG, which will determine if the retina is functional. The opposite eye should be covered while the ERG is being done on the first eye. As the second eye is being done, there is no reason to protect the eye already tested. Bright examining lights used prior to dark-adaptation can reduce ERG voltage and should be delayed until the ERG has been performed.
2. In-depth ERG for research or differentiation of retinal degeneration - this requires general anesthesia, precise illumination source alignment and a detailed protocol. The protocol would typically consist of single and multiple light flashes with various red, blue and white light stimuli and intensities, variable periods of dark adaptation and flicker fusion.

Genesis of the ERG

The ERG is the total response of the retina to light (Fig 1-58). The initial deflection is negative and termed the a-wave. This is followed by a positive deflection, the b-wave, which has a higher potential and lasts longer than the a-wave. In addition to the a- and b-waves, there is usually a second positive deflection, the c-wave, which is more prolonged. The origin of the wave components is complex and poorly understood.

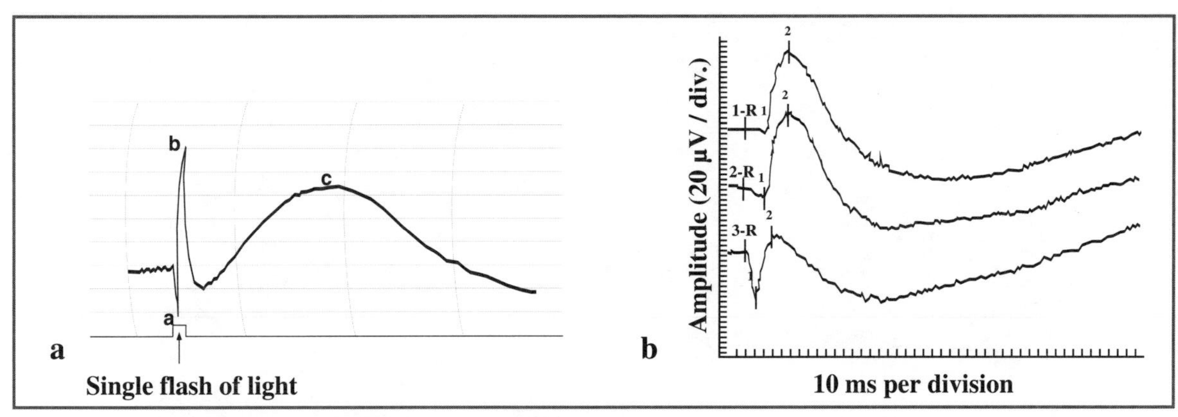

Figure 1-58. Electroretinographic recordings.
a. Tracing made by a direct writer ERG of the response to a single flash of light.
b. Computer-averaged response from the right eye of an awake dog to six light flashes for each tracing. 1-R red, 2-R blue, and 3-R white light.

1. a-wave - the leading edge of the a-wave is generated by the rods and cones when exposed to light. The resultant phenomenon is a complex one but in general it is proposed that light initiates isomerization of the visual pigments, and their products initiate a specific biochemical reaction which concludes in hyperpolarization of the rods and cones.
2. b-wave - has been associated with the Müller cells in the inner nuclear layer. The Müller cells are glial cells rather than neurons.
3. c-wave - originates in the pigment epithelium and may reflect an ion diffusion potential

Evaluation of the electroretinograph

1. Character of the wave pattern - the waves should show sharp deflections and not be slurred
2. Latency values - time period starting with photostimulation to the beginning and end of each wave pattern
3. Wave amplitude values: a- and b-wave amplitudes are examined with greatest emphasis on b-wave changes. In general, an abnormally depressed or lacking b-wave indicates pathologic change in the retina.

Clinical uses of the ERG

1. Diseases where the retina cannot be visualized
   a. Corneal opacity
   b. Cataract
   c. Vitreous opacities
   d. Hyphema
2. Inherited retinal diseases
   a. Generalized progressive retinal atrophy - response varies with type of PRA
   b. Hemeralopia - malamutes: normal rods, absent cone response
   c. Nyctalopia (night blindness) - Appaloosas: decreased b-wave; severe cases may have a totally reduced ERG
   d. Retinal dysplasia - changes will be seen only if lesions are severe
3. Other diseases
   a. Sudden acquired retinal degeneration - decreased or absent ERG can be observed before ophthalmoscopic signs are present
   b. Inflammatory retinal degeneration - focal lesions do not produce significant change. Diffuse lesions will produce a depressed ERG.
   c. Optic nerve disease and cortical blindness - normal ERG
   d. Glaucoma - early glaucoma will have a normal ERG. Chronic glaucoma can have a decreased ERG as the retina undergoes atrophy.

OCULAR AND ORBITAL ULTRASONOGRAPHY

Ultrasonography is useful to determine ocular dimensions, evaluate deeper ocular structures when the optical media are opaque, and identify orbital disease.

Types

1. A-scan gives an anterior-posterior image with peaks reflecting tissues of different densities. It is useful in determining ocular dimension.
2. B-scan provides a two-dimensional image of the eye and orbit (Fig 1-59). The transducer can be positioned to give horizontal, vertical, and oblique scanning of the eye.

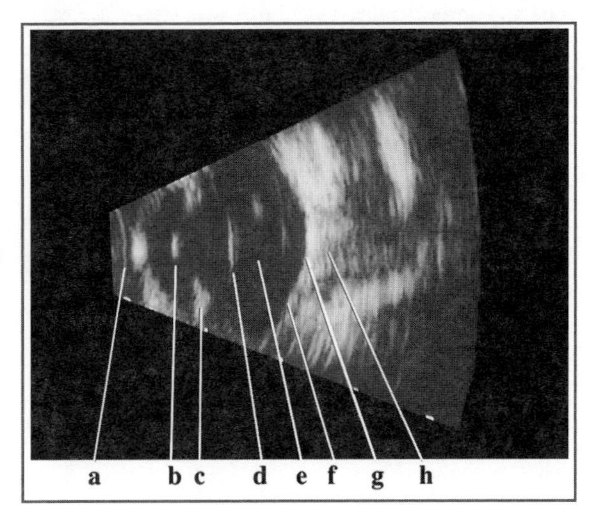

Figure 1-59. B-scan ultrasound image of normal canine eye.
- a. Stand off pad
- b. Anterior lens capsule
- c. Ciliary body
- d. Posterior lens capsule
- e. Vitreous, normally nonechoic, occasionally echos are seen in older dogs
- f. Posterior globe (retina, choroid, sclera)
- g. Optic disk
- h. Optic nerve

Indications

1. Evaluate deeper structures when obscured by opaque tissue or hemorrhage
2. Differentiate tumors from cysts
3. Prescreen cataract patients for retinal detachment
4. Identify foreign bodies and orbital masses

Probe placement

1. Water bath for anterior segment
2. Direct, using coupling for deeper structures

OCULAR AND ORBITAL RADIOGRAPHY

Skull radiographs (plain film) - may be informative if there is bone involvement

Contrast radiographs

1. Dacryocystorhinography - contrast is infused into the nasolacrimal duct to allow visualization and evaluation of obstruction location
2. Orbital angiography - rarely used, but of potential value in assessment of vascular or neoplastic orbital disease
3. Orbitography - contrast can be injected into the extraocular muscle cone to allow determination of whether a mass is within or outside the muscle cone. The images from this technique are difficult to evaluate.
4. Thecography - injection of radiopaque dye into the CSF can be used to outline the optic nerves from the chiasm to the posterior pole of the globes. Largely replaced by CT and MRI.

OCULAR AND ORBITAL COMPUTED TOMOGRAPHY (CT) AND MAGNETIC RESONANCE IMAGING (MRI)

These techniques have largely made other radiographic studies obsolete. Excellent detail of the orbital and intraocular structures is possible. Lesions can be mapped with three-dimensional perspective. Biopsies can be harvested from small targets normally inaccessible.

BIOMICROSCOPY

Biomicroscopy is the examination of an eye with magnification and a light source that may be diffuse or focused (round or slit beam). The slit lamp allows localization of lesions in the cornea, anterior chamber, iris, lens and anterior vitreous. An Aruby lens will permit fundus examination.

Instrumentation

1. Biomicroscope (slit lamp) - Magnifications of 5 to 15x are used for routine examinations.
   a. Handheld models (Fig 1-60) - mobility makes them well suited for veterinary medicine; $3,000 to $5,000.
      1) Zeiss H50-10 - excellent optics, fixed 12.5x lenses
      2) Kowa II - 5x to 20x zoom lenses. This is a very useful instrument. No longer manufactured, therefore hard to find.
      3) Kowa SL-14 cordless, 10x or 16x magnification. Excellent instrument.
   b. Table models - 6 to 40x, lack of mobility limits their use primarily to research
2. Slit lamp alternatives
   a. Light sources - slit penlight, direct ophthalmoscope slit beam, Welch Allyn focusing penlight
   b. Magnification source - binocular loupes 2.5 to 5x

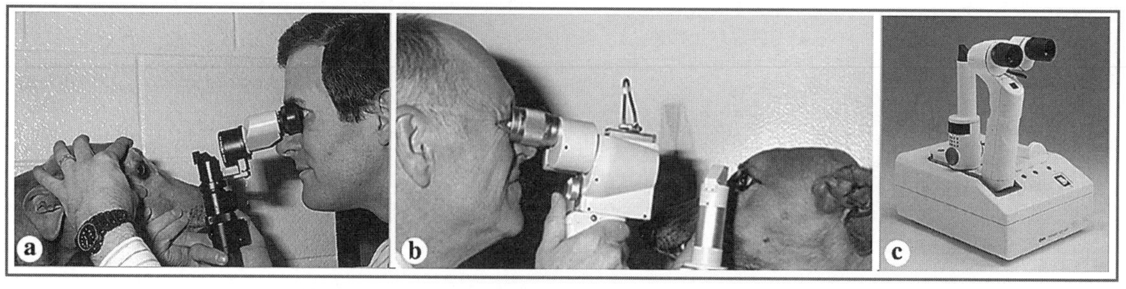

Figure 1-60. Handheld biomicroscopes (slit lamps).
a. Zeiss H50-10
b. Kowa II fiberoptic zoom
c. Kowa SL-14 cordless

Principles of slit illumination

1. *Reflection of light.* When light travels between media of differing refractive indices, there will be reflection of light at that surface. For the eye these surfaces are: air-tear, tear-corneal epithelium, corneal endothelium-aqueous, aqueous-anterior lens capsule, and posterior lens capsule-vitreous.
2. *Relucency* - As light passes through transparent tissues there is relucency (the internal dispersion of light) resulting in opalescence proportional to the density of the tissue.
3. Slit beam appearance of a normal eye at 25x (Fig 1-61)
   a. Air-tear surface = bright line
   b. Corneal epithelium = clear (dark) zone. These cells are mostly fluid, low in cellular solids. Need 10x or greater to visualize.
   c. Corneal stroma = frosted (opalescent) appearance. This is brighter than the lens because of greater density.
   d. Corneal endothelium - aqueous surface = bright line

e. Aqueous = dark space. Insignificant solids in normal aqueous to reflect light.
f. Aqueous-anterior lens capsule surface = bright line
g. Lens stroma = frosted (opalescent) appearance. Least in the cortex and greatest in the nucleus
h. Posterior lens capsule - vitreous surface = bright line
i. Vitreous = clear (dark). Planes between vitreous layers and vestiges of the hyaloid canal can be seen.

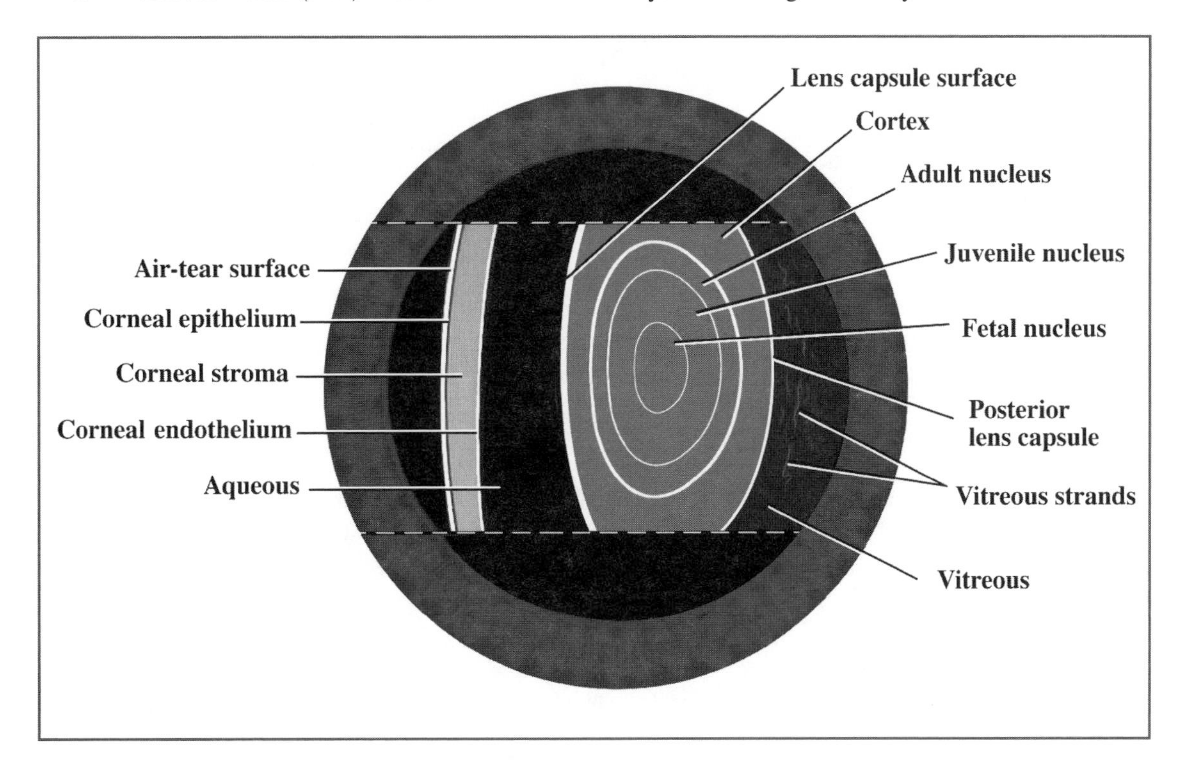

Figure 1-61. Drawing of slit beam appearance of normal eye. All layers are shown in focus. During actual examination, cornea and posterior capsule would be indistinct when focus is on anterior lens capsule.

VISUAL TESTING

TERMS

Amblyopia - decreased vision from any cause
Amaurosis - total blindness from unknown cause

Objective signs of total blindness

Objective signs of total blindness with sudden onset are usually associated with slow or cautious movement. The owner is aware the patient has become blind.

Objective signs of gradual or congenital blindness

Many of these patients appear to have a small amount of sight because of increased perception of the other senses (hearing and smell). The patient will memorize its surroundings and move around well. Some blind horses will lead or respond so well to a bridle that an observer would never know they are blind.

Determination of degree of blindness

1. Menace reflex - will occur from sudden movement near the eye. Be sure that hand motion does not cause air movement that would cause blinking (therefore waving the hand in front of the eye is not acceptable). Use a sheet of glass or plastic between the patient and the moving hand to eliminate air movement. Moving the hand toward the eye from different directions may determine visual field deficits:
   a. Directly toward the eye
   b. Coming in from dorsal, temporal, ventral and nasal
2. Moving object - dropping cotton or rolling tape in front of the patient. The object should not make any noise. Domestic animals are more sensitive in the detection of motion than we are. A good way to check for night blindness is dropping a cotton ball and gradually reducing room light until the patient does not see it.
3. Maze testing - use normal and reduced light
   a. Small animals
      1) Works well for dogs. Unpredictable for cats because of their tendency to seek a secluded area.
      2) Procedure - select an unfamiliar area with objects randomly placed. Start with normal room light (photopic vision) and gradually reduce the light to near darkness (scotopic vision).
   b. Horses
      1) Preferably an inside barn runway where the light can be reduced with obstacles randomly placed (e.g. bales of straw or hay)
      2) Lead the horse through the obstacles starting with normal light and then gradually reducing the light
4. Dazzle reflex - A bright light flashed into an eye with a functional retina and optic nerve will stimulate a photophobic blink reflex. This disappears when function of either ceases. This is useful if:
   a. The fundus cannot be seen
   b. There is acute optic nerve or retinal disease that has not resulted in funduscopic examination changes (e.g. sudden acquired retinal degeneration syndrome, retrobulbar optic nerve disease)

Unilateral blindness

Unilaterally blind horses often develop temperament changes. In time, they adapt and may appear almost normal. Unilateral blindness in cats and dogs may be detected by a very observant owner. Unilateral blindness can be determined by the menace blink reflex or bandaging one eye and then maze testing the animals.

Dogs usually are not disturbed by bandaging the blind eye, but when the good eye is bandaged, they immediately attempt to remove the bandage rather than work through a maze obstacle course.

Visual fields (Fig 1-62)

The visual fields of animals vary significantly and can be categorized into two main groups: predatory (e.g. carnivore—need binocular vision), and nonpredatory (need to be aware of their entire environment and have less need for a large binocular field but a nearly 360° visual field to alert them of impending danger).

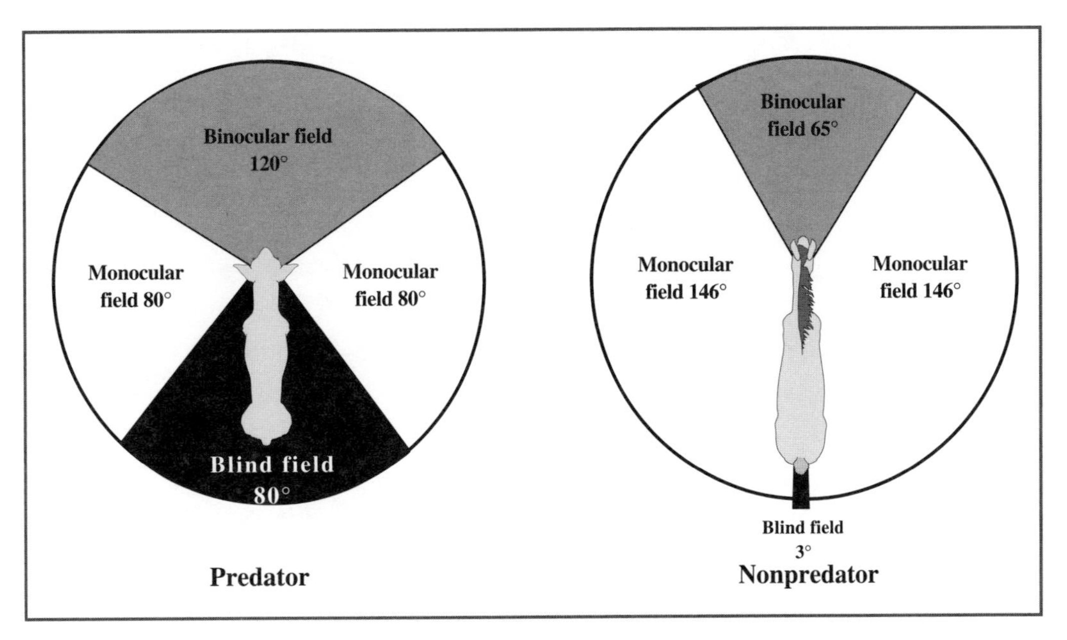

Figure 1-62. Visual fields.
a. Predator (e.g. canine)
b. Nonpredator (e.g. horse)

CHAPTER 2 - OCULAR THERAPEUTICS

METHODS OF MEDICATING AN EYE

Topical administration
Subconjunctival injection
Retrograde arterial perfusion
Intraocular injection
Systemic administration

TOPICAL ADMINISTRATION

Factors affecting penetration

1. Drug characteristics
   a. Chemical characteristics of the drug. Drugs penetrate the cornea by differential solubility and not by simple diffusion (Fig 2-1). This is the most important factor affecting drug penetration of a healthy cornea.
      1) Epithelium - it is the main corneal barrier to drugs. It is readily penetrated by fat soluble (nonionized) compounds and relatively impermeable to electrolytes.
      2) Substantia propria (stroma) - readily penetrated by electrolytes (ionized solutions) and relatively impermeable to fat soluble compounds
      3) Endothelium - same characteristics as the epithelium. Endothelium is not as effective a barrier as epithelium.
      4) *Comment* - Drugs that readily penetrate the cornea are those that exist in equilibrium between the ionized and nonionized forms. Examples are chloramphenicol and alkaloids. Water soluble drugs such as most antibiotics, sulfas and fluorescein will not penetrate the epithelium, but will readily penetrate the stroma if an ulcer is present.
   b. Size of the molecule - the larger the molecule, the poorer the penetration.
   c. Drug concentration - the higher the concentration, the greater the penetration.

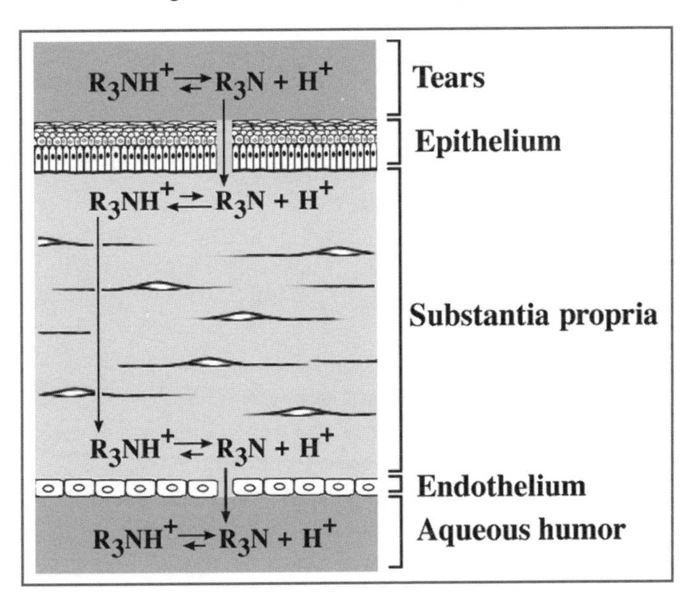

Figure 2-1. The transfer of homatropine through the cornea.
R_3NH+ represents ionized (water soluble) homatropine
R_3N represents nonionized (fat soluble) homatropine

2. Vehicle for the medication
   a. Types of vehicles - drops and ointments are most frequently used, but polymerizing gels, ocular inserts and powders are available
      1) Solutions - less wound healing interference and most rapid absorption
         a) Aqueous buffered electrolyte solutions
         b) Artificial tear bases have greater viscosity (methylcellulose, hydroxyethyl cellulose, polyvinyl alcohol and artificial mucin)
         c) Oil base preparations - vegetable oils (corn, peanut, olive) and mineral oil
      2) Suspensions - similar to solutions and persist in tear film longer than solutions
      3) Ointments (emollients) - petrolatum, lanolin or combinations
      4) Polymerizing gels - 4% pilocarpine is available in a polymerizing gel that remains in the tear film for hours
      5) Solid medication inserts - these dissolve slowly and can be placed in the inferior conjunctival sac (e.g. Lacrisert-Merck & Company, a hydroxypropyl cellulose insert for keratoconjunctivitis sicca)
      6) Continuous delivery membranes - are ocular inserts that provide timed release of medications (e.g. Ocusert Pilo 20 and 40 - Alza, for glaucoma).
      7) Powders - have been used for food animals because of convenience of administration but they are so irritating it is difficult to justify their use.
   b. Properties of vehicles
      1) pH - most human preparations are stabilized near pH 7. Dogs have a tear pH near 6.5. The cornea tolerates a pH of 5 well. pH can affect the penetration and/or shelf life of some medications. Buffers are used to modify the pH when this will not cause incompatibility or affect shelf life of the primary medication.
      2) Tonicity - ideally drops should be isotonic with the tear (1.4% NaCl in man). Normal saline is excellent for animals. Unfortunately, some drugs must be in high concentration to be effective, thus resulting in irritation. High concentration drugs are often less irritating in ointments.
      3) Electrolyte composition
      4) Wetting effect (reduction of surface tension) of quaternary ammonium preservatives - all quaternary ammonium compounds are surface tension reducing agents, therefore they will increase the penetration of water soluble drugs through intact cornea. The most common quaternary ammonium compound used as a preservative is benzalkonium (Zephiran).
      5) Effect of vehicle on drug stability
      6) Sterility of preparation - all FDA approved ophthalmic medications are sterile
   c. Effect of vehicle on therapeutic response (Table 2-1)
      1) Viscosity of the vehicle - viscous vehicles prolong contact time and thereby increase absorption, especially ointments
      2) Oil vehicles - increased contact time but compete with corneal epithelium for fat soluble medications and may retard absorption. Increasing drug concentration will offset this. Less nasolacrimal loss, therefore less systemic absorption.
      3) Duration of medications on the eye
         a) Maximal topical effect for drops is five minutes. A second drop after 30 seconds washes out 45% of the first drop. After two minutes, 17% will wash out and after five minutes, no significant washout occurs. Therefore, five minutes is optimal and two minutes the minimal interval between multiple drop medications. If artificial tear and oil base drops are used, administer the oil base drop last.
         b) Maximal topical effect for an ointment is 20 minutes. If drops and ointments are prescribed, apply the ointment last.
      4) Delaying effect - the ointment bases available today DO NOT have the delaying effect on corneal epithelial healing that was seen in the past
      5) *Comment* - There is considerable debate concerning pros and cons of drops versus ointments. I believe that getting the medication in the eye as directed is more important than the vehicle used. Most small animal owners prefer drops and most large animal owners have greater success with ointments.

Table 2-1. Comparison - Drops versus ointments

	Drops	Ointments
Ease of application	Easiest: small animal	Easiest: large animal
Control of dosage	More precise	Variable
Toxicity intraocular administration	Minimal	Toxic
Dilution by tears	Yes	No
Contact time	Short (frequent medication needed)	Longer (less frequent medication needed)
Systemic absorption	High	Minimal
Drug release from vehicle	Rapid	Slower
Lubricate/protect	Short	Longer
Shaking required	Suspensions only	Not needed
Soils hair	No	Yes (longhaired breeds)

Fate of drugs after topical administration

1. Means of removal - up to 50% of the medication in drops can be absorbed
    a. Passage down the nasolacrimal duct - in man about 80% of an eyedrop-applied drug leaves the cul-de-sac via lacrimal drainage and does not enter the eye
        1) To the surface of the nose where it can drop off or be licked into the mouth
        2) Into the nasal cavity where it can be absorbed or move on into the pharynx
    b. Penetrate the conjunctiva, then enter the sclera or venous return
    c. Penetrate the cornea, then absorb into the anterior uvea and lens, or flow out the filtration angle
    d. *Comment* - Drugs that rapidly enter the conjunctiva and cornea may develop clinical levels in the blood stream very quickly. Apomorphine in the conjunctival sac may result in vomiting in minutes. Because of this, drugs that are highly toxic, have an accumulation effect, or can produce adverse reactions should not be used indiscriminately or without warning the owner of danger.
        1) Cholinesterase inhibitors have been known to cause toxicity and death in cats when used to treat glaucoma. The danger is increased if animals are wearing flea collars.
        2) 1% and stronger atropine ophthalmic solutions when applied frequently or continuously to horses for mydriasis/cycloplegia can produce slowing of intestinal motility.
        3) Occasionally dogs may develop systemic side effects to topical prednisolone or dexamethasone, resulting in signs of Cushing's disease
2. Special affinity for tissues
    a. Atropine has a special affinity for anterior uveal melanin resulting in a prolonged effect
    b. Silver chloride will produce a black precipitate in cornea
    c. Platinic chloride will produce a black precipitate in cornea

Methods of topical ocular therapy

Periodic administration
Continuous irrigation with indwelling medication tubes
Iontophoresis
Massage
Contact lenses
Extended delivery membranes and gels

Periodic administration of solutions and ointments

1. Drops
   a. Small animals - the three-finger technique works very well (Fig 2-2). A righthanded person positions to the left of the patient (lefthanded on the right). The medication bottle is held in the right hand similar to holding a pencil. The patient's mandible is cradled in the medicator's left hand, raising the head until the patient looks upward. Using the same hand, the lower eyelid can be stabilized with the thumb or middle finger, depending on the eye medicated. The medicating hand is placed on the patient's forehead near the eye and moved posteriorly, tensing the skin, thus preventing the dog from blinking the upper eyelid. The tip of the dropping bottle is held directly above the eye, allowing medication to drop on the eye when pressure is applied to the bottle. This technique allows medicating with minimal menace to the dog and avoids accidental contact of the eye with the tip of the dropping bottle. Animals that are difficult to treat at home may be easier to manage when placed on a table, countertop, or held in the owner's lap.

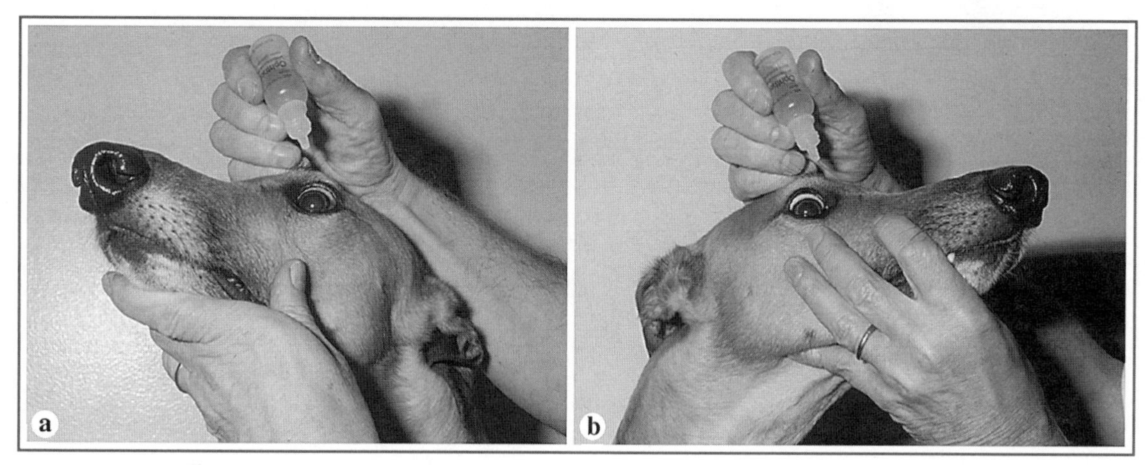

Figure 2-2. Three-finger technique for administering drops to small animals.
a. Left eye
b. Right eye

   b. Large animals - are difficult to treat with dropping bottles. A small syringe with the hub of a 25 gauge needle that has had the needle broken off can be used to direct a fine stream of medication across the cornea (Fig 2-3). This is especially useful during examination when instilling topical anesthesia or fluorescein solution.

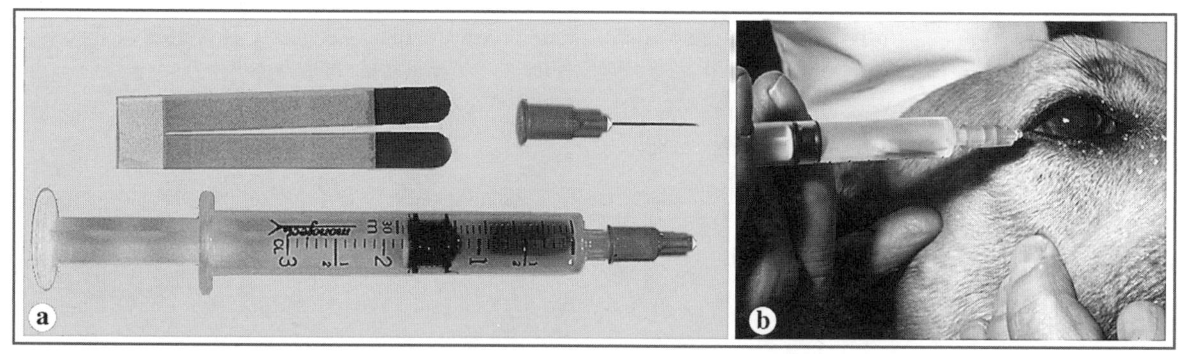

Figure 2-3. Applying fluorescein with a syringe and hub of a 25 gauge needle.
a. Three ml syringe, 25 gauge needle and fluorescein strips before and after preparing for administration
b. Applying stream of fluorescein solution gently to the cornea from the temporal canthus

2. Spray - Ophthalmic solutions can be sprayed on the eye but considerable waste may occur. Sprays provide uniform application to the surface and may reduce the amount of medication needed. Cattle with pink-eye can be treated two to three times daily with minimal handling by using 1:25 to 1:50 Betadine in

a spray bottle. An atomizer can be used for dogs that will not allow the owner to administer drops or ointments.

3. Ointments (Fig 2-4)
   a. Small animals - ointments can be applied by holding the tube in a similar manner as described for applying drops and placing a 0.5 to 1 cm thread of ointment across the cornea. An alternate technique is to pull the lower eyelid away from the globe and apply the line of ointment into the conjunctival sac.
   b. Large animals - pulling the lower eyelid down and placing the ointment in the conjunctival sac works well in quiet animals. If the eye is extremely sensitive or the animal is throwing its head, it may be preferred to apply the medication to a fingertip, force the eyelid open and place the medication between the eyelids at the nasal canthus. As the animal blinks, medicine will be distributed across the cornea.

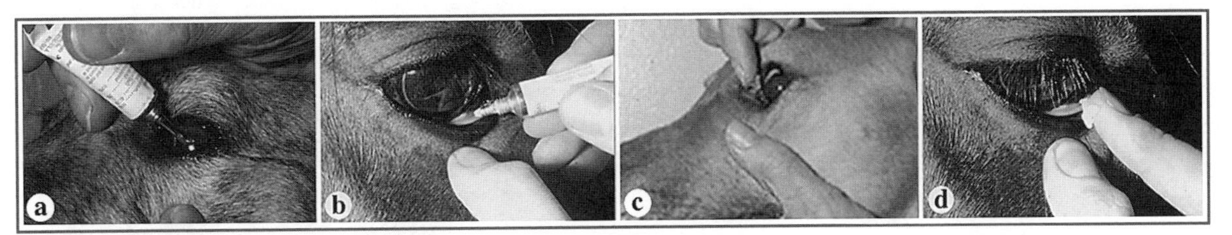

Figure 2-4. Application of ointment to the eye.
a. Applying ointment holding the tube similar to a dropping bottle
b. Applying ointment into the cul-de-sac
c, d. Applying ointment with a finger in a dog and horse

Indwelling medication tubing

The use of subpalpebral or nasolacrimal delivery systems are the most common methods of providing intensive topical medication. After placement, the tubing can be connected to a bottle for gravity flow or a micrometered medication delivery system for continuous therapy. Continuous flow rate of 0.25 to 0.33 ml (6 to 8 drops) hourly is suggested. If intermittent therapy is indicated, a syringe can be used. Indwelling tubing is used most frequently in horses.

1. Indicated when
   a. Continuous or frequent medication is required
   b. The eyelids have been sutured together and topical medication cannot be administered
   c. The animal is difficult to treat or attempting to medicate the eye with drops or ointment would be hazardous to the eye or the person performing the treatment
2. Subpalpebral tubing
   The first subpalpebral medication tubing was the Hessberg Subpalpebral Lavage Apparatus designed to treat *Pseudomonas* corneal ulcers in humans. This apparatus worked fine for small animals but the tubing and technique had to be modified for horses.

   Subpalpebral systems are easiest to place and are preferred for continuous medication but have disadvantages that include slippage of the tubing with corneal irritation, and infection or irritation of the eyelid wound. Sedation and local anesthesia are usually adequate for placement of subpalpebral systems.
   a. Single passage tubing - several modifications of subpalpebral delivery have been used (Fig 2-5). Tubing can be prepared with a flanged bell tip, or by gluing silicone tubing to silicone sheeting with silicone adhesive. For fluted tubing, select the largest polyethylene tubing that will pass through a 12 or 14 gauge needle. Smaller tubing can be used for the other techniques. Silicone tubing and round tip is by far the best subpalpebral medication tubing. It is well tolerated with minimal eyelid reaction and if pulled snugly into the superior fornix does not irritate the globe. A silicone subpalpebral medication delivery system is available from Mila International.

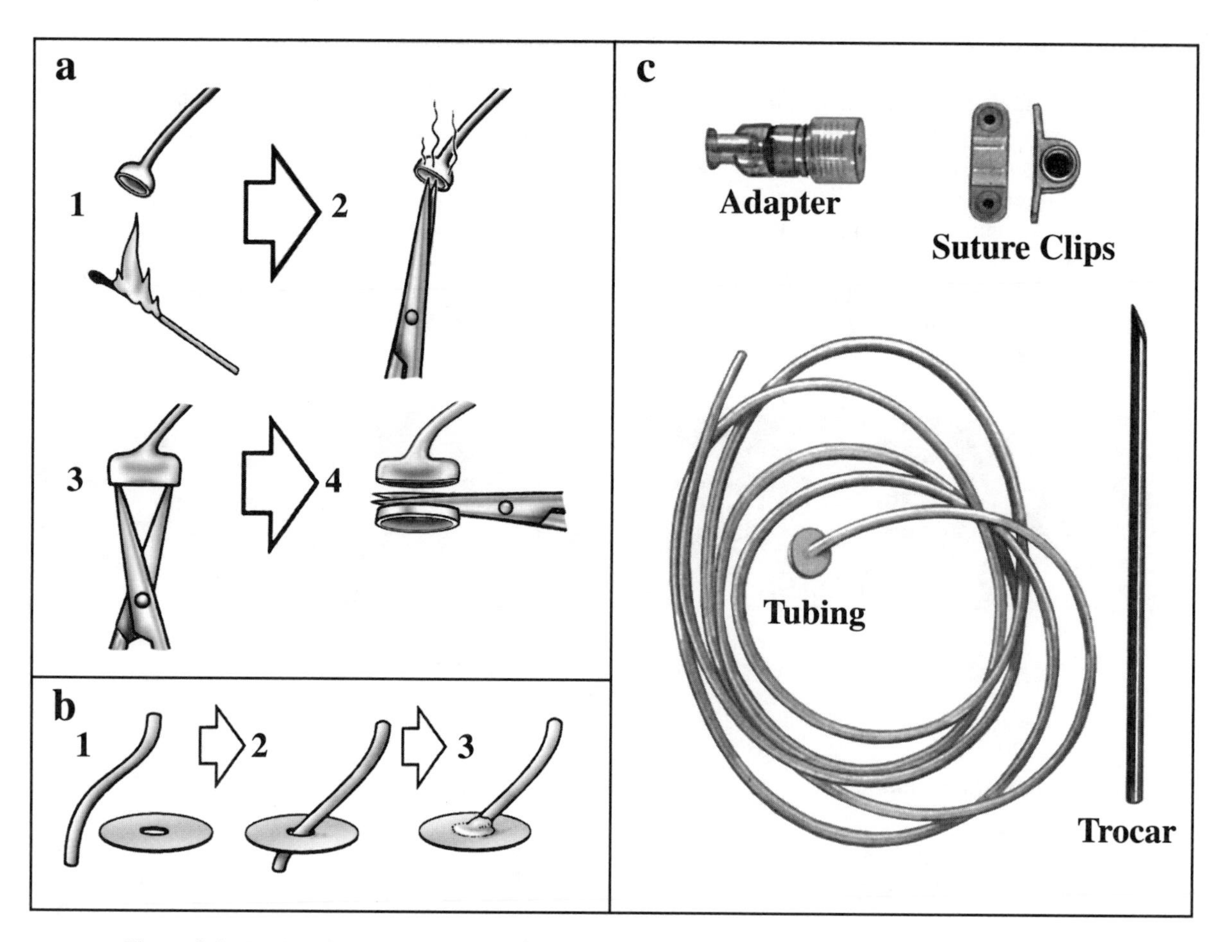

Figure 2-5. Single passage subpalpebral delivery systems.

a. Fluted medication tube using polyethylene
   1. Tubing heated over a flame
   2. Scissors inserted into the bell tip of the hot tubing
   3. Scissors opened to form fluted tip
   4. Edge trimmed if needed

b. Silicone tubing glued to silicone sheeting with silicone adhesive. Allow several days for silicone adhesive to set up. This has the fewest complications.
   1. Silicone tubing and strip of silicone sheeting with small hole
   2. Tubing slipped through hole in sheeting
   3. Appearance after applying adhesive and excess tubing trimmed.

c. Silicone tubing (Mila International) with trocar, skin suturing clips, and infusion adapter. Continuous infusion units available but not shown.

1) Technique for placement (Fig 2-6) - the eye is prepped for sterile surgery. A needle large enough to accommodate the tubing is introduced through the upper lid with the needle penetrating the conjunctiva at the fornix. Next the tubing is threaded into the needle and the needle withdrawn. The tubing is pulled through the wound until the tip is securely located in the upper fornix. A butterfly of adhesive tape is placed around the tubing where it comes through the skin, the tape is sutured to the skin, and the tubing covered with tape over the forehead. Next the tube is secured to a halter or the mane. The tubing is then ready to be connected to a syringe or continuous infusion device.
2) *Comment.* Single passage tubing is very easy to position but must be fabricated in advance of actual use. It may shift during the therapy period, either working down over the cornea and causing irritation or pulling into the eyelid, resulting in medications being delivered intrapalpebrally.

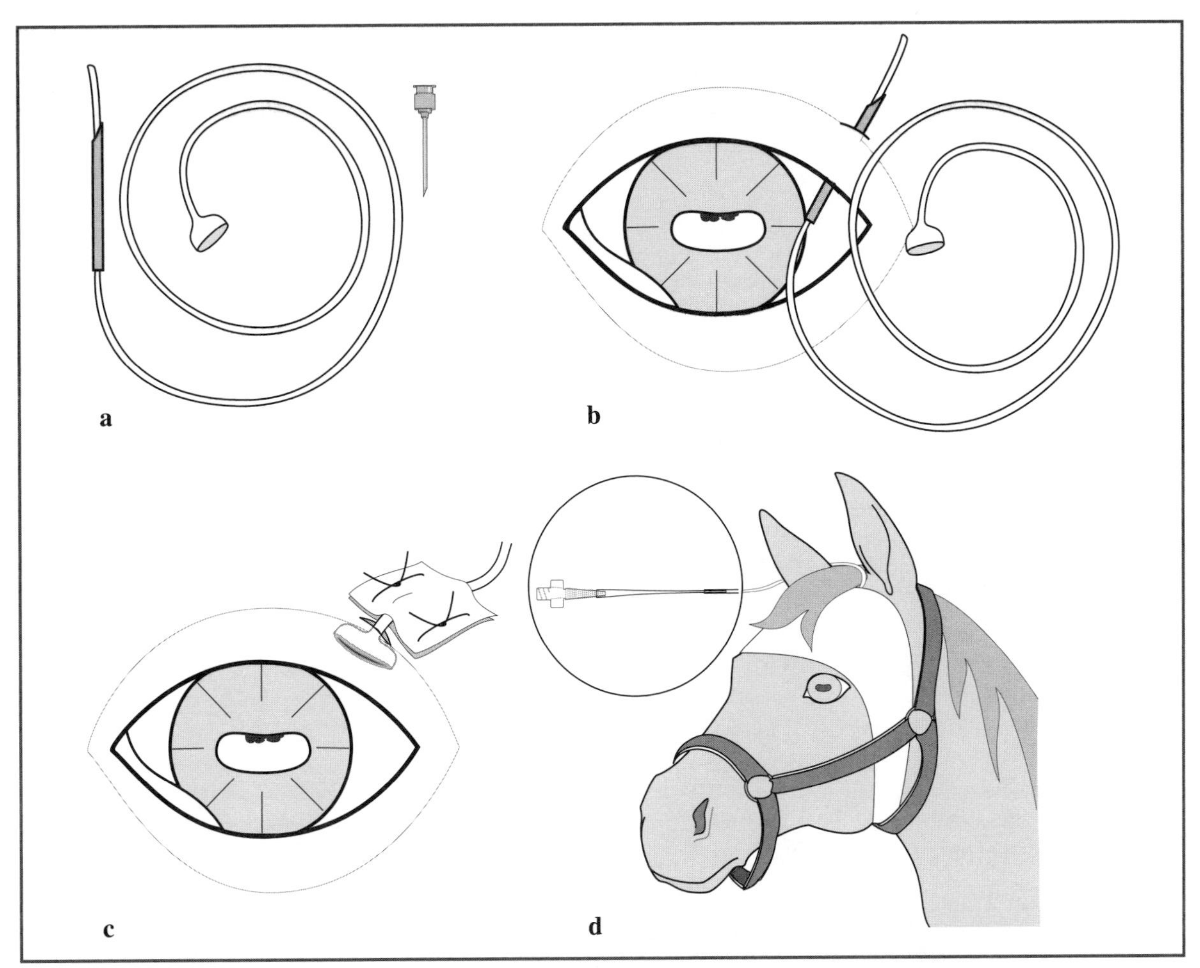

Figure 2-6. Placement of single passage subpalpebral medication tube.
a. Fluted tubing, 12 gauge needle with hub removed, needle to cannulate tubing
b. Passing needle and tubing through upper fornix
c. Medication tube seated in superior fornix and anchored to the skin with butterfly tape
d. Medication tube covered with tape

b. Double passage of tubing - any form of medical plastic tubing can be used (Fig 2-7).
   1) Technique for placement - position a needle large enough to accommodate the tubing in its lumen
   2) At the fornix, above the temporal canthus, insert the needle through the conjunctiva and upper eyelid, pass the tubing through the needle, and then withdraw the needle.
   3) Next the needle is introduced through the upper eyelid near the nasal canthus. Make sure the needle penetrates the conjunctiva at the fornix. The tubing is threaded through the needle and the needle withdrawn, leaving the tubing in the eyelid. This threads the tubing through the eyelid and positions it in the upper fornix. A knot is tied near the end of the tubing at the nasal canthus. A small hole is cut in the tubing in a location such that when the tubing is pulled until the knot is secure against the skin, the hole in the tubing is in the middle of the superior fornix. If small tubing is used, punctures with a 20 gauge needle are satisfactory. Adhesive tape butterflies are placed on the tubing where it comes through the skin at the temporal canthus and near the knot at the nasal canthus. The tape is sutured to the skin to secure the tubing.
   4) Lavach modification (*Large Animal Ophthalmology*, Mosby, 1990) - Lavach simplified this procedure by passing the needle through the eyelid and conjunctiva near the canthus and then back out near the opposite canthus as a single step. The tubing is then passed through the needle and when the needle is withdrawn, the tubing is in the superior fornix ready for securing in place.

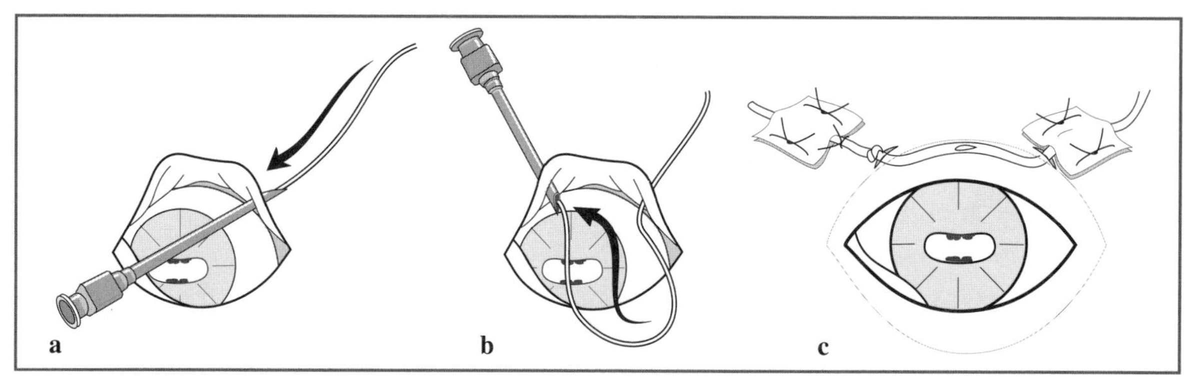

Figure 2-7. Double passage tubing
a. Needle through conjunctiva and upper eyelid at the temporal fornix. Tubing has been placed in needle before withdrawing needle.
b. Needle passed through eyelid entering nasal fornix, and tubing placed before withdrawing needle
c. Small opening made in tubing before secured with butterfly tapes and suturing

5) *Comment* - Double passage systems are easily positioned, will work with any type of medical tubing, and are less prone to slippage than fluted tubing. Unfortunately, they are more likely to cause severe eyelid swelling due to tissue irritation or infection, thus requiring removal before the ulcer is healed. Small tubing is more apt to break but is less likely to cause tissue response.

3. Nasolacrimal tubing - Nasolacrimal systems are more difficult to position but cause less irritation, allowing them to remain in place for weeks. Depending upon style of tubing and tip placement location, larger volumes of medication may be needed to adequately treat the ocular surface. A commercial nasolacrimal medication tube is available from Jorgensen Labs. If this is not available, feeding tubes or urinary catheters can be used (Fig 2-8).

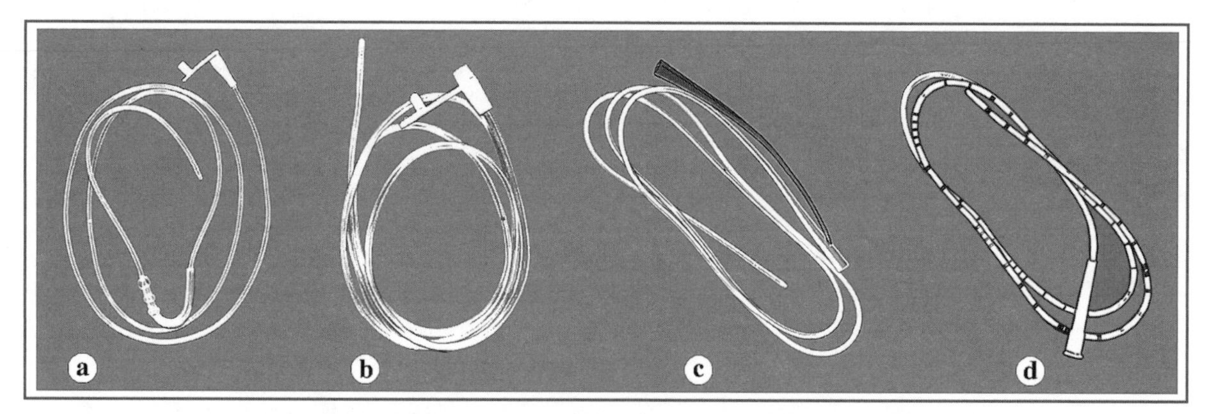

Figure 2-8. Types of tubing (catheters) for nasolacrimal delivery systems.
a. Tubing available from Jorgensen Labs
b. Eight French nasal feeding tube
c. Five French nasal feeding tube
d. Five French canine catheter

a. *Nasolacrimal medication tube using an 8 French nasal feeding tube* (Fig 2-9). In calm horses, tubing can be positioned using local anesthesia and chemical restraint. General anesthesia is preferred if the horse resents manipulation involving the nostril.

The hair is clipped from a small area on the poll, over the dorsal limit of the false nostril and if necessary, inside the nostril on the lateral wall near the nasal punctum. These areas are prepared for aseptic surgery. If the animal is not anesthetized, these sites should be infiltrated with anesthetic. Using a #11 Bard Parker blade, a stab incision is made through the skin over the false nostril and into the nasal vestibule. A visible subcutaneous vein is often present in the area and should be avoided. A 10 gauge or 8 French hubless needle is forced through the wound. Next a feeding tube is passed through the needle into the nasal vestibule and the needle removed, leaving the tubing coming out the nostril. The feeding tube is passed through the nasal punctum up the nasolacrimal canal until marked resistance is met at the beginning of the osseous nasolacrimal canal. This is usually 8 to 10 inches. The depth on the tube should be identified and the tube withdrawn. The tubing is then dried thoroughly.

Using wetproof tape, a butterfly is positioned on the tubing at the point where it was advanced into the nasolacrimal duct. Reposition the tubing in the nasolacrimal duct so the butterfly is at the nasal punctum and with monofilament nonabsorbable suture (nylon), using a figure eight pattern, suture the butterfly to the ventrolateral wall of the nostril at the level of the punctum. Additional butterflies are placed on the tubing for suturing to the skin at the wound over the false nostril and poll. Medium skin clips can be used instead of tape and sutures to secure the tubing in the nose.

Protect the tubing with Elasticon tape over the nostril to the poll. Stabilize the tape ends with tape going around the muzzle and around the head. The delivery tubing can be further protected by bandaging the head with stockinette or using a hood.

Secure the capped end of the feeding tube to the horse's mane or a halter.

This type of delivery system does not adapt well to continuous delivery techniques because there will be backflow of medication around the tubing at the nasal punctum. It works well with intermittent injections but frequently requires large volumes to deliver medication to the ocular surface (1-5 ml). If backflow becomes a problem, it can be reduced by placing a finger where the tube enters the nasal punctum during administration of medication.

Backflow will also be a problem with the commercial delivery system unless the suture molding is snugly positioned against the nasal punctum.

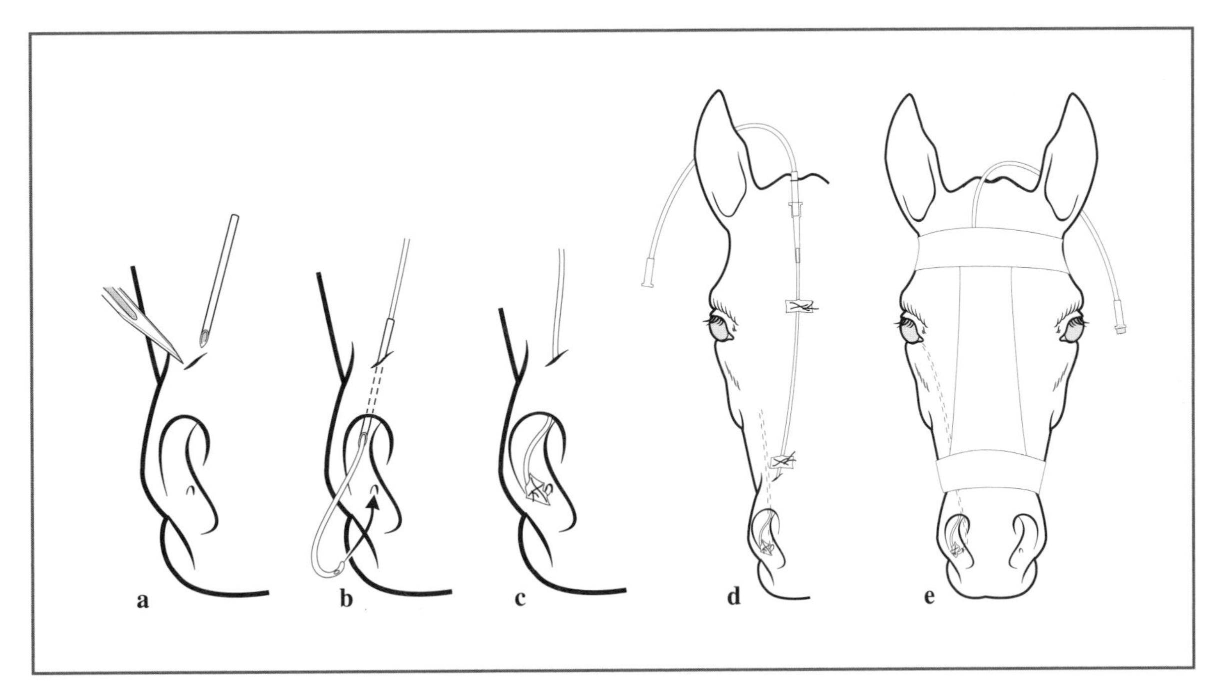

Figure 2-9. Placement of an 8 French nasal feeding tube as a medication delivery system.

a. Incision made over false nostril with scalpel blade
b. Ten gauge hubless needle passed through incision allowing 8 French feeding tube to be drawn through needle
c. Needle withdrawn. Feeding tube passed up nasolacrimal duct. Butterfly tape placed on tube and secured at nasal punctum with nonabsorbable figure 8 suture
d. Tubing secured to skin with additional butterfly tape
e. Tubing covered with Elasticon tape

b. *Nasolacrimal medication tube using 5 French, 36 inch feeding tube extending to the palpebral punctum (Fig 2-10).* This delivery system eliminates the medication backflow problem and can be used with continuous delivery. Pass a 5 French feeding tube through the nasolacrimal duct from either the palpebral or nasal punctum. Insert a 12 gauge needle through the false nostril, thread the nasal end of the feeding tube into the needle and withdraw the needle, leaving the tubing emerging through the skin over the false nostril. Secure the tubing in the nostril with medium skin clips. Next trim the tubing flush with the palpebral punctum. The tubing coming through the skin over the false nostril can be secured to the face and covered with Elasticon tape as previously described for the 8 French tubing. Cannulate the tubing with a 20 gauge needle or cap with a Luer lock tubing adapter.

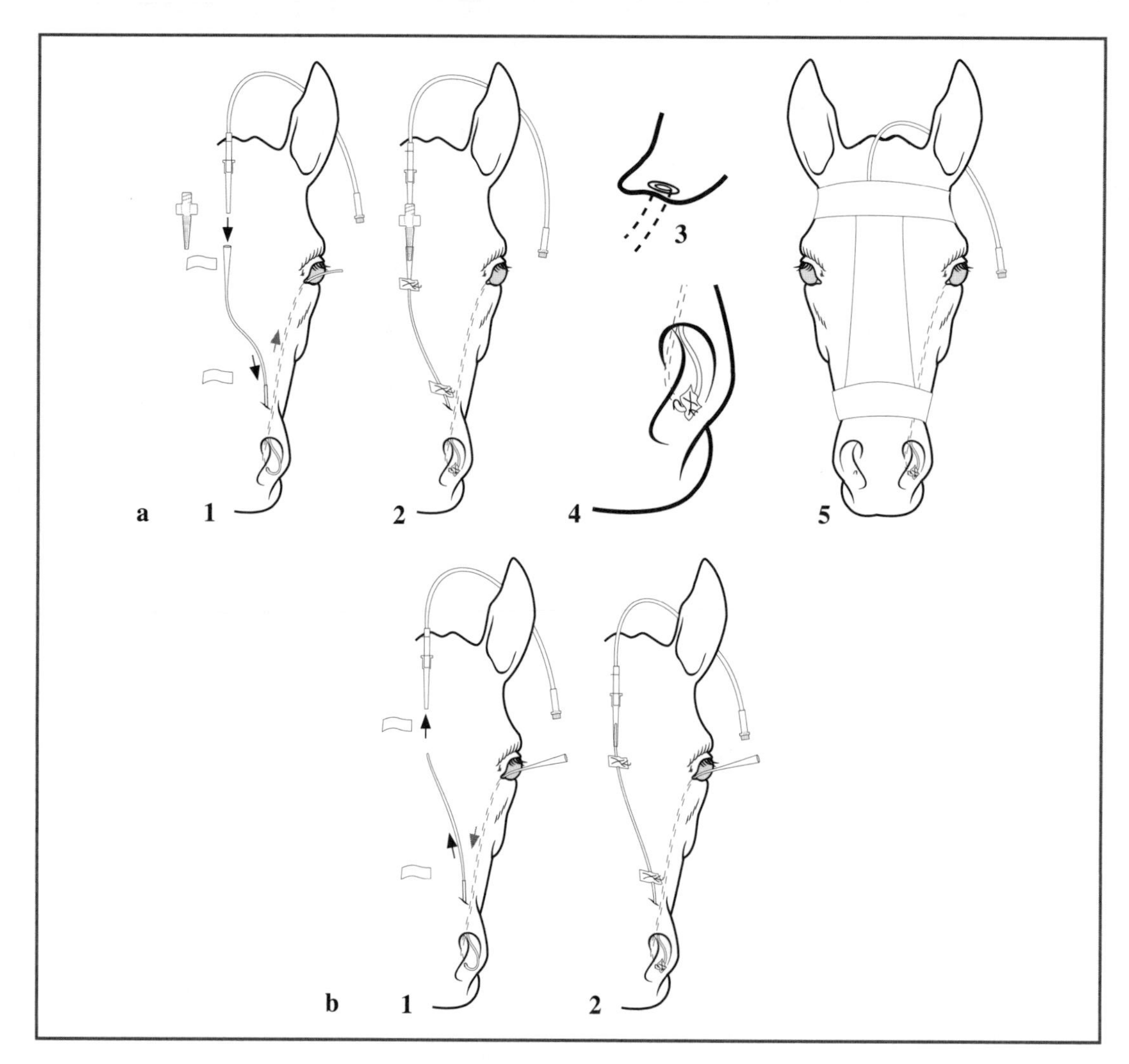

Figure 2-10. Placement of 5 French nasal feeding tube as a medication delivery system.

a. Retrograde passage from nasal to palpebral punctum
   1. Using the technique described for placing an 8 French feeding tube, a 5 French nasal feeding tube is passed retrograde from the nasal punctum until it emerges at the palpebral punctum. A Christmas tree adapter and IV extension tube may be needed for additional length.
   2. Final positioning and securement of the tubing with butterfly tapes
   3. Tubing end removed flush with palpebral punctum
   4. Position of tubing and butterfly tape after sutured in nostril
   5. Tubing covered with Elasticon tape is ready for use

b. Passage of tubing through upper palpebral punctum if retrograde passage is unsuccessful
   1. Tubing passed and blunt end of feeding tube cut off and ready to be forced into catheter adapter for connection to IV extension
   2. Final placement of tubing before tubing cut flush with palpebral punctum. Tubing will be covered with Elasticon tape as shown in a.5. above

c. *Nasolacrimal medication tube using a 5 French Stillman urinary catheter extending to the palpebral punctum.* A Stillman urinary catheter is more rigid than the 5 French feeding tube and can be passed the entire length of the nasolacrimal duct more readily than a feeding tube. It is shorter and therefore after passage it should be attached to other tubing and secured in the same manner as described for the 5 French feeding tube.

Iontophoresis

Uses a medication lens and a direct electrical current to force medication through the cornea. The medication to be used must be ionized and either acid or basic compound. The medication is placed in the lens and a low amperage passed through the lens to force the medication into the cornea. The chemical characteristic of the medication determines the polarity to be delivered to the lens. This method of medication is not applicable to clinical veterinary medicine.

Massage

Place medicine on the eye and then rub the eye through the eyelids. This will increase the penetrability of the cornea and conjunctiva, but is painful and rarely indicated in veterinary medicine.

Extended wear soft contact lenses

1. Uses
   a. To deliver medications - soft contact lenses have the capability to absorb and then slowly release medication. Absorption and release varies with chemical composition of the lens and the drug involved. Lenses typically have a drug delivery half-life of 20 minutes.
      1) The lens may be medicated by presoaking up to 30 minutes before placing on the cornea, or by,
      2) Applying topical medications to patients wearing the soft contact
   b. As a corneal bandage - corneal erosions, stromal ulcers or injuries and corneal bullae
   c. Cosmetic - color tinted lens to conceal corneal, iris or lens blemishes
2. Sources
   a. Human soft lenses - have been used extensively in small animals but success has been limited due to corneal differences between man and animals which frequently results in lens displacement.
   b. Animal soft lenses - (The Cutting Edge Ltd)
3. Limitations
   a. Losing contacts because of:
      1) Poor fit due to breed variations in base curvature and diameter of the cornea
      2) Third eyelid dislodging the lens
      3) Animals blink less frequently than humans, resulting in drying of the lens, which predisposes to the lens coming out when the patient blinks
   b. Extended wear contacts may limit corneal oxygenation and thereby delay epithelial healing
4. *Comment* - A temporary tarsorrhaphy will prevent lens loss. Because the cornea cannot be directly examined, the patient should be observed closely for complications such as sudden development of pain, increase or change in appearance of ocular discharge, swelling of the eyelids, or suture irritation. If complications occur, the tarsorrhaphy should be removed and the eye examined. In tarsorrhaphy patients, medication can be placed between the eyelids at the nasal canthus

Extended delivery membranes and lipid vesicles

1. Ocular inserts - ocular inserts have been made from polypeptides, polysaccharides or cellulose, which slowly release medication
   a. Collagen shields (Fig 2-11) - made from porcine scleral tissue (Soft Shield®. Oasis)
      1) Indications - for the relief of corneal discomfort and acceleration of corneal epithelialization after surgery, traumatic and nontraumatic conditions. Professional judgement in the use of shields must be exercised by the practitioner when the patient has evidence of acute external ocular infection.
      2) How supplied - packages of six lenses with instructions and a forceps for installation
   b. Antibiotic treated collagen inserts have been investigated
   c. Pilocarpine delivery systems (Ocusert - Alza) - for glaucoma
   d. Artificial tear inserts (Lacrisert - Merck & Co) - made from hydroxypropyl cellulose
2. Polymerizing gels - polymerizing gels have been developed that will stay in the conjunctival sac and slowly release medication (Pilopine 4% gel - Alcon Labs)
3. Liposomes - Liposomes are laboratory preparations of lipid vesicles generally containing a water soluble drug that is slowly released. They can be used for topical, subconjunctival, intracranial and parenteral administration. They are relatively large particles and tend to remain at the site of administration or within the circulation for prolonged periods. In addition to this prolonged activity, drug penetration is increased and toxicity is reduced.

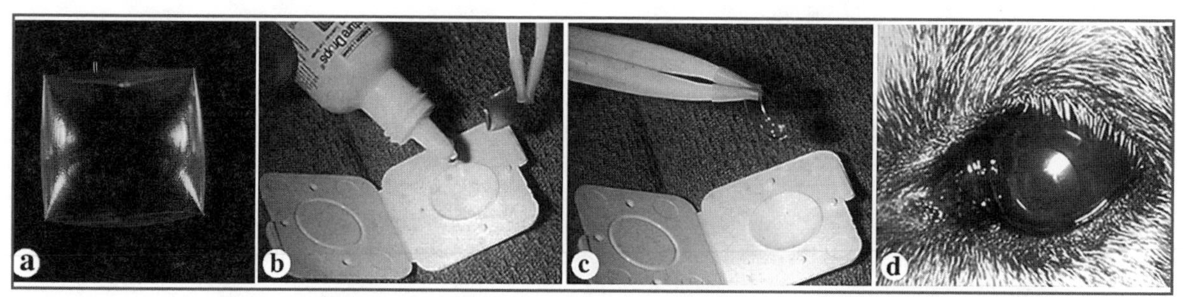

Figure 2-11. Collagen shields
- a. Dehydrated collagen shield
- b. Filling collagen shield tray with antibiotic ophthalmic solution
- c. Removing hydrated solution with forceps
- d. Collagen shield placed on cornea

SUBCONJUNCTIVAL INJECTION

Subconjunctival injection can be made under either the bulbar or palpebral conjunctiva. Subpalpebral conjunctival injections have been used in cattle because of the ease in making the injection. The efficacy of this site is questionable because most of the medicine will be carried away by the palpebral blood supply. Therefore this technique cannot be recommended.

The following remarks pertain to subbulbar conjunctival injection.

Pharmacokinetics

1. Penetration
   a. Direct trans-scleral absorption by passing the selective barrier of the corneal and conjunctival epithelium
   b. Leakage into the tear film to provide transcorneal medication
2. About 1 to 2% enters the eye. Water soluble compounds that penetrate the cornea poorly are especially beneficial. Penetration is greater in inflamed eyes. Injection near the lesion is recommended.

3. Duration varies from one day to several weeks, depending on the agent administered.
4. Tissue affected - anterior segment (cornea, sclera, anterior uvea) and vitreous

Indications

1. Water soluble drugs that penetrate the epithelium poorly (e.g. most antibiotics, especially penicillin)
2. Depot drugs that have slow absorption characteristics (e.g. repository corticosteroids)
3. To achieve a high intraocular drug level for a short period of time with minimal systemic effect (e.g. emergency treatment of acute anterior segment disease)
4. When topical medications cannot be properly administered

Disadvantages

1. Do not inject drugs that might be damaging later or contraindicated if the status of the eye changes
2. Temporary pain at the site of injection (e.g. some antibiotics)
3. Introduction of infection at the site of injection
4. Repository (depot) injections may leave residue at the injection site (e.g. methylprednisolone acetate)

Restraint - most animals can be injected without general anesthesia

1. Dogs - topical anesthesia is usually adequate
2. Cats - topical anesthesia is often inadequate, therefore chemical restraint may also be needed
3. Horses - topical anesthesia and a twitch is satisfactory in calm animals. If the horse is hard to handle, chemical restraint is also recommended.
4. Cattle - topical anesthesia and nose tongs

Injection technique - the dorsal limbus is the most accessible area **(Fig 2-12)**

1. Small animals - with the dog in sternal recumbency, elevate the nose to enhance the downward rotation of the eye. This will improve exposure of the injection site. Stabilize the upper eyelid. About 3 to 5 mm from the limbus, pass a 25 to 27 gauge needle, bevel up, through the conjunctiva and parallel with the sclera. There should not be any resistance to the injection and the conjunctiva should bleb up. If there is any resistance to passing the needle or to the injection, the needle is too deep (either in Tenon's capsule or the episclera). A maximum of 1 ml can be injected. The swelling from the injection disperses in several hours.
2. Large animals - in horses, the upper eyelid can be retracted with an eyelid retractor (Desmarres size 2) or the surgeon's finger. If retraction is not successful, a palpebral nerve block may be needed. In cattle, the area can be exposed by pushing the upper eyelid between the rim of the orbit and the globe. The injection site and technique is the same as for small animals. Up to 2 ml of medication can be injected.

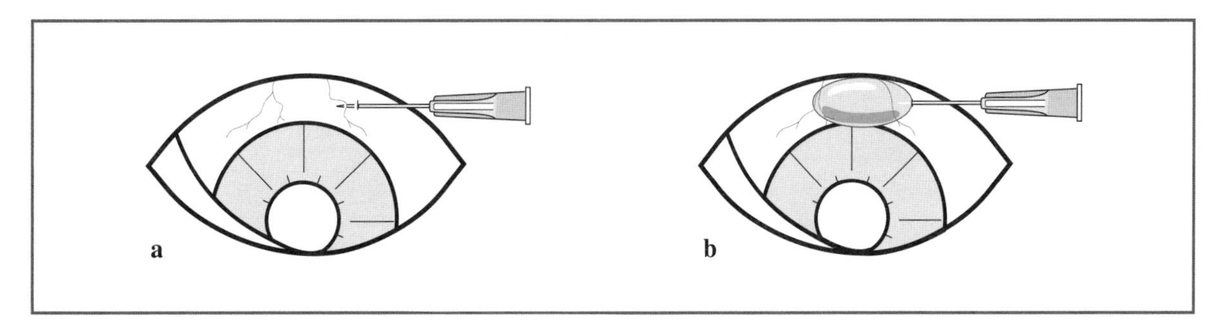

Figure 2-12. Subconjunctival injection.
a. Needle passed beneath the conjunctiva, bevel up
b. Conjunctiva blebs during injection. Fluid will disperse rapidly.

Drugs injected

1. Antibacterial/antimycotic
2. Serum (alpha macroglobulins and endogenous growth factors)
3. Mydriatic/cycloplegics
4. Anti-inflammatory agents

Compatible drugs can be mixed before injection

Comment - Subconjunctival injection should not be used indiscriminately, but if in your judgement it is the best way to treat a specific patient, it is indicated as a supplement to other routes of administration. Many patients can be treated as effectively with systemic and topical treatment. If a drug can penitrate the epithelium, higher tissue drug levels will be achieved by frequent topical rather than subconjunctival administration.

RETROBULBAR INJECTION

Retrobulbar injections diffuse rapidly behind the eye and are used for:

1. Anesthesia and immobilization of the eye and/or eyelids
2. To deliver drugs to the posterior segment of the eye (vitreous, posterior sclera, choroid, retina and optic nerve) and retrobulbar tissues
3. In inflamed eyes, retrobulbar and sub-bulbar conjunctival injection result in similar vitreous drug penetration.

Drugs injected

1. Infiltration anesthetics
2. Antibiotics - intraocular and retrobulbar infection
3. Corticosteroids - trauma (proptosed eyes) or muscle inflammation
4. Contrast media - orbital radiography

Technique - chemical restraint or general anesthesia is recommended

1. Small animals - several techniques can be used (Munger and Ackerman, J Am Anim Hosp Assoc 14:490, 1978)
    a. The author prefers the technique described by Gelatt, whereby a 20 gauge needle is inserted behind the orbital ligament and above the zygomatic arch, and directed medially and slightly caudad behind the eye into the muscle cone to a depth of about one inch, depending on the size of the animal.
    Injection can also be made below the zygomatic arch along a line perpendicular to the lateral canthus with the needle directed medial and slightly posterior.
    b. Technique after repositioning and tarsorrhaphy of a proptosed eye. A repository corticosteroid can be injected into the retrobulbar space by inserting a one inch, 20 or 22 gauge needle through the upper eyelid next to the dorsal rim of the orbit and directing the needle posteriorly between the globe and the orbit.
2. Large animals - chemical restraint is recommended. Retrobulbar injection or aspiration can be made above or below the zygomatic arch. The author prefers the site above the zygomatic arch and caudal to the temporal process of the malar bone. A 20 gauge needle can be directed downward and anteromedial 1.5 to 2 inches behind the eye into the orbital cone.

INTRAOCULAR INJECTION

Intraocular injections may be made into the anterior chamber (intracameral) or intravitreal.

Intracameral injection

This is generally used during intraocular surgery and less frequently if there is severe intraocular infection or inflammation. If possible, use drugs that are specifically prepared for intraocular use. Preservatives, buffering agents or other additives may be present that will damage the eye.

1. Indications
   a. Irrigation during intraocular surgery - sterile 0.9% saline solution, Ringer's solution, or intraocular balanced salt solution (BSS) can be used to maintain the anterior chamber and irrigate out fibrin or blood.
   b. Control pupil size during surgery
      1) Sterile epinephrine 1:10,000 will dilate the pupil and decrease hemorrhage from the anterior uvea. 1:20,000 will dilate but is not as effective for hemorrhage
      2) Intraocular acetylcholine (Miochol) or carbachol (Miostat-Alcon) to constrict the pupil when there is vitreous present in the pupil.
   c. Control excessive fibrin in the anterior chamber - Fibrin formation secondary to ocular surgery or severe anterior uveitis can result in synechia or filtration angle closure that may lead to complications, especially glaucoma.
      1) Heparin, 1,000 units per liter of intraocular irrigating solution will prevent fibrin formation
      2) Tissue plasminogen activator (tPA) can be injected to dissolve existing clots from anterior uveitis or after surgery (See page 124).
2. Injection technique (See Chapter 1, Fig 1-41, page 38) - topical and general anesthesia is recommended. Stabilize the eye with forceps placed near the limbus. Using a 25 to 27 gauge needle on a 2 cc syringe, position the needle with the bevel up and introduce it subconjunctivally about 4 mm from the limbus. Advance the needle until the point is 1.5 mm from the limbus and then force it through the sclera so the needle will enter the anterior chamber in front of and parallel to the iris. Forcing the needle through the limbus takes more pressure than anticipated and can be made easier by rotating the syringe between your fingers. Advance the needle to about 1/4 to 1/3 the distance across the anterior chamber. If the eye is soft, up to 0.15 ml of fluid can be injected without aspirating aqueous. If the pressure is normal, a two-syringe technique is recommended. The first syringe and needle is used to enter the anterior chamber and withdraw as much fluid as you intend to inject. Next remove the aspiration syringe from the needle and attach the second syringe containing the medicine. After the injection, grasp the conjunctiva and needle with a forceps at the site where the needle entered the conjunctiva. After the needle is withdrawn, hold the conjunctiva for a few seconds to seal the wound so that any backflow through the sclera will build up as subconjunctival fluid.

Intravitreal injection

Intravitreal injection is seldom used in veterinary medicine but should be considered when a patient presents with acute endophthalmitis or if an oculotoxic injection of a painful eye with irreversible blindness is desired. The procedure is easily performed.

1. Acute endophthalmitis - The vitreous is poorly penetrated by drugs, therefore even in the inflamed eye, intravitreal injection of antibiotics may be necessary to control a severe posterior segment infection. The dosage of drugs is very critical because overdose may result in toxicity to the retina and ciliary body epithelium (Table 2-4, page 83). The duration drugs remain in the vitreous after injection is variable and when selecting a drug, knowledge of pharmacokinetics of that drug is important.

2. Oculotoxic injection of gentocin - usually results in a pain-free cosmetic eye. Indicated in patients with irreversible blindness due to chronic glaucoma or horses with painful nonresponsive equine recurrent uveitis. The dosage is an estimate, therefore if underdosed, reinjection may be necessary or if overdosed, phthisis bulbi may result.
3. Technique (Chapter 1, page 38, Fig. 1-41)
   a. Small animals - Topical and general anesthesia is recommended. Two tuberculin syringes with 25 to 27 gauge needles are used. One syringe and needle is used to tap the anterior chamber and withdraw a volume of aqueous humor equal to the volume of medication to be injected. This results in a soft eye. The injection site is over the pars plana about 8 mm posterior to the limbus. Using the second syringe with medication, the needle is directed through the conjunctiva and sclera toward the optic papilla to a depth of 1 to 1.5 cm. After the needle is withdrawn, pressure should be applied at the injection site for at least one minute to reduce leakage.
   b. Equine - Topical anesthesia and chemical restraint is usually adequate. If the animal is hard to handle, a short general anesthesia is recommended. The injection site is 1 to 1.5 cm from the limbus over the area of the pars plana. A 25 gauge needle is directed toward the center of the eye and advanced 2.0 cm. If the eye is glaucomatous or the injection to be given exceeds 0.25 ml, it is recommended to aspirate first using a two-syringe technique.

RETROGRADE ARTERIAL PERFUSION

Retrograde arterial perfusion of the eye by catheterization of the infraorbital artery has been experimentally done in the dog (Fig 2-13). Clinical data on its effectiveness is lacking in veterinary medicine.

Comment - This method of treatment is rarely used, but is indicated when:

1. Toxic drugs are needed to treat intraocular lesions (e.g. injection of cytotoxic agents in neoplastic diseases). High intraocular drug levels can be accomplished and the drug is diluted to harmless levels in the venous return to the heart.
2. To achieve unusually high blood levels of drugs in the eye (e.g. antibiotics for panophthalmitis)

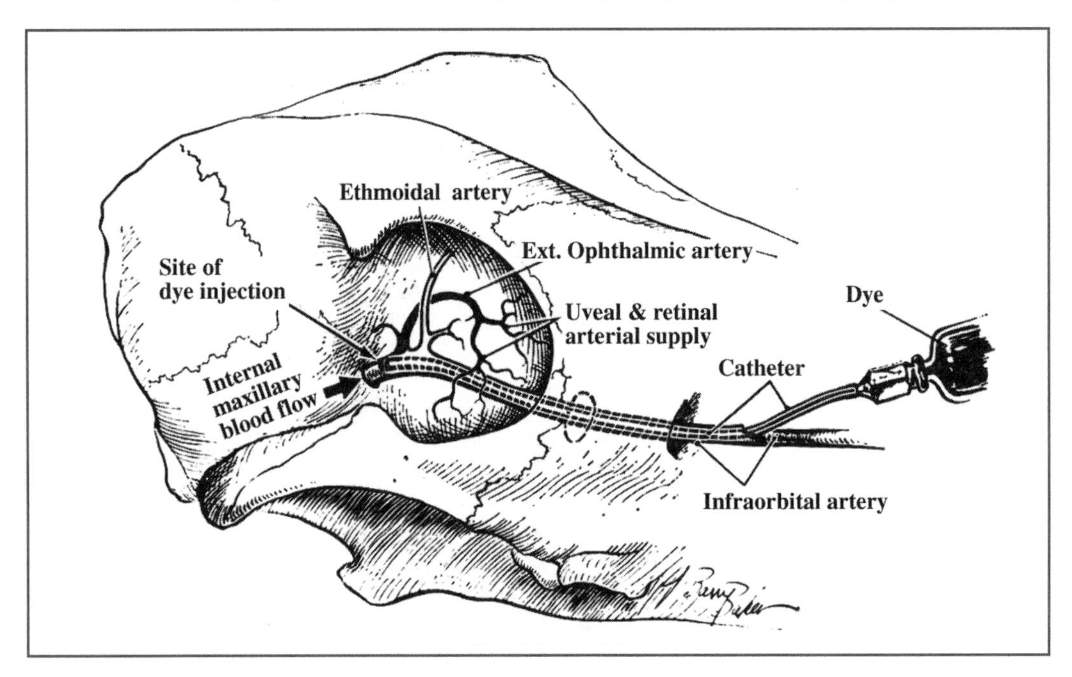

Figure 2-13. Retrograde arterial perfusion.
Injection of infraorbital artery in the dog. Modified from Pinkerton R. Am J Ophthalmol, 1963.

SYSTEMIC ADMINISTRATION

This is the preferred way to treat diseases of the posterior segment. The normal blood-aqueous barrier keeps many antibiotics out of the eye. It is penetrated best by chloramphenicol. Uveal inflammation reduces the blood-aqueous barrier, thus allowing drugs and large molecules to penetrate into the eye. As the inflammation subsides, impermeability returns.

CHOOSING ROUTE OF ADMINISTRATION (Table 2-2)

Choosing the route of administration will be determined by:

1. Drug characteristics
   a. Corneal penetration
   b. Stability of the drug
   c. Duration of activity
2. Convenience of application
3. Location of the lesion
4. Concentration of drug in the tissue needed to be effective

Indications for routes

1. Topical - lids, conjunctiva, cornea, sclera, anterior uvea
2. Subconjunctival - cornea, sclera, anterior uvea, vitreous
3. Retrobulbar - posterior sclera, optic nerve, retrobulbar muscle cone
4. Systemic - eyelids, sclera, anterior and posterior uvea, vitreous, retina, optic nerve, retrobulbar disease and selected conjunctival and corneal diseases
5. Route combinations will often increase drug efficacy (e.g. topical, systemic and subconjunctival when treating severe anterior uveitis in horses)

Table 2-2. Indications for route of administration

	Topical	**Subconjunctival**	**Retrobulbar**	**Systemic**
Eyelids	+			+
Conjunctiva	+	+		*
Cornea	+	+		*
Sclera	+	+	**	+
Anterior uvea	+	+		+
Vitreous		+		+
Choroid and retina			+	+
Optic nerve			+	+
Orbit			+	+

* Selected conjunctival and corneal diseases
** Posterior episcleritis

ANTIBIOTIC AGENTS

Selection of an antibiotic agent is governed by:

- Location of the infection - determined by a thorough examination
- Cause of the infection - presenting signs may be adequate to make a presumptive diagnosis. Complicated cases may require diagnostic tests (cytology, fluorescent antibody staining, serology, and culture/sensitivity). Culturing is not recommended unless the infection is an immediate danger to the eye, or is chronic and not responding to treatment.
- Knowledge of drug properties

KNOWLEDGE OF DRUG PROPERTIES (PHARMACOKINETICS) (Table 2-3)

Knowledge of drug properties is necessary so a drug can be selected that will get to the infection and control it. The drug barriers of the eye are corneal, blood-aqueous and blood-retinal. These barriers are dependent on the tightness of the epithelial and endothelial junctions. There is no pharmacokinetic barrier between the conjunctiva, sclera or choroid. The conjunctival epithelium has the same characteristics as corneal epithelium. Inflammation breaks down the blood-aqueous and blood-retinal barriers.

Corneal barrier - As previously discussed, cornea has very tight epithelial and endothelial junctions, thereby requiring drugs to be lipid soluble to pass through the epithelial and endothelial cell membranes.

Blood-aqueous barrier - The endothelium of the ciliary body capillaries is very porous but the junctions of the nonpigment epithelium are tight, forming the blood-aqueous barrier. Iris capillary endothelium is relatively nonporous and accounts for its blood-aqueous barrier. Prostaglandins are probably the major cause for breakdown of the blood-aqueous barrier. Drugs can pass easily from aqueous into the iris.

Blood-retinal barrier - is formed internally by the nonporous endothelium of the retinal capillaries and externally between the retina and choroid by the tight intercellular junctions of the retinal pigment epithelium.

Comment

1. The blood-aqueous and blood-retinal barriers severely limit nonlipid drugs such as penicillin from the vitreous, aqueous and lens.
2. Plasma protein binding of antibiotics renders them biologically inactive and the blood-aqueous and blood-retinal barriers exclude the protein-bound antibiotic from entering the eye. Acute inflammation reduces the barriers and protein-bound antibiotics can pass into the eye.
3. For topical use in treatment of minor ocular inflammation, it is ***prudent*** to avoid antibiotics that are commonly administered systemically. This reduces risk of developing resistant strains and/or the possibility of patient sensitization to the antibiotic.
4. Synergistic topical combinations can be helpful (i.e. neomycin, polymyxin B, and gramicidin drops, or neomycin, polymyxin B, and bacitracin ointment).

Table 2-3. Intraocular penetration of antibacterial agents

Agents	Systemic	Topical	Subconjunctival
Amikacin	Systemic	Topical	Good
Amoxicillin	Good	Poor	Good
Ampicillin	Poor	Poor	Good
Azithromycin	Poor	Good	Good
Bacitracin	--	Poor	Poor
Cephalosporins	Poor	Poor	Good
Chloramphenicol	Poor/fair	Good	Good
Colistin	Poor	Poor	Good
Erythromycin	Poor	Good	Good
Gentamicin	Poor	Poor	Good
Kanamycin	Poor	Poor	Poor
Lincomycin	Good	--	--
Methicillin	Good	--	Good
Minocycline	Good	--	Good
Neomycin	--	Poor	Poor
Penicillin	Fair	Poor	Good
Polymyxin B	--	Poor	Poor
Rosoxacin	Poor	Good	Good
Sulfonamides in general	Good	Fair	Good
Tetracyclines	Poor	Good	Good
Tobramycin	Poor	Poor	Good
Trimethoprim / sulfa-diazine	Good	--	--

Intraocular penetration of antibacterial agents, courtesy of Charles Martin, *Veterinary Ophthalmology Notes,* University of Georgia, 1994.

ANTIBACTERIALS (Table 2-4)

Too many preparations are available for the practitioner to stock more than a few selected antibiotics. Prescriptions can be written or mixtures formulated as needed. Minimal hospital pharmacy could include:

1. Broad-spectrum mixtures
   a. Ointment - neomycin and polymyxin B with or without bacitracin
   b. Solution - neomycin and polymyxin B with or without gramacidin
2. Gentamicin ointment and solution
3. Terramycin ointment such as oxytetracycline with or without polymyxin B

Aminoglycosides - are effective against many gram-positive and gram-negative organisms, rapidly bactericidal, water soluble, have poor penetration of the blood-aqueous barrier, and are synergistic with penicillins. They are the preferred antibiotic for *Pseudomonas* infections. The suggested order of choice of aminoglycosides for treating *Pseudomonas* ulcers is tobramycin, gentamicin, and amikacin. Cross resistance to aminoglycosides can occur, therefore sensitivity testing is recommended for all *Pseudomonas* ulcers.

1. Amikacin (acetylated kanamycin) - indicated as an *"ace-in-the-hole"* for resistant infections (e.g. *Pseudomonas*. No ophthalmic form is available, therefore a 1% solution can be made in artificial tears. It is the antibiotic of choice for intravitreal injection for panophthalmitis.
2. Gentamicin - is one of the more frequently used antibiotics in veterinary medicine, therefore resistant strains are becoming more common. It is anticipated to be effective against *Staphylococcus, Streptococcus, Pseudomonas* (resistant strains are increasing), *Proteus* and *E. coli*. Gentamicin may cause topical allergy, especially in cats. The concentration in commercial preparations is 3 mg/ml. Concentrated ophthalmic solutions can be prepared up to 15 mg/ml and are indicated in very acute corneal disease. Intravitreal injection is very toxic. As little as 0.1 mg in rabbits may result in retinal toxicity.
3. Neomycin - is not used much systemically, therefore there is little chance of encountering a previously sensitized patient, but it may produce local sensitization with long-term topical use. It is frequently combined with polymyxin and bacitracin in ointments, and polymyxin and gramacidin in solutions. It is indicated for *Proteus vulgaris* and *Staphylococcus* species.
4. Tobramycin (Tobrex, Alcon Laboratories) - is commercially available as drops or ointment containing 3 mg/ml (fortified solutions up to 12 mg/ml can be used). It is similar to gentamicin and not used as much. Therefore, it is a ***first choice drug*** for the management of serious gram-negative infections, especially *Pseudomonas*. Topical irritation can occur with concentrations greater than 6 mg/ml when used with extended wear contact lenses.

Bacitracin - is a water soluble bactericidal antibiotic, with a range similar to penicillin. It is effective chiefly against gram-positive organisms. There are a very few resistant strains because systemic toxicity limits it to topical usage. Sensitization of the tissues to topical use is uncommon.

Cephalosporins - are broad-spectrum antibiotics closely related in structure to penicillin and similar in their mechanism of action. They are not available in ophthalmic preparations. The major indication is probably systemic administration for systemic disease with ophthalmic manifestations, or presurgical for intraocular surgery.

Chloramphenicol - is the smallest molecule of the broad-spectrum antibiotics. It is available in 1% drops and 0.5% ointment. 10% solutions can be used without irritation.

1. It is effective for gram-positive and gram-negative organisms. *Rickettsia, Spirochetes* and *Chlamydia*. It does not affect *Pseudomonas*, and for this reason, combinations are available with polymyxin B. It is bacteriostatic.
2. Because of its biphasic structure, it is lipid and water soluble and therefore penetrates intact cornea. When given systemically, it penetrates the blood-aqueous and blood-retinal barriers.
3. Chloramphenicol cannot be used in food animals because of the possibility of tissue residues.
4. Adverse reactions are rare in animals, and when seen, are transient fever, anorexia, and mydriasis.

Clindamycin - is the chlorinated analogue of lincomycin. It is effective against both gram-positive and gram-negative microorganisms, *Mycoplasma* and *Toxoplasma*. Clindamycin hydrochloride, 0.2%, is the most lipid-soluble form and will penetrate the cornea better than other forms (phosphate and palmitate do not penetrate as well). Systemically-administered clindamycin is selectively concentrated in the retina and choroid. Subconjunctival injection penetrates well, up to 35 mg may be used without irritation. Large doses, 150 mg,

Table 2-4. Concentrations and doses of principle antibiotic agents (from multiple sources)

Drug Name	Topical (commercial)	Topical (fortified for ulcers)	Subconjunctival	Intracameral	Intravitreal
Amikacin	--	6-10 mg/ml	25 mg	250 µg	400 µg
Ampicillin	--	50 mg/ml	50-150 mg	--	500 µg
Bacitracin	500 units/gm	10,000 units/gm	5,000-19,000 units	500-1000 units	--
Carbenicillin	--	4-6 mg/ml	100 mg	--	250-2000 µg
Cefazolin	--	30-50 mg/ml *	100 mg	--	2.25 mg
Cephaloridine	--	32 mg/ml	100 mg	--	250 µg
Cephalothin	--	--	50-100 mg	--	2 mg
Chloramphenicol	5-10 mg/ml	--	50-100 mg	1-2 mg	1-2 mg
Chlortetracycline	10 mg/gm	--	2.5-5 mg	2.5-5 mg	2.5-5 mg
Ciprofloxacin (Ciloxan)	3.5 mg/ml	--	--	--	--
Clindamycin	--	50 mg/ml	15-50 mg/ml	1 mg	1 mg
Colistin	3 mg/ml	10 mg/ml	15-25 mg	100 µg	100 µg
Erythromycin	5 mg/gm	10-50 mg/ml	50-100 mg	1-2 mg	500 µg
Gentamicin	3 mg/ml or gm	8-15 mg/ml *	10-20 mg	--	100-200 µg
Imipen/Cilastatin	--	5 mg/ml	--	--	--
Kanamycin	--	30-50 mg/ml	30 mg	--	--
Lincomycin	--	--	150 mg	--	--
Methicillin	--	50 mg/ml	50-100 mg	1 mg	1-2 mg
Moxalactam	--	100 mg/ml	50 mg	--	1250 µg
Neomycin	3.5-8 mg/ml	33 mg/ml	125-250 mg	2.5 mg	--
Norfloxacin (Chibroxin)	3 mg/ml	--	--	--	--
Ofloxacin (Ocuflox)	3 mg/ml	--	--	--	--
Oxacillin	--	66 mg/ml	--	--	--
Penicillin G	--	100,000-333,000 units/ml	0.5-1.0 million units	1000-4000 units	--
Polymyxin B	10,000 units/ml	--	100,000 units	100 µg	--
Streptomycin	--	--	50-100 mg	0.5-5 mg	0.5-5 mg
Tetracycline	10 mg/gm	--	2.5-5 mg	2.5-5 mg	2.5-5 mg
Ticarcillin	--	6 mg/ml	100 mg	--	--
Tobramycin	3 mg/ml or gm	5-15 mg/ml *	10-20 mg	500 µg	100-200 µg
Vancomycin	--	20-50 mg/ml *	25 mg	--	1000 µg

* Available Wedgewood Pharmacy

cause corneal and conjunctival edema and inflammation. Prolonged oral administration may lead to intestinal overgrowth from nonsusceptible organisms.

Colistin (Colimycin, Polymyxin E) - is effective for gram-negative organisms, especially *Pseudomonas*. Topically it does not penetrate the normal eye or systemically the blood-aqueous barrier. It will penetrate the inflamed eye (0.12% drops) or the normal eye by subconjunctival injection (10 to 20 mg). It is less nephrotoxic than polymyxin B when given systemically. Commercial ophthalmic preparations are not available.

Erythromycin - is available in 0.5% ophthalmic ointment. It is not frequently used but is effective against gram-positive organisms, especially *Staphylococcus* and *Mycoplasma*. Bacterial resistance may develop rapidly. It exhibits poor penetration of the blood-aqueous barrier. It is used primarily when sensitivity tests reveal that it will be effective.

Azithromycin (Zithromax powder for suspension - Pfizer & Wedgewood, or suspensions - Sussex) - it is similar to erythromycin. Broad-spectrum antibacterial, including *Chlamydia*. Dosage for cats with *Chlamydia* 5 mg/kg daily or every other day for 2-3 weeks.

Fluoroquinolones - Active against aerobic gram-positive and gram-negative organisms, including *Staphylococcus*, *Streptococcus*, and *Pseudomonas*. Used in human ophthalmology to treat betalactams or aminoglycoside-resistant organisms.

1. Ciprofloxacin 0.35% (Ciloxan - Alcon)
2. Norfloxacin 0.3% (Chibroxin - Merck)
3. Ofloxacin - 0.3% (Ocuflox - Allergan)
4. Orbifloxacin (Orbax - Schering Plough) - dogs and cats 2.5 mg/kg daily. It crosses the blood-brain barrier very well.

Fusidic acid 1% (Conoptal - Leo) - Fusidic acid is used extensively outside the United States. It has a wide range of susceptible organisms, including *Staphylococcus*, *Streptococcus*, *Corynebacterium* and *Moraxella*. It is in a viscous base that gives prolonged contact with a BID recommended frequency of administration.

Penicillins - are water soluble and vary considerably as to how they affect the eye.

1. Pharmacokinetics
   a. They are seldom used topically because of poor epithelial penetration
   b. When given subconjunctivally, they penetrate well
   c. Poor penetration of blood-aqueous and blood-retinal barriers because they are not lipid soluble. The degree of plasma protein binding also excludes passage through the blood-aqueous barrier. Ampicillin penetrates best; amoxicillin and hetacillin next; penicillin G, methicillin, carbenicillin, and cloxacillin exhibit poor penetration; and dicloxacillin does not penetrate.
2. Indications
   a. Topical - is seldom used because of poor penetration of epithelium and high incidence of local allergic responses, which would sensitize the patient for later systemic use
   b. Systemic - is excellent for adnexal infections, especially amoxicillin-clavulanic acid (Clavamox). Ampicillin's penetration of blood-aqueous barrier makes it a good choice for elective presurgical medication. Amoxicillin is the next choice.

Polymyxin B - cannot be used systemically because of nephrotoxic characteristics. It does not penetrate intact epithelium or blood-aqueous barrier. Subconjunctival injection is irritating and not recommended. It is effective against gram-negative organisms, especially *Pseudomonas* (about 60% effective) and for this reason is included in ophthalmic antibiotic combinations. It is available as a 0.2% ointment or in mixtures with other antibiotics.

Tetracyclines - a large molecule and will penetrate the cornea only if abraded. It works well in the treatment of ulcers and is good for simple conjunctivitis. Not used as much as some of the other antibiotics. Poor penetration of the blood-aqueous and blood-retinal barriers and many resistant strains have developed. It is effective against many gram-positive and gram-negative organisms, *Rickettsia, Actinomyces* and *Chlamydia*; 0.5% Terramycin ointments are available and is the drug of choice for treating *Chlamydia* conjunctivitis.

1. Oxytetracycline (Terramycin) - available with polymyxin B
2. Chlortetracycline (Aureomycin)
3. Demeclocycline (Declomycin)
4. Tetracycline (Achromycin)
5. Doxycycline (Vibramycin) - long acting broad spectrum. Good choice for *Chlamydia*

Trimethoprim sulfate 0.1% and polymyxin sulfate 10,000 units (Polytrim-Allergan) - is a broad spectrum antibiotic combination. Very effective for *Staphylococcus*, *Streptococcus* and *Pseudomonas*.

Sulfonamides - are bacteriostatic and work by preventing bacterial utilization of para-aminobenzoic acid. The newer sulfas and potentiated sulfonamide combinations have a broad antibacterial range.

1. Topical use - topical anesthetics are also esters of para-amino benzoic acid and inhibit sulfa's effectiveness. Their major advantage is low allergenicity. Sulfas are infrequently used except in minor infections or long-term therapy in patients with antibiotic sensitivity. Sulfas penetrate intact cornea poorly, therefore high concentrations are used to increase penetrability.
    a. Sulfisoxazole diolamine (Gantrisin) - 4% ointment or solution has a very broad antibacterial spectrum
    b. Sulfacetamide sodium - 10 to 30% ointments and solutions are available. It is an excellent topical sulfa. It penetrates the eye well in rabbits; poorly in the dog.
2. Systemic sulfas - are seldom used by themselves except when treating specific infections, for which they are the drug of choice. Potentiated sulfonamide combinations with broad-spectrum and prolonged blood levels are used frequently. These are trimethoprim with sulfamethoxazole (Septra) or sulfadiazine (Bactrim/Tribrissen) and ormetroprim with sulfadimethoxine (Primor).

    Systemic sulfadiazine and sulfasalazine have been documented to cause keratoconjunctivitis sicca in dogs, which usually occurs from long term usage but occasionally can be observed within several days, suggesting a sensitization response. Sulfa combinations are useful when treating blepharitis, but, because of the danger of KCS, tear production should be monitored when sulfas are administered. Problems with decreased tear production have not been observed after topical therapy.

Nitrofurazone (Furacin) - is safe and effective topically. It is especially useful for the pretreatment of eyelid lacerations prior to surgical repair. It does not penetrate intact cornea. ***It should not be used in food animals.***

1. Furacin dressing 0.2%. When applied to an eyelid laceration and covered with a bandage overnight will prepare the wound for suturing and first intention healing.
2. Furacin soluble powder. Can be dissolved in physiologic saline solution or artificial tears (5 gm in 10 cc) and used as an eye drop.

ANTIVIRAL AGENTS (Table 2-5)

Ophthalmic herpesvirus infection is common in cats. The human antiherpes drugs available are metabolic inhibitors and if given for an extended period of time may be epithelial toxic and delay corneal healing. Their effectiveness is variable in the cat with the best response seen early in the disease. When prescribing, one should follow the human directions for frequency and duration of treatment. Owners should be advised that these drugs are expensive.

Adenine arabinoside (Vidarabine, Vira-A) - an antiherpes agent that is believed to inhibit DNA polymerase. Available in 3% ophthalmic ointment. Use five times daily.

Idoxuridine (generic - Wedgewood Pharmaceuticals) - 0.1% opthalmic solution. Idoxuridine resembles thymidine and when substituted in virus molecules will result in a virus that cannot function as an infection-producing virus. Initially use every two hours, then reduce to t.i.d. or q.i.d. (moderate price).

Acyclovir (Zovirax) - Effective topically and systemically in man. Acyclovir functions as a substrate for viral thymidine kinase but does not affect host cells. Therefore, it interferes only with the DNA synthesized by virus. Available only for systemic use but 3% ointments have been investigated.

1. Systemic administration - oral suspension, 40 mg/ml
2. Dosage - 5 mg/lb BID
3. Course of therapy - two weeks recommended; four weeks maximum

Povidone-iodine - Povidone-iodine 10% used as an ophthalmic drop is clinically effective in chronic feline herpes keratitis in dilutions of 1:10 (1%) or 1:20 (0.5%). This is an alternate choice when treating recurrent herpesvirus ulcers and keratitis. This preparation does not work with DNA inhibition but interacts with the virus during the brief extracellular phase. Continued treatment with daily Betadine drops may be beneficial as prophylactic therapy in patients with a history of recurring ulcers.

Lysine - Oral lysine is beneficial in some cats as treatment and prophylaxis for recurrent herpesvirus corneal ulcers. Lysine ties up arginine, making it unavailable for herpesvirus replication. BID treatment: kittens 250 mg., adults 500 mg.

Interferon (Intron A, Interferon Alpha-2b, Recombinant - Schering Plough) - Appears to reduce the severity and shorten the course of ocular feline herpes infections when given concurrent with antiherpes medication.

1. Intron A - Solution concentration of 3 million IU per 0.5 ml vial. Costs about $30.00
2. Preparation and storage
   a. Dilute vial contents (3 million IU) to 100 ml with sterile saline = 30,000 IU/ml. Place 1 ml in sterile vial and store at -70° C. (Can store for 10 months)
   b. Reconstitute 1 ml added to 1000 ml with sterile water = 30 IU per ml. Then refrigerate.
3. Dosage - 30 IU per os daily
4. ***Comment*** - an alternative to freezing would be to immediately use. Make several 100 ml vials of 30 IU/ml and store short term in refrigerator.

Table 2-5. Antiviral agents

Name	Topical	Systemic
Idoxuridine (Wedgewood)	0.1% ophthalmic solution	
Vidarabine (Vira-A)	3.0% ophthalmic ointment	
Povidone-iodine (Betadine)	0.5-1.0% in saline	
Acyclovir (Zovirax)		Cats: 5 mg/lb BID
Lysine		250-500 mg BID
Interferon (Intron A)		30 IU/os daily

ANTIFUNGAL DRUGS (Table 2-6)

Limited veterinary literature is available stating the effectiveness of ocular antifungal agents. Treatment should be continuous delivery or every or every 1-2 hours for the first 3 to 6 days depending on response to treatment.

Natamycin (Natacyn - Alcon Laboratories) - 5% ophthalmic solution. This is the only antifungal agent approved as an ophthalmic preparation. Very expensive.

1. Characteristics
   a. Insoluble in water and heat stable
   b. Nonirritating
   c. Poor corneal penetration. Excellent for ulcers but will not penetrate to deep epithelialized corneal lesions
   d. Of no value subconjunctivally
2. Preparations - topical 5% suspension, 15 ml glass dropper bottle. Very viscous, therefore difficult to administer through some ocular delivery systems.

Amphotericin B (Fungizone) - systemic use is limited because of toxicity. It can be used topical, subconjunctival, or intralesional. Topical 1.0 - 1.5% solution can be prepared with water for injection or dextrose 5% in water.

Clotrimazole

1. Characteristics - absorbable orally, nontoxic, will maintain blood levels, and penetrate the blood-aqueous barrier
2. Preparations
   a. Topical dermatologic preparation (Lotrimin) can be used on the eye
      1) 1% solution in oil - less irritating than ointment
      2) 1% ointment
   b. Systemic 60 to 100 mg/kg/day

Fluconazole (Diflucan - Roerig)

1. Systemically effective for *Aspergillus*, *Blastomyces*, *Candida*, *Coccidioides*, *Cryptococcus*, and *Histoplasma*
2. Available in 50, 100, and 200 mg tablets; and IV solution, 2 mg/ml. Administer 2.5 to 5 mg/kg divided BID. Systemic administration does not increase corneal concentration.
3. Fluconazole ophthalmic solution 2 mg/ml (Generic - Wedgewood Pharmacy).

Flucytosine

1. Characteristics - water soluble, nonirritating topically, absorbed orally, nontoxic and will cross the blood-aqueous barrier
2. Preparations
   a. Topical 1 to 1.5% aqueous drops can be prepared
   b. Systemic 200 mg/kg/day

Itraconazole (Sporanox - Janssen) - a very good antifungal for topical use.

1. Systemic
   a. Characteristics - absorption is dependent on gastric pH and presence of food.
   b. Preparation - 100 mg capsules
   c. Dosage: dogs and cats, 5 mg/Kg daily or BID. Horses, 3 mg/Kg BID
2. Topical - commercial preparations not available
   a. Drops - 1% solution can be prepared using artificial tears.
   b. Ointment - itraconazole 1%, dimethyl sulfoxide (DMSO) 30% (Ball, Rebhun, Garder and Patten -1977).
      1) Preparation
         a) One gm itraconazole added to 33.3 ml 90% dimethyl sulfoxide. Mixture heated slowly to 80° C.
         b) 66.6 ml of white petrolatum heated to 80° C.
         c) Solutions mixed as cooled slowly to form ointment.
         d) Ointment can be placed in 6 or 12 ml syringes to facilitate administration.
      2) Administration - QID

Miconazole - readily available as OTC vaginal creams and ointments. This is a good choice when waiting for culture results or delivery of special order ophthalmic preparations. Compounded (Wedgewood Pharmacy) - 1% ophthalmic solution and 2% ophthalmic ointment.

Table 2-6. Antifungal agents

Name	Route of Administration	Dosage	Spectrum
Amphotericin B (Fungizone)	Topical	1.0 -1.5% solution, dilute with water or dextrose 5% in water	*Blastomyces* *Candida* *Coccidiodes* *Histoplasma* *Penicillium*
	Subconjunctival	0.8-1.0 mg	
	Intravitreal	5 µg	
Clotrimazole (Lotrimin-OTC)	Topical	1% solution 1% cream 2% ointment	*Alternaria* *Aspergillus* *Candida* *Mucor*
Fluconazole (Diflucan)	Topical	0.2% IV solution	*Aspergillus* *Blastomyces* *Candida* *Cryptococcus* *Histoplasma*
	Systemic	2.5-5 mg/kg daily	
Fluconazole (Wedgewood)	Topical	0.2% solution	
Flucytosine (Ancobon)	Topical	1% solution	*Candida* *Cryptococcus*
Itraconazole (Sporanox)	Systemic	5 mg per kg daily or BID	*Aspergillus* *Blastomyces* *Candida* *Cryptococcus* *Histoplasma*
	Topical	1% solution	
Itraconazole/ DMSO (Wedgewood)	Topical	1% itraconazole/ 30% DMSO ointment	
Ketoconazole (Nizoral)	Topical	1-2% suspension	*Aspergillus* *Blastomyces* *Candida* *Cryptococcus* *Histoplasma* *Mucor* *Sporothrix*
	Systemic	200 mg tablets 4.5 mg/lb daily or BID	
Miconazole (OTC vaginal preparations)	Topical	1% ointment or cream	*Aspergillus* *Candida* *Cryptococcus*
Miconazole (Wedgewood)	Topical	1% solution 2% ointment	
Natamycin (Natacyn-Alcon)	Topical	5% solution	*Aspergillus* *Candida* *Cephalosporium* *Fusarium* *Penicillium*
Povidone-iodine	Topical	0.2%	
Silver sulfadiazine	Topical	1%	
Thiabendazole	Topical	1-4% solution	*Cladosporium* *Fusarium* *Penicillium* *Phialophora*

Ketoconazole (Nizoral - Janssen)

1. Ketoconazole is systemically effective for arresting systemic mycoses and has been reported to be effective topically for mycotic keratitis.
2. Topical administration
   a. Nizoral 2% dermatologic cream, is in an aqueous vehicle and available in 15 and 30 ml
   b. 1 to 2% ophthalmic drops can be prepared from 200 mg oral tablets; it is poorly water soluble but solubility is increased in a weak acid base
3. Systemic administration (4.5 mg/lb) concurrently with topical may be beneficial in rapidly progressing corneal ulcers

Thiabendazole

1. Characteristics - poorly soluble in water, penetrates cornea well, and is nonirritating topically and systemically
2. Preparations
   a. Topical use - dilute oral worming mixtures to 4% with artificial tears or water
   b. Orally for systemic administration, 25 mg/kg/day

Other antifungal agents

1. Silver sulfadiazine 1% burn ointment - apply q4h
2. Povidone-iodine 0.2% (1:50)
   a. Irrigate corneal foreign body tracts after removal
   b. Topical for mycotic ulcers q2h

IODINE PREPARATIONS

Ionized iodine preparations are potent antimicrobial agents. When used topically, inorganic iodides exhibit epithelial toxicity (cauterizing agents, page 114), whereas organic iodine (povidone-iodine) has minimal epithelial toxicity.

Tincture of iodine - too irritating to recommend for topical use on the eye unless use air-dried swab.

Lugol's solution - less toxic than tincture of iodine because of the absence of alcohol from the solution. Cannot be recommended for topical use.

Povidone-iodine (Betadine, Efodine) - Suggested reading: Roberts, Severin, Lavach. Antibacterial activity of dilute povidone-iodine solutions used for ocular surface disinfection in dogs. Am J Vet Res 1986;47:1207-1210.

The author has worked only with Betadine disinfectant solution (10% povidone-iodine containing 1% available iodine) and all comments and dilutions refer to this product.

1. Pharmacokinetics - Betadine solution 10% has a low pH, which can cause ocular side effects. Full strength Betadine solution applied on the eye and adnexa, followed with saline rinse in three to five minutes, will cause eyelid edema and a transient conjunctivitis in all species. In addition, horses often develop mild leukoma and are predisposed to corneal desquamation. When Betadine 10% is diluted 1:10 with saline solution, the low pH is corrected and side effects are eliminated. The toxicity of iodine to bacteria is increased in an ion-rich environment. Therefore, Betadine solution diluted with saline will kill bacteria more rapidly than full strength Betadine or if diluted in distilled water.
2. Suggested dilutions of 10% Betadine solution in PSS
   a. Presurgical disinfection - 1:50 dilution (0.2% povidone-iodine)
   b. As an ophthalmic solution - 1:20 to 1:10 dilution (0.5% to 1.0% povidone-iodine)
      1) Feline herpes conjunctivitis and ulcers

2) Infectious bovine keratitis (IBK)
3) Nonspecific keratoconjunctivitis

3. Anticollagenase activity - ionized iodine preparations have been observed to be of value in ulcer healing. An anticollagenase activity has been proposed.

ASTRINGENTS, ANTISEPTICS AND DISINFECTANTS

Ophthalmic astringents and antiseptics

1. Boric acid (ointments and drops) - frequently used in man but when used repeatedly in dogs it tends to cause tissue sensitization. It is astringent and antiseptic.
2. Yellow oxide of mercury ointment (astringent)

Skin disinfectants for ocular surgery preparation - The eyelids and conjunctiva are very sensitive to trauma and chemicals, resulting in severe edema if prepared for surgery with routine skin preparation procedures.

1. Betadine disinfectant solution - diluted 1:50 with normal saline solution is an effective skin disinfectant and does not irritate the conjunctiva or eyelids. Do not use Betadine Surgical Scrub for preparing the adnexa. It contains a detergent that will cause corneal and conjunctival epithelial toxicity and/or acute edema of the eyelids.
2. Benzalkonium (Zephiran) - is a popular quaternary ammonium compound that can be used for conjunctival irrigation at 1:5000. Concentrations stronger than 1:750 will cause ocular irritation and more concentrated solution can result in immediate corneal desquamation. Quaternary ammonium compounds are wetting agents and will enhance corneal penetration by drugs.

Ophthalmic instrument disinfectants - ophthalmic instruments are more apt to rust or deteriorate in cold disinfectant solutions than are other surgical instruments. Solution used at CSU is Lysol I.C.

1. Lysol I.C. (distributed by National Laboratories) - phenolic based ready to use instrument disinfectant. This is excellent for ophthalmic instruments. Rapid action. Germicidal, fungicidal, and virucidal. Toxic to mucous membranes, therefore rinse instruments with sterile saline or water before use. This was formerly called Lehn-Fink instrument disinfecting solution.
2. Nolvasan solution (chlorhexidine diacetate - Fort Dodge Laboratories) - Nolvasan solution is used as an instrument and premises disinfectant. It is a very effective virucide. It does not have the antirust and cleaning properties.
3. Amerse (Rhone Merierux) - Amerse is a concentrated disinfectant to be used in a 1:32 water dilution for cold disinfection of precleaned instruments.
4. Cidex (Surgikos) is a 2% glutaraldehyde solution. Can be used for disinfection (10 min soak) or sterilization (10 hrs soak). Avoid contact with skin or mucous membranes. If contact occurs, wash promptly with water.

ANTI-INFLAMMATORY DRUGS

Ocular diseases associated with inflammatory and/or immune-mediated responses are common in animals. In recent years, the medical management of some of these diseases has changed with the introduction of new drugs. In addition to the new drugs, some of the older ones have been re-evaluated and found to be useful.

Ocular inflammation is a protective mechanism but can also threaten visual functions. The use of anti-inflammation agents reduces this response but does not remove the primary cause. Therefore, an accurate diagnosis is necessary to control the inciting cause.

MECHANISM OF OCULAR INFLAMMATION

Suggested reading: Mediators of ocular inflammation. Millichamp and Dziezyc. Progress in Veterinary and Comparative Ophthalmology 1991;1:41-58; and Regulation of intraocular immune responses. English RV. Progress in Veterinary Comparative Ophthalmology 1992;2;41-49.

Injury to a cell membrane releases arachidonic acid that is incorporated in the phospholipid layer of the cell membrane. In the cell, this initiates a cascade of events forming pro-inflammatory mediators that result in the formation of leukotrienes, prostaglandins and free radicals. Corticosteroids inhibit the release of arachidonic acid by liberating an enzyme, lipomodulin, that inhibits phospholipase A_2 from releasing arachidonic acid. Antiprostaglandins inhibit cyclooxygenases that form prostaglandins from arachidonic acid (arachidonic cascade, see Fig 2-14). Prostaglandins are considered the primary mediators of ocular inflammation.

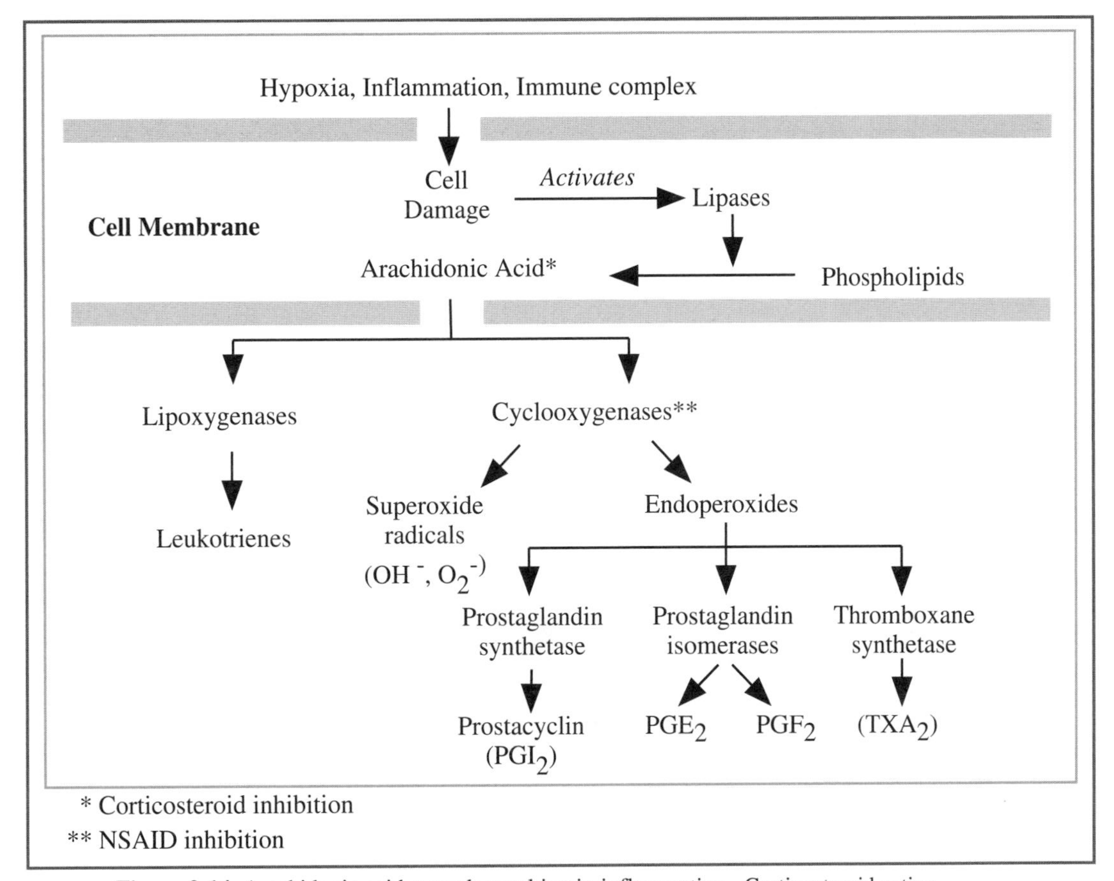

Figure 2-14. Arachidonic acid cascade resulting in inflammation. Corticosteroid action inhibits the release of arachidonic acid from the damaged cell membrane. Nonsteroidal anti-inflammatory drug inhibition occurs by inhibiting the action of cyclooxygenase, thus preventing the formation of prostaglandins (modified from Millichamp and Dziezyc).

CORTICOSTEROIDS

Corticosteroids are usually more effective in acute rather than chronic conditions, and are not effective in degenerative diseases.

Depending on the severity and location of the lesion, corticosteroid administration can be topical, subconjunctival, systemic, intralesional or a combination of these routes of administration.

Beneficial effects of corticosteroids

1. Anti-inflammatory effect
   a. Most of the anti-inflammatory effect is inhibition of the release of arachidonic acid from injured cell membranes
   b. Blocks degranulation of neutrophils, mast cells and basal cells
   c. Prevents the release of proteases, histamines and bradykinin, in turn reducing tissue necrosis
2. Decreased vascular response
   a. Reduces capillary permeability, vasodilation and postinflammatory vascularization
   b. Reduces fluid accumulation in tissues
   c. Reduces cellular exudation
3. Decreased cellular response
   a. Reduces leukocyte infiltration of lesions
   b. Inhibits fibroblast response
   c. Suppression of lymphocyte proliferation

Adverse effects of corticosteroids

1. Corneal changes due to topical administration
   a. Retards epithelial and endothelial corneal regeneration
   b. Potentiates corneal collagenase in ulcers by a factor of 15 times. Systemic administration does not affect corneal collagenase.
   c. Long term (years) frequent administration can result in stromal and epithelial degeneration
   d. Long term administration can lead to discomfort and occasionally conjunctival hyperemia. This occurs more frequently with prednisolone than dexamethasone.
2. Cataract formation - is extremely unlikely but has been suspected in cats from long term systemic administration.
3. Systemic changes
   a. Topical administration in dogs (prednisolone 1% or dexamethasone 0.1%) can suppress the pituitary adrenal axis and have hepatotoxic changes. These changes are reversible when medication is discontinued.
   b. Long term topical administration of prednisolone 1% and dexamethasone 0.1% may occasionally cause mild Cushing's like changes. This does not appear to be patient size or dosage frequency related.
   c. Polydipsia/polyuria in dogs can be seen after subconjunctival depot preparations.

Indications

Because of the anti-inflammatory effect of corticosteroids, they are often used indiscriminately. Therefore, an accurate diagnosis is necessary to determine when they will be truly beneficial.

1. Anti-inflammatory effect in nonpyogenic disease - If infection is properly controlled, concurrent corticosteroids can be helpful, especially feline chlamydial conjunctivitis, *Staph* blepharitis, ocular toxoplasmosis and intraocular mycotic infections.
2. Allergic conditions
3. Reduction of scarring during healing

Of no value in the following diseases

1. Most infections
2. Old scars
3. Degenerative diseases
   a. Cataracts
   b. Corneal dystrophy

Contraindications

1. Infected corneal wounds or ulcers
2. Suppurative eye disease
3. Infectious granulomas

Topical corticosteroids - The effectiveness of topical corticosteroids depends on the potency of the corticosteroid and its ability to penetrate the cornea. Suspension formulations of acetate and alcohol derivatives exhibit biphasic solubility and, therefore, penetrate the cornea better than water soluble phosphate solutions. In addition, the suspension particles may remain in the cul-de-sac longer than solutions. Generic preparations are less expensive.

1. Prednisolone acetate 1% suspension is the most potent topical corticosteroid available; 1/8% suspension can be used when maximum potency is not needed. Ointments containing 0.25% and 0.5% are available only in combination with antibiotics or sulfas.
2. Prednisolone phosphate 1% and 1/8% solutions are often less expensive than prednisolone acetate and are a satisfactory substitute for prednisolone acetate.
3. Dexamethasone is available as 0.1% suspensions and solutions, and 0.05% ointment. Ointments and the alcohol suspension have the greatest penetrating ability. Dexamethasone sodium phosphate solution does not penetrate as well. Combinations with antibiotics are available (Maxitrol).
4. Fluorometholone is an alternative when prednisolone or dexamethasone sensitivity is present. It does not cause the IOP increase seen in man with prednisolone and dexamethasone. Clinical potency is less than prednisolone 1%. Available in 0.1% suspension (FML - Allergan; Flarex - Alcon; eFLone - Ciba Vision), 0.25% suspension (FML Forte - Allergan), and 0.1% ointment (FML S.O.P. - Allergan).
5. Less potent (mild) corticosteroid-antibiotic combinations are available for treating mild inflammatory reactions with or without infection.
   a. Chlorasone (0.25% prednisolone acetate and 1.0% chloramphenicol - Evsco).
   b. Gentocin durafilm (0.1% betamethasone and gentocin 0.1% - Schering-Plough).
   c. Neopredef (0.1% isoflupredone and neomycin 0.5% - Pharmacia & Upjohn).
6. Indications for use of topical corticosteroid preparations
   a. Blepharitis
   b. Conjunctivitis
   c. Corneal diseases - inflammatory and immune-mediated
   d. Episcleritis - usually as an adjunct to systemic medications
   e. Anterior uveitis - usually as an adjunct to systemic medication
7. Generic sources for ophthalmic preparations, especially corticosteroids, can result in significant savings. Some of these companies are Akorn, Schein, Sussex and Wedgewood.

Subconjunctival corticosteroids

1. Short term effect (one to two days) can be achieved with:
   a. Prednisolone acetate suspension: small animals 2.5 to 10 mg, equine 25 to 50 mg
   b. Dexamethasone: small animals 0.5 to 1.0 mg; equine 2 mg
2. Depot effect (7 to 21 days) can be achieved with:
   a. Betasone (Schering-Plough) - 5 mg betamethasone diprorionate for slow absorption and 2 mg betamethasone sodium phosphate for rapid per ml. Dosage: cats and small dogs 0.1 ml (.7 mg), medium dogs 0.2 ml (1.5 mg), large dogs 0.3 ml (2 mg). Horses 1-2 ml (7-14 mg).
   b. Depo-Medrol (methylprednisolone 40 mg/ml). Dosage: cats and small dogs 0.1 ml (4 mg), medium dogs 0.15 ml (6 mg), large dogs 0.2-0.25 ml (8-10 mg). Horses 0.5-1 ml (20-40 mg).

    c. Triamcinolone, 40 mg/ml. Dosage: same as methylprednisolone.
3. Indications
    a. Keratitis
    b. Episcleritis
    c. Anterior uveitis

Systemic corticosteroids

Systemic corticosteroids are indicated when topical and/or subconjunctival routes of administration cannot reach the diseased tissues in adequate amounts to produce the desired anti-inflammatory response. The drug of choice depends upon the clinician's previous experience with systemic corticosteroids. Prednisolone/prednisone or dexamethasone are most frequently used. The choice may vary depending on the disease or circumstances requiring systemic corticosteroids.

Prednisolone is the author's first choice.

1. Small animals - Prednisolone/prednisone administration schedule: start with a loading dosage, then reduce dosage and frequency according to patient response. 1 to 2 mg/kg BID or TID, five to seven days, then daily for five to seven days, then QOD 10 to 14 days, and then 0.5 to 1 mg/kg QOD as needed for long term control of the disease. If patients respond rapidly to initial treatment, the dosage schedule can be shortened to reduce undesirable side effects.
    a. Inflammation of the sclera, uvea and/or retina should be treated with systemic corticosteroid
    b. Emergency intraocular surgery without pre-existing inflammation. Intravenous dexamethasone sodium phosphate, 0.25 mg/lb or prednisolone sodium phosphate or succinate, 0.25 to 0.5 mg/lb can be used for loading dosage. Then oral prednisolone postoperatively.
    c. Elective intraocular surgery that can result in anterior uveitis (lens removal, glaucoma cyclocryosurgery). Precondition one to three days with oral prednisolone. Continue medication after surgery as previously described.
    d. Peracute immune-mediated or traumatic inflammation of uvea, retina and optic nerve. *Pulsed corticosteroid therapy* should be considered when an immediate response to treatment may be necessary to avoid irreversible complications in severe uveitis or presurgically in eyes with uveitis. Pulse therapy using suprapharmacologic doses followed by maintenance prednisolone dosage may provide immediate symptomatic relief but avoid the side effects seen with prolonged high dosage. Initial high dosage of corticosteroid is safe but repeated dosage may cause hemorrhage.

        Methylprednisolone sodium succinate (Solu-Medrol). The dosage recommended for acute spinal cord injuries and disk problems is 30 mg/kg IV; may repeat q6h for 24 hours. For ophthalmic emergencies, we use 5 to 20 mg/kg IV depending on severity of the disease with a second injection in 12 to 24 hours if needed.
2. Equine - prednisolone preferred over dexamethasone because of the problem seen with laminitis due to dexamethasone
    a. Prednisolone. Initial dosage (immunosuppressive) is 0.5 mg/lb per day up to two weeks. Maintenance dosage (anti-inflammatory) is 0.25 mg/lb per day up to three weeks.
    b. Dexamethasone 2 mg/ml administered IM only or dexamethasone sodium phosphate 4 mg/ml IV only. Dosage 5 mg/100 lbs (0.05 mg/lb).
3. Indications
    a. Blepharitis
    b. Episcleritis/scleritis
    c. Anterior uveitis
    d. Chorioretinitis
    e. Optic neuritis
    f. Orbital inflammation

PROGESTERONE-LIKE COMPOUNDS

Some progesterone-like compounds have anti-inflammatory activities that are beneficial when corticosteroids are contraindicated. No generally accepted explanation for the anti-inflammatory activity has been advanced. Indications are corticosteroid-responsive inflammation of the palpebral and bulbar conjunctiva, cornea and anterior segment of the globe.

Systemic - Megestrol acetate (Ovaban - Schering) is the most specific treatment of eosinophilic keratitis in cats. Owners should be advised that untoward actions can occur, i.e. personality changes (calming, antiandrogenic), diabetes mellitus, adrenocortical suppression, increased appetite, lethargy, depression, and mammary development (fibroadenomatous hyperplasia). Do not administer megestrol acetate to animals with suspected liver disease.

ANTIPROSTAGLANDINS (NONSTEROIDAL ANTI-INFLAMMATORY DRUGS - NSAID)

Prostaglandin is a major mediator of acute and chronic ocular inflammation. Prostaglandins have been shown to be mediators of certain kinds of intraocular inflammation. They produce disruption of the blood aqueous barrier, vasodilation, increased vascular permeability, leukocytosis and an initial increase in intraocular pressure followed by decreased intraocular pressure. They also play a role in the miotic response produced during intraocular surgery. Antiprostaglandins can be used singularly or in combination with corticosteroid therapy. They are especially indicated systemically to supplement topical or subconjunctival corticosteroids when systemic corticosteroids could cause problems.

Topical - Topical antiprostaglandins are indicated: 1) for intraoperative miosis, especially during cataract surgery; 2) when topical corticosteroids are contraindicated.

1. **Ocufen (flurbiprofen sodium, 0.03%).** In small animals it is useful as an adjunct to preoperative mydriatics for elective intraocular surgery. Recommended dosage: 1 drop every 30 minutes beginning two hours before surgery.
2. **Suprofen 1% (Profenal-Alcon).** Indicated for the inhibition of intraoperative miosis. Recommended dosage - on the day of surgery, two drops in the eye hourly for three hours before surgery.
3. **Voltaren (diclofenac, 0.1%).** Indicated for preoperative miosis, and postoperative prophylaxis and treatment of ocular inflammation.
4. **Indomethacin** - no commercial preparation in the USA. An ophthalmic solution can be made using Indomethacin powder for solution (#1-7378; 5, 10, 25 gm - Sigma). Prepare a 1 or 2% solution by diluting 150 to 300 mg of powder in 15 ml of artificial tears. Used two to four times daily in treatment of anterior uveitis and as a pre- and postcataract anti-inflammatory agent. Commercially available in Canada, Indocid ophthalmic suspension 1% (Merck & Co).
5. **Acular (Ketorolac 0.5% - Allergan)** - has been approved for allergic conjunctivitis

Systemic administration is the most frequent route for antiprostaglandins

Precautions. All antiprostaglandins except for Carprofen interfere with platelet aggregation and therefore increase bleeding time.
Do not use if gastric or intestinal ulcers exist. Bleeding is enhanced if used with prednisolone. Aspirin will have a synergistic action on gastrointestinal hemorrhage. Full dosage of prednisolone combined with a full dosage of either aspirin or Banamine can cause intraocular hemorrhage during intraocular surgery. If a full dosage combination is given for several days, fatal gastrointestinal hemorrhage can result. Banamine prior to cataract surgery predisposes to transient postoperative glaucoma.

1. **Flunixin meglumine (Banamine)** - indicated with acute diseases and is an excellent drug to control ocular pain in animals.
    a. Small animals - the dosage in small animals is 0.2 to 0.5 mg/kg (suggested dose 0.33 mg/kg) intravenously daily. Some veterinarians use a dosage as low as 0.1 mg/kg daily. Do not exceed five days in small animals. Intramuscular injection has delayed action and causes pain. It can be used as a premedication one to two hours prior to elective surgery to reduce postsurgical swelling and pain. When given at the time of surgery or postoperatively, there is good pain control but is less effective for controlling swelling.
    b. Equine - follow manufacturer's directions for dosage (1 mg/kg IV)
2. **Aspirin** - is indicated in chronic uveitis, episcleritis and chorioretinitis. Buffered aspirin is indicated in small animals that show digestive tract irritation to regular aspirin. Available in 1.25 and 5 grain tablets for small animals and 60 and 240 grain boluses or powder for horses. Aspirin powder applied on the grain is accepted better than crushing the boluses. When using powder, occasionally a sweet mix is needed for acceptance. One pound jars of powdered aspirin can be purchased from chemical supply houses. At CSU we order from Baxter Scientific.
    a. Dosage
        1) Dogs - 10 mg/kg BID (1.25 gr/15 lbs or 5 gr/60 lbs). Reduce dosage later if possible.
        2) Cats - 10 mg/kg q48h. Reduce to one-half dosage later if possible.
        3) Equine - 25 mg/kg (1.1 gm/100 lbs) BID. After one to two months, reduce to daily treatment. If daily dosage does not give desired effect increase daily to 35 mg/kg (1.3 gm/100 lbs) for a couple of weeks before returning to BID.
        4) Eleven grams of aspirin powder is a slightly rounded tablespoon; 13 gm is a rounded tablespoon, 15 gm is a heaping tablespoon.

3. **Butazolidin (phenylbutazone)** - recommended for horses. Butazolidin is not as effective for acute uveitis as Banamine but it can be quite effective in subacute cases, especially refractory cases after Banamine has been used for a maximum period.
   Dosage for adult horses - 2 gm BID PO or intravenously for subacute and acute ocular inflam-mation, up to two weeks; 1 gm BID for chronic inflammation
4. **Ketofen (ketoprofen 10% IV solution).** Indicated for inflammation and pain associated with musculoskeletal disorders in horses. Ocular effects have not been established. Proposed mechanism of action is inhibition of both cyclooxygenase (antiprostaglandin) and lipoxygenase (antileukotriene) arms of the arachidonic acid cascade.
5. **Carprofen (Rimadyl-Pfizer)** - Very good inhibition of uveitis flare. ***Unlike other antiprostaglandins, it does not affect bleeding.*** Adverse reactions are rare, the most common being hepatopathy. Labrador retrievers reported most frequently. Canine dosage is 1 mg/lb b.i.d.

ANTIHISTAMINES

Histamine release is an important factor in ocular and adnexal inflammation, allergic response, and the initial inflammatory reaction occurring with adnexal and intraocular surgery. For topical use, antihistamines are available individually or in combination with vasoconstrictors and/or decongestants.

Topical antihistamines

1. **Levocabastine HCl (Livostin-Ciba Vision) - 0.05% ophthalmic suspension.**
2. **Olopatadine HCl (Patanol-Alcon) - 0.1% ophthalmic solution.**

Topical antihistamine/decongestant combinations - The antihistamines used are pheniramine maleate and antazoline. The decongestants are phenylephrine HCl, naphazoline, and tetrahydrozoline. Artificial tear bases result in increased viscosity and thereby increased contact time. Some over-the-counter preparations are listed below (modified from Ophthalmic Drug Facts, Wolters Kluwer Company, St. Louis).

	Decongestant	**Antihistamine**	
Naphazoline HC1 & Pheniramine Maleate Solution (Various, e.g., Moore)	naphazoline HC1 0.025%	pheniramine maleate 0.3%	In 15 ml.
Naphazoline Plus Solution (Parmed)			In 15 ml.
Naphcon-A Solution (Alcon)			In 15 ml. Drop-Trainers
Opcon-A Solution (Bausch & Lomb)	naphazoline HC1 0.027%	pheniramine maleate 0.315%	In 15 ml.
Naphazoline HC1 & Anta-zoline Phosphate Solution (Various, e.g., Moore, Schein, Steris)	naphazoline HC1 0.05%	antazoline phosphate 0.5%	In 5 & 15 ml.
Vasocon-A Solution (Ciba Vision)			In 15 ml.

Systemic antihistamine

Systemic antihistamines are very useful premedications when administered 20 minutes prior to decompressing the eye during intraocular surgery (lens removal, iris surgery) and cyclocryosurgery for glaucoma. The clinical effect of antihistamine peaks 20 to 30 minutes after administration and then maintains significant blood levels for another hour. Injection should be repeated in surgery lasting more than two hours.

MAST CELL STABILIZERS

Mast cell stabilizers inhibit the degranulation of mast cells and, therefore, the release of histamine from these cells. The drug is relatively untested in veterinary medicine. There is limited clinical data in animals but in man it is very beneficial for controlling allergic keratoconjunctivitis, and is especially indicated when long-term treatment is needed.

1. Cromolyn sodium (Crolon-Bausch & Lomb) - 4% solution. Dosage: 1-2 drops 4-6 times daily.
2. Lodoxamide tromethamine (Alomide-Alcon) - 0.1% solution. Dosage: 1-2 drops q.i.d.

IMMUNOSUPPRESSIVE AGENTS

Immunosuppressive agents can be useful in some immune-mediated diseases that are not responsive to corticosteroids or in patients that are responding adversely to corticosteroids. Synergistic activity with corticosteroids may occur, thereby controlling a disease with reduced amounts of both drugs. In turn, this will reduce undesirable effects of both drugs.

Topical cyclosporine A

1. Sources
   a. Optimmune (0.2% cyclosporine ophthamlic ointment - Schering-Plough) - available for use in dogs.
   b. Formulation - 1-2% solution
      1) In hospital using Sandimmune (10% cyclosporine oral solution or capsules).
      2) Commercial pharmacy - by prescription to local pharmacy or veterinary pharmacy (e.g., Wedgewood Pharmacy).
      3) Cyclosporine will oxidize after it is exposed to air. Shelf life of oil suspension is 60 days.
   c. Formulation of 0.5% ointment - a 0.5% ointment can be prepared by liquefying ophthalmic ointment or U.S.P. petrolatum in a warm water bath, then adding the cyclosporine and placing this mixture in a 6 ml syringe for administration to the eye.
2. Pharmacology - cyclosporine is a strong immunosuppressive for which the exact mechanism of action is not known. Its primary use in man is prophylaxis of allogeneic organ transplants. Research suggests the effectiveness includes:
   a. Specific and reversible inhibition of immunocompetent lymphocytes
   b. T cells are preferentially inhibited
   c. It inhibits lymphokine production and release, including interleukin-2
3. Indications - Immune-mediated disorders of the adnexa and anterior segment of the eye. Very beneficial in keratoconjunctivitis sicca. We have had success treating punctate keratitis and German shepherd pannus, some cases of episcleritis and nodular granulomatous episclerokeratitis (NGE), and staphylococcus blepharitis. Other immune-mediated diseases with corneal vascularization should benefit but benefits are yet to be determined.
4. Contraindications - In active feline herpesvirus, keratoconjunctivitis may be exacerbated by topical cyclosporine or active infection may be prolonged.
5. Administration - Usual recommendation is one drop BID until improvement is noticed. Response usually noticed in three to four weeks. Maximum effect by eight weeks. As patient improves, dosage can be reduced to daily and possibly every other day. Treatment is continued as needed. Can be used concurrently with other medications.
6. Adverse reactions - No systemic reactions have been observed from topical use. Local reactions are occasional eyelid changes (redness and hair loss) and conjunctival irritation. This is probably due to vehicle irritation and can be controlled by discontinuing for two to three days and then using:
   a. Drops freshly prepared with castor oil
   b. Reducing frequency of administration to daily or QOD
   c. If 1% solution was used, reduce concentration to 0.5%

Azathioprine

1. Description - Azathioprine (Imuran - Burroughs Wellcome) is a derivative of mercaptopurine that has immunosuppressive characteristics. The mechanism for this action is obscure. The drug suppresses hypersensitivities of the cell-mediated type and causes variable alteration in antibody production. Azathioprine is a slow-acting drug and effects may persist for a week or more after the drug has been discontinued.
2. Indications - NGE, episcleritis and uveitis

3. Adverse reactions - The most common adverse reaction in man is hematologic suppression with leukopenia and anemia. This has rarely been observed by the author in dogs.

   In dogs, the most frequent observation has been gastrointestinal signs with vomiting, diarrhea, and/or depression occurring three to seven days after starting therapy. Liver enzymes are usually elevated, indicating hepatotoxicity. When the drug is stopped, the patient improves very rapidly. As soon as the patient returns to normal, Imuran can usually be reinstituted at one-half the dosage that produced toxicity. One dog was observed that was so hypersensitive that a therapeutic level of Imuran could not be established.

   A complete blood count and chemistry profile are recommended before starting therapy in older animals.
4. Dosage - initial dosage of Imuran is 0.5 to 1 mg/lb daily. As the lesion improves, reduce to the minimal dosage that will control the disease. This may be as little as 0.5 mg/lb every 7 to 10 days.
5. Synergistic with corticosteroid therapy. When used with prednisolone, alternate day therapy with both drugs at reduced maintenance levels is often successful.

CHEMICAL RESTRAINT AND ANESTHESIA

CHEMICAL RESTRAINT

May be necessary for minor ophthalmic procedures on patients and as a supplement to topical or local anesthesia. Especially useful in horses.

Horses - examination and minor surgical procedures

1. Chemical restraint with xylazine, detomidine and if necessary supplemented with butorphanol
2. Recommended dosages
   a. Xylazine 10% (Rompun - Miles Inc) - 0.5 to 1.0 mg/kg IV will generally give 30 minutes of restraint
   b. Detomidine 1% (Dormosedan - Smith Kline Beecham) - 10 to 40 μg/kg will give 45 minutes to one hour restraint
   c. Butorphanol 1% (Torbugesic - Fort Dodge) - 4 to 8 mg for an adult horse can be given and, if necessary, can be repeated. Because of its analgesic nature, using it in combination with either of the previous two drugs is very beneficial.
   d. A combination of 150 mg xylazine and 5 mg butorphanol will result in excellent restraint for the 900-1000 pound horse for 20 to 30 minutes. This can be repeated if needed.

Dogs

1. Tranquilizers cause protrusion of the third eyelid which complicates the examination
2. Oxymorphone 1.5 mg/ml (P/M Oxymorphone HCl - Mallinckrodt, Vet. Inc.) - 0.05-0.1 mg/lb IV or IM will sedate these animals and provide analgesia. Maximum dose 4.5 mg.
3. Propofol 1% (Diprivan - Zeneca Pharmaceuticals) - 10 mg/ml - ultrashort general anesthetic, 4-6 mg/kg to effect. Anesthesia lasts about five minutes. Good for short procedures; can be repeated if needed.
4. Butorphanol (Torbugesic, Torbutol) - 0.1 to 0.4 mg/kg
5. Combination of xylazine and oxymorphone. Premedicate with subcutaneous atropine and wait 10 to 15 minutes. Xylazine 0.6 mg/kg IV and oxymorphone 0.06 mg/kg IV. This can be reversed with yohimbine 5 mg and naloxone 400 μg subcutaneously.

TOPICAL ANESTHETIC AGENTS

Indications

1. To simplify examination and/or treatment
2. To differentiate superficial from deep pain

Precautions against indiscriminate use

1. May increase chances of further injury, especially if an adnexal foreign body is present
2. May cause sensitization with continued use
3. May be epithelial toxic or delay corneal epithelial healing with continuous administration

Application

1. Normal eyes - 2 to 3 applications 30 seconds apart are recommended. Corneal anesthesia begins in seconds but the conjunctiva takes longer. Anesthesia lasts 10 to 20 minutes.
2. Acute conjunctivitis - interferes with the efficiency of conjunctival anesthesia and shortens its duration. One or two additional applications are beneficial.
3. Topical anesthetic paralyzes smooth muscles that control conjunctival capillaries, thereby causing vascular injection that will be self-limiting when the anesthetic wears off.

Cocaine 1 to 4%

1. Rarely used because of corneal epithelial toxicity
2. Can be used for epithelial debridement

Proparacaine hydrochloride 0.5% (Alcaine, Ophthaine, Ophthetic)

Proparacaine is the most popular anesthetic. It will cause a transient corneal irregularity (roughening) that may make ophthalmoscopic examination difficult. This lasts 30 to 60 minutes. Therefore, do a screening ophthalmoscopic examination before putting it on the eye. After a bottle of proparacaine has been opened, it will deteriorate at room temperatures in several months resulting in brown discoloration. Discard when this color change occurs. Refrigeration will slow deterioration.

Tetracaine hydrochloride 0.5% (AK-T Caine, Pontocaine)

Tetracaine is less toxic to corneal epithelium than proparacaine but will cause tissue sensitization with repeated use.

Lidocaine 4% (Xylocaine)

Four percent ophthalmic lidocaine solutions are available in Canada and many other countries. 4% topical solution for oral mucous membranes and 2% solutions for injection can be used on the eye. Compared to proparacaine it is more irritating on first instillation and slower for conjunctival anesthesia. Lidocaine is stable when exposed to light and temperature extremes, making it a good choice for ambulatory services.

Topical anesthetic and fluorescein mixtures

1. Fluracain (Akorn)
2. Fluress (Pilkington, Barnes Hind)
3. Flurate (Bausch Lomb)
4. Flu-Oxinate (Pasadena)

INFILTRATION ANESTHESIA

Indications - infiltration anesthesia is injection of anesthesia into the area where surgery will be performed, such as:

1. Eyelid infiltration for tarsorrhaphy and minor surgery
2. Retrobulbar injection to augment general anesthesia
3. Multiple injections into a muscle cone and eyelid infiltration can be used for eye removal in cattle

Infiltration anesthetic agents - used at CSU

1. Lidocaine hydrochloride (Xylocaine) 2%, onset 4 to 6 minutes, duration 60 to 90 minutes (2 hrs with epinephrine)
2. Mepivacaine (Carbocaine) 2%, onset 3 to 5 minutes, duration 90 to 120 minutes

Local infiltration of eyelids for tarsorrhaphy (Fig 2-15)

Most frequently used in horses but can be done in small animals when general anesthesia is considered dangerous.

1. Starting 1 cm above the lateral canthus, pass a 23 or 25 gauge 2.5 inch spinal needle SQ to the nasal canthus, keeping 1 cm from the eyelid margin. These needles are flexible and can be guided to follow the curvature of the eyelid. If difficulty is experienced as the needle is passed nasally, inject a small bleb

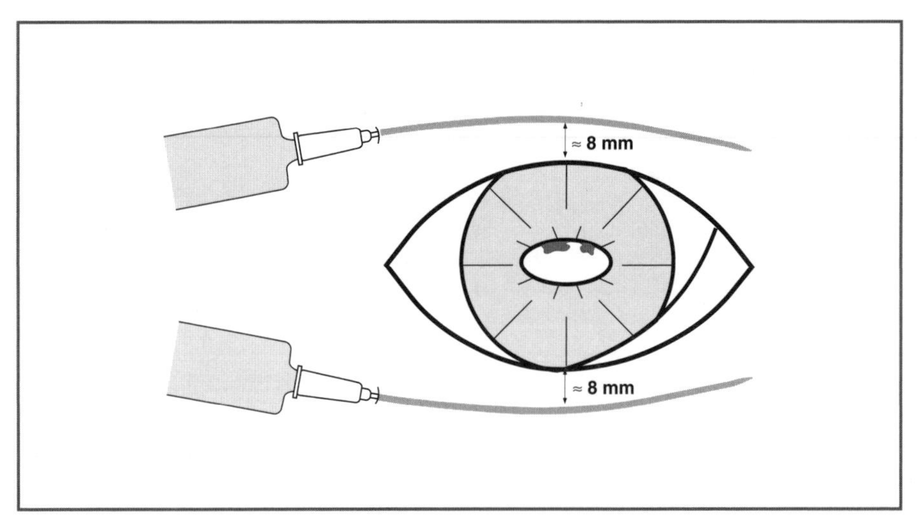

Figure 2-15. Local infiltration anesthesia, eyelids. Schematic of placement of 23 or 25 gauge spinal needles from the temporal canthus.

of anesthetic to facilitate advancement.

2. As the needle is withdrawn, inject 3 to 6 ml of anesthetic along the upper eyelid.
3. The lower eyelid is injected in the same manner.

Retrobulbar anesthesia

Retrobulbar anesthesia can be used as an adjunct to anesthesia in horses and dogs to reduce nystagmus and enophthalmos during corneal and intraocular surgery. When combined with eyelid infiltration it can be used for eye removal in cattle.

1. Dogs - rarely needed. Paralysis of the extrinsic muscles with systemic atracurium is preferred in patients under gas anesthesia and assisted ventilation.
   a. The author's preferred retrobulbar site is the notch caudal to the orbital ligament and above the zygomatic arch. A 20 gauge needle is directed medially and slightly downward into the retrobulbar tissues to a depth of 1 to 1.5 inches. 1 to 2 ml of anesthetic is injected.
   b. An alternate technique would be to enter the skin on a vertical line perpendicular to the lateral canthus, below the zygomatic arch and anterior to the coronoid process of the mandible. Direct the needle medially for a distance of 1 to 1.5 inches.
2. Horses - blocking individual muscles or a 4-point block can be helpful during anesthesia (Fig 2-16)
   a. Each quadrant of the muscle cone is injected with 5 to 10 ml of lidocaine through a 3 inch 20 gauge needle.
   b. The superior quadrant is injected by directing the needle through the center of the upper eyelid parallel to the globe.
   c. The temporal quadrant is injected by passing the needle through the temporal canthal skin following the globe posteriorly.
   d. The inferior quadrant is injected by passing the needle either through the lower eyelid or directly into the conjunctiva parallel to the globe. To avoid the optic nerve it is necessary to direct the needle slightly nasal.
   e. The nasal quadrant is injected by elevating the third eyelid and directing the needle through its base parallel to the globe.
   f. *Comment* - Failure to inject anesthetic into the muscle cone or injecting it in front of the orbital septum will cause the drug to migrate forward under the conjunctiva. The swollen conjunctiva will then limit corneal exposure.

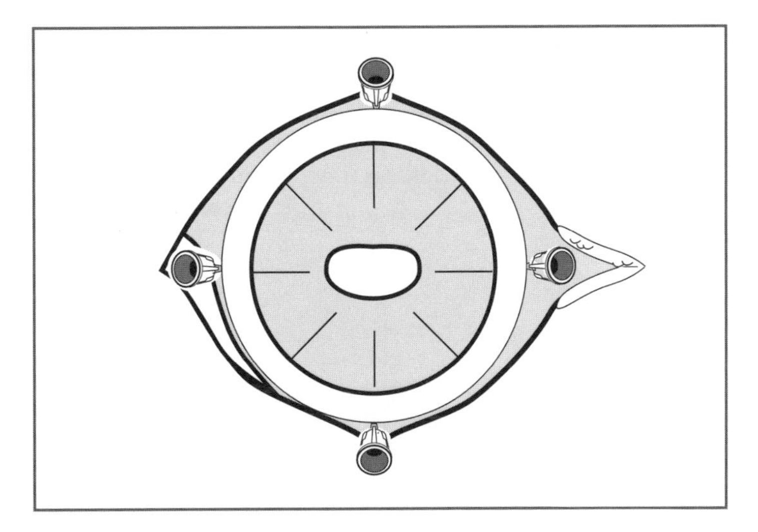

Figure 2-16. Four-point block for large animals. Needle positions for transconjunctival injection in an animal with a canthotomy. Transpalpebral injection can be used except at the nasal canthus.

REGIONAL ANESTHESIA - Blocking of a nerve trunk to a specific region. It is most frequently used in horses and cattle, and less frequently in the dog. With the advent of improved drugs for chemical restraint and analgesia, the necessity for regional blocks has been reduced. After completing a block, it is advisable to massage the site well to increase anesthetic penetration of the nerve. Motor nerves are harder to block than sensory.

Equine regional anesthesia - the auriculopalpebral branch of the facial nerve is motor to the orbicularis oculi. The frontal, zygomatic, lacrimal and infratrochlear branches of the trigeminal nerves are sensory.

1. Auriculopalpebral nerve block has been used for many years and results in paralysis of the orbicularis muscle of the upper eyelid and variable paralysis of the lower eyelid. It can be performed at three sites (Fig 2-17).
   a. Auriculopalpebral block - Using a 20 gauge 1 1/4 inch needle, infiltrate 5 ml of anesthetic subfascially in the depression just anterior to the base of the ear where the caudal border of the coronoid process of the mandible meets the zygomatic process of the temporal bone. At this point, the nerve emerges from the parotid salivary gland and becomes subcutaneous on the lateral aspect of the dorsal tip of the coronoid process.
   b. Palpebral branch at dorsal process of zygomatic arch - Palpate the most dorsal border of the zygomatic arch. Place a 22 gauge needle beneath the skin until it contacts bone and infiltrate 3 to 5 ml of anesthetic subfascially along the upper border.
   c. Palpebral branch over zygomatic arch near lateral canthus - The nerve can be palpated over the zygomatic arch posterior to the lateral canthus. Infiltrate 3 to 5 ml of anesthetic over the nerve with a 22 gauge needle.
2. Frontal (supraorbital) nerve block - This nerve is sensory to the upper eyelid. The supraorbital foramen is located in a depression where the supraorbital process widens medially. The depression is usually palpable. Two ml of anesthetic can be injected into the foramen in the depression and an additional 2 ml can be deposited subcutaneously over the area.
3. Zygomatic nerve block - This nerve can be blocked by injecting 2 ml of anesthesia along the ventral rim of the orbit below the temporal canthus.
4. Lacrimal nerve block - This nerve can be blocked by injecting 2 ml of anesthesia along the dorsal rim of the orbit medial to the lateral canthus.
5. Infratrochlear nerve block - This nerve can be blocked by palpating the notch in the dorsal rim of the orbit above the nasal canthus and injecting 2 to 3 ml of anesthesia deep and slightly rostrad to the notch.
6. *Comment* - To block all of these nerves would take much more time than eyelid infiltration, but if one is dealing with just one small area of the eyelid that is to be anesthetized, these individual blocks could be useful.

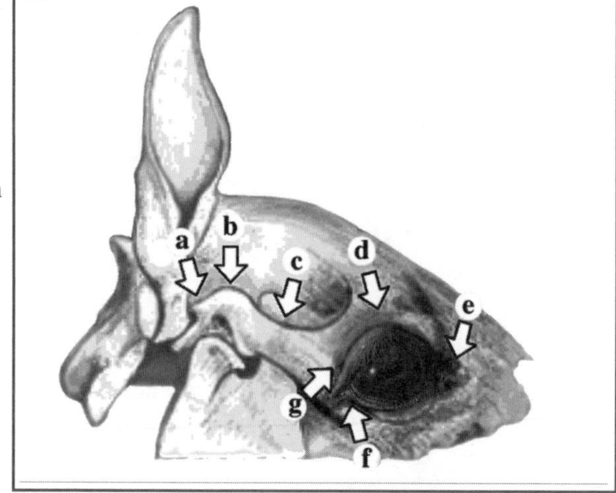

Figure 2-17. Sites for equine regional anesthesia blocks.
- a. Auriculopalpebral n.
- b. Palpebral n. over dorsal process zygomatic arch
- c. Palpebral n. over zygomatic arch near lateral canthus
- d. Frontal n.
- e. Infratrochlear n.
- f. Zygomatic n.
- g. Lacrimal n.

Small animal palpebral nerve block

The palpebral branch of the facial nerve is located in the subcutaneous fascia along the dorsal border of the caudal one-half of the zygomatic arch and is accompanied by the small artery and vein. The nerve is often palpable. The nerve can be blocked by injecting 1 to 2 cc of anesthetic with a 22 gauge needle in a line over the dorsal border of the caudal half of the zygomatic arch. If the nerve is palpable the injection is made at the spot where palpated (Fig 2-18).

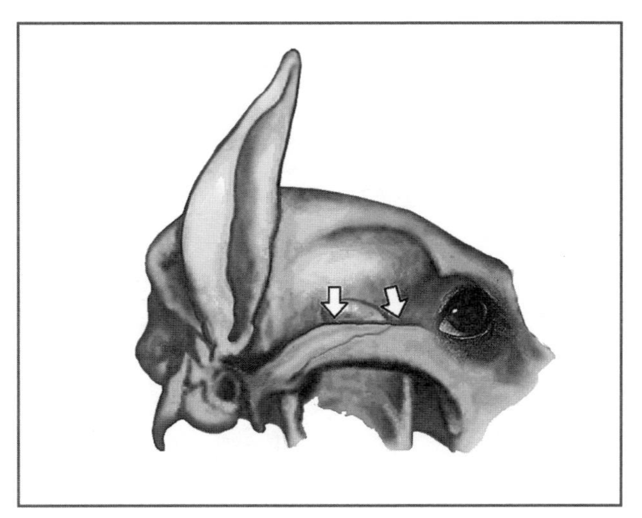

Figure 2-18. Canine palpebral nerve block. Choice of injection sites (arrows).

Peterson regional block - This block is designed specifically for cattle but has also been modified for the horse and the dog.

1. Bovine - In cattle the block anesthetizes the whole side of the head except for the tongue and the lower jaw and consists of two parts.
    a. With at least a 5 inch, 18 gauge needle, locate the V notch formed by the zygomatic arch and the supraorbital process of the malar bone just posterior to the lateral canthus of the eye. Then parallel to the frontal bone and perpendicular to the jaw, pass the needle straight into the coronoid process of the mandible. Walk the needle tip off the anterior edge of the mandible and pass it on to the deep site of the foramen orbitorotundum. Avoid hitting the pterygoid crest and infuse the large bundle of nerves with approximately 20 ml of anesthetic. Several motor nerves (abducens, trochlear, oculomotor) pass into this foramen with two branches of the trigeminal nerve (the maxillary and the ophthalmic), which are the main objectives of this block. They are sensory for the orbit, lower eyelid, upper lid, frontal area, horn, face, upper lip and teeth (everything except the lower jaw and tongue).
    b. The second part of the Peterson block passes the needle posterior along the zygomatic arch before the needle is withdrawn from the skin to block the auricular palpebral branch of the facial nerve at a palpable notch just anterior to the ear. This part of the block takes care of the motor innervation of the upper eyelid and facilitates surgery and orbit manipulation, especially in big bulls and adult cattle.
2. Similar regional blocks are described for the horse and dog.

PARASYMPATHOMIMETIC DRUGS (MIOTICS)

Miotics act at the myoneural junction, mimicking the effect of acetylcholine on parasympathomimetic postganglionic nerve endings in the eye. They constrict the pupil, cause contraction of the ciliary muscle that produces accommodation and opens the filtration angle, and increase the vascular permeability. They are used primarily to treat glaucoma but their miotic and pressure reducing effect decreases with chronic therapy (Table 2-7).

Table 2-7. Topical miotic agents

Cholinergics (direct acting)	**Trade Name**	**Percent**	**Duration of Miosis**
Carbachol	Carbacel Isopto Carbachol	0.75-3.0	~2 hours
Pilocarpine	Many	0.25-10	~4-8 hours
Anticholinesterases (indirect acting)			
Physostigmine	Many	0.25-0.5	~12-36 hours
Demecarium bromide	Generic/Wedgewood	0.125-0.25	~days
Echothiophate iodide	Phospholine iodide	0.03-0.25	~days
Isoflurophate (DFP)	Floropryl	0.025	~days

CHOLINERGIC MIOTICS - have direct acting effect on the muscarinic receptors of the eye

Pilocarpine

1. Uses
   a. Glaucoma therapy
      1) Topical 0.25% to 10% solutions (1% preferred); 1 drop q4-8h
      2) Pilopine-HS gel 4% gel. Extended contact hydrophilic gel. Reduces sensitization reactions. Apply daily in PM or BID.
   b. Lacrimator - oral and/or topical to stimulate lacrimation
   c. As a diagnostic agent in normotensive eyes with mydriasis
2. *Comment* - Immediate intraocular pain from spasm of iris and ciliary body muscle can occur in normal animals. Prolonged topical application may produce tissue sensitization, resulting in acute pain and redness. This is most likely to occur with concentrations of greater than 1%. Because of this tissue sensitization, topical solutions must be diluted or discontinued. Duration of miotic activity about 4 hours. Drops, especially when mixed with epinephrine 1% result in ***red*** discoloration of the tears.

Acetylcholine 1% (Miochol-E - Ciba Vision) - used intraocular during surgery, very effective. Duration of miotic activity 10 to 20 minutes. Follow with topical pilocarpine when surgery complete.

Carbachol

1. Topical 0.75-3.0% (Isopto Carbachol - Alcon) - used for glaucoma therapy. Administer 1 to 2 drops one to four times daily.
2. Intraocular 0.01% in 1.5 ml vials (Miostat-Alcon) - 0.25-0.5 ml used for miosis during surgery. Miosis maximal in 2 to 5 minutes. Longer lasting than Miochol-E.

CHOLINESTERASE INHIBITORS

Have an indirect effect by inhibiting enzymatic hydrolysis of acetylcholine at the nerve ending. Therefore there will not be any effect on denervated structures where there is not production of acetylcholine. The binding of cholinesterase may be reversible (short acting) or irreversible (long acting).

Physostigmine salicylate (Eserine) 0.25% and 0.5% (reversible) and duration of miotic activity about 4 hours. Short action limits use. May be used as a diagnostic agent in normotensive eyes with mydriasis.

Echothiophate (Phospholine iodide) 1/32%, 1/16%, 1/8%, or 1/4% ophthalmic solution (irreversible) - excellent in small animals. 1/16% is usually adequate given BID initially, then daily. Cataracts have been reported as toxic reaction with long term therapy in man, but not described in animals.

Demecarium (Generic/Wedgewood) 0.125% and 0.25% ophthalmic solution (irreversible) - fairly long acting, does not cause much iris congestion. Irritating in man but seldom causes discomfort in dogs.

Caution - Long acting cholinesterase inhibitors should be used with caution:

1. Use the lowest effective concentration
2. Monitor animals with flea collars
3. Cats are more sensitive to cumulative poisoning than dogs

MYDRIATICS

Are either parasympatholytics or sympathomimetics
Parasympatholytics paralyze the iris sphincter (mydriatic) and the ciliary body muscles (cycloplegic)
Sympathomimetics stimulate the iris dilator muscle (mydriatic)

PARASYMPATHOLYTIC (CYCLOPLEGIC) MYDRIATICS

Atropine

1. Forms available
   a. Topical ointments and drops, 0.5 to 4%
   b. Solutions for injection, 0.5, 2 and 15 mg/ml
2. Pharmacology
   a. Penetrates cornea and conjunctiva readily
   b. Blocks acetylcholine-innervated postganglionic cholinergic nerves
   c. Has special affinity for pigmented tissue of iris and ciliary body, resulting in prolonged mydriasis. It may take 10 to 14 days before the drug disappears from the eye in small animals, three weeks in horses.
3. Clinical indications to maintain long term cycloplegia and mydriasis
   a. Cycloplegia - reduces pain from ciliary spasm caused by corneal ulcers and anterior uveitis
   b. Mydriasis
      1) Control miosis of anterior uveitis
      2) Dilate pupil before and after intraocular surgery
      3) Facilitate vision with central corneal opacity and nuclear cataract
   c. Break down synechia - This is more effective if used in combination with phenylephrine
4. Administration
   a. Topical 1% solution or ointment - four times daily and then reduce to minimal frequency needed to control miosis. Prolonged frequent administration may lead to colic in horses as a result of systemic absorption.
   b. Subconjunctival injection - is usually limited to horses with severe uveitis or synechia. Injection of 1 to 2 mg will result in high uveal concentration without systemic effect. After the pupil is dilated, topical application one to three times daily should maintain mydriasis. Injection of an atropine-neosynephrine mixture (see phenylephrine discussion) will result in more rapid and profound mydriasis.

Homatropine HBr - 2% and 5% topical. may take three days before pupil returns to normal. Rarely used clinically. Indicated for short term therapy.

Scopolamine 0.3% topical

1. Topical - 4-7 days duration. May be combined with phenylephrine in difficult to dialte patients or for early synechia. Murocoll 2 (phenylephrine 10% and scopolamine 0.3% - Muro). These drops are irritating and it may be preferred to use a topical anesthetic prior to the Murocoll 2 if the eye is painful.
2. Parenteral - 1/200 grain subcutaneously as a preanesthetic instead of atropine will give profound mydriasis in the average size dog.

Cyclopentolate (Cyclogyl) - 0.5%, and 1%. Onset .5 to 1 hour; lasts one day. Used for ophthalmic examinations and short term therapy such as minor injuries.

Tropicamide (Mydriacyl/generic available) 0.5 to 0.1% - maximum effect in 20 minutes. Completely gone in four to six hours. This is the best dilating agent available for examination. 1.0% is the preferred strength to use.

MYDRIATIC FOR BIRDS

Suggested reading: Mikaelian I, Paillet I, Williams D. Comparative use of various mydriatic drugs in kestrels. Am J Vet Res 1994;55:270-272 and Ramer JC et al. Effects of mydriatic agents in cockatoos, African gray parrots, and blue fronted Amazon parrots. J Am Med Assoc 1996;208:227-230.

Topical vecuronium bromide - a curare-like neuromuscular blocking agent

1. Kestrels - two to three drops of 4 mg/ml three times at 15 minute intervals produces mydriasis in 30 minutes, maximal at 60 minutes and lasting four hours. No side effects were noted.
2. Cockatoos, African gray parrots, and blue fronted Amazon parrots - 2 drops of 0.8 mg/ml is an effective mydriatic. Side effects from adsoption were observed, therefore caution should be used when applying vecuronium bilaterally.

Intracameral - pancuronium and atracurium have been used. Administer 10% of systemic dose.

SYMPATHOMIMETIC DRUGS

These drugs may be direct acting (phenylephrine, epinephrine) or indirect acting (hydroxyamphetamine).

Phenylephrine

1. Topical preparations
   a. Topical vasoconstrictor, 0.125% - to constrict conjunctival blood vessels. Often incorporated in ophthalmic drops prescribed for simple and allergic conjunctivitis.
   b. Mydriatic for examination in dogs, 2.5 to 10% (AK-Dilate, Mydfrin, Neo-Synephrine). Dilation in 10 to 60 minutes, recovery in three hours. May be used as an adjunct to tropicamide in dogs(especially puppies) that are hard to dilate. 10% solution is irritating. Combination available: Murocoll 2 (10% phenylephrine and 0.3% scopolamine - Muro). Dilation may last 3 to 7 days.
   c. Diagnostic agent
      1) Location of lesion in Horner's syndrome. 1% used in man, results in mydriasis with postganglionic Horner's syndrome. 2.5% suggested for dogs.
      2) As vasoconstrictor to differentiate superficial (conjunctival) from deep (episcleral) blood vessels
2. Subconjunctival injection in horses - Phenylephrine 1% solution for injection when combined with atropine for injection is synergistic
   a. Preparation - using a 1 cc syringe add 1 mg atropine for injection to 5 mg neosynephrine
   b. Injection - depending on the severity of miosis or duration of the synechia, inject 1/2 or all of the mixture
   c. Onset of mydriasis - begins in 15 minutes and maximal one hour

Hydroxyamphetamine HBr 1% (Paredrine - Pharmics Inc.)

Indirect-acting adrenergic agonist. Causes release of norepinephrine from postganglionic adrenergic nerve terminals. Mydriatic activity compares to 2.5% phenylephrine. Maximum dilation in 45 to 60 minutes, lasts 4 to 6 hours. Will not dialte a pupil with postganglionic Horner's syndrome.

Epinephrine

1. Topical - a weak mydriatic
   a. Epinephrine 0.5 to 2% topical solution (Epitrate, Epinal, Eppy/N, Epifrin, Glaucon)
      1) Open angle glaucoma
      2) Control hemorrhage from debulked eyelid tumors after cryosurgery

3) Diagnostic to differentiate superficial from deep vascular injection. Within 15 to 30 seconds after a drop of epinephrine, superficial (conjunctival) blood vessels will be constricted while deep (episcleral) will be slightly affected or unchanged.

b. Sterile epinephrine diluted to 1:10,000. To control hemorrhage during conjunctival and corneal surgery.

c. Diagnostic agent in Horner's syndrome

2. Intraocular - to dilate the pupil and reduce hemorrhage from the anterior uvea during surgery.
   a. Preparations available for preparing sterile 1:10,000 to 1:20,000 dilution for intraocular use
      1) Preparations with preservatives, e.g. epinephrine for injection 1:1,000 or Eppy/N topical solution 1%
      2) Sterile preservative-free epinephrine USP 1:1000 (American Reagent Laboratories)
      3) *Comment* - Preparing dilute epinephrine with products containing preservatives has a transient detrimental effect to the corneal epithelium and will result in temporary corneal edema. The surgeon must decide whether the temporary corneal change is more serious to the patient than the hemorrhage or the miotic pupil the epinephrine will control. By using preservative-free epinephrine, this complication can be avoided.
      4) Precaution - Ventricular fibrillation may result from intraocular epinephrine. Concentrations stronger than 1:10,000 can be tolerated in dogs but are dangerous in the equine. This danger is greatest with Fluothane (halothane) anesthesia.
3. Subconjunctival - subconjunctival 1:10,000 epinephrine can be used in adnexal surgery to control hemorrhage

Dipivefrin (Propine - Allergan) 0.1%

1. Pharmacology - Propine is a prodrug of epinephrine that requires biotransformation to epinephrine before therapeutic activity occurs. It has enhanced absorption and therefore a lessened concentration (0.1%) has a pharmacodynamic effect on the anterior uvea greater than 1% epinephrine drops. The duration is longer and fewer side effects occur. There is minimal mydriasis.
2. Indications - open angle glaucoma
3. Dosage - 1 drop BID
4. *Comment* - used as an adjuvant with other drugs in the medical management of glaucoma

BETA ADRENERGIC BLOCKING AGENTS (ALPHA 2 ADRENERGIC ANTAGONISTS)

Pharmacology - These medications work by blocking beta-2 adrenergic sites, decreasing aqueous production (as much as 50% in man) and, thereby decreasing intraocular pressure. Unfortunately, they are less effective and require higher concentration in dogs and cats. Slight pupillary constriction occurs in the treated eye in dogs and cats, and even the untreated eye in dogs. Systemic absorption may result in respiratory and cardiovascular complications.

Products available

1. Timolol maleate 0.25 and 0.5% (Timoptic - Merck & Co)
2. Levobunolol 0.25 and 0.5% (Betagan - Allergan)
3. Betaxolol 0.25% (Betoptic - Alcon)
4. Carteolol hydrochloride 1% (Ocupress-Otsuka)
5. Metipranolol 0.3% (Opti Pranolol-Bausch & Lomb)

Dosage - 1 drop BID

Comment - These drugs, if used alone, are probably not adequate to treat glaucoma but when used in combination with others have a synergistic effect.

PILOCARPINE-EPINEPHRINE COMBINATIONS

Pharmacology - Pilocarpine by enhancing outflow, and epinephrine by reducing production and increasing aqueous clearance values are synergistic and will lower pressure more effectively than the individual drugs.

Combinations available

1. Pilocarpine 2%-epinephrine 1% (P_2E_1) - this has been the most effective combination
2. Pilocarpine 1%-epinephrine 1/2% ($P_1E_{1/2}$) is indicated if sensitivity develops to P_2E_1.

Frequency of administration - QID

Red discoloration of the tears and staining of facial hair is common. The owner may believe the stain is blood.

Comment - Combinations of these drugs were popular in human glaucoma treatment but are now being replaced by the beta blocking agents. Because of this, they are less available.

CARBONIC ANHYDRASE INHIBITORS

Carbonic anhydrase inhibitors are nonbacteriostatic sulfonamides and are indicated in the medical management of glaucoma. They are poor diuretics and have been replaced for that purpose by superior diuretics (e.g. furosemide). Furosemide is NOT a carbonic anhydrase inhibitor, therefore does not affect intraocular pressure. Dosage and frequency of administration must be monitored carefully because they will produce electrolyte disturbances resulting in metabolic acidosis, panting, vomiting, diarrhea, anorexia and hypokalemia. As a general rule, if the patient has a two to three hour period beyond the duration of drug effect, electrolyte balance will be re-established and adverse side effects can be reduced. For this reason, BID treatment is preferred to TID for extended treatment.

$$H_2O + CO_2 \underset{}{\overset{\text{Carbonic anhydrase}}{\rightleftharpoons}} H_2CO_3 \rightleftharpoons H^+ + CO_3^-$$

MECHANISM OF ACTION ON AQUEOUS PRODUCTION

About 40 to 60% of the aqueous secretion is related to carbonic anhydrase activity in the ciliary body epithelium. The exact mechanism as to their effect on formation of aqueous is not known.

It has been proposed that the bicarbonate (HCO_3) thus formed combines with sodium and other cations and moves into the posterior chamber carrying water with it, thus producing aqueous. The H^+ ion returns to the ciliary circulation.

DRUGS AVAILABLE

When prescribing carbonic anhydrase inhibitors, the dosage should be titered to the minimal amount necessary to maintain the desired intraocular pressure.

Acetazolamide (Diamox) 125-500 mg tablets, 500 mg time released spansules, and 500 mg parenteral vials

1. Dosage - 10 mg/kg BID or TID
2. Acetazolamide is a poor choice for continuous therapy because it can cause electrolyte disturbance and nausea in 24 hours

Dichlorphenamide (Daranide) 50 mg tablets

1. Dosage - 2.5 mg/kg BID or TID
2. Fewer side effects than acetazolamide. This is the preferred carbonic anhydrase inhibitor by many veterinarians.

Methazolamide (Neptazane) 50 mg tablets

1. Dosage - 5 mg/kg BID or TID
2. Dosage can be exceeded without adverse effect. Therefore, well suited for cats and small dogs (less than 40 pounds).

Dorzolamide HCl (Truspot - Merck) - 2% ophthalmic solution.
Maximum effect up to 5 hrs. When used with other topical medicines it definitely prolongs the efficacy of conservative management.

1. Dosage: 1 drop TID in affected eye(s). Can be used concomitantly with other topical medications. Allow 10 min between medications.
2. Concomitant administration with oral carbonic anhydrase inhibitors is not recommended.

Brinzolamide (Azopt-Alcon) - 1% ophthalmic solution

1. Dosage - 1 drop TID to the affected eye(s). Can be used concurrently with other topical drugs.
2. In man, less discomfort upon instillation than dorzolamide.
3. Concurrent administration with oral carbonic anhydrase inhibitors is not recommended.

CARBONIC ANHYDRASE INHIBITOR/BETA-ADRENERGIC BLOCKING AGENT

Dorzolamide hydrochloride - Timolol maleate (Cosopt-Merck) - 2% dorzolamide, 0.5% timolol.

1. Dosage - 1 drop in affected eye BID.
2. If used with another topical drug, administer 10 minutes apart.

PROSTAGLANDINS

Lantanoprost (Xalatan-Upjohn) - 0.005% ophthalmic solution

1. Pharmacology - prostaglandins $F_2\alpha$ analogue that reduces intraocular pressure by increasing scleral outflow. It absorbs quickly into the cornea and is released slowly into the aqueous. It is effective in dogs and should be in horses. No pressure change occurs in normal cats. Miosis occurs in dogs and cats. Maximum response in 6 hrs. Some effect up to 4 days in normal dogs. Use in acute inflammation is discouraged.
2. Dose: 1 drop daily BID
3. Most effective in treating primary glaucoma and post-surgical ocular pressure increases following lens phacoemulsification.

SYSTEMIC OSMOTIC AGENTS

Systemic osmotic agents reduce intraocular pressure by reducing aqueous ultrafiltration and drawing fluid directly from the eye (aqueous and vitreous). Their osmotic effect is diminished in inflamed eyes because of reduction of the blood aqueous and blood vitreous barriers. Water should be withheld for two to four hours because rehydration will reduce osmotic activity. These agents are most effective at decreasing the IOP on the first administration. If the IOP does not decrease after the second dose, consider alternative treatments.

INDICATIONS

Glaucoma - the most frequent indication

1. Acute high pressure glaucoma
2. Chronic glaucoma not responding to topical medications and/or carbonic anhydrase therapy
3. Glaucoma secondary to hyphema

Retinal edema - with impending or beginning detachment

Cataract surgery - as a premedication for open sky techniques to avoid vitreous presentation. Not indicated as a premedication in phacofragmentation.

Perforating corneal injuries - with vitreous swelling leading to collapse of the anterior chamber

AGENTS MOST FREQUENTLY USED

Mannitol - 15 to 25% IV solutions. Mannitol is not absorbed orally.

1. Osmotic of choice for initial acute glaucoma therapy
2. Dosage - 1 to 2 gm/kg IV over 10 to 20 minute period
3. Onset - 30 to 60 minutes, depending on rate of infusion
4. Duration - 6 hours; can be repeated
5. 20% solution will precipitate when cold; warm in hot water bath if crystals are present
6. 50 ml bottles from generic sources (25% mannitol - Lyphomed); convenient and economical

Glycerol (Glycerin USP/Glyrol 75%, Osmoglyn 50% - Alcon). Glycerin is tasteless and viscous. Glyrol and Osmoglyn are flavored. Metabolized into glucose.

1. Not as effective as mannitol - good drug for home therapy or short term maintenance
2. Dosage - 1 to 2 cc/kg oral BID or TID
3. Onset in 10 to 30 minutes. Duration 4 to 5 hours. Can be repeated.
4. Limited value after 5 to 7 days continuous therapy
5. If vomiting occurs, dilute 50/50 with skim milk

Isosorbide (Ismotic 45%, Alcon). It is not metabolized and would be an alternative to glycerin.

1. Dosage - 1.5 gm/kg oral
2. Onset 30 minutes, duration 5 to 6 hours

Comment - Mannitol is drug of choice for immediate effect. Oral glycerin best for continued administration.

Sodium ascorbate - IV 1 to 2 gm/kg for immediate effect. This osmotic is not confined to the vascular compartment and is less effective than mannitol, especially in the presence of anterior uveitis.

CORNEAL DEHYDRATING AGENTS

Topical hypertonic (hyperosmolar) solutions and ointments osmotically attract water through corneal epithelium or exposed stroma. They are applied to reduce corneal edema for diagnostic and therapeutic purposes.

DIAGNOSTIC PROCEDURES

Glycerin assists ocular examination by reducing corneal edema. Topical anesthesia may be indicated to reduce irritation from glycerin drops.

USP Glycerin

Ophthalgan (Wyeth-Ayerst) - sterile glycerin solution

THERAPEUTIC PREPARATIONS

Indications

1. Reduce corneal edema and bullae development due to corneal endothelial disease. This is especially beneficial in horses.
2. An adjunct in the treatment of refractory and recurrent corneal ulcers with concurrent stromal edema near the regenerating epithelium. The beneficial effect on ulcer healing is not fully understood. Even when ointments are used, the tears return to normal osmolality in minutes.

Preparations

1. Hypertonic salt preparations
    a. 2-5% sodium chloride solutions (AK-NaCL - Akorn; Adsorbonac - Alcon; Muro 128 solution - Bausch & Lomb)
    b. 5% sodium chloride ointment. The author's first choice. Usually the least irritating hypertonic preparation.
2. Glucose 40% ointment (IOLAB Corp)

CAUTERIZING AGENTS AND INSTRUMENTS

Chemical and thermal cautery are used.

CHEMICAL CAUTERIZATION

Severe - Dangerous to use because precise depth of activity is difficult to control

1. Liquid phenol (carbolic acid) - acid precipitates corneal protein and is therefore self-limiting. The preferred choice of severe cauterizing agents.
2. Trichloracetic acid
3. Lunar caustic (silver nitrate sticks) - a strong base and must be neutralized with NaCl to precipitate the silver as silver chloride. If this is not neutralized, it will continue to react with the cornea until there is the possibility of irreversible damage. Silver chloride may precipitate in the cornea as a permanent black residue. This is the most dangerous cauterizing agent.
4. Tincture of iodine 7% - seldom used on eyes now, but popular many years ago

Mild

1. Iodine preparations
   a. Tincture of iodine 3.5% - alcohol in tincture is very irritating
   b. Air-dried tincture of iodine on a cotton applicator can be used to cauterize superficial indolent ulcers.
   c. Lugol's solution - this is the only form of inorganic iodine that should be used on the unanesthetized eye.
2. Copper sulfate crystals (cupric sulfate is a clear blue crystal) - large clear crystals can be used to scrape lymph follicles from the inner surface of the third eyelid. Be careful not to excessively cauterize or leave bits of the crystal in the tissues. Either will result in an extremely severe conjunctivitis and serious corneal damage.
3. Dilute silver nitrate solution on a cotton applicator. Then neutralize with physiologic saline solution.

Comment - Chemical cauterization is sometimes used to remove proliferative lesions from the adnexa and cornea.

HEAT CAUTERIZATION

Type

1. Disposable ophthalmic cautery - two types are available; one for coagulation (1350°) and the other for cutting (2200°F). Concept - disposable cauteries, boxes of 10. Vetroson pocket cauteries (Summit Hill Labs) use replaceable AA batteries.
2. Change-A-Tip cautery kit (MDS)
3. Electrocautery units - many are available

Uses

1. Very useful to control hemorrhage by coagulation
2. Treat surgical site after tumor removal
3. To treat blood vessels entering the cornea from the limbus (peritomy). These blood vessels will return if the stimulus that caused the vessel to enter the cornea persists. If the initial stimulus has disappeared, the blood vessel will not return.
4. To treat glaucoma
5. Making incisions in conjunctiva, sclera and iris

HYPERTHERMIA

Hyperthermia is moderate heating of tissue compared to the searing heat of cautery.

TYPES OF HYPERTHERMIA

Whole body

Regional - involves a large mass such as the liver

Localized - only type of hyperthermia readily available to the practitioner

INSTRUMENTATION - localized hyperthermia **(Fig 2-19)**

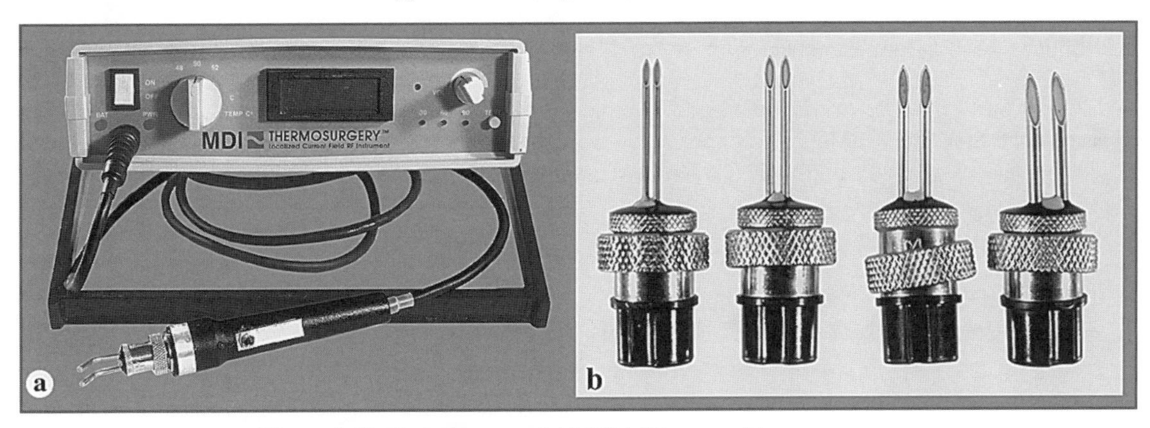

Figure 2-19. Hypertherm model MV04 (Thermotech).
a. Hyperthermia unit with surface probes on handle
b. Four penetrating probes

Local field hyperthermia units produce a radiofrequency (rF) current that passes through tissue between electrode tips developing a localized current field (LCF) that results in hyperthermia of the tissue between the probes. A thermistor in the probe senses the tissue temperature and when the selected temperature is reached, a modulator reduces the rF current to maintain the temperature and a timer is activated. A time and temperature relationship of 50 ± 1°C for 30 seconds is the desired temperature. Higher temperatures (55°C) result in cautery that kills both normal and abnormal cells. Hyperthermia is more selective, resulting in death of tumor cells with minimal damage to normal cells. Surface and penetrating probes are available depending on the tissue to be treated. Heating occurs between the probes and to a distance of 3 to 4 mm from the probe (Fig 2-20).

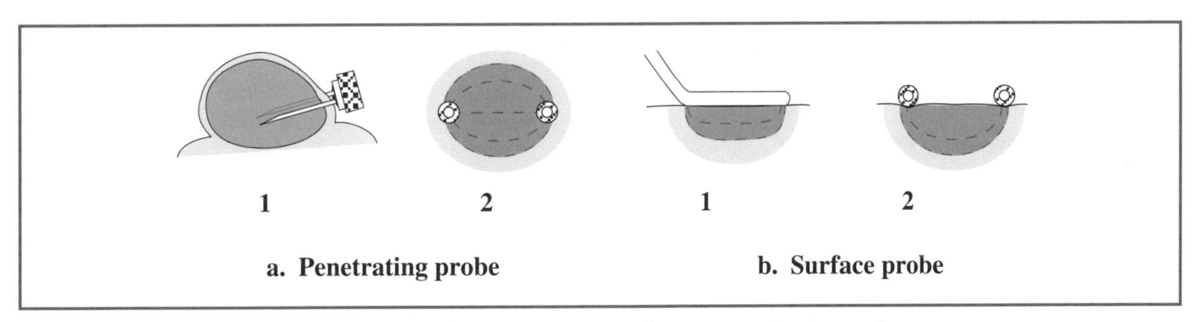

Figure 2-20. Schematic demonstrating tissue response according to type of probe used.
a. Penetrating probe
   1. Penetrating probe in tumor
   2. Transverse view illustrating current flow (broken lines) and area of tissue heated by current (shaded area)
b. Surface probe
   1. Lateral view showing depth of tissue heating
   2. Cross section view representing current flow (broken lines) and heated area (shaded area)

TREATMENT PROTOCOL

Site preparation - clip hair and apply topical antiseptic

Biopsy - if tumor type has not been identified

Anesthesia - local anesthesia with adequate restraint, or general, depending on location of the lesion and species

Probe choice - depends on the size and location of the lesion

1. Superficial lesion - surface probe for lesions less than 4 mm thick or after debulking larger lesion
2. Deep lesions - combination of surface and penetrating probes

Technique - treat the entire lesion twice

1. Thin lesions - multiple overlapping surface applications covering the lesion. Second application applied across the first treatment in a grid pattern.
2. Larger lesions - a grid pattern with surface and piercing probes is helpful to ensure adequate treatment

Reevaluation

1. Recheck in three to four weeks
2. Multiple treatments may be needed

Comment. Comparison of hyperthermia to cryothermia.

Advantages	**Disadvantages**
Portable	Large lesions time consuming
Simple technique	Limited access to deep lesions
Few adverse effects	Possibility of multiple treatments

CRYOTHERMIA

Cryothermia is subjecting a cell system to subfreezing temperatures that remove available water and biotransfer it into ice crystals.

PATHOPHYSIOLOGY

Direct cellular death - This occurs in the first few minutes after freezing and results from ice crystal disruption of cell membranes, electrolyte changes, alteration of cellular proteins and thermal shock.

Vascular collapse - Small blood vessels, particularly capillaries, are irreversibly damaged, leading to hypoxia and infarction.

Factors affecting cell death

1. Fast freeze-slow thaw
2. The number of freezes - two minimum; three for large or malignant tumors
3. Minimum temperature necessary at the edge of the lesion. When possible, thermocouple needles should be placed at the periphery of the lesion.
   a. -20°C for cryosensitive tissues (tarsal glands)
   b. -25°C most neoplasms
   c. -30°C for squamous cell carcinoma in all species
4. Approximately 70 to 80% of the frozen tissue will slough

EQUIPMENT

Liquid nitrogen (N_2) - 196°C, cost $800 and up **(Fig 2-21)**

1. Advantages
   a. Most effective (coldest)
   b. Best for large tumors
   c. Rapid freeze
   d. Variable methods of application (spray, probe)

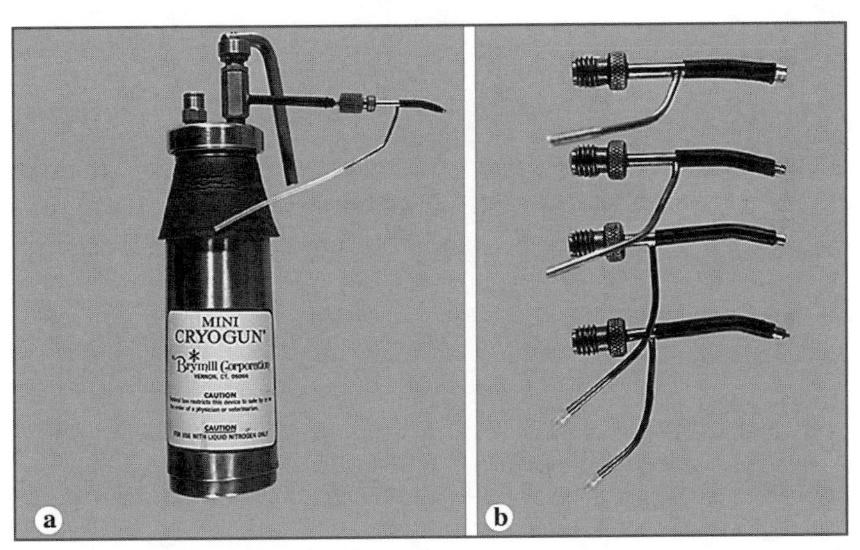

Figure 2-21. Mini Cryogun® (Brymill) liquid nitrogen unit and ophthalmology probes.
a. Mini Cryogun® unit
b. Ophthalmology probes (general surgery probes and spray aperatures not shown)

2. Disadvantages
    a. Short shelf life for cryogen
    b. ***Run-off*** at spray site can be ***dangerous*** to normal tissues

Nitrous oxide (N_2O) - 89°C, cost $1500 and up **(Fig 2-22)**

1. Advantages
    a. Long shelf life
    b. Variety of probes available
    c. Immediate defrost of probe if it inadvertently contacts adjacent tissue
2. Disadvantages
    a. Slower freeze
    b. Limited to smaller lesions
    c. Immediate defrosting of probe results in rapid thaw if hemostatic clamps are not used

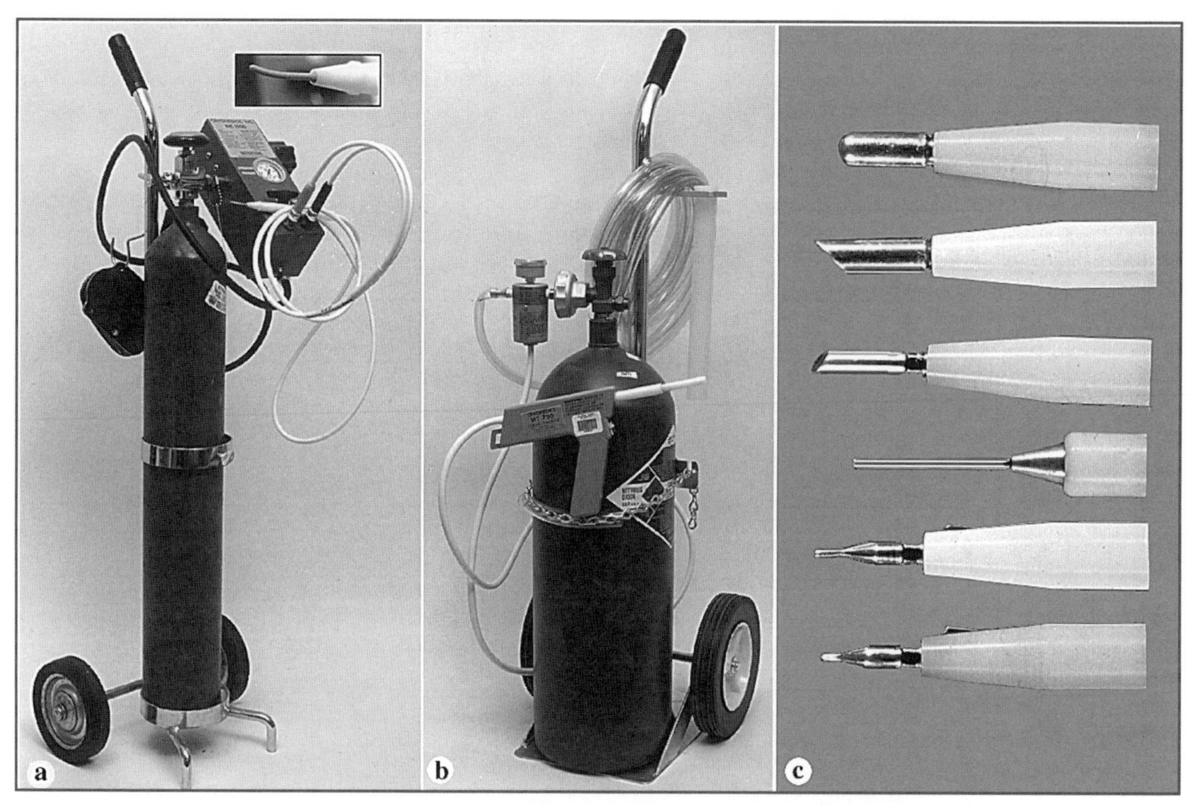

Figure 2-22. Nitrous oxide cryosurgery units.
a. Cryomedics MC 1000 (Cabot) with lens tip (inset)
b. Cryomedics MT750 with scavenger system
c. Tips adaptable to ophthalmology

TECHNIQUE

Site preparation - clip hair and apply topical antiseptic

Anesthesia - local with adequate restraint, or general, depending on the lesion location and species

Biopsy - before freezing

Freezing - debulking and freezing margins is usually preferred

1. Probes
   a. Size should approximate size of lesion
   b. Can be used in cavities
   c. Liquid nitrogen probes defrost slowly, leading to a slow thaw. Therefore, tap water or physiologic salt solution should always be available when using liquid nitrogen to defrost a probe that inadvertently contacts adjacent tissues. Nitrous oxide probes defrost immediately.
   d. Probes will adhere better to moist tissues
2. Spray
   a. Faster freeze, but also faster thaw
   b. Easier to apply to nonspherical lesions

INDICATIONS

Neoplasia

Corneal vascularization

Proliferative tissues

Cysts - after incision and draining

Epilation - distichiasis/trichiasis

Glaucoma - transcleral freezing of the ciliary body

Luxated lens - removal of lens with small cryoprobe that adheres to the lens

TISSUE RESPONSE

Mild postfreezing discomfort and absent in 12 hours. The tissues darken and may bleed slightly until they scab over in a few days.

Scab falls off in 10 to 20 days

Depigmentation of skin - healed skin lesions will be pink in two weeks and slowly repigment in three to six months

White hair - will be a permanent change

Minimal scarring and deformity

ANTINEOPLASTIC AGENTS

Antineoplastic drugs used in general oncology are also indicated in ophthalmic oncology.

CYCLOPHOSPHAMIDE (Cytoxan) - Cyclophosphamide is antineoplastic and immunosuppressive. It can be used individually or in combination with other drugs.

Indications

1. Adnexal tumors - especially histiocytomas
2. Ocular changes associated with malignant lymphoma

Dosage - 1 to 2 mg/kg daily, then reduce to QOD as lesions improve. Maintenance dosage will depend on disease treated.

Precautions - monitor WBC after five days. Medication must be altered with severe leukopenia.

CISPLATIN

Cisplatin is an inorganic heavy metal complex that has properties similar to alkylating agents by producing interstrand and intrastrand crosslinks in DNA. It can be used systemically and intratumorally. Expensive.

Indications in horses (Theon A, et al. Intratumoral chemotherapy with cisplatin in oily emulsion in horses. J Am Vet Med Assoc 1993;202:261-265)

1. Intratumoral - as an alternate to other modalities in the treatment of adnexal tumors
2. Equine sarcoid and squamous cell carcinoma - excellent sensitivity response
3. Can be used independently or in combination with surgical removal.

Preparation - prepare a 2 mg/ml water-oil emulsion

1. Dissolve 10 mg cisplatin in 2 ml sterile distilled water
2. Emulsify with 3 cc sterile sesame oil (can be autoclaved) by mixing between two sterile syringes using a three-way stopcock.

Injection technique

1. Chemical restraint or general anesthesia is recommended
2. Disinfect injection site with 1:50 Betadine saline solution
3. Inject the tumor with a dosage of 0.5 ml (1 mg) cisplatin emulsion per cm^3 of tumor
4. Multiple injections are made as the needle is withdrawn and continued until mixture exudes, ensuring saturation of the tumor. Parallel or crossing patterns can be used. Injections should extend 1 cm beyond lesion margins.
5. Bandage the lesion

Precautions - Extreme effort should be taken to prevent contamination of personnel, equipment or the patient. Follow directions on the physician's package insert.

1. Disposable gloves should be worn
2. Cisplatin leakage should be wiped clean immediately and materials disposed of in a sealed plastic bag

Aftercare

1. Systemic antibiotic and tetanus booster is recommended
2. Change the bandage in 24 and 48 hours (wear gloves and dispose of bandage in a sealed plastic bag)

Reinjection

1. A series of four injections two weeks apart is recommended. Reinjection can be delayed if there is severe tissue reaction.
2. If the tumor recurs, injections can be repeated.

VINCRISTINE SULFATE

Indications - angiosarcomas

1. The author has had limited success in treating ocular and/or adnexal angiosarcomas in horses.
2. Consult with an oncologist before prescribing this drug.

Dosage

1. 0.5 to 0.75 mg/m^2 body surface. For a 1000 pound horse, 0.75 mg/m^2 would be 2.6 mg administered IV.
2. Repeat weekly 8-10 weeks. When effective, improvement begins in about one month.

Precautions

1. Colic and neurotoxicity has been reported after administration.
2. Extremely toxic to tissues. ***Use a catheter.*** Even when a catheter is used, vasculitis may occur.

CIMETIDINE (Tagamet - Smith Kline and French)

Description - Cimetidine is a histamine H_2-receptor antagonist. During recent years it has been recognized as a biologic response modifier with antitumor properties effective in treating some tumors, including melanoma in horses and dogs.

Mechanism of action - Unknown. It may be beneficial by inhibiting suppressor T cells which could enhance contrasuppressor T cell antitumor influence on macrophage function.

Horses - In horses it may manifest its optimum effect after three to four months of treatment. Tumors disappear or regress and become static.

Dogs - The author has used cimetidine therapy on a dog with severe multiple melanoma of all eyelids and the muzzle. The lesions were so severe that surgical removal or cryotherapy would have resulted in severe eyelid and muzzle deformity. After four months the larger tumors were reduced to about 30% of their original size and small tumors had disappeared. At that time the owner chose to discontinue treatment, with the option to treat the remaining tumors with cryotherapy if they started to grow or recur.

Dosage

1. Dogs - 2.5 mg/lb TID
2. Horses - 2.5 mg/kg TID

ANTIMETABOLITES FOR LOCAL INJECTION

Two drugs have been recommended as fibroblast inhibitors when injected around glaucoma anterior chamber shunt implants, thus reducing fibrous encystment (of the valve) that would interfere with valve function.

Fluorouracil (5-fluorouracil, 5-FU) - inhibits thymidylate synthetase resulting in inhibition of DNA synthesis, thus inducing cell death in cells growing at a more rapid pace.

Mitomycin, MTC (Mutamycin - Bristol Labs) - is an antibiotic that selectively inhibits the synthesis of DNA. Using sterile water, dilute 5 gm vial to 0.2-0.4 mg/ml. Soak a sponge with soultion and apply to the area. Stable for 60 days if frozen.

IMMUNOSTIMULANTS

Activation of macrophages by immunostimulants leads to a release of a variety of cytokines. The cytokine response enhances the immune response in a variety of ways. As a result this boosts the immune system and an animal is better able to overcome chronic infections or enhance resistance to tumors.

Table 2-8. Immunostimulants licensed for use in domestic animals

Product Name	Active Principle	Indications	Route of Administration
Immunoregulin[R] (ImmunoVet)	Killed *Propionibacterium acnes*	Adjunctive therapy for pyoderma in dogs	Subcutaneous
Nomagen[R] (Fort Dodge Laboratories)	Mycobacterial cell wall fraction	Treatment of equine sarcoid or bovine ocular carcinoma	Intralesion
Regressin[R]-V (Vetrepharm Research)	Mycobacterial cell wall fraction	Treatment of equine sarcoid or canine mammary tumors	Intralesion
Ribigen[R]-B (Ribi Immunochem Research)	Mycobacterial cell wall fraction	Treatment of bovine ocular carcinoma	Intralesion
Ribigen[R]-E (Ribi Immunochem Research)	Mycobacterial cell wall fraction	Treatment of equine sarcoid	Intralesion
Staphage Lysate (SPL)[R] (Delmont Laboratories)	*S. aureus* components with bacteriophage	Treatment of canine pyoderma	Subcutaneous

ANTICOLLAGENASE (ANTIPROTEASE) DRUGS

Excessive amounts of corneal collagenase (proteases capable of disrupting corneal collagen) will break down stromal collagen, creating a progressive ulcer that may progress slowly or if severe, perforate in a matter of hours.

SOURCES OF CORNEAL COLLAGENASE (See also page 293)

In normal cornea, small amounts of collagenase are produced constantly to maintain normal turnover of collagen fibrils.

Endogenous sources - Endogenous corneal collagenase production takes about five to seven days after injury to become significant.

1. Regenerating corneal epithelium produces excess collagenase. If the subepithelial proteoglycan layer is damaged, collagenase can enter the cornea; if it is intact, the cornea remains protected.
2. Budding endothelium associated with corneal vascularization
3. Migrating neutrophils liberate latent collagenase that is activated by plasmin

Exogenous sources

1. Bacteria - especially *P. aeruginosa*
2. Fungi

COLLAGENASE (PROTEASE) INHIBITORS - are drugs that will prevent the breakdown of corneal collagenase by proteases

Chelating drugs (See also page 125) - Collagenase requires calcium and zinc ions to work. Therefore, any chelating drug that ties up these ions will temporarily render collagenase harmless (e.g. Na, EDTA). Clinical value would depend on continuous topical administration.

Acetylcysteine

1. Sources: 10 to 20% solution (Mucosil 20% - Dey Laboratories). Available from pharmacy distributors or by prescription.
2. Concentration - dilute to 5% in artificial tears or other drug combinations (e.g. ulcer solution, page 320). Concentrations exceeding 5% are irritating. If 5% concentration causes irritation, a 2% dilution can be used.
3. Indications
    a. Anticollagenase - stromal ulcers
    b. Mucolytic - to dissolve mucus in dry eye patients

Serum - Fresh serum has been known to be effective in ulcer management for over 100 years. This beneficial effect is due to the anticollagenase activity of alpha-2-macroglobulins and endogenous epithelial growth factors. Equine tetanus antitoxin can also be used.

1. Stability
    a. Alpha-2-macroglobulins are stable, therefore fresh and immune serum are satisfactory sources
    b. Epithelial growth factors are less stable. Fresh serum should be refrigerated and discarded after seven days if their benefit is desired.
2. Routes of administration - topical and subconjunctival (see pages 298, 319).

Penicillamine (Cuprimine - Merck Sharpe & Dohme) - Ophthalmic drops made suspending 1-2% penicillamine have been tried with limited success.

Antiplasmin agents - Aprotinin is an effective inhibitor of plasmin and possibly collagenase. High levels of tear plasmin frequently are seen in human chronic ulcers. Plasmin interferes with fibronectin, the glycoprotein that anchors regenerating epithelial cells to the corneal basement membrane, thereby predisposing epithelial cell detachment. It has been shown to be helpful in man. Benefits in animals are questionable. The author observed variable results when treating indolent ulcers in dogs and horses with a solution containing 50 IU/ml 4 to 6 times daily.

Dilute Betadine 0.2% (1:50) is of value in topical treatment of refractive ulcers.

Polysulfated glycosaminoglycan - PSGAG (Adequan IM 100 mg/ml - Luitpold Pharmaceuticals Inc.) - Inhibits plasmin and plasminogen activators. Ophthalmic drops, made by diluting to 1:1 with artificial tears to make a 50 mg/ml solution, have been reported to be 70-80% effective when treating canine persistent corneal erosion (Willeford, Miller and Abrams: in Proceedings 28th Annual ACVO Meeting 1997; p.18).

COLLAGENASE POTENTIATORS

Corticosteroids increase the activity of collagenase by 14 times, therefore are contraindicated in corneal lesions with collagenase activity. See corneal healing (Chapter 10, page 289) and treatment of ulcers (Chapter 10, page 319).

SURGICAL ENZYMES

After injury, fibrin stops hemorrhage and produces a matrix for healing. After this matrix serves its purpose, fibrinolysis occurs as a result of plasminogen being converted to plasmin by plasminogen activators. Systemic plasminogen activators, such as streptokinase, have been used to help disperse swelling and hemorrhage after trauma but were too toxic to use intraocularly. Recombinant tissue plasminogen activator (tPA) can be safely used intraocularly to dissolve fibrin and blood clots. It does not have any toxic effects.

STREPTOKINASE - This has had a limited effect on dispersing swelling and hemorrhage after trauma. 5,000-10,000 units IM or IV divided BID to TID.

TISSUE PLASMINOGEN ACTIVATOR (tPA)

Suggested reading: Martin C et al. Ocular use of tissue plasminogen activator in companion animals. Vet Compar Ophthalmol 1993;3:29-36.

In man, tPA is used intravenously to dissolve blood clots associated with myocardial infarction. When it is injected intravascularly, it will break down fibrin and blood clots. It does not have any toxic effects when injected at recommended levels (75-100 µg injected intravitreally in rabbits will cause retinal toxicity). The sooner fibrin forms, the better the response to tPA. It is usually ineffective after seven days.

Sources

1. tPA 0.1% (100 µg/0.1 ml) solution prepared 0.25 ml/syringe (Wedgewood Pharmacy).
2. In hospital formulation is possible but very expensive (50 mg vial costs $1,300). Prepared by dissolving 50 mg in 200 ml of sterile water to prepare 250 µg/ml solution, then draw 0.3 ml (75 µg) into a TB or insulin syringe and freeze at -70° C. until needed.

Preparation and storage

1. Dissolve 20 mg in 20 ml sterile water and dilute further with 60 ml sterile physiological saline solution to a final concentration of 250 µg/ml (25 µg/0.1 ml).
2. Reconstituted tPA has a short half-life at room temperature but is stable at -70°C. Therefore we draw 0.3 ml (75 µg) into tuberculin or insulin syringes and freeze at -70°C until needed.

Intracameral (anterior chamber) administration

1. Indications
   a. Synechia from recent inflammation or surgery
   b. Large fibrin clots with endothelial and/or iris attachment
   c. Postoperative glaucoma
   d. Stabilized hyphema - clots more than 5-7 days old do not respond well.
2. Technique (anterior chamber centesis, Chapter 1, page 38)
   a. If glaucoma is present, tap the anterior chamber using an empty syringe with a 27 or 30 gauge needle and remove 0.1 ml aqueous. The syringe with the tPA can be switched to the needle in the anterior chamber or the needle can be withdrawn and the anterior chamber retapped with a tPA syringe and needle.
   b. If the pressure is normal, the aspiration of aqueous is not necessary and the original tapping should be done with the tPA syringe and needle.
   c. Inject into the anterior chamber: small animals 25-50 µg; equine 50-150 µg.
   d. Using the needle as a probe, carefully attempt to relieve some of the fibrin or blood clot adhesions
   e. Injection can be repeated in 7 to 10 minutes

Intravitreal administration - to dissolve blood clots. There is potential for retinal toxicity, therefore use cautiously. The current recommendation in man is 3 to 12.5 µg.

Topical administration (Gerding PA, Eurell T. Evaluation of intraocular penetration of topically administered tissue plasminogen activator in dogs. Am J Vet Res 1993;54:836-839).

Clinical effectiveness has not been determined. Gerding reported one drop tPA 1.0% yielded the same intraocular level as one drop tPA 0.5% administered three times at 10 minute intervals but levels were much lower than recommended intracameral injection.

VISCOELASTICS

Viscoelastic agents sodium hyaluronate and hydroxypropyl methylcellulose are used for ocular surgical procedures including lens extraction, intraocular lens implantation, and perforating keratoplasty to protect corneal endothelium and maintain the anterior chamber. A common unlabeled use is to protect the cornea in "dry eye" patients.

Sodium hyaluronate

1. For lens implantation (Healon, Amvisc, AMD Vitrax)
2. For treating joint disease (Equron - Solvay; Hyalovet - Fort Dodge; Hylartin - American Equine; Synacid - Schering Plough)

Sodium hyaluronate and chondroitin sulfate. For intraocular surgery (Viscoat - Alcon)

Hydroxypropyl methylcellulose (HPMC) 2% (Ocucoat - Storz)

Hylashield (Imed - Canada) - can be used as a tear replacement. Also helps reduce the irritation caused by topical antiviral agents.

CHELATING AGENTS

Topical application of chelating agents has been helpful in the management of some chronic corneal diseases.

Suggested uses

1. Stromal lipid keratopathies - characterized by calcium cholesterol or lipid substrates
2. Reducing corneal plaque - formation that may develop following parotid duct transposition
3. Anticollagenase - effective for corneal ulcers by tying up calcium present in the tears and cornea

Source - Sequester-Sol (13.4% dipotassium ethylenediamine tetra acetate - K^2EDTA), Baxter #2948

Preparation - dilute to 1-2% with artificial tears

Administration - 1 drop QID, reduce as needed when eye improves

INTRAOCULAR IRRIGATING SOLUTIONS

Normal saline solution (PSS)

Normal saline solution can be used but has been associated with postoperative corneal edema as a result of endothelial damage. It is satisfactory for emergency procedures but is discouraged for long term procedures.

Lactated Ringer's solution

This is superior to PSS because it contains calcium ions that are important for maintaining corneal endothelial cell junctions. It is satisfactory for emergency and long term procedures.

Balanced Salt Solution (BSS - Alcon Labs)

BSS is a sterile physiologic balanced salt solution that is isotonic to the tissues of the eye. It is the preferred intraocular irrigating solution.

1. **BSS** - electrolytes only. Recommended for short term surgeries.
2. **BSS Plus** - electrolytes enriched with bicarbonate, dextrose, and glutathione. Recommended for all intraocular surgeries, especially long term infusion surgeries.

Anticoagulant for intraocular irrigation solution

Anti-inflammatory premedication before intraocular surgery reduces but does not eliminate fibrin formation during intraocular surgery. To control this, heparin solution can be added to the irrigating solution to give a concentration of 1 unit/ml of irrigating solution. Greater concentrations can be irritating to intraocular tissues.

EYE WASHES (COLLYRIA)

An eye wash (collyrium) is a very beneficial part of ocular therapy.

ISOTONIC SALINE SOLUTION

This is the most available irrigating solution but lacks a bacteriostatic agent and can become contaminated.

COMMERCIAL IRRIGATING SOLUTION

These are sterile isotonic solutions sold over the counter. They contain balanced electrolytes and bacteriostatic agents to maintain sterility.

Ak-Rinse, Aqua Flow, Dacriose, Eye-Stream

ARTIFICIAL TEARS (Demulcents)

Natural tears, because of their complex layers (outer lipid, inner serous, and deep mucus) cannot be totally replaced by a tear substitute. Tear replacements contain large molecules that will remain on the cornea longer than aqueous electrolyte preparations.

INDICATIONS

1. Symptomatic treatment for dry eyes
2. As a vehicle for preparing topical ophthalmic medication

MAJOR COMPONENTS OF ARTIFICIAL TEARS

Ethyl- and methylcellulose derivatives

Some examples are Lyteers, Tear Gard, Isopto Tears, Lacril, Tearisol, Methulose, Murocel
Preservative-free preparations are available for patients showing sensitivity, e.g. Cellufresh and Celluvisc (Allergan)

Polyvinyl alcohol

Some examples are Akwa Tears, Liquifilm Tears and Forte and Tears Plus. Two products in this group do not have the traditional preservatives (Refresh, Hypotears PF).

Other polymeric systems

These contain complex compounds such as an artificial mucin (polyvinylpyrrolidone) in Adsorbotear and Tears Naturale. Some other examples are Comfort Drops, Dual Wet, Tears Renewed.

OCULAR EMOLLIENTS (Lubricants)

Emollients are ocular ointments that are used to form an occlusive film over the eye to lubricate and protect it from drying. They do not require prescriptions.

INDICATIONS

General anesthesia - prevent drying and secondary ulceration

Postophthalmic surgery lubricant

Lagophthalmos - from palpebral paralysis and exophthalmos

Decreased corneal sensation - trigeminal paralysis

KCS - when drops cannot be administered at frequent intervals and as a nighttime medication

Recurrent corneal erosion

TYPES

Emollients

Some examples are: Akwa Tears ointment, Duolube, Duratears, Hypotears ointment, Lacri-Lube S.O.P., Refresh P.M., Tears Renewed ointment

Medicated ophthalmic ointments - an inexpensive substitute for true emollients

1. Boric acid ophthalmic ointment - may induce hypersensitivity reactions in dogs
2. Antibiotic ointments - choose an inexpensive single antibiotic preparation (e.g. Bacitracin ophthalmic ointment) to reduce the chance for antibiotic hypersensitivity and the development of resistant bacteria

CHAPTER 3 - OPHTHALMIC INSTRUMENTS AND SUTURES

OPHTHALMIC SURGICAL INSTRUMENTS

ADEQUATE SET FOR MOST OPHTHALMIC PROCEDURES WOULD BE:

	Instrument	Price range - 1994
1.	Needle holder	$60-350
2.	Corneal forceps	155-350
3.	Fixation forceps	125-180
4.	Cilia forceps	5-50
5.	Arruga capsule forceps	80-125
6.	Corneal scissors	90-130
7.	Utility (iris) scissors	45-90
8.	Cyclodialysis cannula	20

Comment. Good quality curved mosquito hemostatic forceps can be substituted for fixation forceps.

NEEDLE HOLDERS

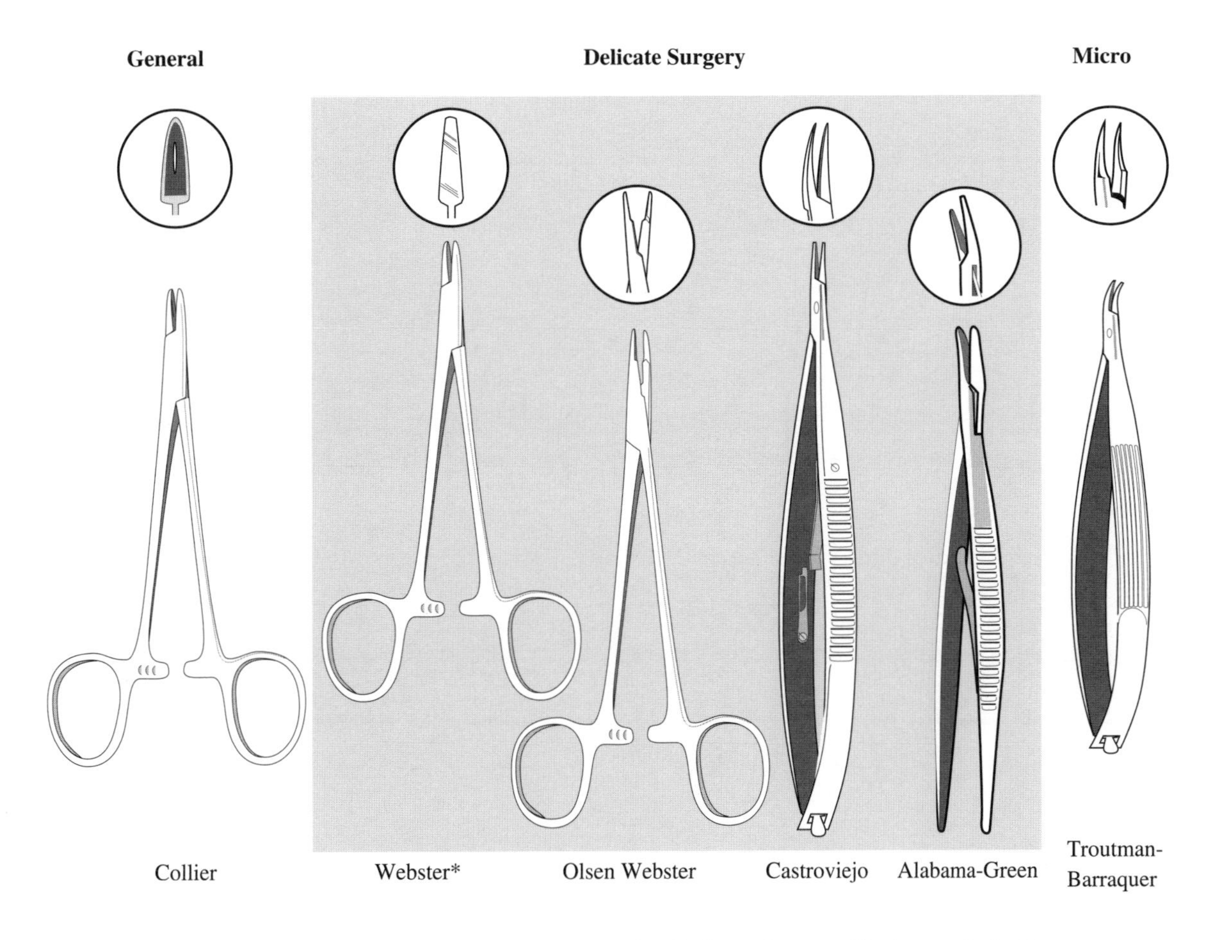

*Good Quality mosquito hemostatic forceps, straight or curved, with fine points are effective needle holders.

SCISSORS

Corneal | **Corneal** | **Capsulotomy** | **Iris** | **Iris**

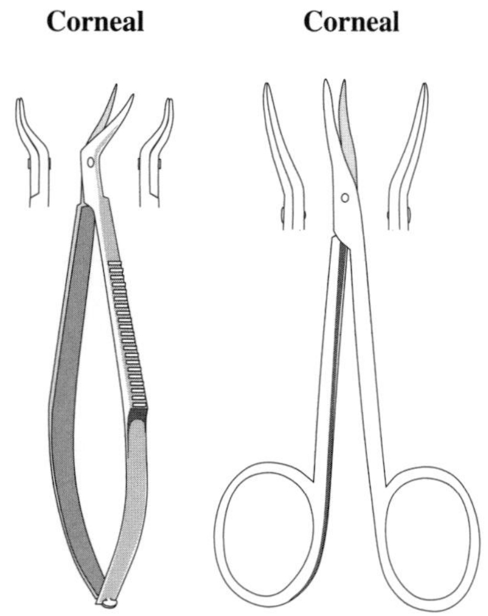

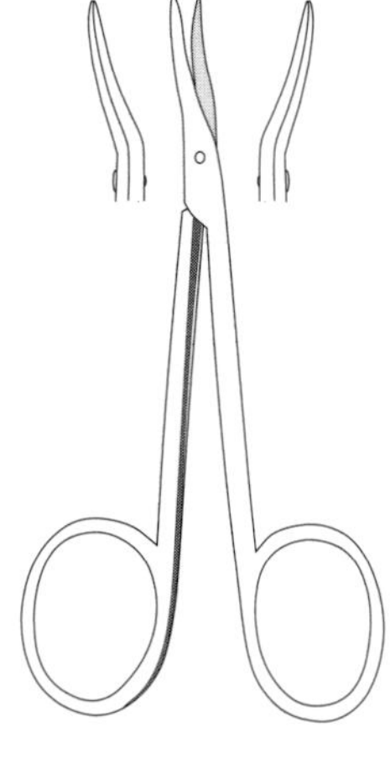

Troutman-Castroviejo R & L (medium blades)

McGuire R & L (moderate curve)

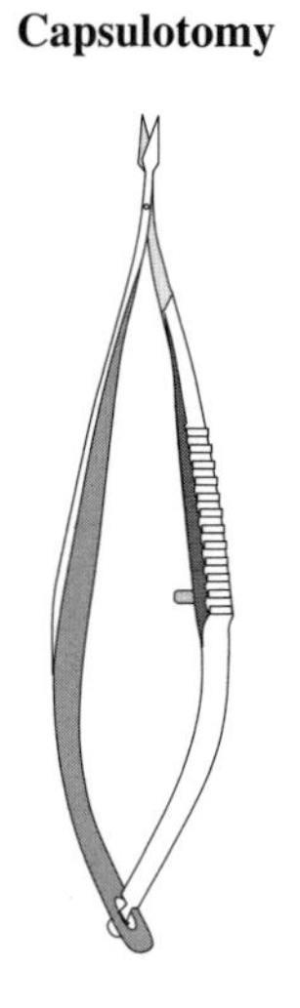

Vannas (sharp tips)

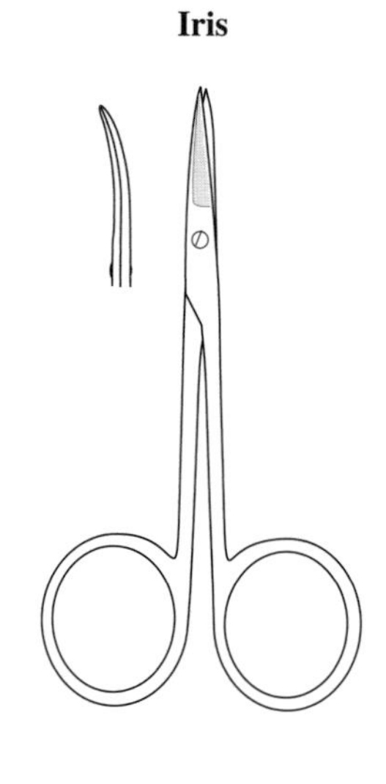

Eye scissors (large rings, general purpose)

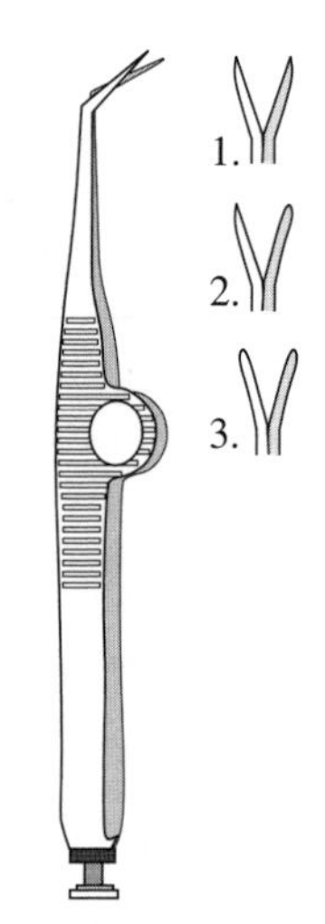

DeWecker
1. sharp/sharp
2. sharp/blunt
3. blunt/blunt

Tenotomy | **Strabismus** | **Enucleation** | **Suture**

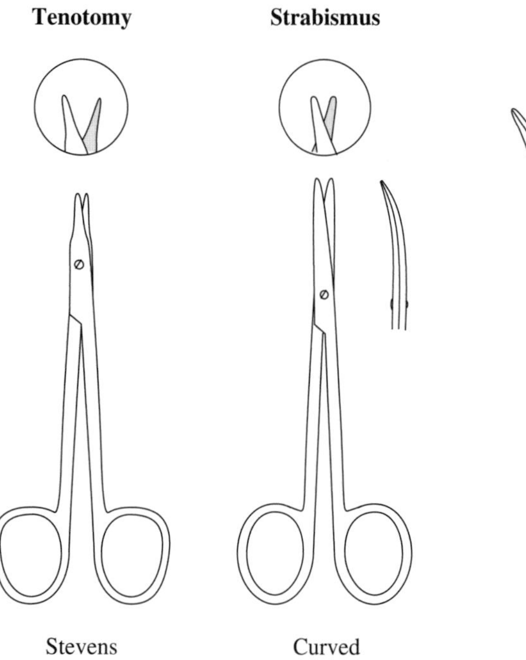

Stevens

Curved

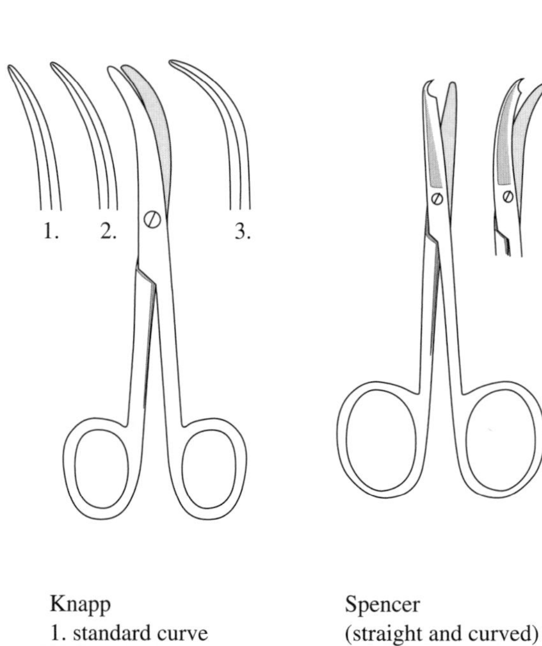

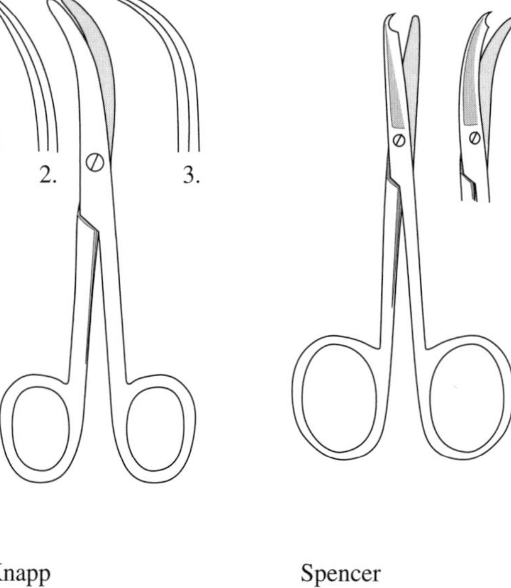

Knapp
1. standard curve
2. medium curve
3. strong curve

Spencer (straight and curved)

SUTURING FORCEPS WITH TYING PLATFORMS

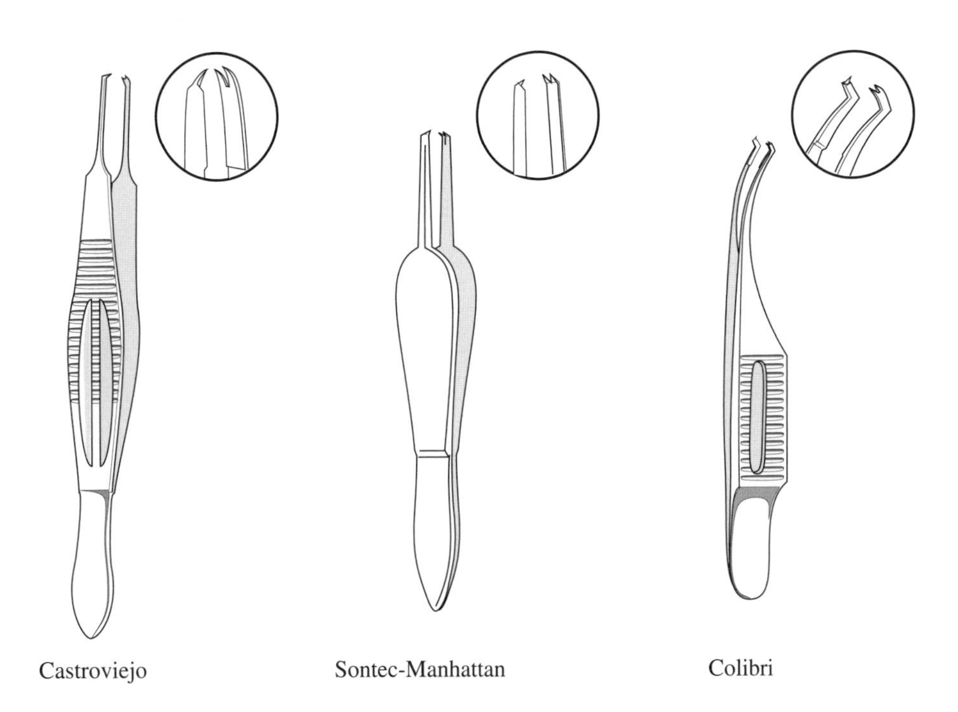

0.12 mm teeth-healthy cornea
0.30 mm teeth-edematous cornea and conjunctiva
0.50 or 0.60 mm teeth-sclera and eyelids

TYING PLATFORM FORCEPS

FIXATION FORCEPS

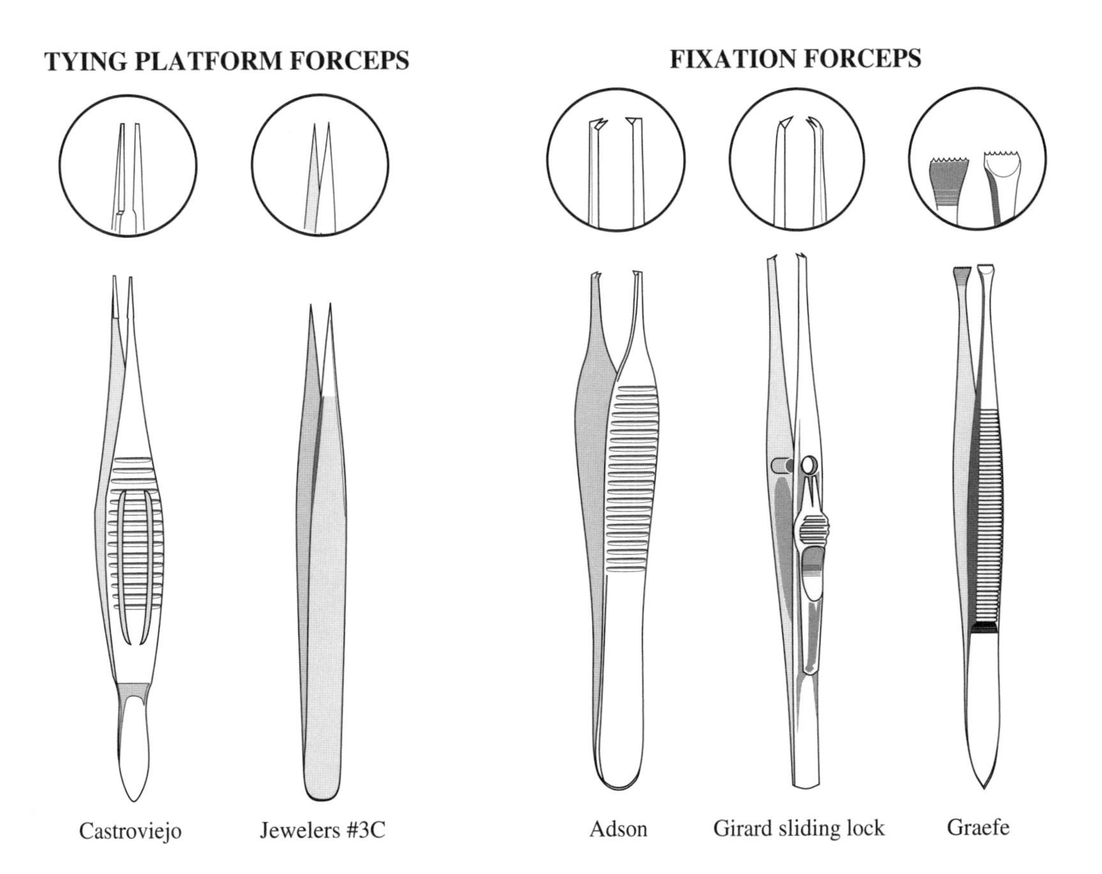

CILIA FORCEPS

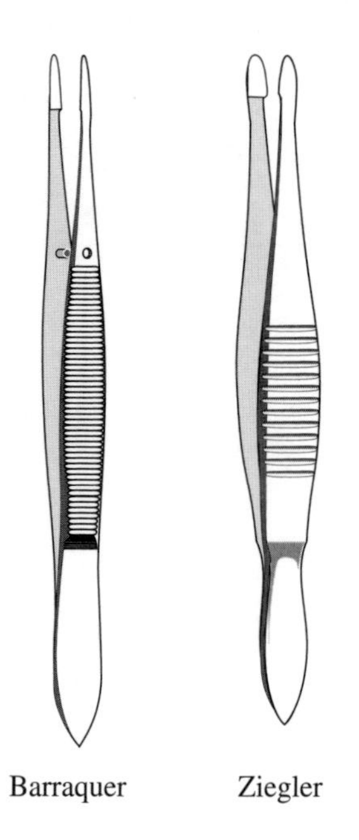

Barraquer   Ziegler

LENS CAPSULE FORCEPS

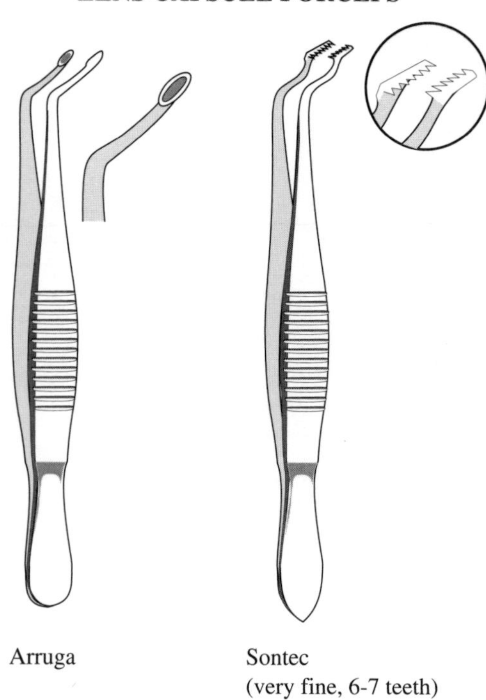

Arruga

Sontec
(very fine, 6-7 teeth)

EYELID STABILIZATION FORCEPS

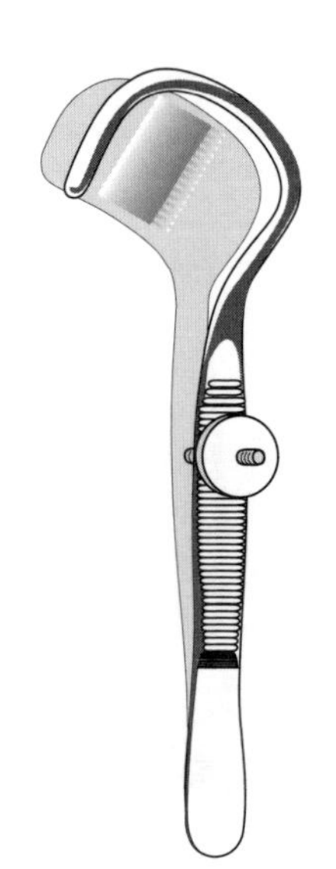

Snellen
entropion

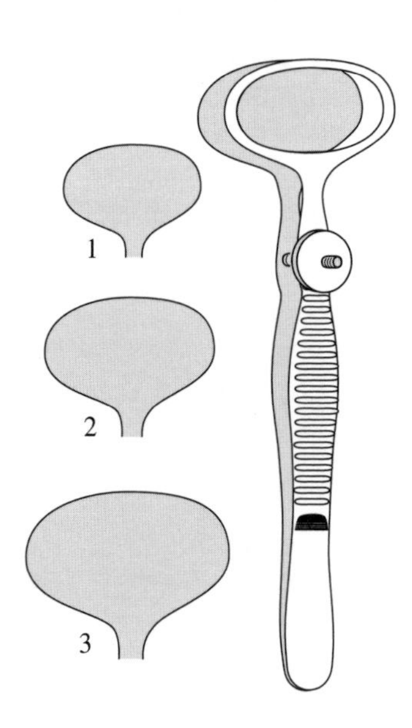

Desmarres chalazion

1. Small	16 mm
2. Medium	20 mm
3. Large	26 mm

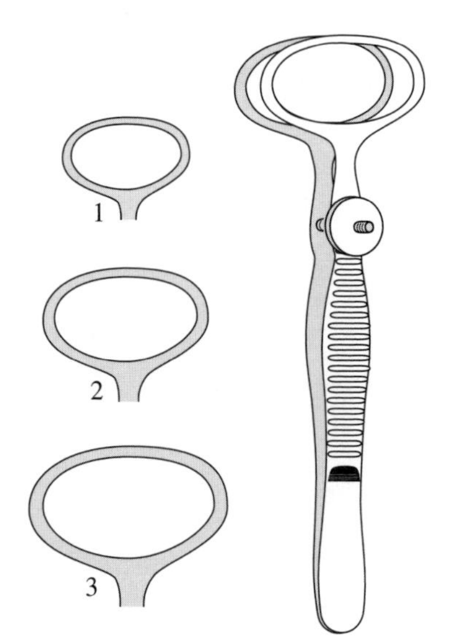

Sontec tumor forceps

1. Small	16 mm
2. Medium	20 mm
3. Large	26 mm

EYELID SPECULA

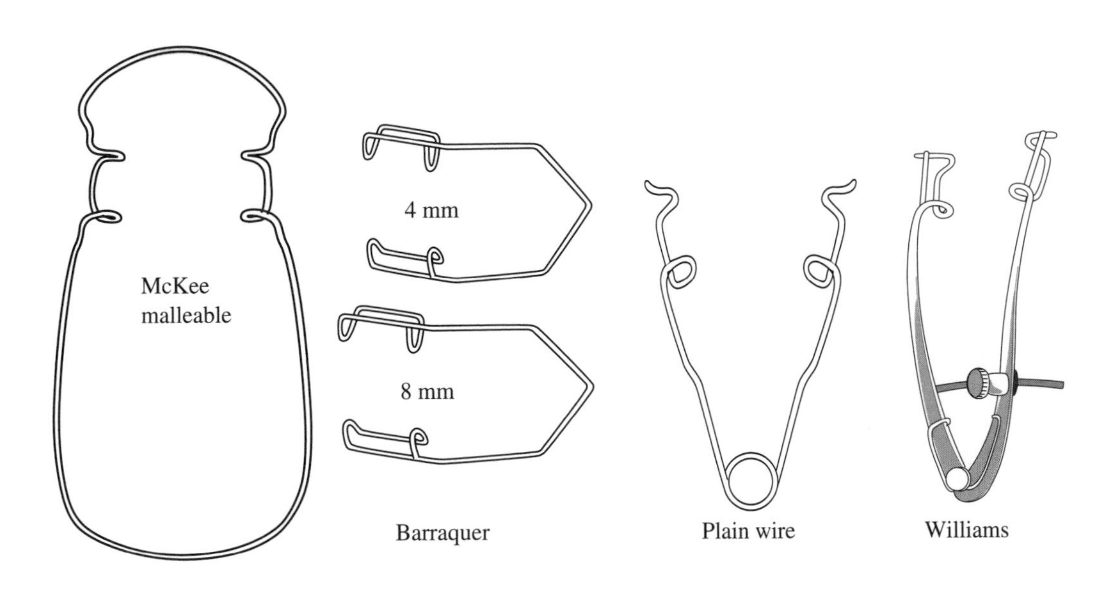

Barraquer

Plain wire

Williams

EYELID RETRACTORS

LID PLATE

LACRIMAL CANNULAS

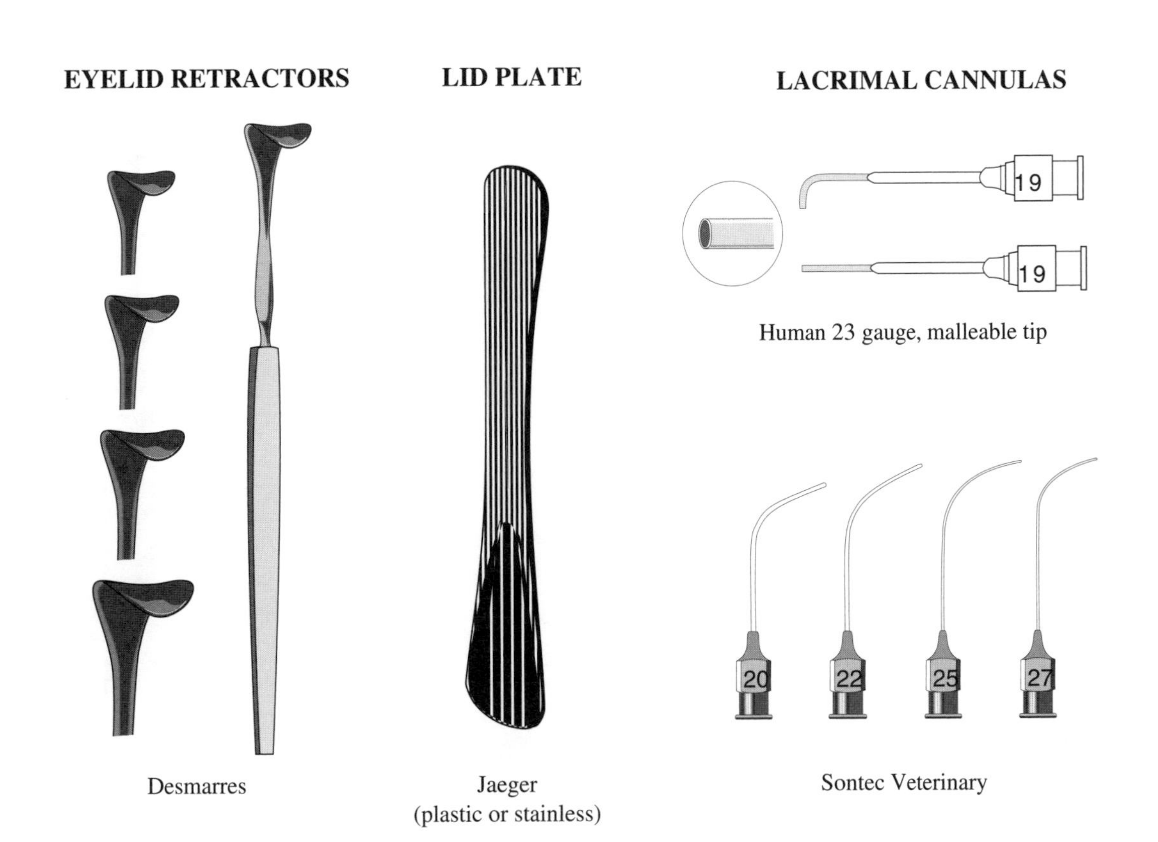

Human 23 gauge, malleable tip

Desmarres

Jaeger
(plastic or stainless)

Sontec Veterinary

CUTTING INSTRUMENTS

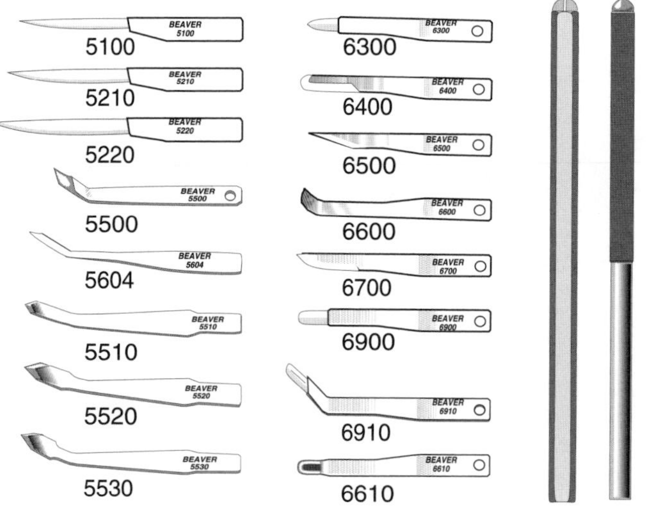

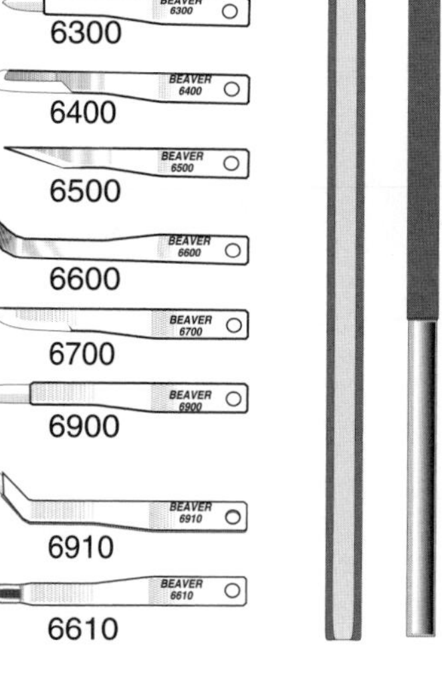

Beaver blades

Beaver handles

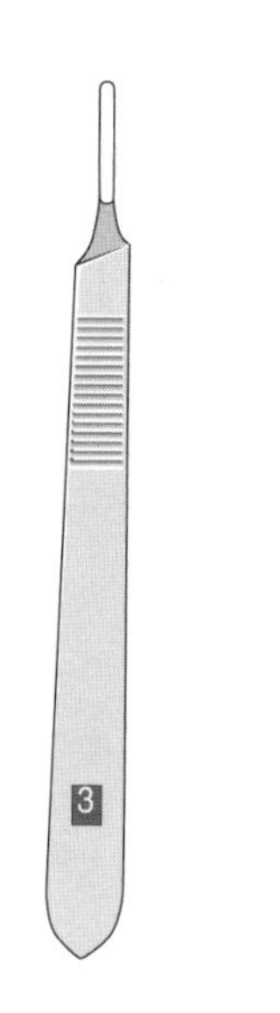

Bard-Parker
#3 handle

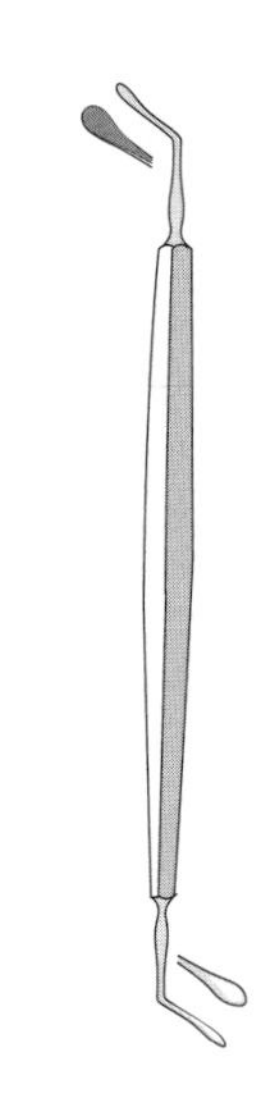

Martinez
corneal dissector

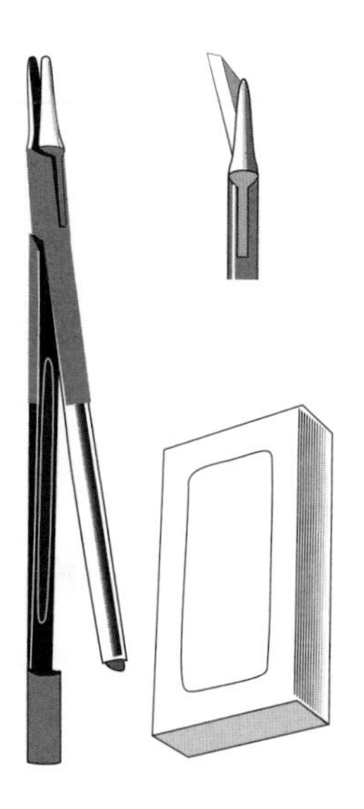

Swiss blade breaker
and special blades

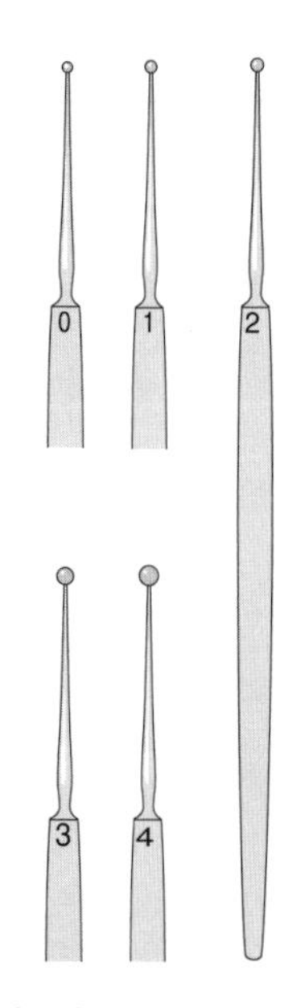

Meyerhoefer chalazion curet
12-1300 size 0, 1.50 mm dia
12-1310 size 1, 1.75 m m dia
12-1320 size 2, 2.25 mm dia
12-1355 size 3, 2.50 mm dia
12-1365 size 4, 3.50 mm dia

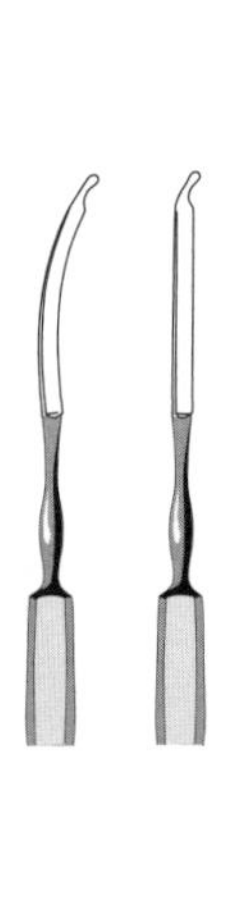

Weber
canaliculus
knives

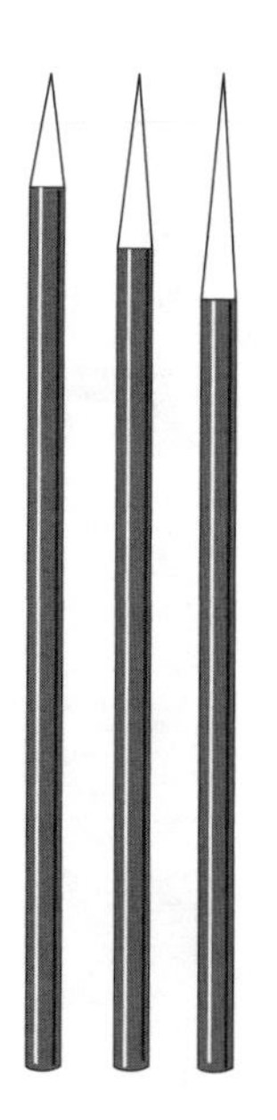

Welder lacrimal
dilators
#1 fine
#2 medium
#3 heavy

MISCELLANEOUS

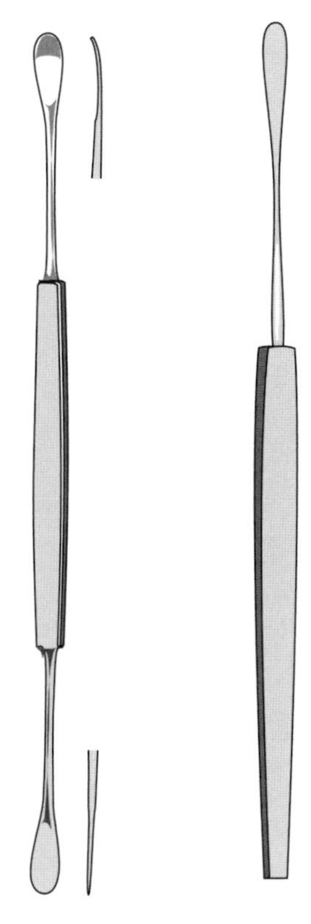

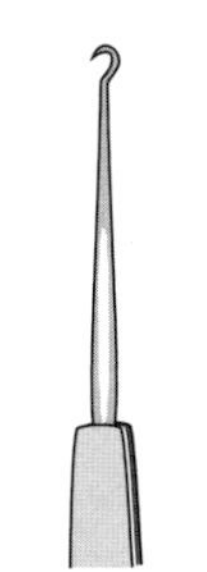

Tyrell
iris hook

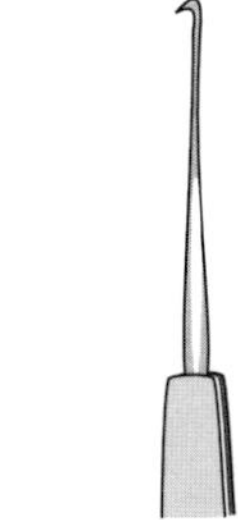

Wilder
cystostome

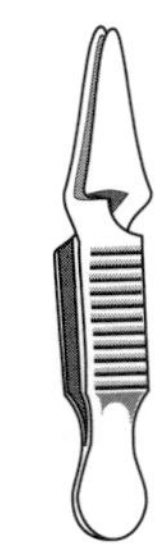

Serrefine
clamp

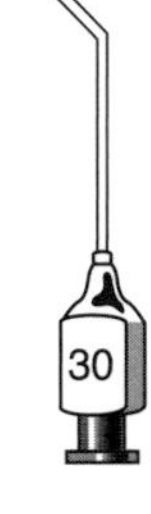

Green spatula

Kimura platinum
spatula

Castroviejo
cyclodialysis
spatula

Culler
iris spatula
2 mm wide

Air injection
cannula - 30 gauge

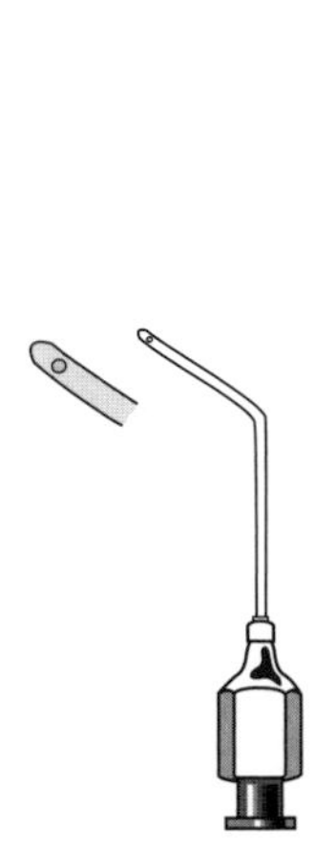

Gans cannula
cyclodialysis
with side port

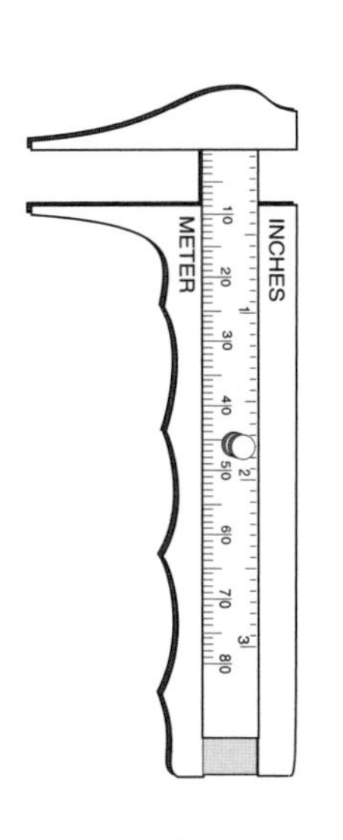

Jameson
calipers

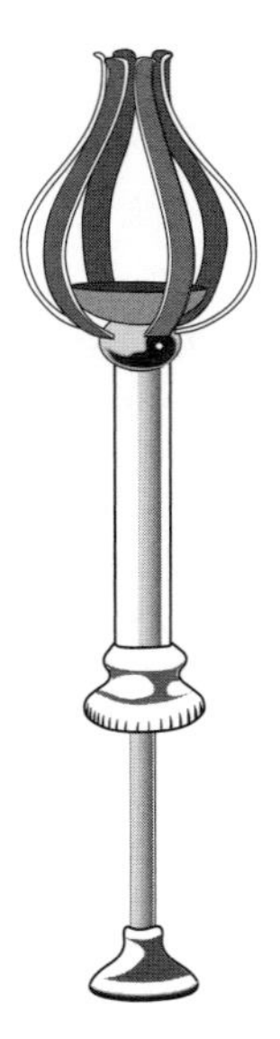

Carter sphere
introducer

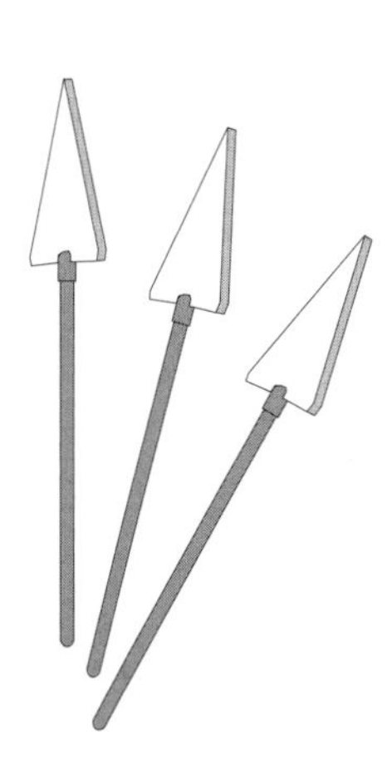

Surgical cellulose
spears

SUTURES

Many specialized sutures and needles are available for ophthalmic surgery. The cornea and sclera are very dense and cannot be easily sutured unless proper ophthalmic needles (reverse cutting or spatula) are available (Table 3-1).

Absorbable suture may be used to eliminate the need for suture removal.

CORNEAL SUTURE REACTION IN DECREASING SEVERITY

Surgical gut and collagen - most severe reaction
Silk - for many years the most popular ophthalmic suture
Polyglactin 910 (Vicryl) and polyglycolic acid (Dexon) - If silk is removed from the cornea at two weeks, the reaction will be about the same as seen with Vicryl and Dexon when they come out at 3.5 weeks.
Polyglyconate (PDS or Maxon) - least reaction of absorbable suture
Nonabsorbable synthetic sutures - results in the least tissue reaction

SILK - can be used in all ocular tissues

Excellent for short term procedures (eyelid and globe stabilization during surgery, and third eyelid flaps). Very easy to work with, has the softest exposed ends. Has been replaced in corneal surgery by synthetic sutures.

COLLAGEN AND SURGICAL GUT - can be used for buried suture in conjunctiva and eyelids. Not as easy to handle as silk. Synthetic absorbable sutures are preferred by most surgeons.

SYNTHETIC ABSORBABLE SUTURES - are used in all tissues, especially cornea. Can be used in the skin when nonabsorbable sutures would be difficult to remove. Suture ends are stiffer than silk and can cause irritation. Absorption occurs in two phases: loss of tensile strength during early postoperative period, followed by loss of mass when most of the tensile strength is gone.

Dexon and Vicryl - will remain in tissues about 3.5 weeks. Currently the most popular corneal suture in veterinary medicine.
Maxon and PDS - absorb more slowly and produce less tissue reaction

SYNTHETIC NONABSORBABLE SUTURE

Monofilament nylon (Dermalon, Ethilon) - excellent skin and corneal suture. It can be buried. Suture tips are stiff, therefore suture should be trimmed closely to avoid irritation.

Fine sutures (8-0 and smaller) can be left in the cornea without causing irritation if suture tips are cut short or the knot buried. More difficult to work with and requires special knot.
Braided nylon (Norolon, Surgilon) - same indications as monofilament nylon but does not have stiff ends.
Polypropylene (Prolene/Surgilene) - same indications as nylon
Polybutest (Novafil) - least resistive suture available and has same indications as nylon

Table 3-1. Sutures and needles for ophthalmic surgery

Suture size	Silk		Nylon		Polygly-colic acid	Polyglactin 910	Gut and collagen	
	D & G	Ethicon	D & G (Dermalon)	Ethicon (Ethilon)	D & G (Dexon)	Ethicon (Vicryl)	D & G	Ethicon
STANDARD SUTURES								
2-0	--	--	CE-10*	FS	--	--	--	--
3-0	--	--	CE-6	FS-1	PRE-6	PS-1	PRE-6	PS-2
4-0	PR-4	PS-2	CE-4	FS-2	PRE-4	PS-2	PRE-4	FS-4
5-0	--	--	PRE-2	P-3	PRE-2	P-3	PRE-2	PS-4
OPHTHALMIC SUTURES								
6-0	CE-21	G-1	PRE-1	P-1	P-1	C-3	CE-21	PS-6
7-0	LE-2	TG-140-8	LE-2	TG-175-8	LE-2	TG-175-8	--	--
8-0	LE-1	TG-140-6	LE-1	TG-175-6	LE-1	TG-175-6	--	--
9-0	--	TG-140-4	LE-1	TG-175-4	LE-1	TG-175-6	--	--

*Indicates needle size and type.

CHAPTER 4 - GENERAL PRINCIPLES OF OCULAR SURGERY

A wide variety of ophthalmic problems require surgical correction. Prior to any surgical procedure, it is imperative to evaluate the ocular condition, select the most appropriate surgical procedure, and pay strict attention to proper surgical technique to assure best results.

RESTRAINT, SEDATION AND ANESTHESIA

The degree of restraint or type of anesthesia will depend on the procedure being considered, the species, and temperament of the patient. Minor adnexal procedures may often be completed with topical and/or local anesthesia, while major eyelid surgeries necessitate general anesthesia. Minor surgeries of the globe (e.g. biopsy, cytology, and epithelial debridement) can be performed in small animals with only topical anesthesia, whereas sedation is indicated in large animals. General anesthesia is recommended for major ocular surgery. The choice varies with the species. As a general rule, intravenous anesthesia is often satisfactory for short term procedures and inhalation for longer term and intraocular surgeries. Isoflurane is the preferred inhalation anesthetic. With isoflurane there is smooth induction and recovery, it is safe, and provides adequate muscle relaxation. Halothane is acceptable if relaxation of extraocular muscles is not needed, however it predisposes to ventricular fibrillation if epinephrine is used topically or intraocularly. If ocular immobilization is needed, assisted respiration and atracurium are recommended.

Cats

1. Minor manipulation and surgery - ketamine and acepromazine combinations
2. General eyelid and ocular surgery - inhalation anesthesia (isoflurane is preferred)

Dogs

1. Examination and minor manipulations - topical anesthesia is usually adequate. If the animal will not allow examination, oxymorphone or butorphanol (a non narcotic sedative) is preferred over tranquilizers because tranquilizers cause protrusion of the third eyelid.
2. Minor surgery
    a. Adnexa - local anesthesia and/or chemical restraint (tranquilizer, butorphanol)
    b. Painful procedures less than 10 minutes - preanesthesia and ultrashort barbiturates or profenal
    c. General surgery - inhalation anesthesia - isoflurane is preferred

Equine

1. Examination and minor manipulations
    a. Topical anesthesia
    b. Palpebral nerve block - if severe blepharospasm
    c. Chemical restraint
        1) Procedures up to 15 to 20 minutes - xylazine with or without butorphanol
        2) Procedures greater than 20 minutes - detomidine and butorphanol
2. Surgery
    a. Minor surgery
        1) If can be done standing - chemical restraint and appropriate local anesthesia
        2) If cannot be done standing - intravenous anesthesia - combination of ultrashort barbiturates, glyceryl guaiacolate, xylazine and/or detomidine.
    b. General surgery
        1) If eye motion is not a problem - halothane
        2) If eye motion needs to be controlled - isoflurane

PREPARING THE PATIENT

Premedication

1. Elective procedures - do not do elective surgery on an infected eye
   a. Topical
      1) Antibiotics
         a) Adnexal surgery - if the eye appears normal premedication is not needed. If there is conjunctivitis or blepharitis, control the infection before doing elective surgery. When culture results are available, it is safe to concurrently start specific antibiotic treatment and perform surgery.
         b) Intraocular surgery - a topical broad spectrum antibiotic three to five days before surgery may reduce the chance for postoperative infection. A good presurgical disinfectant preparation should destroy all organisms present, thereby negating the need for presurgical antibiotic. Do not use oil base ointments less than 24 hours before surgery.
      2) Mydriatics - indicated prior to intraocular surgery if a dilated pupil is observed. Atropine beginning 12 to 24 hours prior to surgery.
   b. Systemic
      1) Antibiotics - preoperative are not needed for adnexal surgery but are recommended several hours prior to intraocular or orbital surgery
      2) Anti-inflammatory
         a) Adnexal surgery - flunixin 4 to 12 hours presurgically to reduce postsurgical edema or discomfort
         b) Intraocular surgery - systemic and topical anti-inflammatory drugs may be beneficial three to five days prior to surgery
         c) Antihistamines 20-30 minutes prior to incising the eye.
2. Emergency procedures
   a. Topical - premedications are not routinely administered before emergency surgery. If administered, do not use oil base ointments prior to intraocular surgery. If they have been used, thoroughly clean the eyes after anesthesia.
   b. Systemic - usually administered immediately after examination
      1) IV antibiotics are recommended immediately before or after surgery in patients with severe adnexal injuries or those requiring intraocular surgery
      2) Anti-inflammatory - intravenous rapid acting corticosteroids for patients requiring intraocular surgery

Presurgical preparation

1. Protect the cornea - A non-oil base such as Surgilube (E. Fougera & Co) can be instilled in the conjunctival sac, over the cornea, and along the edge of the eyelids to reduce the hair that may collect on the eye during clipping.
2. Clipping - The size of the area to be clipped is determined by the surgery to be performed. It may be minimal for some adnexal procedures or extensive for intraocular surgery or eye removal.
   If cornea perforation is present, clipping the eyelids of a recent corneal wound that has not had time to seal with fibrin should be done cautiously, if at all, to avoid manipulation that will result in further iris prolapse or contamination of the anterior chamber.

Skin and adnexal preparations

The author prefers 1:50 (0.2%) Betadine as an irrigating and disinfectant solution. The conjunctival sac should be irrigated thoroughly to remove all hair, debris and traces of ointments. The skin should be thoroughly cleansed with sponges soaked in Betadine. Irrigating and cleaning should be continued for two minutes. At that time Betadine-soaked sponges are placed on the eye and prepared skin, to remain for a minimum of two more minutes before removal for surgery.

PRINCIPLES OF SURGERY OF THE GLOBE

Exposure

A good exposure is necessary. It generally requires canthotomy and eyelid stabilization. Excessive manipulation or tension to expose the eye makes ocular surgery more difficult and decreases the chances for successful surgery.

Prolapsing the eye is the alternative to canthotomy and eyelid stabilization. Prolapse is easily done in cattle and is a satisfactory method of exposure and eye stabilization for ocular procedures such as superficial keratectomy. It can be performed in dogs with a shallow orbit and large eyelid openings. It cannot be used for intraocular procedures because the pressure to prolapse the eye would force intraocular tissue out through the wound.

1. Canthotomy (Fig 4-1) - required in most animals. Exceptions are cattle, exophthalmic dogs with large eyelid openings and some cats. Cut the entire thickness of the eyelid at the lateral canthus with scissors. An eyelid speculum in the eye at the time of the canthotomy will make this easier. Do not cut the lateral orbital ligament.

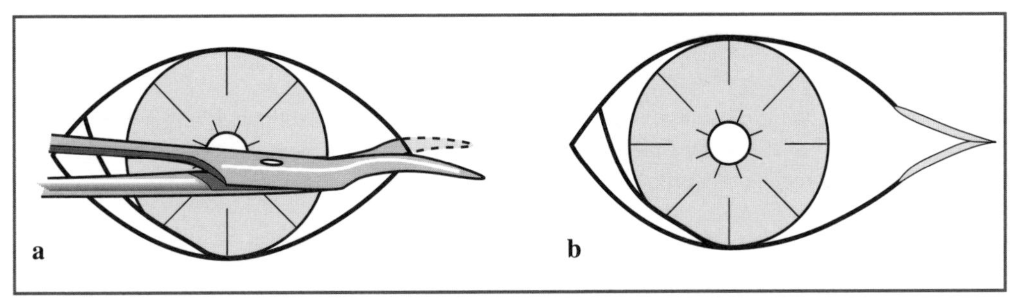

Figure 4-1. Lateral canthotomy.
a. Cutting lateral canthus with scissors
b. Appearance after canthotomy

2. Eyelid fixation (stabilization) - this can be done with a speculum or by suturing the eyelids open. Specula are best for nonperforating surgery but offer the risk of putting excess pressure on the eye with perforating lesions or during intraocular procedures.
    a. Eyelid suturing (Fig 4-2) - suturing the eyelids open takes more time than placement of a speculum and when properly done offers excellent exposure without putting pressure on the eye. Four sutures placed near the edge of the eyelid and anchored to the skin around the eye will stabilize the lids and expose the globe. Because of the looseness of the facial skin, the sutures in the lower eyelid need to be anchored further away from the eye than those on the upper eyelid. Four-0 silk suture is excellent for this procedure.
    b. Eyelid specula (see Chapter 3, page 133) - There are many styles available but lightweight wire specula are available that will stabilize the eyelids without increasing intraocular pressure in small animals. The McKee malleable wire speculum is excellent for horses and can be used on larger dogs.

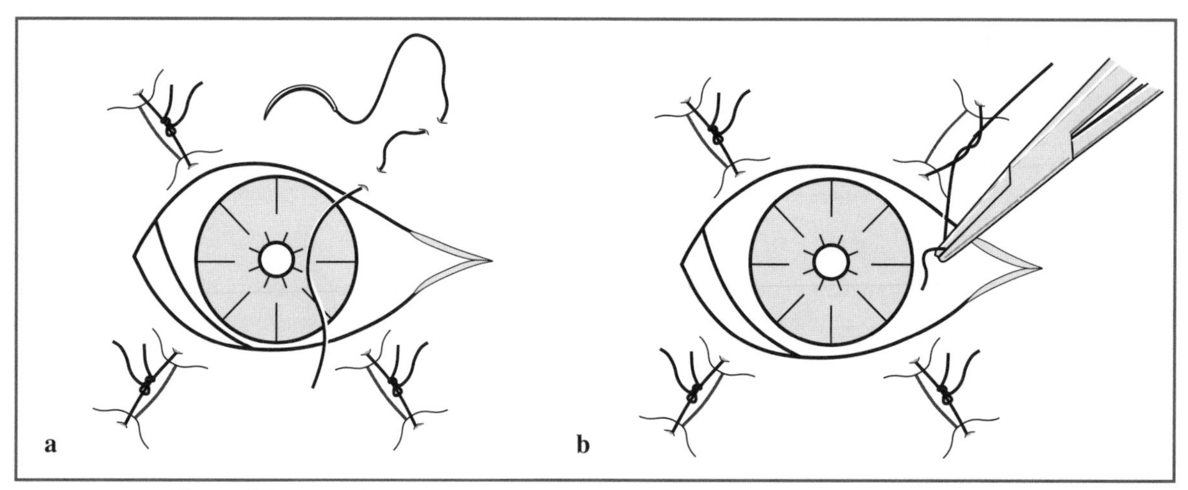

Figure 4-2. Eyelid fixations with sutures.
a. The fourth mattress suture has been placed but not tied. Note the canthotomy to improve exposure of the globe.
b. Sutures are drawn as tight as necessary to provide desired exposure

Globe stabilization

In animals, a downward rotation of the eye is seen with pain, ocular manipulation and light planes of anesthesia. When this occurs, the area of the globe that needs to be accessible during surgery is often inaccessible. Therefore, fixation with forceps or sutures placed in the sclera is needed.

1. Forceps stabilization - fine tip curved mosquito hemostatic forceps placed at the limbus at 9 and 3 o'clock are excellent stabilization for external operative procedures such as superficial keratectomy. They are generally not satisfactory for intraocular procedures because they will distort the cornea and collapse the anterior chamber when the eye is manipulated. Girard fixation forceps with locks can also be used.
2. Fixation sutures (Fig 4-3) - fixation (bridle) sutures can be placed in the sclera 1 to 2 mm from the limbus at 12 o'clock and 6 o'clock positions. Six-0 silk with a sharp ophthalmic needle (e.g. G-1 Ethicon, CE-21 Davis Geck) will cut into the sclera, keeping trauma to a minimum. Sutures placed in the conjunctiva are ineffective. Tie an open loop and attach serrefine artery clamps or hemostats to facilitate ocular positioning.

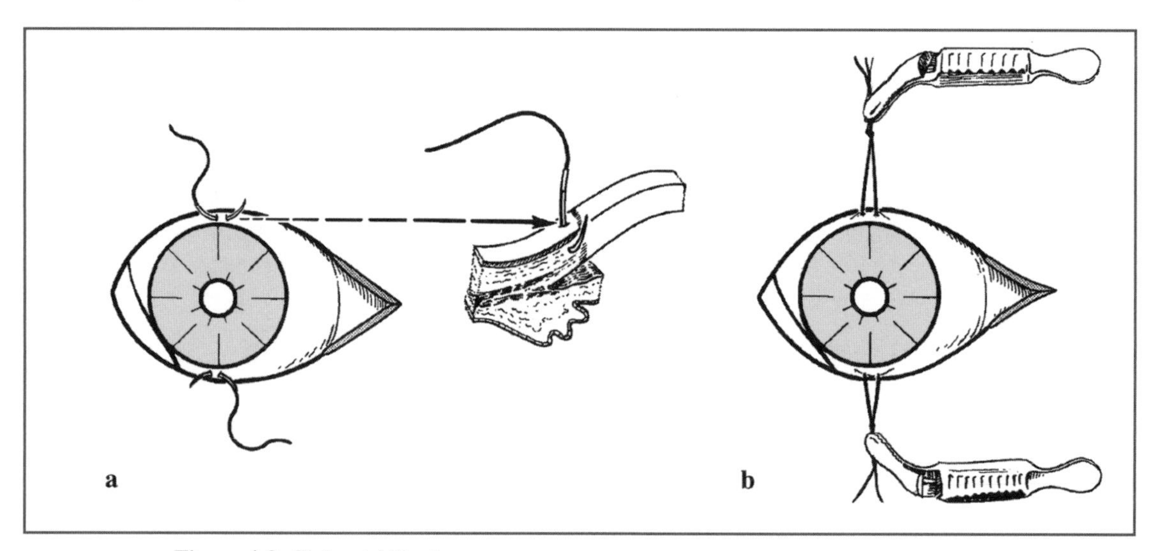

Figure 4-3. Globe stabilization.
a. Placement of 6-0 silk sutures in the perilimbal sclera at 6 and 12 o'clock
b. Sutures tied in open loops and secured with serrefine artery clamps.

Corrective procedure

The eye is now ready for surgery.

The importance of avoiding overmanipulation and excessive pressure on the eye cannot be overemphasized. Therefore, the combination of suturing the eyelids open and bridle sutures to stabilize the eye are the safest for the surgeon with minimal ophthalmic instruments. The eyes of animals do not have enough corneal and scleral rigidity to maintain their shape during intraocular surgery when manipulative pressure is applied.

As previously mentioned, when intraocular surgery is necessary, irrigate the conjunctiva and cornea thoroughly before surgery. Sterile saline is satisfactory. Be sure there is absolutely no oil base ointment that might get into the eye and cause a chemical uveitis. If hemorrhage is a problem during intraocular surgery, balanced salt solution (BSS) or sterile saline with 1:10,000 epinephrine is satisfactory.

Corneal suturing (Fig 4-4)

1. Suture needles - Cornea is very dense and because of this only ophthalmic needles are satisfactory for suturing. Several styles of needles are available; all are cutting points and are very sharp. See Chapter 3 for sutures and needles routinely used. Needle size varies with the suture size being used. Six-0 suture will have a larger needle than 7-0 or 8-0. Edematous cornea will justify a larger needle than healthy cornea.
2. Types of suture - Ophthalmic sutures are available in silk, catgut, collagen, nylon, Mersilene, Vicryl, Dexon, PDS and Maxon. The choice is up to the surgeon. Noncapillary silk can be used in all ocular tissues satisfactorily but for the most part it has been replaced by other sutures, especially Dexon and Vicryl.
3. Suture depth - Corneal sutures should be placed 2/3 to 3/4 the thickness of the cornea. Do not penetrate the endothelium; this can lead to:
   a. Chronic leakage of aqueous and possible intraocular infection
   b. An epithelial granuloma developing in the anterior chamber. As the suture passes through the cornea, epithelial cells may line the wound. If these cells reach the anterior chamber they can develop into granuloma.
4. Suture placement
   a. In small animals, the suture should be placed to incorporate about 1 mm of tissue on each side of the wound. Draw up until it is firm but not cutting in. Always place a third overhand knot to prevent the suture from slipping. Place sutures so they are about 1 to 1.5 mm apart.
   b. In large animals, incorporate about 1.5 mm of tissue on each side of the wound and place sutures 1.5 to 2 mm apart. If the cornea is edematous, more cornea should be incorporated in the suture.

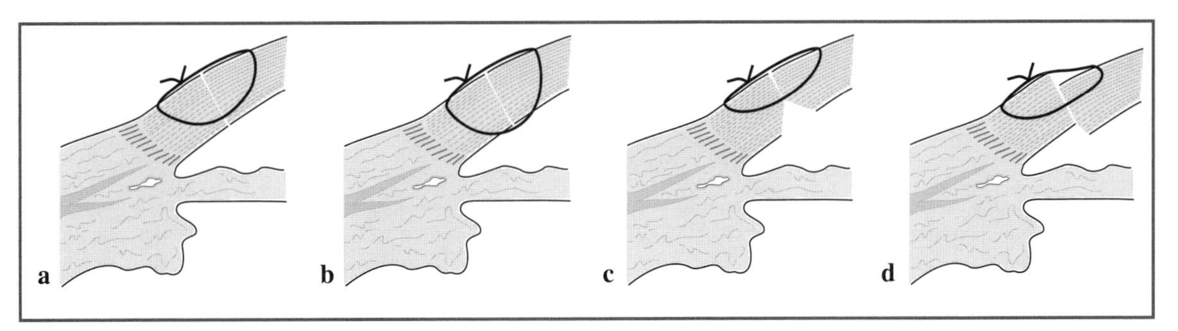

Figure 4-4. Corneal suturing.
- a. Properly placed corneal suture
- b. Suture too deep; perforating into anterior chamber
- c. Suture too superficial; endothelium not sealed properly. This will result in excess corneal edema.
- d. Suture unevenly placed. This results in poor apposition of the wound edge.

Establishing the anterior chamber

Maintain the anterior chamber so that anterior synechia can be avoided.

1. Irrigation - Using BSS or saline, with or without epinephrine. Irrigate when fibrin becomes obvious or when blood fills the anterior chamber.
2. Air injection - Air is useful in maintaining the chamber during surgery and makes it easier to see the cross-sectional appearance of the corneal wound. If the wound is near the limbus, air will remain in the anterior chamber during suturing. If the wound is central, air will escape when corneal sutures are placed. When the wound is closed to the point that only one or two sutures are needed, air will generally remain.
3. At the termination of surgery:
    a. Irrigation - If the anterior chamber is deep and the iris does not have any tendency toward anterior synechia, fill the chamber with irrigating solution. Inject only enough fluid to restore the shape of the eye and depth of the anterior chamber. Leave the eye soft. Let newly forming aqueous restore intraocular pressure.
    b. Air injection (Fig 4-5) - If the anterior chamber is shallow, air can be injected to reduce anterior synechia formation. Inject only enough air to separate the iris from the corneal wound. Do not inflate the anterior chamber completely. Excess air can result in transient interference in aqueous flow. The air is generally injected with a 27 or 30 gauge needle before the last suture is tied.

        If the wound leaks air during injection, air can be injected at the limbus with a 25 to 27 gauge needle. The needle can be used as an iris spatula to break down adhesions as air and/or dilute epinephrine are injected.

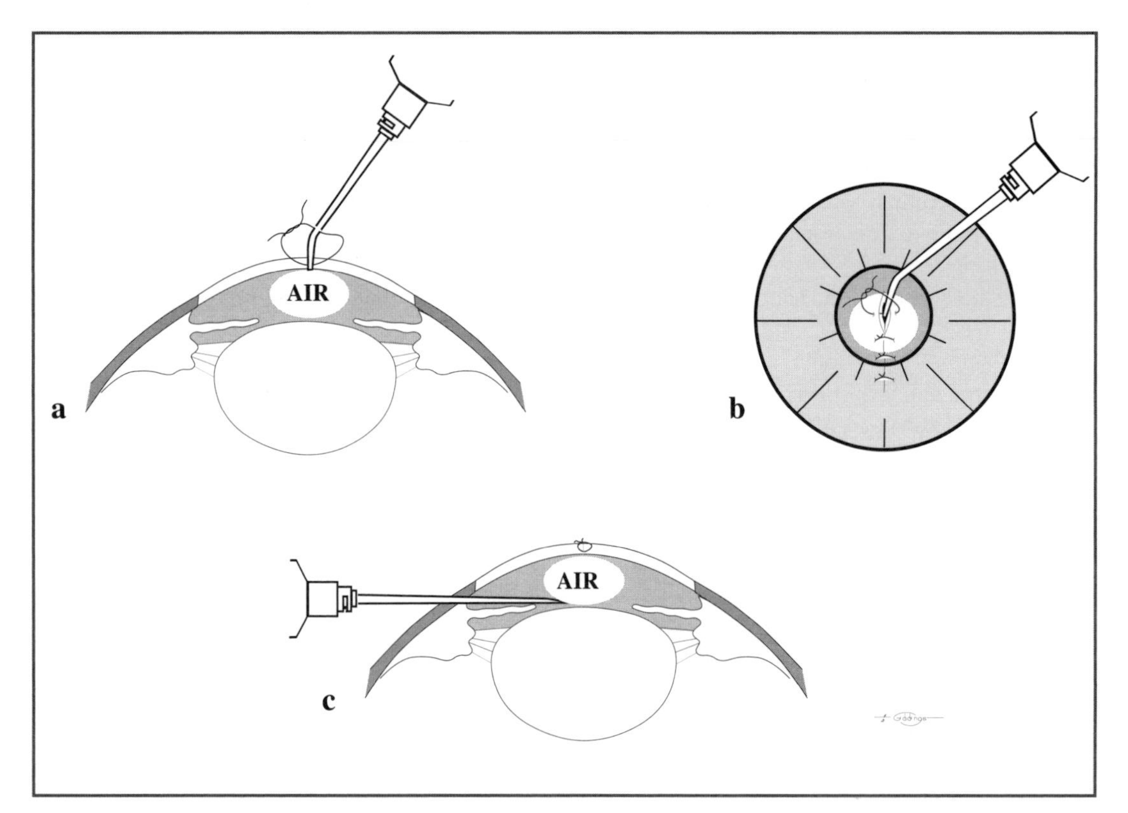

Figure 4-5. Injecting air into the anterior chamber.
- a & b. Lateral and frontal views of injecting air through the wound with a 30 gauge air injection cannula before the last suture is tied
- c. Lateral view of injecting air with a 25 to 27 gauge needle passed through the sclera.

c. Excess fibrin formation - Intracameral injection of 25 μg tissue plasminogen activator (tPA) will dissolve fibrin and relieve synechiae.

4. Canthotomy closure - The canthotomy should be closed with a figure-eight suture and as many interrupted sutures as necessary (see closing eyelid lacerations; Chapter 5, page 177). An absorbable suture versus nonabsorbable is the surgeon's choice.

   After closing the canthotomy, it may be necessary to protect the eye (see methods of protecting the cornea, below) or fit the patient with an Elizabethan collar.

Medical aftercare for intraocular surgery

1. Antibiotics
   a. Topical as long as needed
   b. Systemic
      1) Elective surgery recommended for three to five days. If sterile surgical techniques are maintained, postoperative antibiotics may not be needed.
      2) Emergency surgery - five days or as long as deemed necessary
2. Mydriatics - until uveitis disappears
3. Corticosteroids
   a. Topical - can be used immediately if the cornea is healthy
   b. Systemic
      1) Elective - started immediately postoperatively when sterile technique was maintained
      2) Emergency surgery - started as soon as the danger of intraocular infection passes or appropriate systemic antibiotics are started. The sooner corticosteroids are started after intraocular surgery, the less the chance of problems from postsurgical uveitis.
   c. Subconjunctival - use is determined by the procedure being performed. Do not use in septic eyes.
4. Antiprostaglandins - can be used any time. Usually they are not as effective as corticosteroids, but they do not have any ocular contraindications.

Suture removal (for nonabsorbable sutures)

1. Eyelids - Fourteen days is recommended, especially with sutures that cause minimal tissue reaction.
2. Corneal sutures - nonabsorbable sutures can be removed after 14 days. If the cornea is vascularized, sutures can be removed when the vascularization crosses over the wound.

METHODS OF PROTECTING THE CORNEA (GLOBE)

Bandage over the eye
Collagen shield (see Chapter 2, page 74)
Extended wear contacts (see Chapter 2, page 73)
Third eyelid flaps
Suturing eyelids together (tarsorrhaphy)
Combination third eyelid flap/tarsorrhaphy

Third eyelid suturing techniques

There are two basic ways of suturing the third eyelid: suture the third eyelid to the bulbar conjunctiva or the upper eyelid. These techniques usually require general anesthesia. A previous traumatic proptosis of the eye will be followed by scar tissue formation that will immobilize the third eyelid in the nasal canthus. If at a later date one of these patients should require corneal protection, it may be necessary to do a tarsorrhaphy.

1. Third eyelid sutured to bulbar conjunctiva (Fig 4-6)
   a. Technique - Three overlapping horizontal mattress sutures are placed in the third eyelid and bulbar conjunctiva. An additional simple interrupted suture might be placed at either end of the overlap if the cornea is not adequately covered. When placing the sutures, be sure that the suture goes through the cartilage of the third eyelid and that the conjunctival suture is in the loose fold of conjunctiva, about 5 mm from the limbus. Tie each suture as it is placed. Notice that the bulbar conjunctiva is very mobile and will pull over the cornea. If the suture is placed in the episclera, the conjunctiva will not be mobile. Cut the suture ends at least 5 mm long. The suture is visible and can be easily removed. When sutures are placed in this manner, the eye and third eyelid move as a single structure without movement between them. This is the advantage compared to suturing the third eyelid, the upper eyelid, or tarsorrhaphy. The conjunctiva is so moveable that it covers one-third of the cornea, and the third eyelid the remaining two-thirds.
   b. Small animals - Six-0 silk is used routinely. If a large breed or excessive tension, 4-0 or 5-0 silk. In dogs, this technique will hold for 7 to 21 days; 7 to 10 days in exophthalmic patients, 10 to 14 days in most dogs and up to three weeks if eyes are deep set. Use topical anesthetic drops to anesthetize the adnexa for removing the sutures. In cats the third eyelid may remain in position for longer than four weeks.
   c. Equine - This technique will hold for 3 to 10 days; three to seven days in exophthalmic patients and 5 to 10 days in enophthalmic. Use topical anesthetic drops to anesthetize the adnexa for removing the suture. Three-0 or 4-0 silk is routinely used.
   d. *Comment.* Do not leave the sutures in place too long. If they loosen and rub the cornea, they may cause a corneal epithelial erosion. If this happens, remove the sutures. The corneal erosion will heal in three to five days.

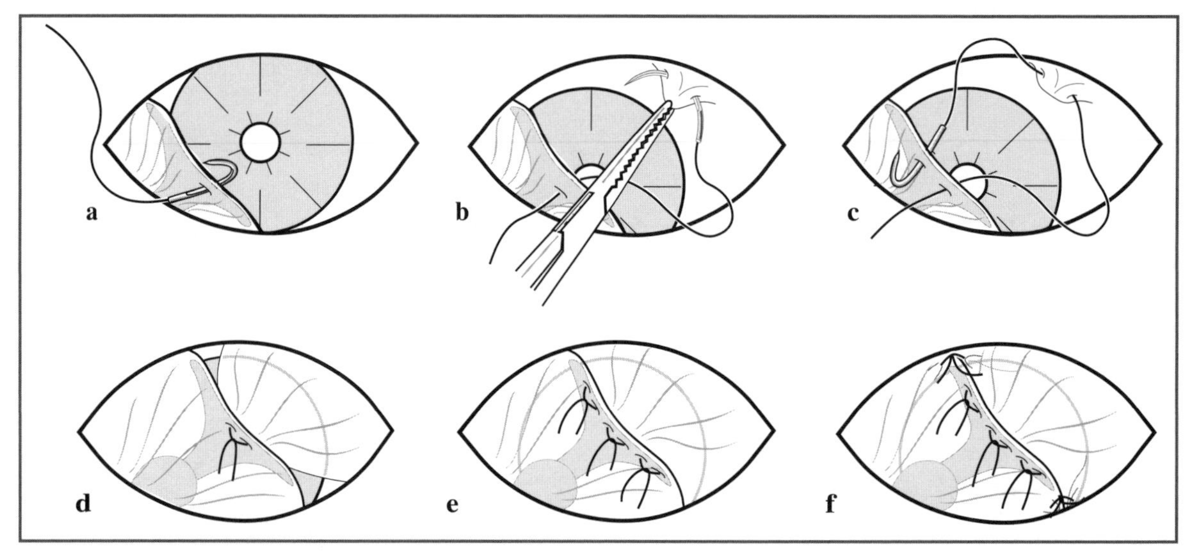

Figure 4-6. Third eyelid sutured to bulbar conjunctiva.
   a. The center suture is placed first. Identify the central portion of the cartilage of the third eyelid and pass the suture needle through the third eyelid, catching the cartilage about 1 mm from its edge.
   b. A horizontal mattress suture placed in the bulbar conjunctiva about 5 to 7 mm from the limbus. Pick up the bulbar conjunctiva with a forceps to be sure it is freely mobile.
   c. The suture needle is passed through the third eyelid from the bulbar side, again catching the edge of the cartilage.
   d. The suture is tied. If the suture has been properly placed, the entire cornea will be covered by the third eyelid as it slides over the conjunctiva.
   e. Second and third sutures are placed in the same manner, catching the nasal and temporal limits of the cartilage.
   f. Additional simple interrupted sutures may be needed to properly cover the cornea of dogs with large eyelid openings or a prominent eye.

2. Third eyelid sutured to upper eyelid (Fig 4-7)
   a. Technique - Overlapping horizontal mattress sutures are used. The suture is started by passing the needle through the upper eyelid at the base of tarsal glands. Next, a horizontal mattress stitch is placed through the anterior surface of the third eyelid, making sure to catch the cartilage. Then the suture is brought back out through the upper eyelid. Preplace three sutures before tying any of them. The suture knots will lie on the outside surface of the upper eyelid. If the eye is exophthalmic or there is extra tension on the sutures, the sutures may pull through the eyelid before the cornea is healed. This rarely occurs but can be prevented by positioning a button, a piece of split rubber tubing, a length of wide rubber band or umbilical tape on the outer surface of the eyelid. Suture through the stent as the suture is placed in the eyelid. This will distribute pressure evenly over the eyelid.

      This technique will hold longer than third eyelid to conjunctiva technique but has the disadvantage of allowing some movement between the eye and the third eyelid.
   b. Small animals - 6-0 silk is used routinely and 4-0 or 5-0 in large breeds. This suture pattern gives longer support to the eye than suturing the third eyelid to the bulbar conjunctiva and will hold for two to four weeks in dogs and four or more in cats.
   c. Large animals - This is preferred method of third eyelid suturing because it lasts one to two weeks. Routinely, use 4-0 silk; 2-0 or 3-0 can be used if there is excessive tension or the tissues are edematous.

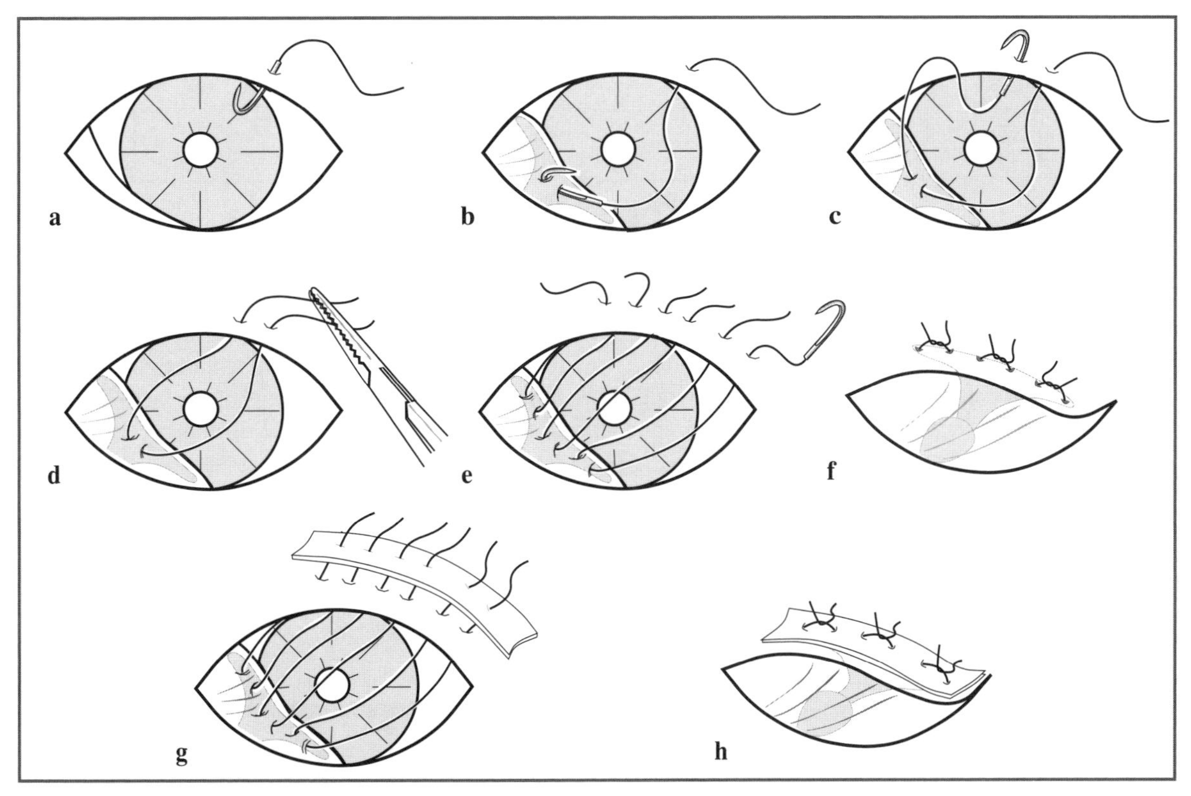

Figure 4-7. Suturing third eyelid to upper eyelid.
- a. Directing the needle through the eyelid immediately above the base of the meibomian glands
- b. Placing the needle in anterior surface of third eyelid incorporating the central portion of the cartilage about 1 mm from its outer edge
- c. Passing the needle through upper eyelid from inside to outside completing sliding horizontal mattress stitch
- d. Free ends of suture are tagged with hemostatic forceps so the remaining two stitches can be preplaced
- e. Three preplaced sutures
- f. All sutures tied
- g. Sutures preplaced through wide rubber band
- h. Sutures tied over wide rubber band

Suturing eyelids together (tarsorrhaphy)

Tarsorrhaphy is the simplest way to protect the eye and requires only a line block (Chapter 2, page 102) for anesthesia. It is most frequently used in horses but is indicated in small animals when the third eyelid is immobile or the eye is extremely exophthalmic. It does not protect the cornea as well as a third eyelid flap because of greater movement between the cornea and the eyelids.

1. Through-and-through suturing (Fig 4-8) - This can be a simple interrupted or horizontal mattress suture pattern. Simple interrupted sutures are the easiest to place. Unfortunately, they rub the cornea and often produce irritation leading to ulceration. Horizontal mattress sutures give better support, but still may rub the cornea.

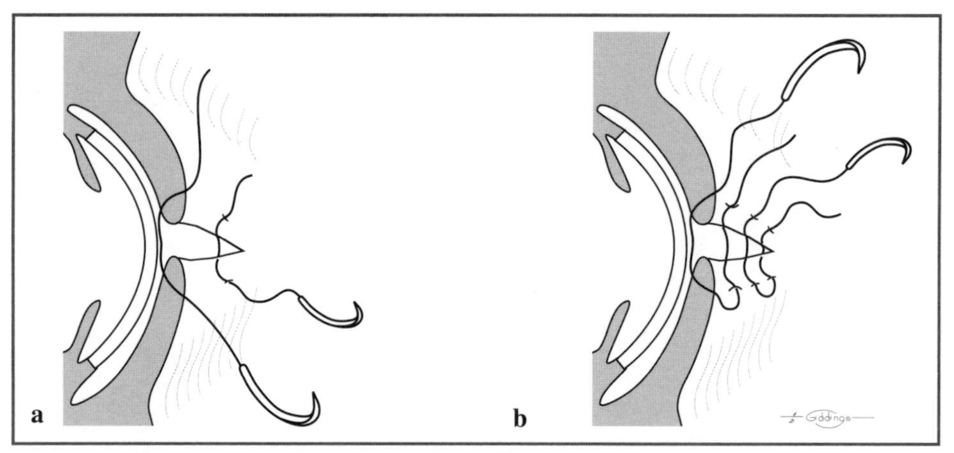

Figure 4-8. Through-and-through eyelid sutures.
a. Cutaway diagram showing position of simple interrupted suture
b. Cutaway diagram of horizontal mattress suture

2. Split-thickness horizontal sutures (Fig 4-9) - This gives the best support and the suture strands between the eyelids do not rub the cornea. Three sutures are adequate in large animals, two or three in small animals, depending on the size of the palpebral opening. The sutures should be placed well behind the tarsal glands and emerge from the edge of the eyelid at or slightly in front of the openings of the tarsal glands. The sutures will hold up to six weeks. It is not unusual for slight separation of the eyelids by three weeks. Monofilament nylon is recommended, 2-0 in large animals, and 4-0 to 5-0 in small animals. Excessive tissue reaction occurs with silk suture.

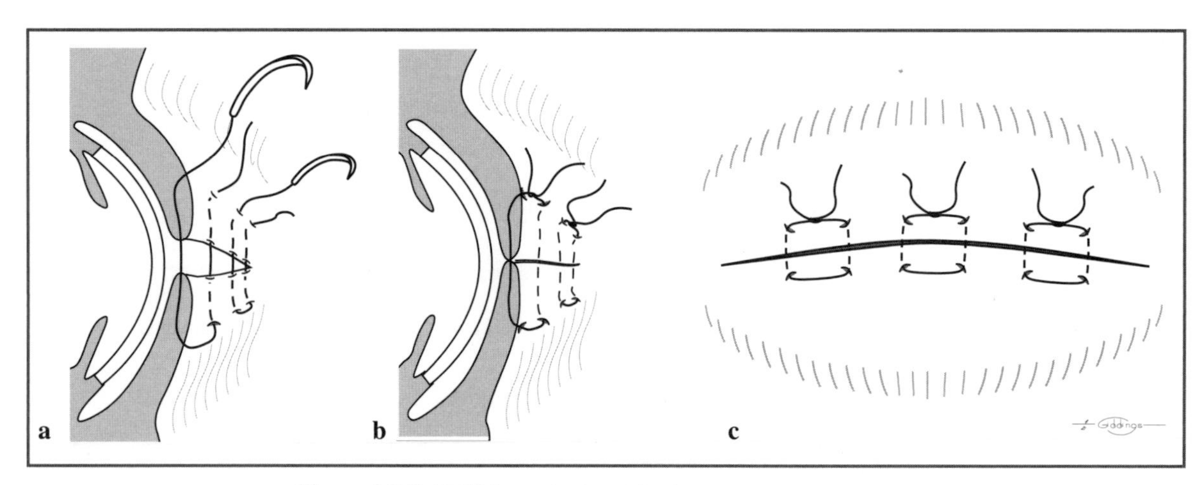

Figure 4-9. Split thickness horizontal sutures.
a. Cutaway diagram of preplaced split thickness sutures
b. Cutaway diagram of tied split thickness sutures
c. Appearance of eyelids sutured together

Bovine techniques

Simplified techniques combining third eyelid and eyelid suturing have been developed for cattle. This protects the cornea from suture erosion that would result from suture going through the eyelid only. Sutures can be placed without anesthesia in an animal restrained in a chute or a calf held on the ground. Protecting the cornea is the most important step in treating deep and severe ulcers in cattle with infectious bovine keratoconjunctivitis (Chapter 8, page 265). The author has seen this suture pattern used in small animals and horses but does not recommend it because there is inherent danger of scarring that would not be cosmetic. Absorbable sutures are recommended so that suture removal will not be needed. Number 1 suture in adults and 2-0 or 3-0 in calves.

1. Multiple suture technique (Fig 4-10) - This consists of a continuous suture placed through the eyelids and incorporating the cartilage of the third eyelid. After placing the suture, it may be cut and tied as are simple interrupted sutures.

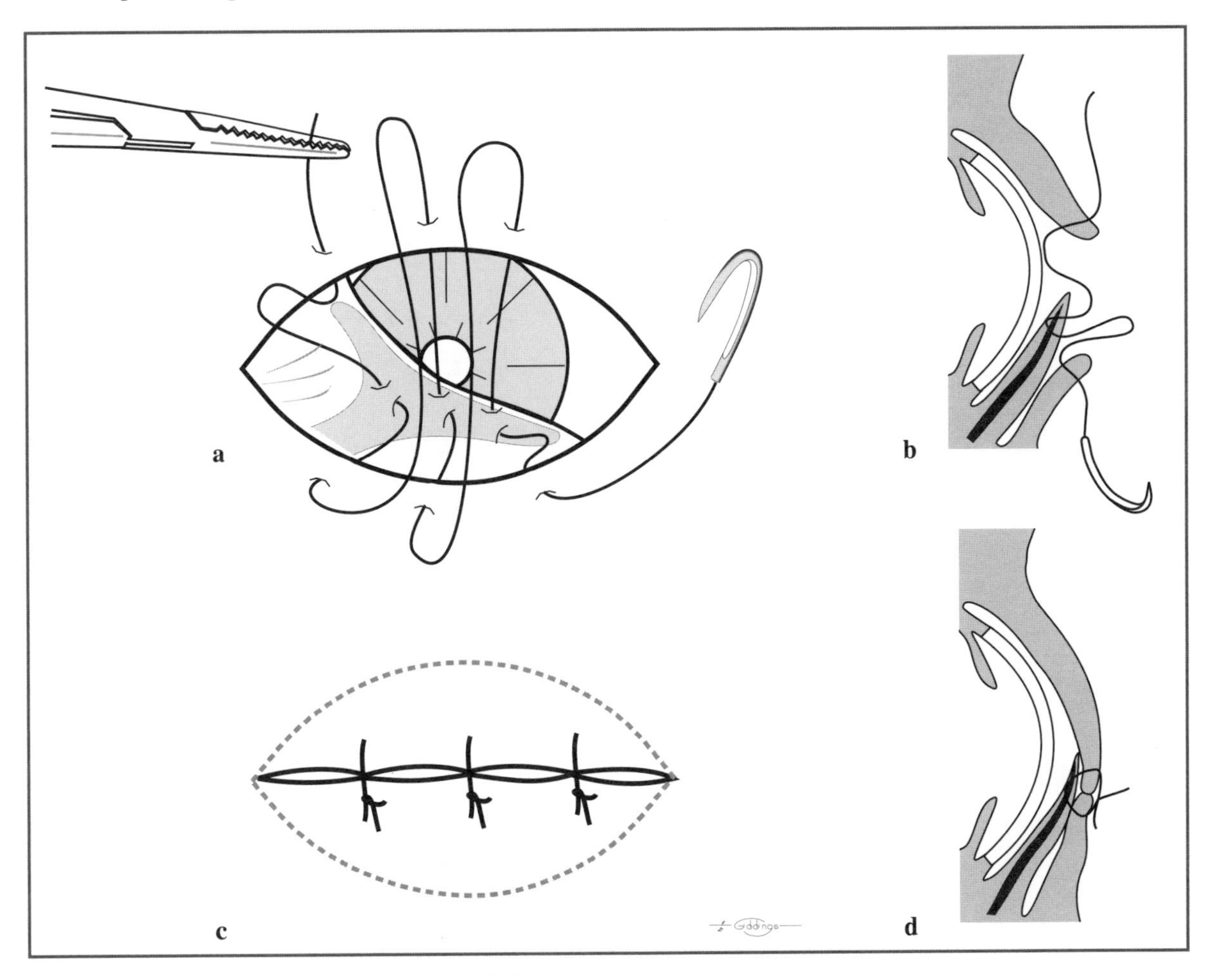

Figure 4-10. Multiple suture technique
a. Diagram of suture passed through the eyelids and incorporating the third eyelid. It can be placed as a continuous suture, then cut and tied simple interrupted
b. Cutaway diagram showing placement of one suture
c. Appearance of eyelids when suturing is complete
d. Cutaway diagram showing one suture tied

2. Single suture technique (Fig 4-11) - This is the fastest and least discomforting to the patient. The pattern is started by passing the suture through the eyelid at least 1 cm below the lateral canthus. Next, the needle is passed through the cartilage horizontal to the border of the third eyelid, and the final stage is to direct the needle from the inside of the eyelid out at least 1 cm above the lateral canthus. When this mattress suture is tied, it will pull the third eyelid toward the temporal canthus as the outer one-third of the eyelid is closed by the suture.

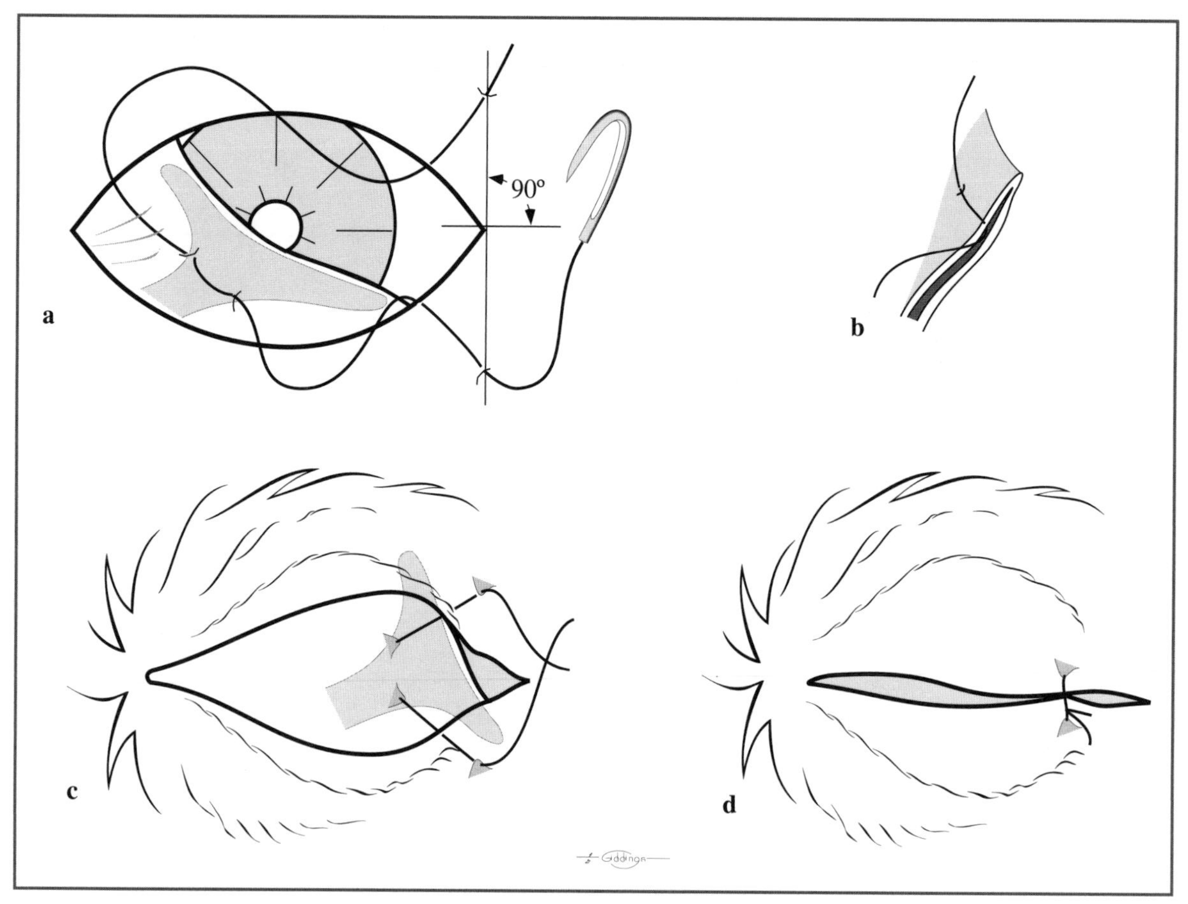

Figure 4-11. Bovine single suture tarsorrhaphy.

a. The suture is passed through the eyelid 1 cm above the lateral canthus. Next the third eyelid cartilage is included and the suture brought out through the lower eyelid 1 cm below the canthus.
b. Placement of the suture in third eyelid cartilage
c. Applying tension to suture draws third eyelid across the cornea
d. Appearance of the eyelids when suture is tied

CHAPTER 5 - EYELIDS

ANATOMY

The eyelids are the major protection for the eye (Fig 5-1).

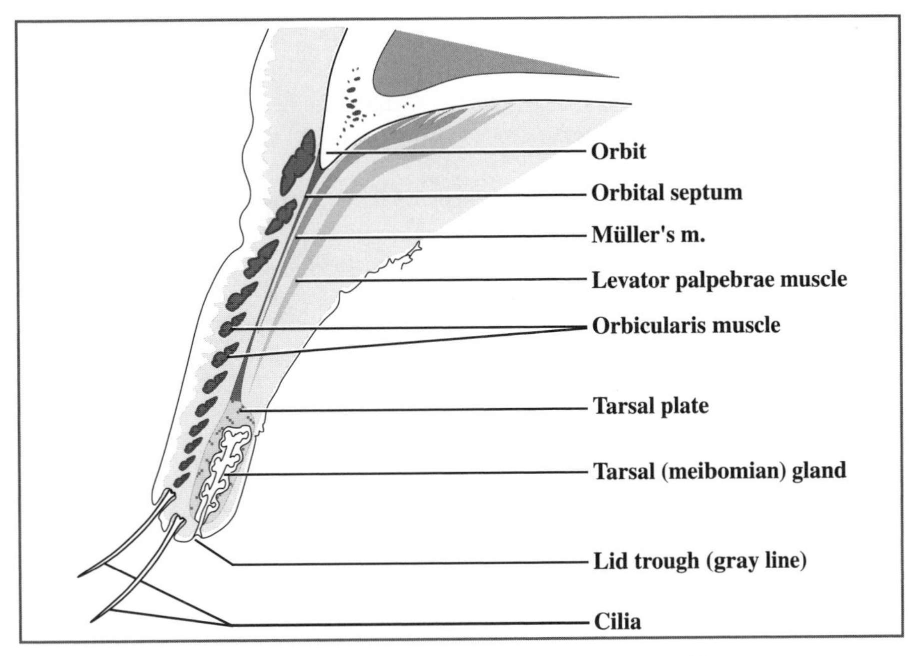

Figure 5-1. Schematic cross-section of upper eyelid.

MUSCLES AND MOTOR NERVE SUPPLY

Orbicularis m. is a sphincter muscle located immediately under the skin that closes the palpebral fissure. It receives its motor supply from the palpebral branch of the facial nerve (CN-VII) and is responsible for the blink reflex and blepharospasm seen with ocular pain.

Levator palpebrae superioris m. originates from inside the orbit and is the main muscle elevating the upper eyelid. It receives its motor nerve supply from the oculomotor nerve (CN-III).

Müller's m. is smooth muscle originating from the levator in the upper lid and the ventral rectus in the lower lid. It is innervated by sympathetic fibers found in the ophthalmic branch of the trigeminal nerve (CN-V).

Three superficial facial muscles innervated by the facial nerve (CN-VII) also contribute to keeping the palpebral fissure open. They are:

1. Superciliaris muscle in the medial upper eyelid
2. Sphincter colli profundus pars palpebralis - has a palpebral portion in the lower eyelid
3. Retractor anguli oculi muscle - draws the lateral canthus laterally and accompanied by orbital fascia, functions as the lateral canthal ligament

SENSORY NERVE SUPPLY - is entirely trigeminal (CN-V)

Maxillary branch - zygomatic, lower eyelid; lacrimal, lateral canthus

Ophthalmic branch - infratrochlear, medial canthus; frontal (supraorbital), midportion upper eyelid

MEDIAL CANTHAL LIGAMENT - a well developed ligament anchored on the orbital rim and originating from the orbicularis oculi

ORBITAL SEPTUM - periosteum at the orbital rim continues as a fascial sheath in the eyelids to join the tarsus, thus acting as a barrier between the orbit and superficial eyelid

GLANDS OF THE EYELIDS

The meibomian glands (tarsal glands) are long sebaceous glands in the tarsal plate. Contribute the oil layer of the tear film. Infection can result in pyogranuloma called chalazion.

The glands of Zeis are modified sebaceous glands connected with the follicles of the eyelashes.

The glands of Moll are sweat glands located in the same area as the glands of Zeis. In man, staphylococcus infection of the glands of Zeis or Moll is referred to as hordeolum or sty.

EYELASHES (CILIA)

Dog - present on upper lid, absent on lower

Cat - poorly developed, not true eyelashes

Equine - many upper lid lashes, few lower

Bovine, ovine and camelids - many upper lid lashes, few lower

FUNCTION OF THE EYELID

To protect the eye via blink reflexes

1. Sensory
    a. Mechanical stimulation of the cilia and vibrissae
    b. Corneal and conjunctival stimulation
2. Optical - menace and dazzle reflexes

Remove foreign matter from the eye

Provide tear components - especially the lipid layer

Redistribute tear film - tear film breakup occurs in 20 seconds or less, resulting in dry areas on the cornea. Evaporation accounts for about 25% of tear loss.

Provide tear removal

1. Blinking propels tears nasally
2. Puncta located in the eyelids at the medial canthus are the entry sites for passage of tears down the nasolacrimal drainage system

When eyelids are closed

1. Provide oxygen for the cornea
2. Remove visual stimuli and light reduction
3. The eyelids exclude 60 to 70% of light from entering the eye

CONGENTIAL CONDITIONS OF THE EYELIDS

AGENESIS

Absence of all or part of the eyelid. Sometimes referred to as coloboma (a congenital cleft or fissure). It occurs infrequently but is seen in small animals more frequently than large animals. Check these patients carefully for concurrent congenital abnormalities in the iris and lens. Inheritance has been proposed in sheep and Burmese cats.

Upper eyelid agenesis in cats

1. Signs are present at birth but many are not presented until several months of age
   a. Bilateral defect in the upper eyelid beginning at the temporal canthus and extending a variable distance toward the nasal canthus
   b. Mild cases may present with mild keratitis with temporal skin hair directed toward the cornea
   c. Severe cases may have blepharospasm, marked trichiasis, keratoconjunctivitis sicca, and advanced exposure keratitis
   d. Examine for concurrent congenital ocular defects (especially iris and lens)
2. Treatments - kittens should be treated conservatively until they are better surgical candidates
   a. Mild cases may require cryoepilation for the misdirected hairs growing out over the cornea
   b. More severe cases are surgery candidates. Several procedures have been used.
      1) Rotating pedicle grafts from the lower eyelid (Figs 5-2, 5-3)

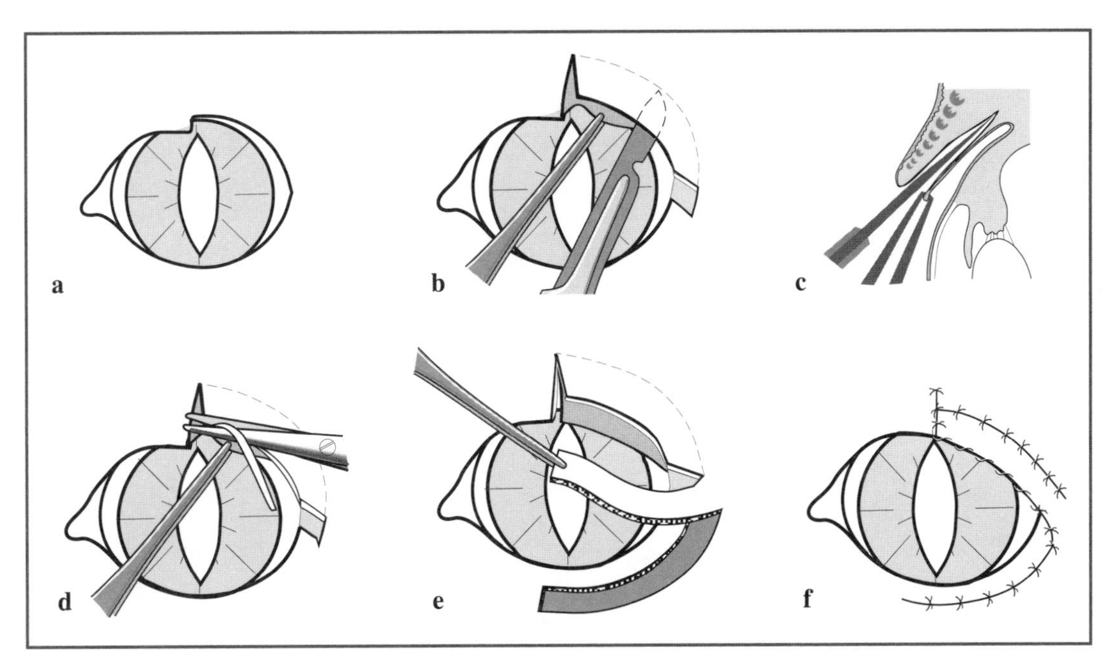

Figure 5-2. Repair of feline eyelid agenesis - pedicle graft from lower eyelid.
- a. Appearance of mild eyelid agenesis
- b. A skin incision is made perpendicular to the eyelid at the medial limit of the defect. The skin is separated from the conjunctiva and undermined to the lateral canthus. A block of skin is removed to allow the graft to line up with the eyelid edge.
- c. Cross-section demonstrating separating skin and conjunctiva
- d. Removal of the skin edge
- e. Donor skin is removed from the lower eyelid and rotated toward the area of agenesis. The conjunctiva is then cut along the length of the perpendicular eyelid incision. This will allow it to be extended down to cover the inside of the pedicle graft.
- f. The pedicle is sutured to the skin with interrupted nonabsorbable suture. Then the conjunctival edge is sutured to the pedicle with continuous suture and lastly the donor site is closed.

2) Rotating pedicle graft from the forehead
3) Blogg technique whereby the lateral canthal portion of lower eyelid is advanced to the medial border of the agenesis area. Then a lateral canthotomy is used to create a new canthus. (Agenesis of the feline upper eyelid. Feline Pract 1985;15:31-35.)

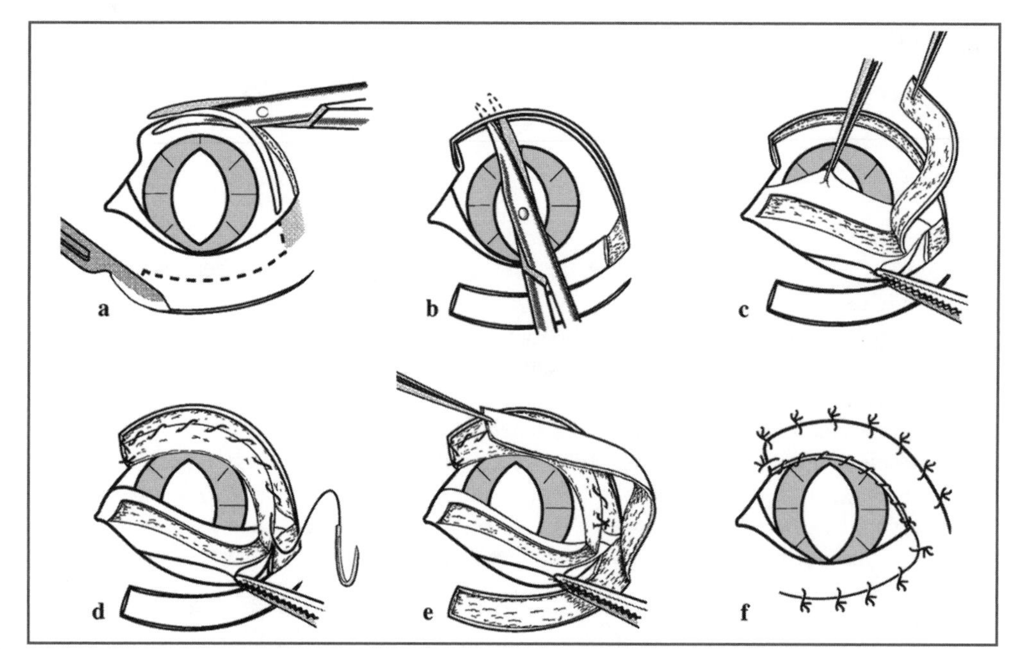

Figure 5-3. Pedicle lower eyelid graft with conjunctival pedicle graft from third eyelid. This technique is indicated when a pedicle skin graft would be inadequate (Dziezyc J, Millichamp NJ. Surgical correction of eyelid agenesis in the cat. Am Anim Hosp Assoc 25:513-516, 1989).

a. Appearance of severe eyelid agenesis
b. Separating skin in the area of the defect away from the globe. The pedicle graft is prepared and a small piece of skin is removed to allow the graft to line up with the recipient skin.
c. The graft is sutured to skin and the donor site partially closed
d. A pedicle of conjunctiva is removed from the third eyelid with the base extending onto the globe
e. The conjunctival pedicle is rotated 180° and sutured to the limbal conjunctiva beneath the skin graft
f. The edge of conjunctival graft is sutured to the edge of the skin graft and the final sutures are placed in the lower eyelid to close the donor site

SPLIT EYELID DEFORMITY IN JACOB SHEEP (FOUR-HORNED NAVAJO SHEEP)

Four-horned (polycerate) sheep may have a genetic eyelid deformity that ranges from a minor notch or complete split in the upper eyelids.

Pathogenesis

Related to division of the horn bud during fetal development. Changes in skull development and horn position may also occur.

Clinical signs

1. Eyelid deformity may vary from a tuft of eyelashes at the side of small notch to a complete split in the eyelid exposing the globe and orbital rim.
2. Tearing as a result of trichiasis from the eyelash tuft
3. Chronic keratitis with corneal scarring
4. Skull changes - incomplete orbit, vertical forehead, forward-growing horns
5. Polled ewes with eyelid lesions are genetically polycerate

Breeding significance

1. Rams with eyelid lesions are not recommended for breeding
2. Breeding two-horned rams to four-horned ewes reduces incidence
3. Breeding four-horned rams to four-horned ewes increases incidence

DERMOID OF THE EYELID Dermoid is the congenital misplacement of skin and its dermal appendages (hair, fat, glands).

Inheritance has been suggested but not defined in the Saint Bernard, German shepherd, Dalmatian, dachshund and Burmese cat.

Signs - Dermoids may involve the eyelids, globe or involve both.

1. The lateral canthus is most frequently involved, characterized by tufts of hair misdirected toward the eye. In addition to the eyelid, bulbar conjunctiva and cornea may be involved. Signs of ocular irritation are often minimal.
2. Small dermoids on the inside of lids may cause only slight epiphora and mild blepharospasm, In this case, eversion of the eyelid is required for diagnosis.

Treatment - Surgical removal is recommended.

1. If no secondary changes (epiphora, keratitis) - treatment would be for cosmetic reasons
2. Dermoids of the lateral canthus may be interpositioned between normally developed eyelids, in which case the dermoid can be removed and the wound closed similarly to a canthotomy.
3. Dermoids with extensive lid involvement usually require blepharoplastic reconstruction.

EYELASH DISEASES

Terminology (Fig 5-4)

1. *Trichiasis* - hair growing from a normally placed follicle directed toward the eye. This can be congenital or occur after eyelid injury.
2. *Distichiasis* - eyelashes growing from the tarsal gland toward the eye. This may vary from a cilium to a complete row of eyelashes. Upper or lower lids may be affected.
3. *Ectopic (atypical - aberrant), distichia* - cilium originating in a tarsal gland and growing through the conjunctiva directly toward the cornea. Rarely an ectopic cilium may come through the conjunctiva from a site beyond the tarsal gland.
4. *Districhiasis* - more than one cilium growing out of a follicle - quite common.

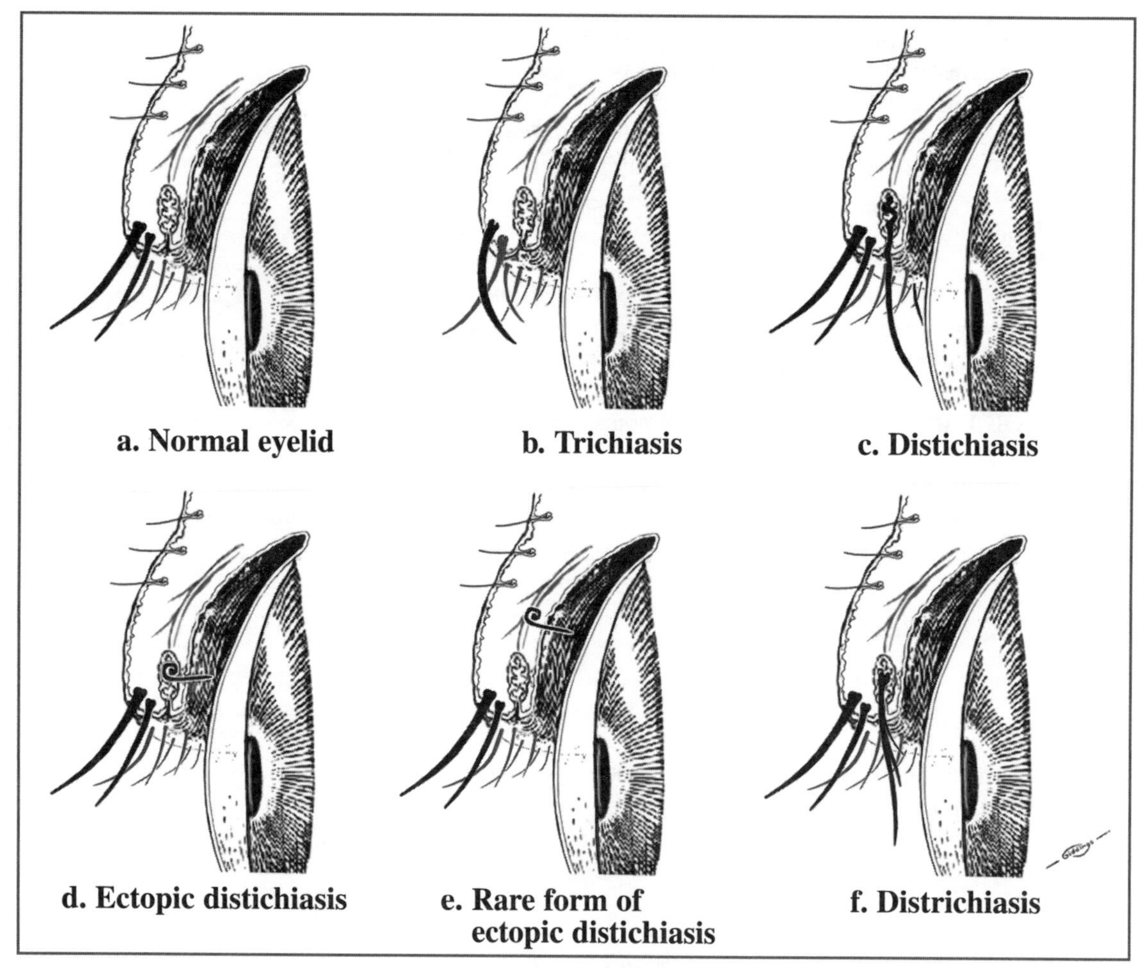

Figure 5-4. Schematic drawings of normal and abnormal eyelashes.

Incidence and clinical significance

1. Dogs
   a. Trichiasis - usually secondary to breed conformation with treatment directed toward correcting the primary cause. In veterinary medicine, all periocular hair touching the globe may be included in this category.
      1) Misdirected cilium - rare
      2) Toy breeds - occasionally seen as a congenital condition involving the temporal portion of the upper eyelid
      3) Brachycephalic breeds with nasal fold and/or caruncle hair contacting the eye
      4) Entropion resulting in hair directed to the cornea
   b. Distichiasis - the common form of eyelash disease. Upper and lower eyelids can be involved. Inheritance is involved. Very common in the cocker spaniel and poodle, and less frequent occurrence in many breeds. On repeated examinations the location and number may vary, indicating lashes fall out and are replaced similarly to skin hair.
      1) Silky lashes may occur that float in the tear film without causing irritation (seen in poodles and cockers). In this case treatment may not be recommended.
      2) Coarse stiff lashes are more common in other breeds. These lashes are irritating if they touch the cornea and often require treatment.
   c. Atypical - uncommon, but is the most painful form of distichiasis. The pain causes blepharospasm, thus the lid applies more pressure on the cornea and in turn can cause a corneal erosion. Generally only one lash is involved but occasionally several will be found. Both eyes are rarely involved. This can be observed in animals of all ages, indicating that the ingrown lash may be present for years before it penetrates the conjunctiva. Close examination of the tarsal gland area may reveal follicles that contain a nonemerged cilium.
2. Cats - primary eyelash disease is uncommon
   a. Trichiasis
      1) Trichiasis - from upper eyelid agenesis
      2) Entropion
      3) Nasal fold trichiasis in Persians
   b. Distichiasis - occurs occasionally; when seen, are coarse stiff lashes
3. Equine - very rare
   a. Trichiasis - acquired after eyelid injury
   b. Distichiasis - rarely seen. Will be coarse stiff lashes that require treatment if they touch the cornea
4. Bovine - not reported but undoubtedly occurs

Signs - chronic irritation

Examination with a loupe and penlight is recommended. Misdirected lashes may be normal in size, but often are very fine, short and pale in color, and therefore are not easily detected. If drops of moisture can be seen on the meibomian border of the eyelid when a penlight is directed on the eyelid, the examiner will find this tear droplet is held by a misplaced cilium.

1. Epiphora
2. Pain - if mild, the owner may notice increased blinking; if severe, blepharospasm may result in entropion
3. Corneal changes as a result of chronic irritation
   a. Scarring
   b. Superficial pigmentation
   c. Ulceration - distichiasis is a common cause for refractory ulcers seen in a referral practice
      1) True distichiasis probably is not capable of causing an ulcer. However, when a corneal epithelial injury occurs, the blepharospasm from the injury will result in the distichia preventing healing of the injury.
      2) Atypical distichia are capable of causing an ulcer.

Treatment of distichiasis - magnification is recommended to identify the abnormal cilia. Premedication with flunixin meglumine two hours before surgery will reduce post-treatment swelling.

1. Cilia forceps epilation - this is a temporary treatment because the eyelash will grow back in four weeks. Indicated for short term relief.
2. Electrolysis
    a. Types - Several types are available, but are tedious to use if there are more than a few lashes. The use of electrosurgical equipment is not advised because severe and irreversible damage to the eyelids can result. An economical epilator is available (Vetko-33 epilator, Vetko) (Fig 5-5).

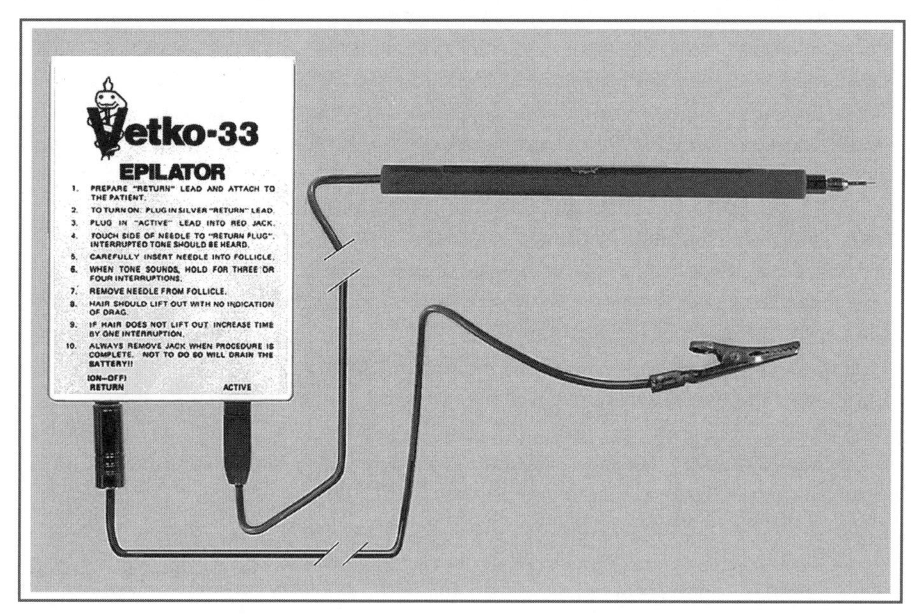

Figure 5-5. Vetko-33 epilator. Has a standardized 2 to 3 milliamperes current and a 3.5 second timing tone.

    b. Technique (Fig 5-6) - The epilation needle is inserted along the root of the cilium. Activation of the current will result in hydrogen bubbles coming out around the needle. The current is continued for 9 to 12 seconds. The cilium may come out when the needle is removed. If it does not, squeezing the tarsal gland with a cilia forceps may express the cilium. If it is still in place, grasp it with the ciliary forceps. Gentle traction should pull it from the follicle. If it is secure, repeat the electrolysis procedure. A broken cilium, or one that is forcefully pulled out, will regrow.

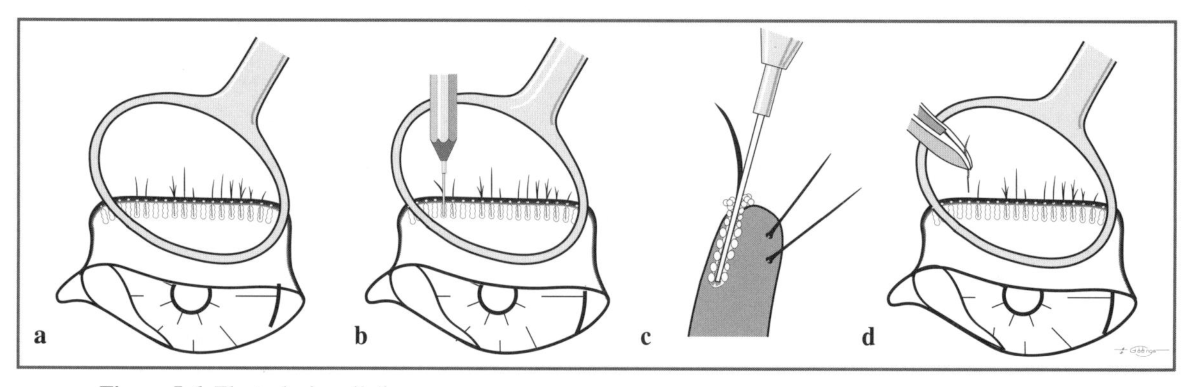

Figure 5-6. Electrolysis epilation.
a. Chalazion clamp in place
b. Electrolysis needle introduced into cilium bearing follicle
c. Apply current 9 to 12 seconds. Bubbles coming out around the needle indicate hydrolysis.
d. Removing cilium with forceps. If there is any resistance, the procedure should be repeated.

c. Complications
   1) Recurrence of lashes. This is the most common problem and occurs from incomplete electrolysis of the cilia-bearing meibomian gland. In young dogs, additional cilia may occur from glands that appear normal at the time of initial treatment.
   2) Eyelid damage from excess current. This can occur if surgical units are used at settings greater than 3 milliamperes.
   3) Damage to the punctum. Stay at least one meibomian gland away from the palpebral puncta. Misplaced lashes in this area usually touch the third eyelid and do not cause irritation.

3. Cryoepilation - this is the author's preferred method of treatment
   a. Equipment - Liquid nitrogen and nitrous oxide units are available. The cilium germinal epithelium is more sensitive to cryonecrosis (- 25°C) than the other eyelid tissues which are resistant to permanent damage from colder freezing temperatures (-30°C).
   b. Technique (Fig 5-7) - A chalazion (or Sontec tumor) lid forceps is placed on the eyelid to stabilize the eyelid and occlude blood flow. This facilitates a rapid freeze and a slow thaw. An appropriate probe is held against the basilar portion of the involved tarsal gland(s). The freeze is continued until the ice ball formed crosses the lid edge 1 to 2 mm. Slow thawing is facilitated by maintaining probe-tissue contact during the thawing period. A second freeze is recommended, especially if nitrous oxide is used. If liquid nitrogen is used, a single freeze may be adequate; this reduces some of the post freezing edema.
   c. Side effects
      1) Transient swelling for several days. Most pronounced in toy breeds. Premedication with Banamine one to two hours prior to treatment will reduce edema formation.
      2) Transient depigmentation of skin involved in the ice ball
      3) Permanent poliosis of eyelid hair
      4) Tissue slough if excessive freeze (-50°C)

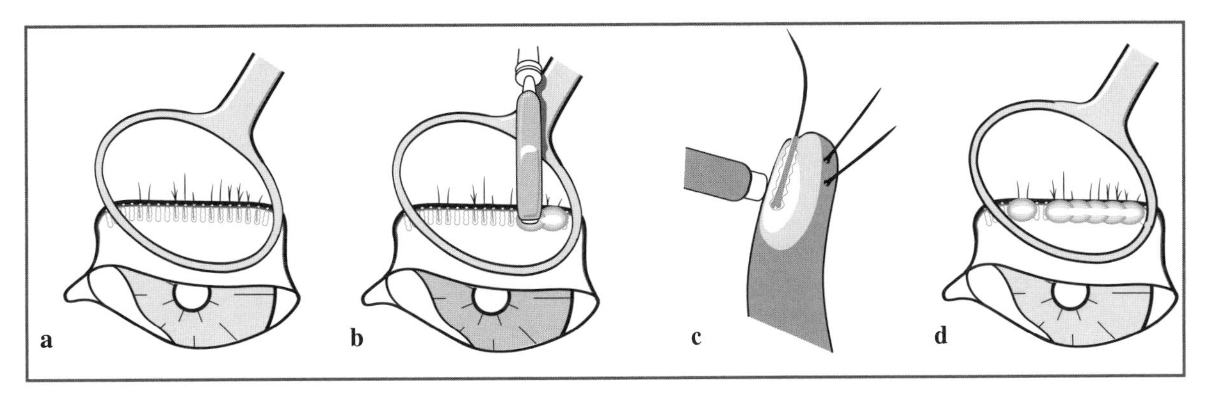

Figure 5-7. Cryoepilation.
- a. Chalazion clamp in place
- b. The cryoprobe is centered over the lower one-half of the tarsal gland
- c. Freezing is continued until iceball crosses eyelid edge 1 to 2 mm
- d. Multiple freezes can be made. When frozen areas thaw, perform a second freeze if using nitrous oxide.

4. Basal tarsal gland cautery (Riis RC. Basal meibomian gland cautery. Proc ASVO, 1982, pp 88-93) (Fig 5-8).
   a. Stabilize the eyelid with a chalazion forceps
   b. Electrocauterize the basilar portion of the tarsal gland containing the germinal epithelium
   c. Potential for complications
      1) Regrowth of cilia
      2) ***Excessive cauterization may result in tissue necrosis***

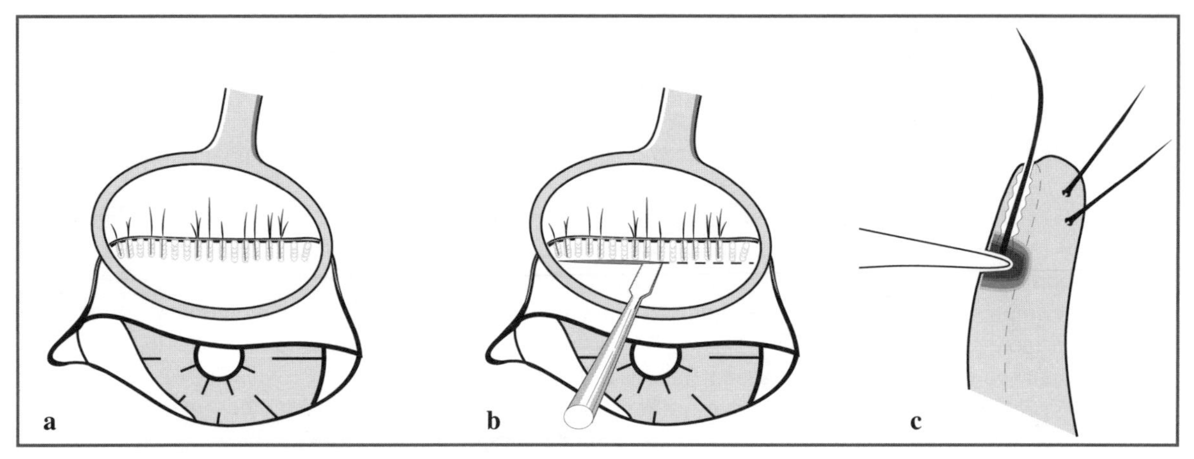

Figure 5-8. Basal tarsal gland cautery.
a. Eyelid stabilized with chalazion forceps
b. Electrocautery blade applied at the base of the tarsal glands containing germinal epithelium for the cilium
c. Cross section showing depth of cauterization

5. Transconjunctival resection of the base of the tarsal gland. Modified from Campbell LH. Conjunctival resection for canine distichiasis. J Am Vet Med Assoc 1977;171:275-277 (Fig 5-9).
   a. Stabilize the eyelid with a chalazion forceps
   b. The first incision is through the conjunctiva 1 to 1.5 mm below the tarsal gland opening parallel to the eyelid margin. The incision is deepened until the lashes have been cut. A second parallel incision is made below the base of the tarsal glands. This strip of tissue between the parallel incisions containing the base of the tarsal gland is removed.

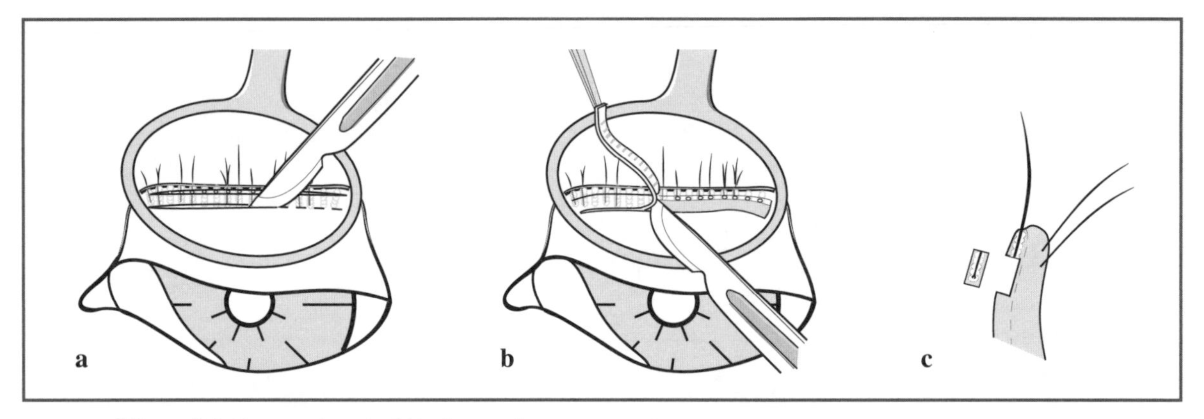

Figure 5-9. Transconjunctival block resection.
a. Eyelid stabilized with chalazion forceps. Incision through middle of tarsal glands.
b. Strip of tissue containing base of tarsal glands can be dissected free with a blade or scissors
c. Cross section showing block of removed tissue

6. Transconjunctival resection of the base of the tarsal gland with CO_2 laser surgery. After stabilization with a chalazion forceps, the base of affected tarsal glands can be individually resected. Excellent results.
7. Eyelid splitting. This procedure should not be done without thorough evaluation of the patient.
   a. Technique (Fig 5-10) - Choose patients with good thick eyelids that do not have any obvious deformities. Remove the cilia bearing meibomian gland with a very sharp blade such as a broken razor blade. The wound does not require suturing. Because of the high occurrence of complications, this technique cannot be recommended for routine use unless the surgeon is experienced.

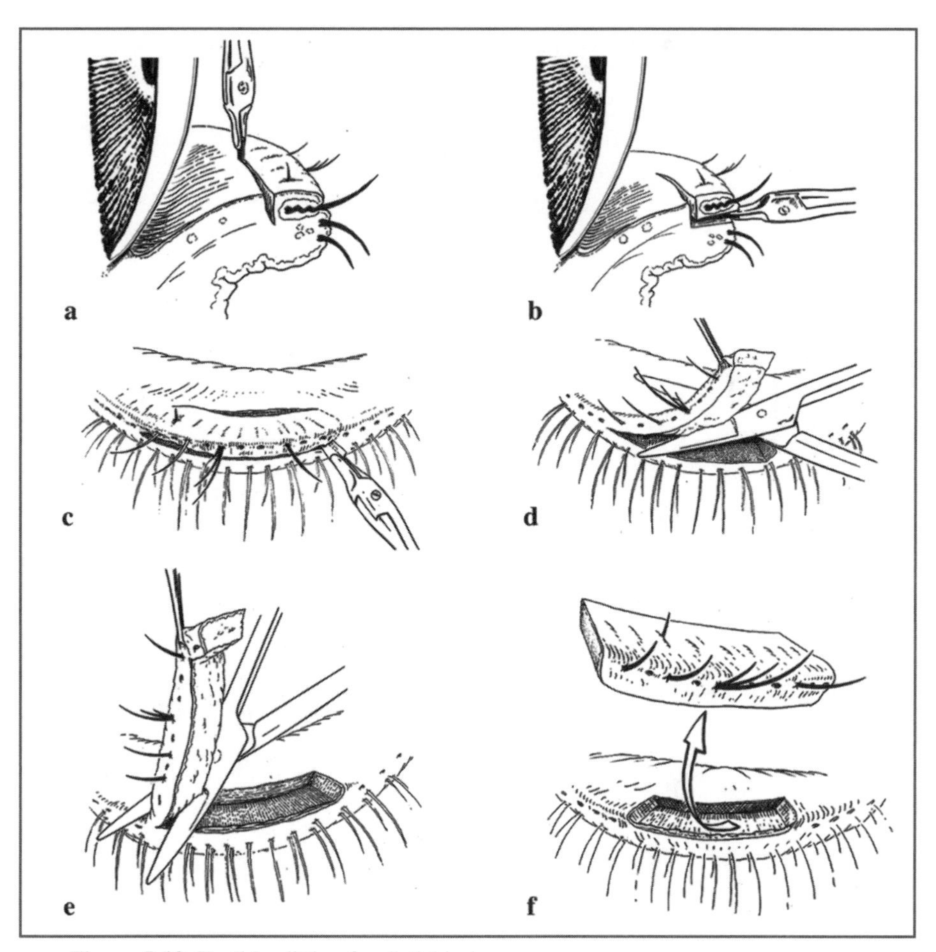

Figure 5-10. Eyelid splitting for distichiasis.

a. Incising the palpebral conjunctiva along the base of the affected meibomian glands
b. Splitting the eyelid to remove the affected meibomian gland
c. Turning the razor blade at a 45° angle to extend the incision toward the palpebral conjunctiva
d. Removing the affected meibomian glands by joining the two incisions
e. Cutting the affected tissue free with scissors. The angle of incision is 45°.
f. Appearance of eyelid after affected meibomian glands have been removed. Removed tissue is shown.

b. Complications

1) Recurrence of lashes. Incomplete removal of the affected meibomian gland will be followed by regrowth of a cilium that causes more irritation than the original lesion.
2) Entropion. If the eyelid is thin, postsurgical scar contraction can cause entropion when 1/2 or more of the lid is split.
3) Notching or shortening of the lid. If the tarsal plate is damaged or fractured prior to surgery, scar tissue contraction will result in a lid deformity.
4) Epiphora. If surgery is performed too near the nasal canthus, the punctum may be inadvertently removed. Keep the punctum visualized, or catheterize it with a nylon suture so that the incision can be stopped one or two meibomian gland openings away from the punctum.

Treatment of ectopic (atypical) distichiasis - Magnification and stabilization with a chalazion forceps is recommended.

1. Wedge resection (Fig 5-11) - Removing an eyelid wedge from the inner surface of the eyelid that contains the affected meibomian gland is a sure way of surgical correction. Fix the eyelid in a chalazion forceps and remove the affected tarsal gland with a sharp blade. The eyelid will heal uneventfully without suturing or medical treatment. If a corneal ulcer is present, examine it for

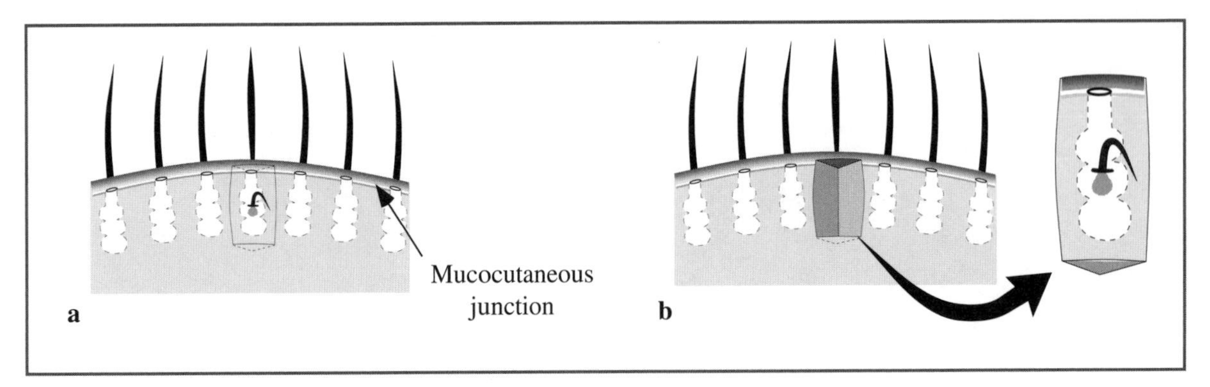

Figure 5-11. Ectopic cilium.
a. Schematic of everted eyelid showing ingrowing cilium. The area to be excised is shown.
b. Affected tarsal gland excised. A notch is present in the lid that will heal in two to three days.

undermining and treat accordingly (see corneal erosion; Chapter 10, page 323).
2. Cryoepilation - make a longitudinal incision in the affected tarsal gland to remove the atypical cilium and then freeze with a small cryoprobe.
3. CO_2 laser epilation - very effective

Treatment of trichiasis

1. Single lashes - cryosurgery or electroepilation
2. Toy breeds with temporal upper eyelid trichiasis - using the Hotz-Celsus entropion procedure, evert the edge of the eyelid until the eyelashes are in normal position.
3. Trichiasis due to conformation (nasal folds, caruncle hair, entropion) - correct the primary condition

CONGENITAL DISEASES OF THE PALPEBRAL PUNCTA

Incidence - Congenital palpebral punctal disease is common in dogs, especially cocker spaniels; infrequent in cats; extremely rare in other species.

Clinical findings

1. The puncta may be small
2. Absent (imperforate)
3. Misplaced (ectopic)

If both puncta are affected, epiphora will result. If the eyelid is normal and one normal punctum is present, epiphora should not occur.

Differential diagnosis of congenital punctal problems - Kittens may develop punctal and canaliculus scarring leading to occlusion as a complication to neonatal herpesvirus conjunctivitis. Thorough examination will differentiate this from congenital problems.

Treatment of small punctum - Chemical restraint and topical anesthetic usually adequate

1. Enlarge punctum with a punctal dilator, canaliculus knife or corneal scissors (Fig 5-12)
   a. Punctal dilator - can be inserted into the small punctum and as the dilator is advanced the punctum will be enlarged
   b. Canaliculus knife - has a blunt tip and a sharp cutting edge. After the blunt tip has been passed into the small punctum, the blade will enlarge the punctum by advancing and levering the sharp blade against the canaliculus wall.
   c. Corneal scissors - the most practical way because it does not require special instrumentation. One tip of the scissors is advanced into the small punctum to the depth desired and then the scissors closed. This incises the canaliculus wall to enlarge the punctum.
2. *Comment* - An enlarged palpebral punctum will not constrict at a later date.

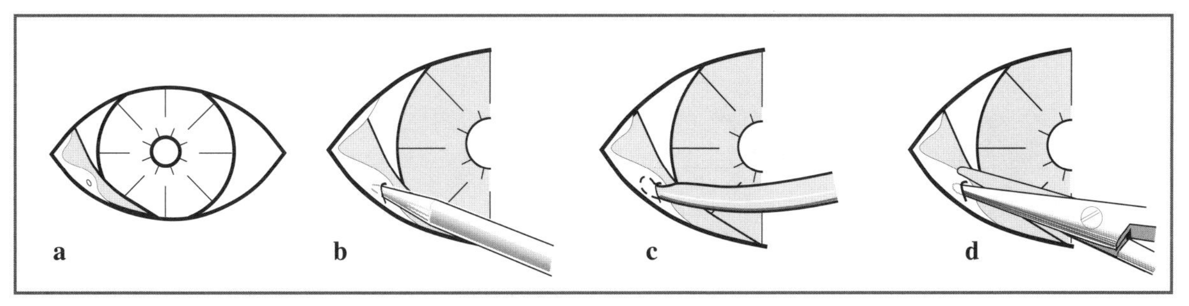

Figure 5-12. Punctum enlargement.
- a. Small punctum exposed by everting lower eyelid at nasal canthus
- b. Punctal dilator
- c. Canaliculus knife
- d. Corneal scissors

Treatment of imperforate palpebral puncta - Chemical restraint with topical anesthesia is often adequate but general anesthesia may be needed.

1. Single palpebral punctum
   a. Flushing other punctum (Fig 5-13) - cannulate the patent punctum with a lacrimal cannula and flush with PSS to produce a bleb at the site of imperforate punctum. Grasp the conjunctiva and incise or remove the conjunctiva with scissors.

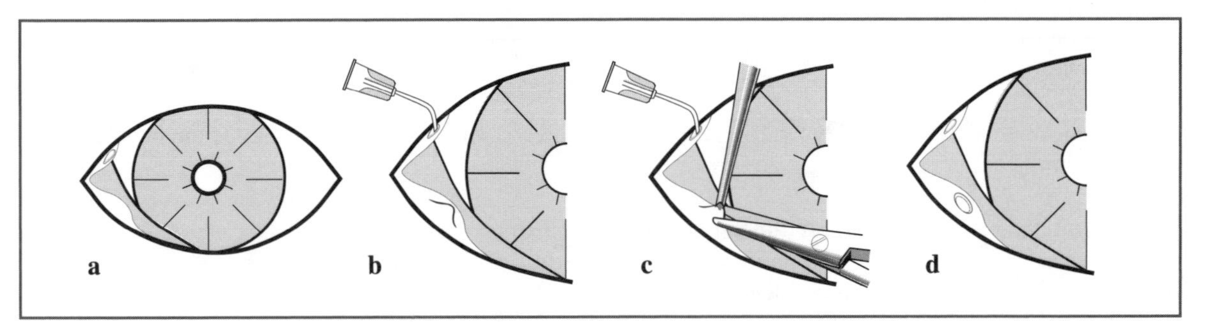

Figure 5-13. Flushing patent canaliculus to raise mucosal bleb over imperforate lower punctum.
- a. Imperforate lower punctum.
- b. Forming bleb by flushing through upper punctum
- c. Grasping bleb with forceps so mucosa over canaliculus can be cut to form new punctum
- d. Appearance after surgery

   b. If flushing the opposite punctum was unsuccessful, the canaliculus can be cannulated with a 25 gauge needle in the same manner as hitting a vein (Fig 5-14). Application of tension on the edge of the eyelid with a fixation or mosquito forceps will usually demonstrate a furrow in the eyelid representing the course of the palpebral canaliculus. If the canaliculus is not visualized, gentle pressure along the anticipated course with a dissecting probe or punctal dilator will usually outline it. Using a 25 gauge needle on a small syringe filled with PSS, the needle can be threaded into the canaliculus in the same manner as hitting a vein. Slowly inject PSS to determine if the canaliculus has been cannulated. After it has been cannulated, a blade can be used to cut the thin layer of conjunctiva over the needle to make a new punctum.

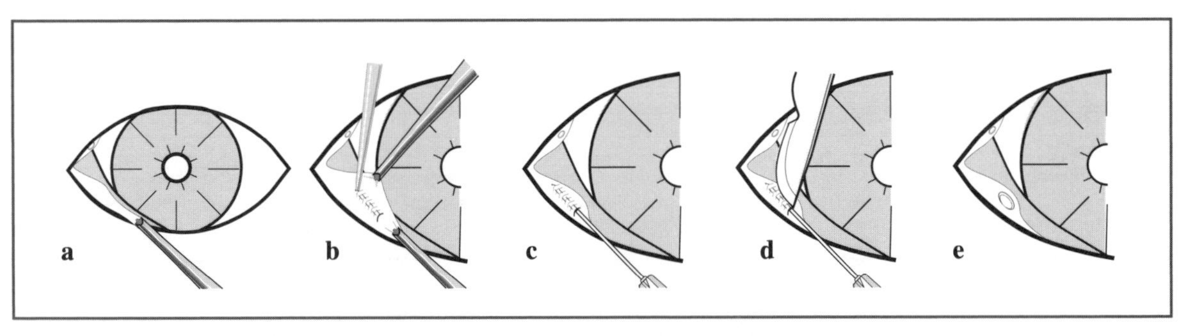

Figure 5-14. Cannulating lower canaliculus with 25 gauge hypodermic needle.
- a. Lower eyelid stabilized and everted with forceps
- b. Course of canaliculus outlined by pressure on it with a dissecting probe or punctal dilator. A second forceps placed on the mobile palpebral conjunctiva may be helpful in identifying the canaliculus.
- c. 25 gauge needle cannulating canaliculus
- d. Cutting down on needle with #15 Bard Parker blade
- e. Appearance of newly formed punctum

2. If both puncta are imperforate - general anesthesia recommended for small animals and llamas. Topical anesthesia and chemical restraint may be adequate for horses.
   a. Nasal punctum cannulation and retrograde flush and retrograde flush with PSS to produce bleb at the site of the imperforate puncta (Fig 5-15). Grasp conjunctival bleb and incise or remove with scissors. Retrograde flushing will not raise a bleb at the imperforate puncta if there is an opening in the nasolacrimal duct over the root of the carnassial tooth into the nostril.

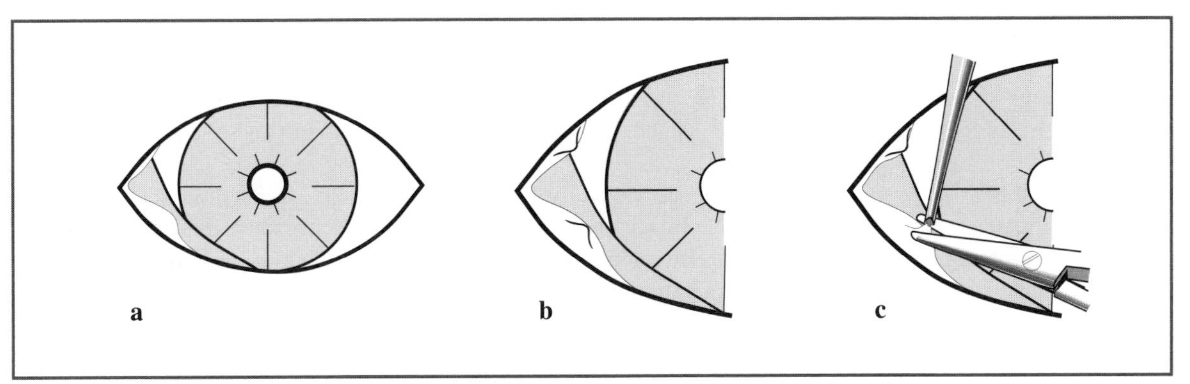

Figure 5-15. Retrograde flushing from nasal punctum when both puncta are imperforate.
a. Lower eyelid everted near canthus exposing area of imperforate punctum
b. Bleb forms over area of imperforate upper and lower puncta when flushing from nasal punctum
c. Grasping lower bleb with forceps so punctum can be formed with scissors

   b. Retrograde catheterization from the nasal punctum with monofilament nylon suture to palpebral canaliculum (Fig 5-16). Apply moderate pressure with the catheter to elevate the conjunctival membrane where the punctum should be. Then cut the membrane with scissors.
   c. If flushing and catheterization are unsuccessful - cannulating the palpebral puncta with a 25 gauge needle as previously described is recommended.
3. *Comment* - Reobstruction of an enlarged puncta has not been observed by the author.

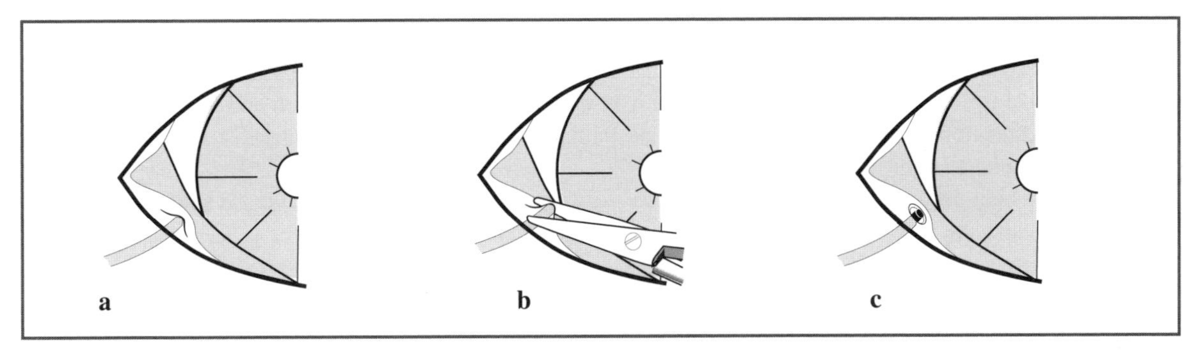

Figure 5-16. Retrograde catheter passed from nasal punctum to identify area of imperforate punctum.
a. Mucous membrane of imperforate punctum "tenting up" over tip of catheter
b. Cutting across "tented" mucosa to form punctum
c. Appearance of new punctum with catheter in place

ANKYLOBLEPHARON

Ankyloblepharon is an adhesion of the edges of the eyelids to each other. Precocious animals have their eyes open at birth. Animals that are not fully developed often open their eyes later.

Large animals - have their eyes open at birth. Premature births may still have ankyloblepharon. If this happens, the eyelids should be opened. If tearing is inadequate, topical antibiotic ointment is administered until tear production is adequate.

Cats and dogs - have congenital ankyloblepharon that persists into the second week of life. If the eyes have not opened by 14 to 16 days they should be opened. A small opening is present at the nasal canthus at birth.

Opening eyelids - Gentle traction on the lids will generally start to separate them. If this does not work, open them with corneal scissors. This can be done by slipping one tip of a corneal scissors into the nasal opening of the lid and forcing the scissors toward the lateral canthus. This will separate the eyelids along their border. If there is evidence of conjunctivitis, topical antibiotic ointments should be administered. DO NOT apply topical corticosteroids until the physiologic corneal edema disappears (1-3 days).

Neonatal conjunctivitis in puppies and kittens with ankyloblepharon

1. **Incidence and signs** - Conjunctivitis can occur in neonatal puppies and kittens before the lids separate. This will result in a noticeable swelling of the lids.
   a. Usually a small accumulation of discharge will be seen at the nasal canthus as a result of the small opening. All of the pups in the litter may be involved. This is usually a bacterial infection transmitted by the bitch prenatally or at birth. Therefore, be sure to check her for genital infection.
   b. Kittens with herpesvirus conjunctivitis can also present with the same signs
2. **Treatment** - If the pup is past seven days old, the lids can be opened with gentle traction; if this does not work, open with corneal scissors as described for ankyloblepharon.
3. **Aftercare** - After the eyelids have been opened, treat the conjunctivitis with topical antibiotic ointments. Do not use a topical corticosteroid in these patients because of the corneal edema present. If tear production is low, use topical ointments until tear production is adequate.
4. *Comment*
   a. If the eyelids are not opened the cornea may ulcerate, leading to perforation and loss of vision. The end result may be secondary glaucoma or phthisis bulbi. Prompt treatment will result in a normal eye and no significant scarring.
   b. Opening the eyelids before the normal time for them to open will not injure the eyes if tear production is adequate.

SMALL PALPEBRAL FISSURE (MICROBLEPHARON) - The size of the palpebral opening normally is related to the size and prominence of the globe.

Etiology

1. Microphthalmia results in small palpebral fissure and a prominent (protruded) third eyelid.
2. Blepharophimosis is congenital narrowing of the palpebral fissure with a normal eye (Akita, chow chow, collie, English bull terrier, Kerry blue terrier, Shar-pei).
3. Contraction of the eyelids after extensive cryosurgery for eyelid neoplasia

Signs - Often does not produce any signs

1. Epiphora - because of poor eyelid fit at nasal canthus
2. May predispose to entropion
3. If the eye is small, the third eyelid will be prominent (protruded).

Treatment - Usually none unless entropion develops. Severe blepharophimosis can be treated by enlarging the palpebral fissure (Fig 5-17).

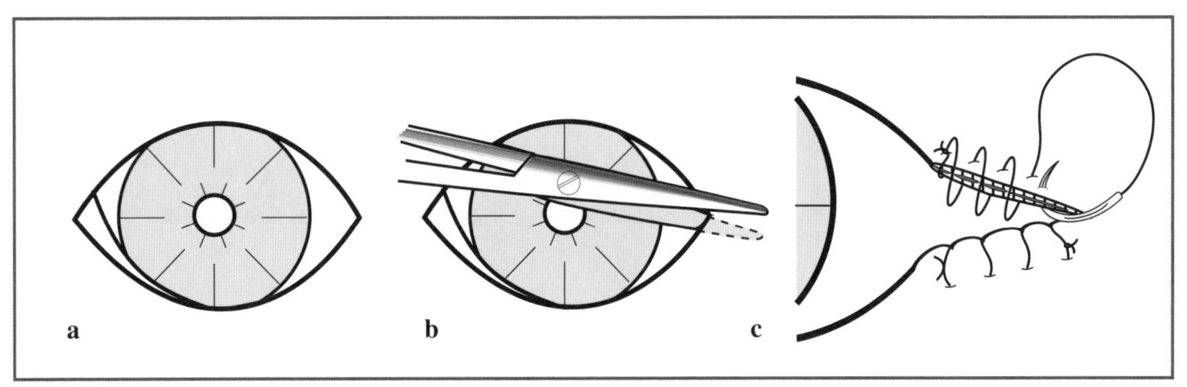

Figure 5-17. Enlarging the palpebral fissure.
a. Small eyelid opening
b. Canthotomy to enlarge eyelid opening
c. Conjunctiva sutured to the skin with 6-0 nonabsorbable suture

Comment

Acquired contraction of the palpebral fissure occurs following phthisis bulbi and occasionally as a complication after severe eyelid disease or injury. If it occurs as a complication, enlarging the fissure may be indicated.

LARGE PALPEBRAL FISSURE (MACROBLEPHARON) - This predisposes to corneal and scleral exposure, and abnormal tear film dynamics.

Incidence

1. Brachycephalic breeds with shallow orbits. These breeds typically have prominent nasal folds that compound the globe exposure with direct irritation of the eye from hair growing on the fold. When questioned, the owner may also be aware the dog has some degree of lagophthalmos when sleeping.
2. Breeds with redundant facial skin (Saint Bernard, some hounds, spaniels). These breeds will be predisposed to ectropion and in the case of the Saint Bernard, possibly entropion.

Signs

Lagophthalmos leading to secondary keratitis. The degree of secondary keratitis is determined by the severity of exposure and nasal fold irritation. Be sure to check tear production.

1. Pigmentary keratitis - this usually starts at nasal limbus and if not controlled may cover the cornea.
2. Superficial corneal vascularization and scarring will accompany the pigment changes.
3. Secondary corneal ulcers

Treatment

A thorough examination is needed to determine if medical and/or surgical treatment is needed. If so, what will be most appropriate in this patient.

1. Mild exposure. If eye is normal, treatment is not needed at this time. Mild changes may be controlled with topical antibiotic/steroid ophthalmic ointment.
2. Globe exposure without nasal fold irritation - lateral canthoplasty may be adequate
3. Globe exposure complicated by nasal fold irritation - nasal canthoplasty with or without lateral canthoplasty

Permanent lateral (temporal) canthoplasty to reduce palpebral fissure

1. Removal of eyelid margins and associated tarsal glands with two-layer closure (Fig 5-18). The author has good results with this technique.

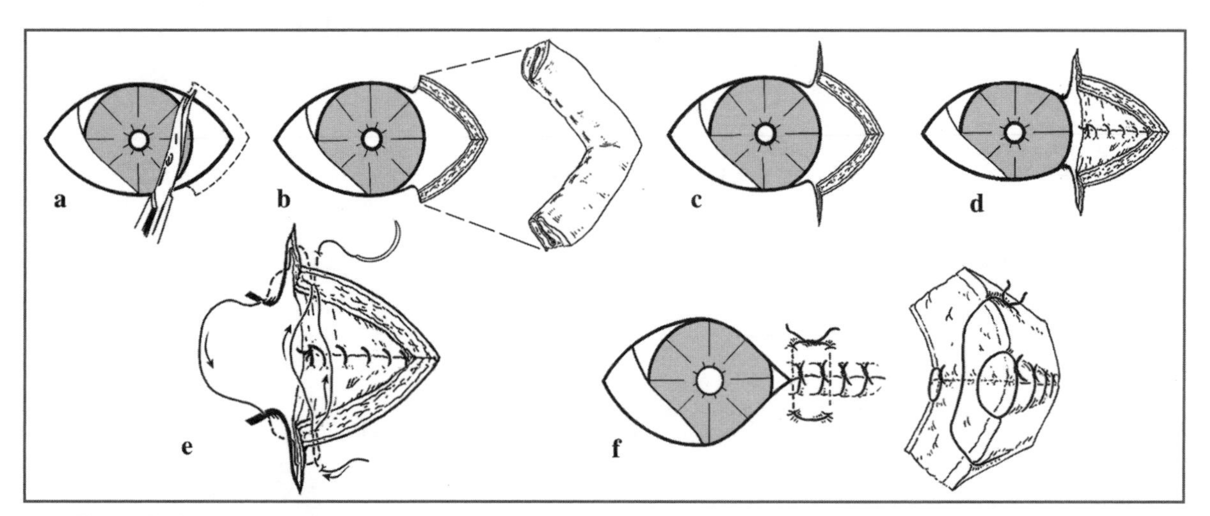

Figure 5-18. Permanent lateral tarsorrhaphy to reduce palpebral fissure (removal of tarsal bearing eyelid margin).

a. The amount of closure at the temporal canthus is determined and the eyelid margin marked (area to be removed indicated by dotted lines)
b. Removed tissue. Note that the tarsal glands are entirely removed to prevent postsurgical cyst formation.
c. The incisions perpendicular to eyelid are extended (1 to 1.5 times original depth). This will allow for more cosmetic lateral canthus after closure.
d. The conjunctiva is opposed with 5-0 or 6-0 absorbable suture using a continuous pattern
e. The new canthus is formed with a split thickness figure-eight nonabsorbable suture
f. The remainder of the skin wound is closed with simple interrupted sutures. A large vertical mattress suture supporting the new canthus is optional.

2. Two-layer closure with skin and conjunctival flap (Fig 5-19)

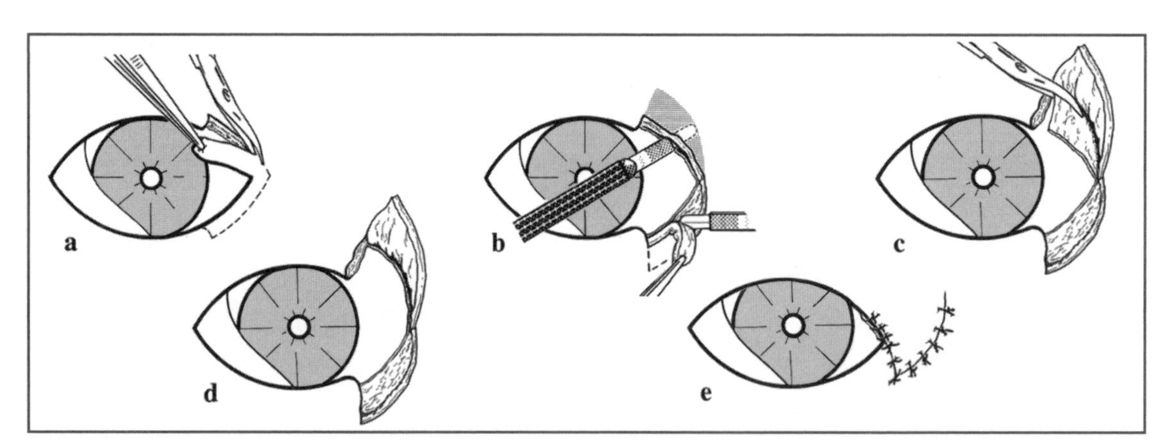

Figure 5-19. Permanent lateral tarsorrhaphy, two layer closure with skin and conjunctival flap. Modified from Atlas of Veterinary Ophthalmic Surgery, Bistner, Aguirre, Batik, WB Saunders, 1977. The amount of eyelid shortening is determined by pinching the eyelids together near the lateral canthus to give the desired appearance.

a. The eyelid margins and associated tarsal glands are excised from the surgical site. Shading indicates areas involved in the skin and conjunctival flaps.
b. A triangle of conjunctiva is undermined. A matching triangle of skin is removed from the lower eyelid.
c. The nasal side of the upper eyelid triangle is cut full thickness so it can be rotated over the conjunctival triangle of the lower eyelid. The triangle of conjunctiva is removed with scissors.
d. Appearance of surgical site after conjunctiva has been removed. Suturing the conjunctival wound with absorbable suture is optional.
e. The skin wound is sutured with 4-0 or 5-0 nonabsorbable suture. The eyelid splitting defect in the upper eyelid can be closed with a continuous suture.

Permanent medial (nasal) canthoplasty to reduce palpebral fissure

1. Splitting eyelids and one-layer closure protect cornea from nasal fold irritation or nasal entropion (Fig 5-20) - this technique preserves both puncta but later the skin may stretch more than with the pocket canthoplasty. This stretching may result in recurrence of globe exposure.

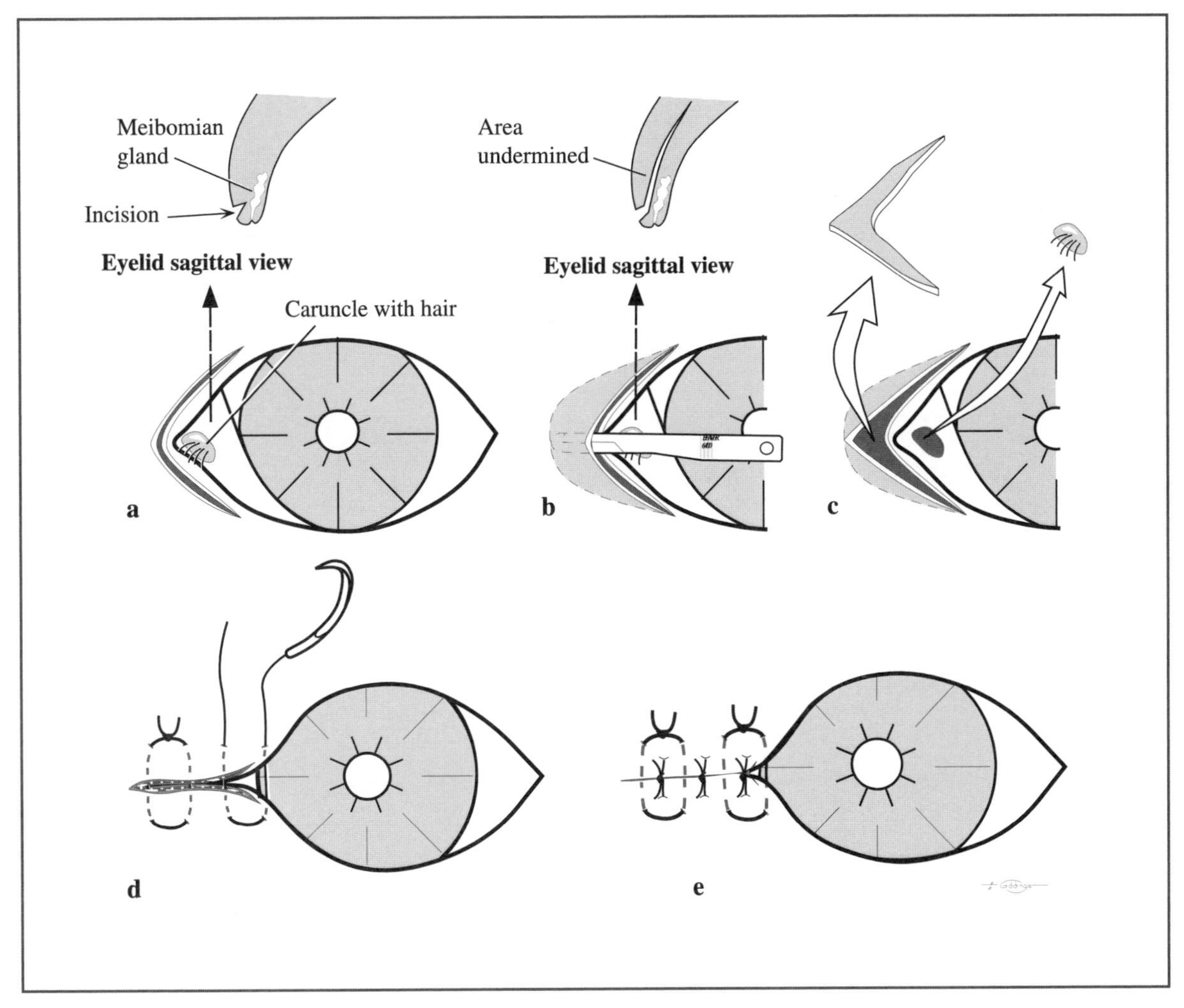

Figure 5-20. Nasal canthoplasty - splitting eyelid and one layer closure.

a. A skin incision is made along the eyelid margin superficial to the tarsal glands. The length of the incision will be determined by the degree of nasal canthus closure desired.
b. The skin is undermined to free it of orbital attachment
c. An arrow-shaped wedge of skin and the caruncle are removed
d. The wound is closed with nonabsorbable mattress sutures. The suture away from the canthus should be split thickness beyond the eyelid wound.
e. Simple interrupted sutures can be placed over the mattress sutures to enhance skin closure

2. Medial canthus pocket flap technique (Fig 5-21) - this technique is stronger but sacrifices the upper punctum

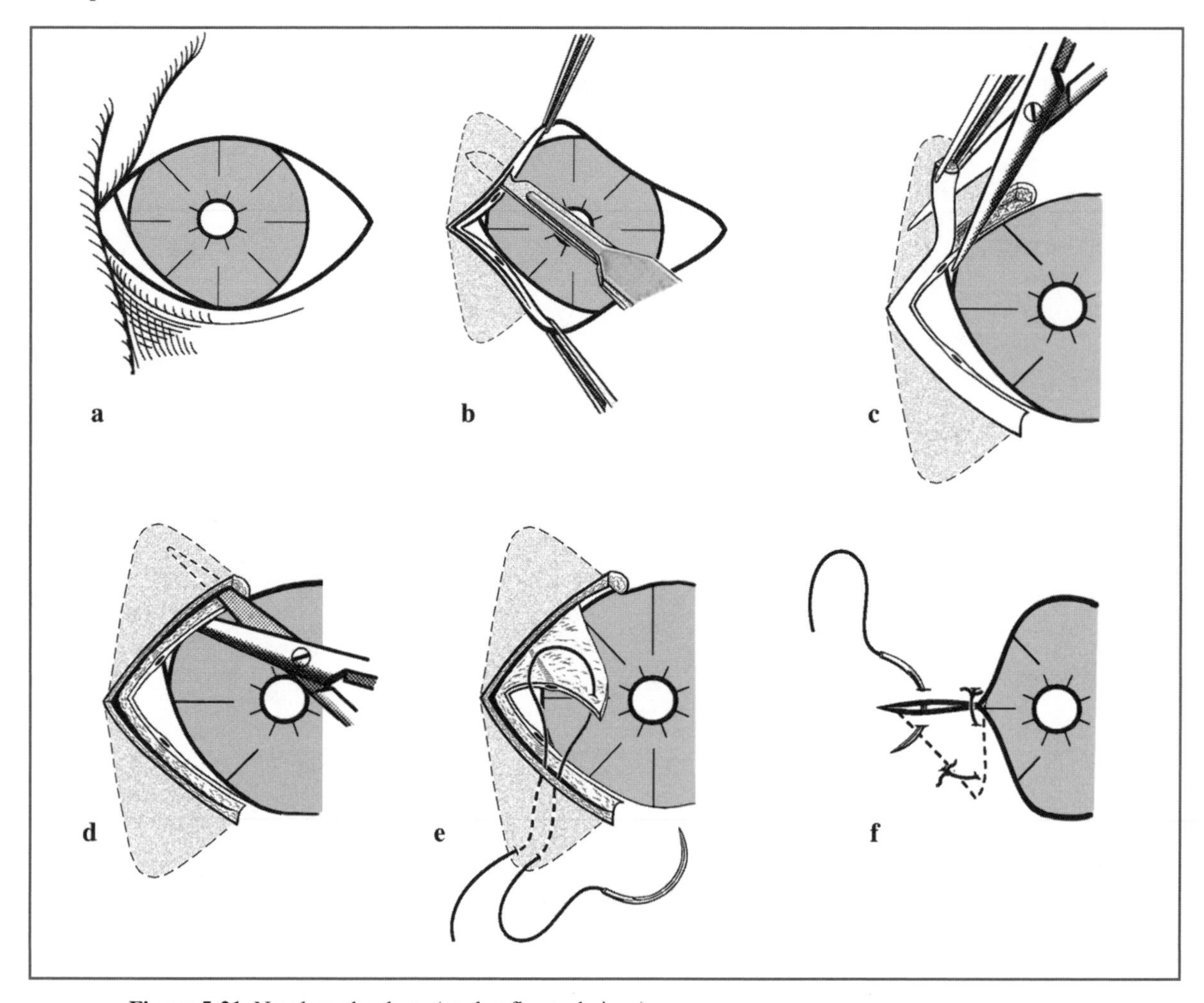

Figure 5-21. Nasal canthoplasty (pocket flap technique).

a. Brachycephalic dog with prominent nasal fold and nasal entropion
b. Splitting eyelids at mucocutaneous junction for length of desired closure. The skin is undermined creating pockets.
c. Removal of eyelid edge
d. Cutting conjunctival surface of upper eyelid to free flap to be pulled into lower pocket
e. Placement of 4-0 or 5-0 suture to pull flap into pocket
f. Skin is sutured to close wound

PROMINENT NASAL FOLDS IN DOGS

Brachycephalic breeds (especially toys) have a prominent nasal fold. If it is excessive, it may cause secondary dermatitis, epiphora, and keratitis.

Signs

1. Epiphora - Tears may result in the furrow between the nasal fold and the eyelids developing a moist dermatitis that will not respond to medical treatment, thus requiring surgical treatment.
2. Corneal changes - may be mild to severe. Severe changes may cause blindness.
   a. Pigmentary keratitis
   b. Superficial vascularization
   c. Interstitial scarring
   d. Ulceration

Treatment - Treatment is not necessary unless secondary problems exist.

1. Medical treatment
   a. Epiphora - oral tetracyclines will reduce the staining of the folds caused by epiphora. This will also reduce some of the irritation seen along the fold that results from the constant moisture.
   b. Blepharitis
      1) Frequent cleaning with 1:50 Betadine solution
      2) Topical treatment with antibiotic/steroid ophthalmic or dermatologic ointment
   c. Corneal changes
      1) Pigment and vascularization - antibiotic/steroid ointment one to three times daily
      2) Corneal ulcers - stop topical steroids if being used. Recommend corrective blepharoplasty as soon as possible. It may be necessary to temporarily protect the cornea with a third eyelid flap.
2. Surgical treatment
   a. If prominent nasal fold is the only problem, partial or complete nasal fold removal will be adequate. Most breed standards desire deep folds for show purposes. Therefore, nasal canthoplasty will be indicated (Fig 5-20 and 5-21).
      1) Partial fold removal (Fig 5-22) - this is the most cosmetic approach because it leaves half of the nasal fold. In this procedure, the side of the fold that touches the nose is removed. The fold is divided along its length and then excised where it touches the nose along its nasal side.

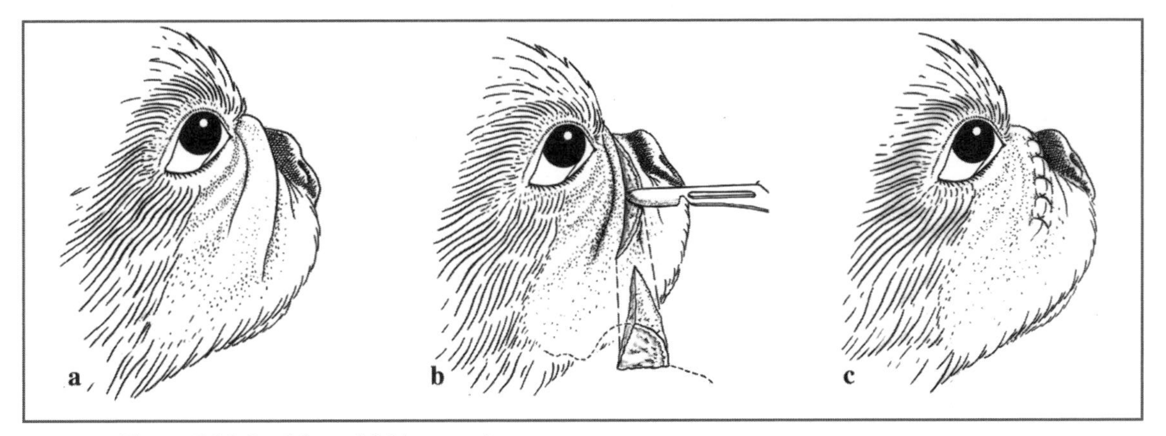

Figure 5-22. Partial nasal fold removal.
a. Lateral view
b. Nasal portion of fold removed. Lateral view of the area. The removed tissue is shown.
c. There is still a small nasal fold after suturing the wound

2) Complete fold removal (Fig 5-23) - this is a better procedure from the dog's standpoint, but changes the appearance of the dog significantly. The entire fold is removed and the wound sutured with nonabsorbable suture. Sharp scissors are the easiest way to remove the fold. Be sure to remove the fold by starting the incision at the lower end (lip end) of the fold and cutting upward toward the forehead.

b. ***If concurrent problems exist (lagophthalmos, nasal entropion, marked corneal changes), a medial canthoplasty should be considered. This also gives a better cosmetic appearance than fold removal.***

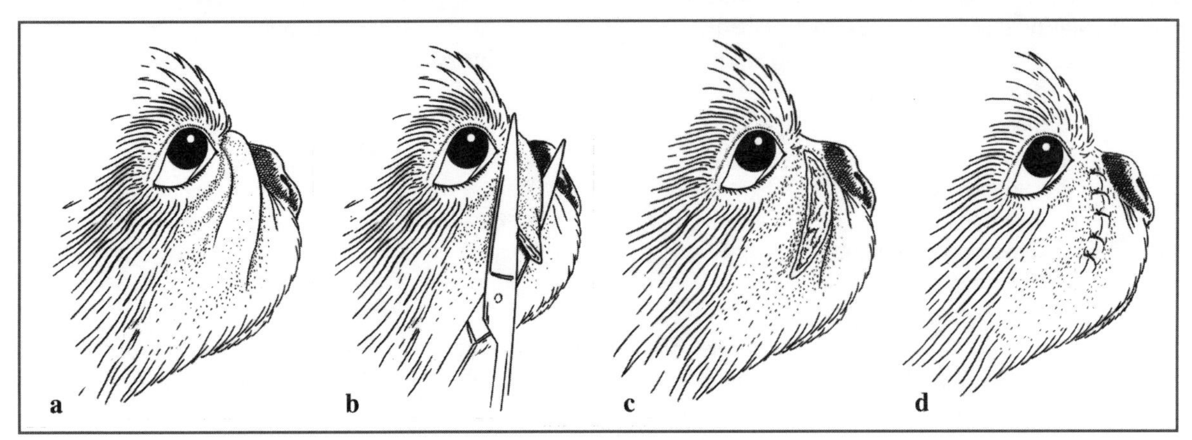

Figure 5-23. Complete nasal fold removal.
a. Lateral view
b. Starting incision with scissors at lower end of fold
c. Entire fold removed
d. Wound after suturing

ACQUIRED DISEASES OF THE EYELIDS

BLEPHARITIS- inflammation of the eyelids (skin, associated glands and stroma). The eyelids represent a skin appendage, therefore blepharitis is often part of a generalized dermatitis and treated as part of the generalized disease.

Causes

1. Bacterial - staphylococcus most common
2. Dermatomycosis - small animals, *M. canis* and *T. mentagrophytes*
3. Parasitic - *Sarcoptes* (dogs, cattle), *Demodex* (dogs, cats), *Notoedres cati* (cats), *Habronema lanae* (horses), *Cuterebra* larvae
4. Allergic reactions - vaccines, angioneurotic edema
5. Immune-mediated skin diseases (atopic blepharitis, drug reactions, pemphigus complex, lupus erythematosus
6. Actinic (solar) - all species
7. Traumatic
8. Neoplastic - early stages of squamous cell carcinoma can simulate inflammation

Signs

1. Vary with etiology - may be unilateral or bilateral, superficial versus deep, acute versus chronic
2. Acute - more blepharospasm, hyperemias, exudation and excoriation
3. Chronic - ulceration, alopecia, and cicatrix
4. May have concurrent conjunctivitis and/or keratitis

Diagnosis is based on:

1. Clinical signs
2. Careful examination
3. Diagnostic tests
    a. Culture
    b. Cytology
    c. Biopsy
    d. Skin testing

Treatment - correct the primary cause

BACTERIAL (PUSTULAR) BLEPHARITIS

Pustular blepharitis in dogs is commonly a *Staphylococcus intermedius* infection observed in young dogs as a part of the juvenile pyoderma complex or in adult dogs as a chronic blepharitis.

Pathophysiology - includes:

1. Staphylococcal organisms produce a dermatonecrotizing enzyme
2. Inflammatory reaction adds to tissue damage as the result of a massive influx of PMNs and subsequent release of their lysosomal enzymes.
3. In man, a poor host macrophage action has been demonstrated against staphylococcus.

Young dogs (juvenile pyoderma)

1. Signs - Generalized pustular dermatitis involving eyelids, face and muzzle. Regional lymph nodes may become enlarged and abscessed. Increased temperature and general malaise may be seen. Conjunctivitis and keratitis may or may not be present.
2. Treatment
   a. Systemic antibiotics - It is advisable to treat locally and systemically with the most effective antibiotic, as determined by sensitivity tests.
   b. Systemic corticosteroids - Should not be used until the infection is under control. Then they are recommended systemically and locally to reduce scarring and shorten the total course of the disease.
   c. Topical antibiotics and corticosteroid combination should be used three to four times daily.
3. Course - Animals will start to respond in four to seven days. Antibiotics should be continued three to four weeks or until all active lesions are healed. Continue systemic cortisone for about one to two weeks past this point.
4. Prognosis - Good if treatment is started early.

Adult dogs

A chronic disease that may be present for months before treatment is started. It is a combination of tissue sensitization and chronic infection, and should be considered to be primarily an immunologic disorder. Hypothyroidism can be a predisposing factor.

1. Signs - Severe thickening of the eyelids with involvement of the tarsal glands. Longstanding cases have local depigmentation and areas with draining abscesses. Eversion of the lids reveals multiple enlargements of the tarsal glands with inspissated purulent material. Conjunctivitis and keratitis are usually minimal, but may be present.
2. Treatment - This is a complex problem and must be treated systemically and topically. Culture and sensitivity are recommended before starting treatment. The disease is chronic, therefore waiting two or three days before starting treatment will not make any difference.
   a. Local treatment - chemical restraint or short general anesthesia is indicated in patients with severe involvement
      1) Incise and curet or express the affected tarsal glands and skin abscesses
      2) Topical antibiotic-corticosteroid combinations and cyclosporine 1% ophthalmic solution
      3) Hot packs for 10 to 15 minutes, two to three times daily until swelling disappears
   b. Systemic treatment
      1) Continue the antibiotics until the lesions disappear (3-6 weeks)
      2) Prednisolone is an important part of the treatment. Start with the anti-inflammatory level BID and continue until there is improvement. This is usually 5 to 10 days. Reduce to daily for a similar period and then continue every other day for a minimum of 10 treatments. Dose can be reduced further in some cases.
3. Course - Most patients respond well to this treatment but some will become recurrent.
4. Recurrent cases - Staphylococcus vaccine is of value in recurring cases. In some cases, vaccine may be needed indefinitely. The author has used a canine staphylococcus bacterin with excellent response but the CSU Diagnostic Laboratory discontinued making the bacterin. A copy of the preparation protocol can be obtained by contacting the author. *Staphylococcus* bacterins or lysates (Staphage Lysate - SPL, Types I and III, Delmont Labs) have been used with variable success.

EYELID CYSTS

Eyelid inclusion cysts are uncommon. If near the puncta or canaliculi, flushing and/or catheterization is recommended to eliminate the possibility of nasolacrimal involvement. Treatment may be either: 1) surgical dissection and wound closure; or 2) lancing followed by cryotherapy of the cyst lining with a cryoprobe and allowing the wound to heal by granulation.

BLEPHARITIS FROM RUBBING

1. Examine carefully to identify and remove cause
2. Symptomatic treatment consists of an Elizabethan collar in small animals or a hood in horses to prevent further self trauma.
   a. Protecting the eyelids - Elizabethan collar for small animals; hood for horses
   b. Anti-inflammatory drugs - flunixin works well to control adnexal pain

HABRONEMA EYELID GRANULOMAS IN HORSES

Habronema granulomas of the eyelids and nasal puncta have been reduced markedly by the use of ivermectin as a wormer. Involvement of the puncta and canaliculi may result in epiphora. Express or curet the inspissated material and treat topically with antibiotic/steroid ointment.

CHALAZION - Chalazion is chronic enlargement of a meibomian gland by obstruction of its duct, and the gland distends with yellow inspissated secretion.

Dogs - Chalazia are usually seen in older dogs and are static. This differentiates them from adenomas, which continue to grow. Treatment is usually not needed; if enlarging, expression may be adequate. Otherwise incise and curet contents. Expressing may result in rupture of the gland. If ruptured, the contents can cause a foreign body reaction in the tissue leading to a granulomatous response.

Cats - Bilateral multiple lipogranuloma, originating from the tarsal glands, can develop along the conjunctival margin of the eyelids. These lead to thickening of the eyelids, epiphora and mild conjunctivitis. Surgical removal has been successful without recurrence.

EQUINE BLEPHAROLITHS

The author has seen horses with mineralized deposits in the area of the tarsal glands. The owners have usually been aware of eyelid swelling that has gradually progressed over months. Surgical removal discloses small rough calculi 1-3 mm in diameter. One horse had a large calculus at the nasal canthus that resulted in epiphora. The general location of these calculi is similar to *Habronema* lesions, suggesting the initiating cause could have been an *Habronema* granuloma.

CAT ABSCESSES

Cat abscesses near the eye may result in severe edema, which will clear up spontaneously when the abscess is drained. Some abscesses can be most easily drained through the inner surface of the eyelid. Do not worry about the pus draining over the eye; if it drains over the eye, treat the abscess and the eye with the same ophthalmic preparation.

SOLAR BLEPHARITIS

Actinic radiation may lead to solar blepharitis in cats, cattle, dogs and horses that lack pigment in the eyelids. These animals, except for dogs, will be predisposed to squamous cell carcinoma. The severity of the reaction is related to environment (high elevation and sunny, dry climates). Housing the animals during the day helps but may not be possible.

Medical treatment - Sunscreen, sun absorbing dyes and antibiotic steroid preparations, and fly masks in horses, provide temporary relief.

Tattooing will provide relief for a minimum of five years

1. Preparation for tattooing
   a. If the eyelids are ulcerated, treat medically and protect from sunlight until the eyelids heal. Ulcerated skin will not retain ink well and is prone to excessive bleeding, which will wash the ink out.
   b. Premedication with flunixin meglumine will reduce postoperative eyelid swelling.
   c. General anesthesia is recommended.
   d. Place newspaper or other disposable material under the patient's head.
   e. Gloves are recommended to protect hands from staining with tattoo ink.
   f. Clipping and scrubbing the area is NOT necessary.
2. Instrumentation
   a. Three needle identification tattoo instruments can be used but are time consuming to use
   b. Multiple needle (8-10) tips are more efficient. The author uses a tattoo instrument with a 10-needle cluster. Sharp needles are necessary for good skin penetration.
   c. Tattoo ink - the author uses the black tattoo ink available for food animal use.
3. Tattoo technique
   a. Stabilize the eyelids by placing a lid plate or B-P handle beneath the area to be tattooed.
   b. Adjust the tattoo instrument so the needle tips will protrude 1-2 mm beyond the needle guard when the instrument is operating. This depth will assure adequate penetration of the needles to carry ink into the skin, yet allow the instrument to slide across the skin without catching or tearing the surface.
   c. Dip the needle cluster into the ink and then tattoo back and forth over the eyelid.
   d. Periodically rinse the skin with water and wipe clean to assess progress. The procedure is repeated until the skin has a uniform black color. This will fade to blue-gray in 30 days.
   e. The edge of the eyelid is difficult to tattoo with the multiple needle tip. The standard three needle tip of an identification tattoo is better suited for this area.
4. Aftercare minimal - horses develop a more severe reaction than dogs
   a. Dogs - usually not necessary. Topical antibiotic/steroid drops or ointment TID for one to three days will control conjunctivitis.
   b. Horses may develop a more severe reaction. May be painful first 24 hours and attempt to rub the eyes. Immediate swelling develops and disappears in two to four days. If areas ulcerate during tattooing, scabs will form. Topical antibiotics (steroid ointment) TID for several days and systemic flunixin meglumine or phenylbutazone for two to four days if needed.

EDEMA OF THE EYELIDS (BLEPHAREDEMA) - Eyelid edema is usually secondary to a primary problem

Etiology

1. Urticaria (diet or post vaccine) occurs bilaterally in upper and lower eyelids and lips. Owner may not be aware of skin welts or swelling of the vulva.
2. Insect bites - unilateral
3. Trauma - direct trauma or self-inflicted from rubbing
4. Infectious - periorbital or retrobulbar
5. Venous congestion of the orbit - retrobulbar tumor

Signs

1. Extreme swelling of the eyelids
2. Pain or itching
3. Urticaria - other skin areas may also be involved

Treatment - identify and correct primary cause

1. Urticaria or insect bite. Systemic corticosteroids or antihistamines.
2. If severe pruritus:
   a. Physical restraint - Elizabethan collar (small animals), cross tying (horses)
   b. Chemical restraint - tranquilizers
   c. Systemic treatment - anti-inflammatory

EYELID LACERATIONS

It is common for the eyelids to be injured, either in accidents or fights. The lids are very vascular and will heal readily even when seriously injured.

Evaluation of the traumatic eye - Do a complete examination of the patient and determine:

1. If only the eyelid is injured - immediate treatment can be performed
2. If there is moderate shock and/or serious injuries to other systems - treatment of the eye can be performed after proper treatment of shock and/or injuries
3. If there is severe involvement of other systems - do not attempt specific treatment of the eyelid until the patient can be safely anesthetized. Local treatment is advisable until surgical repair of the eyelid can be performed.

Wound duration

1. If fresh (< 4 hrs) - repair as soon as possible (immediate treatment)
2. If old (> 12 hrs) - repair at your convenience, in the next 24 hours (delayed treatment)
3. If between 4 to 12 hours - use your own judgement as to immediate or delayed treatment

Immediate treatment, presurgical protocol

1. Premedicate with a systemic antibiotic
2. General anesthesia - usually needed to get precise closure of the palpebral borders of the wound
3. Clean the wound thoroughly with 1:50 Betadine in saline solution
4. Clip hair from edges of the wound
5. Four minute disinfecting prep: clean wound for two minutes and then cover area with Betadine-soaked sponges for two minutes

Delayed treatment, presurgical protocol

1. Start systemic antibacterials
2. Protect the wound and eye with a furacin treated bandage. This is not always possible in small animals, but routinely effective in horses (Fig 5-24). A bandage will control infection, reduce swelling, simplify surgery and assure first intention healing.

Wound closure - most small animal wounds are perpendicular to the eyelid margin; equine wounds tend to extend parallel to the lid margin, forming a flap. A two-layer closure gives the best results. Absorbable buried suture and nonabsorbable skin suture are preferred. Appropriate suture would be 6-0 absorbable suture for the conjunctiva, 4-0 (equine), or 5-0 (small animal) nonabsorbable for the skin and muscle layer. Minimal wound debridement is recommended. The rich vascularity of the eyelid leads to rapid healing. The patient is continued on systemic antibiotic three to five days after surgery. In horses, a postoperative bandage with instructions to the owner that it can be removed in 24 hours will protect the eye during recovery and hauling home. Small animals may try to rub the eye during recovery but usually ignore it after one to two hours. An Elizabethan collar may be indicated if they act like they will rub it. Instruct the owners ***to not manipulate*** the eyelid; avoid ophthalmic medications if possible.

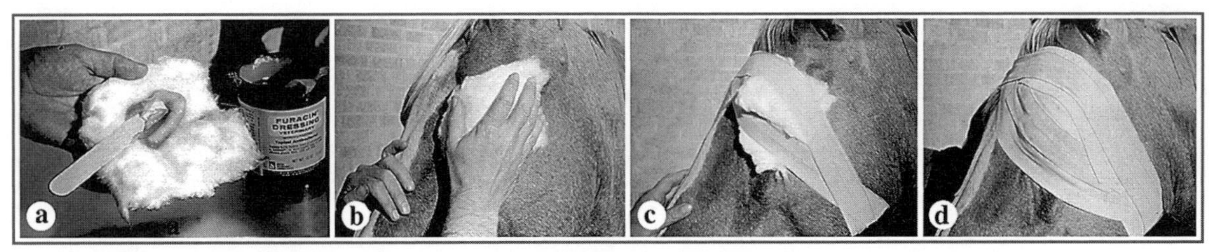

Figure 5-24. Furacin eye bandage for delayed treatment of an eyelid laceration.

a. Topical furacin ointment applied to a four inch cotton pad
b. Cotton pad applied to the eye
c. Elastic tape (Elasticon, Johnson & Johnson) is used to secure the bandage starting on the forehead above the normal eye, covering the anterior portion of the cotton pad, extending over the angle of the mandible, coming up on the other side above the good eye, then covering the posterior portion of the cotton pad and once more encircling the head.
d. Short strips of tape are used to build up the bandage over the injured eye. Covering the tape ends with an encircling strip of white tape will prevent any strips of tape from coming free.

Repair of vertical wound with little tissue loss (Fig 5-25)

Trim edges as little as possible, then appose the tissues carefully. If there is severe swelling and the conjunctiva is pulling away, suture the conjunctiva before placing the skin sutures. Starting away from the edge of the eyelid, place conjunctival sutures so that the knots are buried in the wound and therefore will not rub the eye. Place the first skin suture along the sharp edge of the eyelid, with the suture going through the tarsal glands. Cut the suture ends short so they will not irritate the cornea. This is the appositional suture. The next suture is placed in the skin about 2 mm from the edge of the lid. The suture should be deep (nearly to the conjunctiva) and catch the tarsal plate. This is the tension suture, taking up most of the wound tension. Place as many sutures as needed to finish closing the wound. An eyelid sutured in this fashion will heal with a smooth eyelid edge. A figure-eight suture can be used instead of the first two sutures described. If properly placed, it is preferred. Give systemic antibiotics for four to five days if the wound is severely contaminated or was infected. ***Do not manipulate the lid*** and, if possible, avoid all forms of ophthalmic medications.

Repair of parallel laceration

Because of abundant eyelid circulation, even a narrow band of eyelid tissue can be repositioned. Loss of this tissue can result in cicatrix and secondary trichiasis. When closing this type of wound, the author's preference is to place a figure-eight suture at the palpebral border and then suture the conjunctiva. If the eyelid has marked swelling, several space obliterating interrupted sutures may be placed in the muscle layer before the skin is closed.

Repair of lacerations with major tissue loss

If considerable tissue has been lost, consider the technique described for replacing tissue lost during surgical removal of eyelid tumors. Many blepharoplastic techniques are described in the literature and a technique can generally be found for any situation that might be encountered.

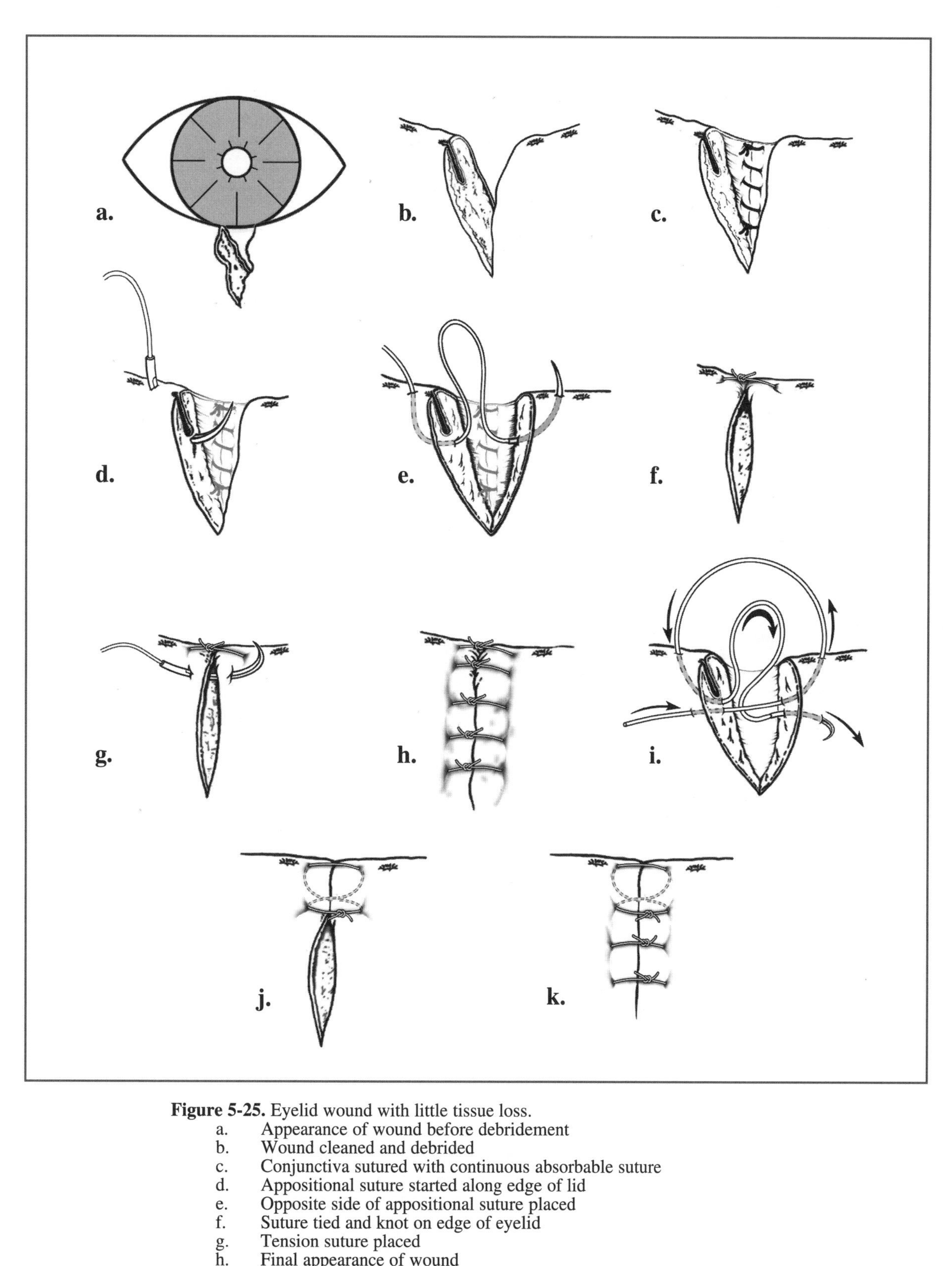

Figure 5-25. Eyelid wound with little tissue loss.

a. Appearance of wound before debridement
b. Wound cleaned and debrided
c. Conjunctiva sutured with continuous absorbable suture
d. Appositional suture started along edge of lid
e. Opposite side of appositional suture placed
f. Suture tied and knot on edge of eyelid
g. Tension suture placed
h. Final appearance of wound
i. Figure-eight suturing pattern can be used as an alternate to the appositional and tension sutures. Final step of suture placement.
j. Suture tied
k. Final appearance of figure-eight suture

EYELID TUMORS

Eyelid tumors are the most frequent form of ocular neoplasia. There is considerable variation in the types observed between species. For this reason, the incidence will be discussed separately. Any tumor occurring in the skin can be seen in the eyelid. As a general rule, every growth removed from the eyelids should be examined histologically for cell type and degree of malignancy. An exception to this would be tarsal gland adenomas in dogs.

Dogs

1. Most common tumors
   a. Tarsal gland adenoma (cystadenoma) - most common eyelid tumor. Will cause conjunctivitis and if touches the cornea, keratitis. If the lid is everted, the diseased gland can be clearly visualized beneath the mucous membrane. They often originate in the ductal region of the tarsal gland and have a "cauliflower" appearance as they emerge on the eyelid margin. Obstruction of the duct may lead to cystic changes with a secondary granulomatous response if glandular secretions escape into the eyelid. They are usually benign. Recurrence is common if treatment is incomplete.
      1) Cryosurgery - is the author's preferred method of treating these tumors (Fig 5-26). Extensive tumors can be treated leaving minimal eyelid deformity.

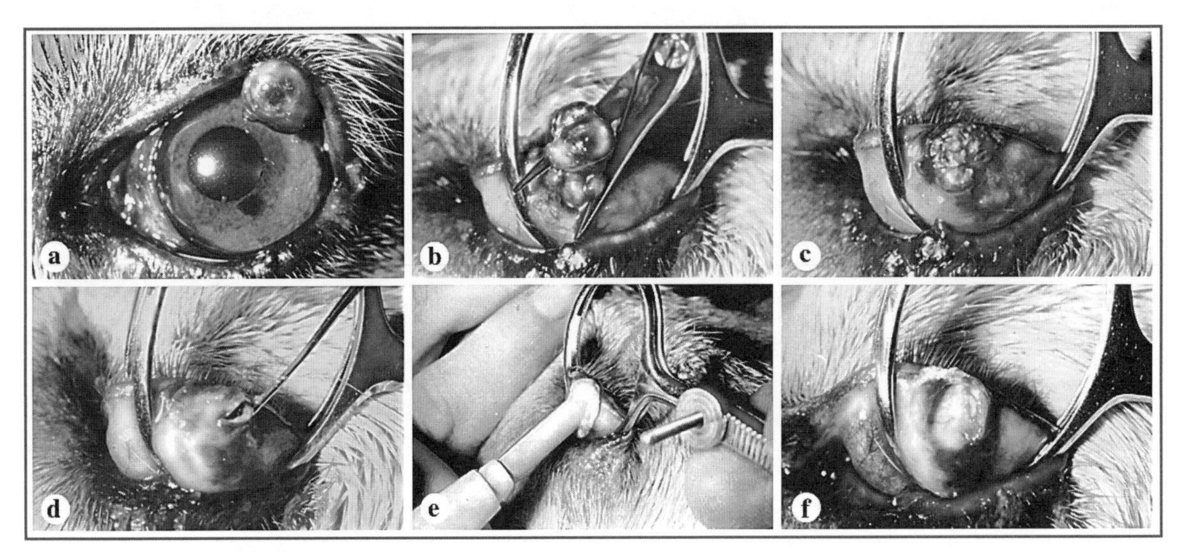

Figure 5-26. Cryotherapy of eyelid tumor.
- a. Ulcerated tarsal gland adenoma
- b. Eyelid stabilized with Sontec tumor forceps and debulking with corneal scissors
- c. Tumor after debulking with scissors
- d. Curettage of remaining tumor
- e. Cryoprobe freezing tumor site. The area will be allowed to thaw and then be refrozen.
- f. Appearance after freezing

      2) Hyperthermia - is also effective
      3) Surgery - some small tumors can be removed from the inner surface leaving eyelid skin intact. The majority will require wedge resection. Large tumors will require reconstructive blepharoplastic techniques. See surgical treatment of eyelid tumors, page 184.
   b. Melanoma - second most common eyelid tumor in dogs (vizsla and Weimaraner predisposed). They are usually benign but even those that are histologically malignant have benign behavior. Respond well to surgical excision, or debulking followed with cryosurgery. Systemic treatment with cimetidine should be considered with multiple melanomas of the eyelids and lip margins.
   c. Papilloma in older dogs - surgical removal is recommended if they are increasing in size. Pedunculated papillomas can often be removed with scissors, without local anesthesia.

2. Tumors less frequently seen - histiocytoma, mast cell tumor, angiosarcoma, basal cell carcinoma, fibroma, and squamous cell carcinoma. Diagnosis is established by cytology or biopsy, which in turn determines choice of treatment.
   a. Histiocytomatosis is usually seen in young dogs and may occur on the eyelids. They may also involve the globe and lips. Even after biopsy, dogs with multiple lesions may be difficult to differentiate from immune-mediated diseases such as discoid lupus or nodular granulomatous episclerokeratitis (collie granuloma). Spontaneous regression can occur after 3 to 12 weeks. Multiple lesions with no signs of regression should be treated with systemic medications.
      1) Single lesions - intralesional injection with depot corticosteroid
      2) Systemic corticosteroids - given at an anti-inflammatory dosage for three to four weeks
      3) Refractory cases (consult an oncologist) may respond to anticancer drugs. Cytoxan - 0.5 to 1 mg/lb once daily until tumors start to regress. This is usually 7 to 10 days. Monitor the white count after the fifth day. If the total white count drops below 6,000, reduce to one-half the dosage. If the count drops to 4,000, discontinue the medication until it increases and exceeds 6,000.
      4) Refractory cases - consult an oncologist
   b. Mast cell tumors - vary depending on cellular activity. If small, wide excision or intralesional corticosteroids. If larger or growing rapidly, the author recommends consulting with or referring to an oncologist for appropriate treatment.
   c. It should be noted that ***squamous cell carcinoma of the eyelid is uncommon***. The author has seen it in young dogs appearing quite similar to viral papillomatosis. Histologic differentiation is necessary.
3. Nonneoplastic lesions of the eyelids
   a. Viral papillomas - can occur on the eyelid, conjunctiva and cornea of young dogs. A clinical variation of oral viral papillomatosis. May be seen concurrently with oral lesions or as a separate entity. If causing secondary conjunctivitis, remove surgically or crush to stimulate immunity. If not causing irritation, it will eventually regress as the animal develops immunity. Cryotherapy is good for refractory cases. Can also be treated medically with Cytoxan.
   b. Hyperkeratosis with pigmentation is occasionally seen and can be easily confused with early melanoma. Biopsy is necessary for differentiation. Treatment may not be needed, but corticosteroid ointments will be beneficial.
   c. Inflammatory granulomas

Cats - eyelid tumors are less common than in the dog and when seen are more difficult to control than in dogs

1. Squamous cell carcinoma is most frequently seen. Occurs in cats with nonpigmented eyelids and should be given a guarded prognosis. It is often mistaken by the owner as blepharitis or a nonhealing injury and because of delay may have become invasive when presented for examination. Examine the face, especially the nose and ears, for additional lesions. Depending on the extent of the lesions, surgical treatment, cryotherapy, hyperthermia, radiation or anticancer drugs can be used. A combination of hyperthermia and radiation has been the most successful method for refractory patients. Eye removal may be needed to get the entire lesion when there is extensive involvement.
2. Other tumors are less frequently observed and cytology/biopsy is needed before treatment can be recommended. Those seen include lymphosarcoma, myxoma, Schwannoma, and basal cell carcinoma.

Horses

1. Squamous cell carcinoma is the most common tumor of the eyelid, adnexa and cornea. The incidence varies geographically with ultraviolet radiation proposed as the primary initiating factor.
   a. Predisposing factors
      1) Lack of skin pigmentation
      2) Breeds - draft horses, especially Belgian
      3) Increases with age
      4) Sex - males more than females and geldings more than stallions

b. Location of lesions - globe and third eyelid more frequently involved than eyelids. All areas can be involved in the same patient.
c. Signs - Lower eyelid and medial canthus are most frequently involved. The lesions may vary in appearance.
    1) Erosive lesion of the eyelid - initially appear as blepharitis, then progressive loss of eyelid. Scabs and a variable amount of mucopurulent discharge will be seen.
    2) Proliferative - beginning with a papillomatous appearance, progressing to rough proliferative mass that will bleed on contact
    3) Extensive tumors with necrosis have a foul odor.
d. Diagnosis - clinical appearance is suggestive; cytology or biopsy is diagnostic
e. Treatment - varies with the extent of the lesion. Modalities available to the veterinarian:
    1) Surgery - excision works well for smaller tumor
    2) Cryotherapy - tissue sparing and often can be done with local anesthetic and chemical restraint. Quickly performed.
    3) Hyperthermia with LRF current - multiple applications are needed for large lesions, thus requiring more time than cryotherapy. Debulking the lesion will reduce hyperthermia time.
    4) Radiation - limited access to practitioner
    5) Chemotherapy - intralesional injection with cisplatin
    6) Immunotherapy - intralesional injection with BCG preparations
f. Prognosis - guarded if involving nonpigmented tissues
    1) Local recurrence is common
    2) Metastasis is low - highest for a lesion involving the nasal canthus and third eyelid

2. Equine sarcoid - is seen frequently in the eyelid and surrounding skin. Local recurrence after treatment is common. ***Metastasis is not a problem.***
    a. Signs
        1) May be single or multiple
        2) Initial - firm dermal and subdermal mass that often grows slowly
        3) Ulceration - as the mass enlarges ulceration is common; when this occurs, the growth rate usually increases
        4) Thin verrucous plaques are sometimes seen around the eyelids. These are often stationary.
    b. Diagnosis - biopsy (this should include skin)
    c. Treatment
        1) Verrucous plaques - if stationary, no treatment; if owner requests treatment, hyperthermia (LRF current) is recommended
        2) Surgery - not recommended because high recurrence rate
        3) Immunotherapy - Mycobacterial cell wall fractions (Nomagen, Fort Dodge; Regressin-V, Vetrepharm). Multiple injections of 1 ml/cm^2 or until the tumor is saturated, repeated at two to four week intervals. Animals that do not respond after four injections should be considered refractory. The author has had excellent results with this treatment until recently when an increase in refractory patients has been experienced.
        4) Hyperthermia - good results, requires multiple treatments three to four weeks apart. Currently the author's preferred treatment.
        5) Cryotherapy - variable results. Author has been disappointed with results.
        6) Chemotherapy - Cisplatin injection is promising. The author has not had time to thoroughly evaluate. This is a hazardous substance that requires special handling.

3. Melanomas - Seen in eyelids of breeds predisposed to melanoma development.
    a. Signs - firm, slow growing, black mass in the eyelid. May mechanically interfere with blinking, irritate the eye, or cause epiphora.
    b. Diagnosis - cytology/biopsy
    c. Treatment - cryotherapy ***without*** debulking has been quite successful.

4. Other tumors - less frequently seen
    a. Fibroma/fibrosarcoma and neurofibroma can be confused with equine sarcoid
    b. Angioma/angiosarcoma - usually appear as a subcutaneous mass with a corded feel on palpation. They tend to grow slowly (months). The skin will usually remain intact. The owner should be cautioned of the possibility of metastasis.
        1) Treatment
            a) Surgical resection - they usually recur
            b) Medical treatment - vincristine weekly until tumor regresses has been successful in some cases
        2) Prognosis - metastasis can be quite early with hemangiosarcoma
    c. Papilloma - seen occasionally in older horses. Surgical removal.

Cattle

The only significant eyelid tumor is squamous cell carcinoma.

1. Contributing factors
    a. Genetic predisposition, especially ocular and periocular skin and haircoat, are important.
        1) Most common in the Hereford and Hereford cross breeds
        2) Seen less frequently in Brahman and Charolais
    b. Ultraviolet radiation seems to be a contributing factor (is an established factor in man)
    c. Viral infection proposed - IBR isolated from 15 of 32 cases in one study.
    d. Nutritional status - high feed levels are predisposing
2. Incidence
    a. Peak incidence 7 to 9 years of age, seldom seen less than four years of age
    b. In one study, 80% of all tumors in cattle were cancer eye; however in another study, 20% of all lesions diagnosed clinically as squamous cell carcinoma were not
    c. 0.1 to 1.6% of slaughtered cattle have cancer eye
    d. Reports of metastasis are from 4.7% to 15% - most are from lid lesions
3. Location of lesions (Witt 1984)
    a. Cornea 60% - lateral limbus more common than medial
    b. Lower eyelid 27%
    c. Upper eyelid 10%
    d. Nictitans 7%
4. Classification of lesions
    a. Limbus lesions are classified as:
        1) Hyperplasia - hornlike eyelid projections (referred to as "wickers" by ranchers) will often develop from the eyelids; excision is effective
        2) Papilloma
        3) Carcinoma
    b. Lid lesions are classified as:
        1) Keratoma
        2) Acanthosis
        3) Papilloma
        4) Carcinoma
5. Treatment
    a. Surgical excision is possible for early lesions, but cryotherapy or hyperthermia are faster, easier, and better. Enucleation or exenteration of the orbit for advanced lesions.
    b. Cryotherapy
        1) Very high cure rate is described by cryotherapy using liquid nitrogen and a double freeze technique (J Am Vet Med Assoc 1976;168:213). Freeze to -25°C, thaw and refreeze to -25°C.
        2) Selection of lesion - the lesion should have distinct borders. You should be able to palpate all edges of the lesion so the thermocouple probes can be placed below the lesion to ensure freezing all of it.

c. Hyperthermia
   1) Very effective on early lesions of the globe and adnexa
   2) Debulking is recommended before treating large lesions. Even with debulking, treatment may be time consuming.
d. Immunotherapy - Nomagen (Fort Dodge) - mycobacterial cell wall fractions. It is quite effective on small lesions (< 2.5 cm diameter) 80%; medium tumors (2.5-7.0 cm diameter) 70%; not recommended for large tumors

Surgical treatment of eyelid tumors

1. Small tumor removal (Fig 5-27) - if animals are brought in early enough, the tumor can be removed without disfiguration of the lid. If it is necessary to cut through all the layers of the lids, small tumors can be treated by removing a small triangular wedge. Use of a foursided excision profile will result in removal of eyelid margin. A two layer closure described for eyelid laceration provides greatest stability. Animals with excess lids (e.g. spaniels and some hounds) can tolerate removal of 1/4 to 1/3 of an eyelid. Animals with small eyelid openings (e.g. collies) will not tolerate much shortening of the eyelid.

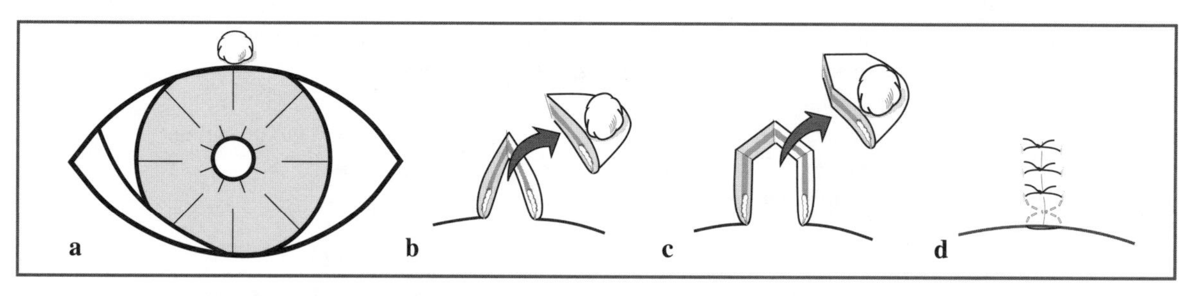

Figure 5-27. Small tumor removal.
- a. Small tumor on upper eyelid
- b. Pie-shaped wedge removed from eyelid
- c. Foursided block removal is indicated for a larger tumor while maintaining a short incision
- d. The wound is sutured the same as described for closing eyelid lacerations (see Fig 5-25)

2. Removal of large tumors - Removal of large tumors may result in considerable eyelid loss. In these cases, sliding flap techniques should be employed. Many techniques have been described. Sliding H-flaps have worked well for the author.
   a. Sliding H-flap (Fig 5-28). This is probably the simplest reconstructive procedure for major eyelid defects. This technique is also valuable in repairing eyelids after major loss from injury.

      Mark the eyelid so that the tumor will be removed with a square or rectangular piece of eyelid. Then mark two equilateral triangles below. Make sure the side of the triangle is of equal length to the vertical side of the rectangle. Remove the section of the eyelid containing the tumor. Do not remove any more of the deeper layers of the eyelid than necessary. Undermining of the skin is started along the incision away from the eyelid edge. This allows dissection toward the edge of the eyelid. If the dissection is started along the edge of the eyelid, it is more difficult to perform.

      Next remove the triangles of skin at the base of the wound. Scissors are excellent for this. Slide the flap into position. If a small tumor has been removed, the flap will move without being undermined. If the flap does not move easily, undermine it. The first sutures should be placed along the border of the eyelid and the next at the dogleg of the wound. Sutures may be removed after 14 days. Eye medication is not indicated unless the animal has conjunctivitis or keratitis.

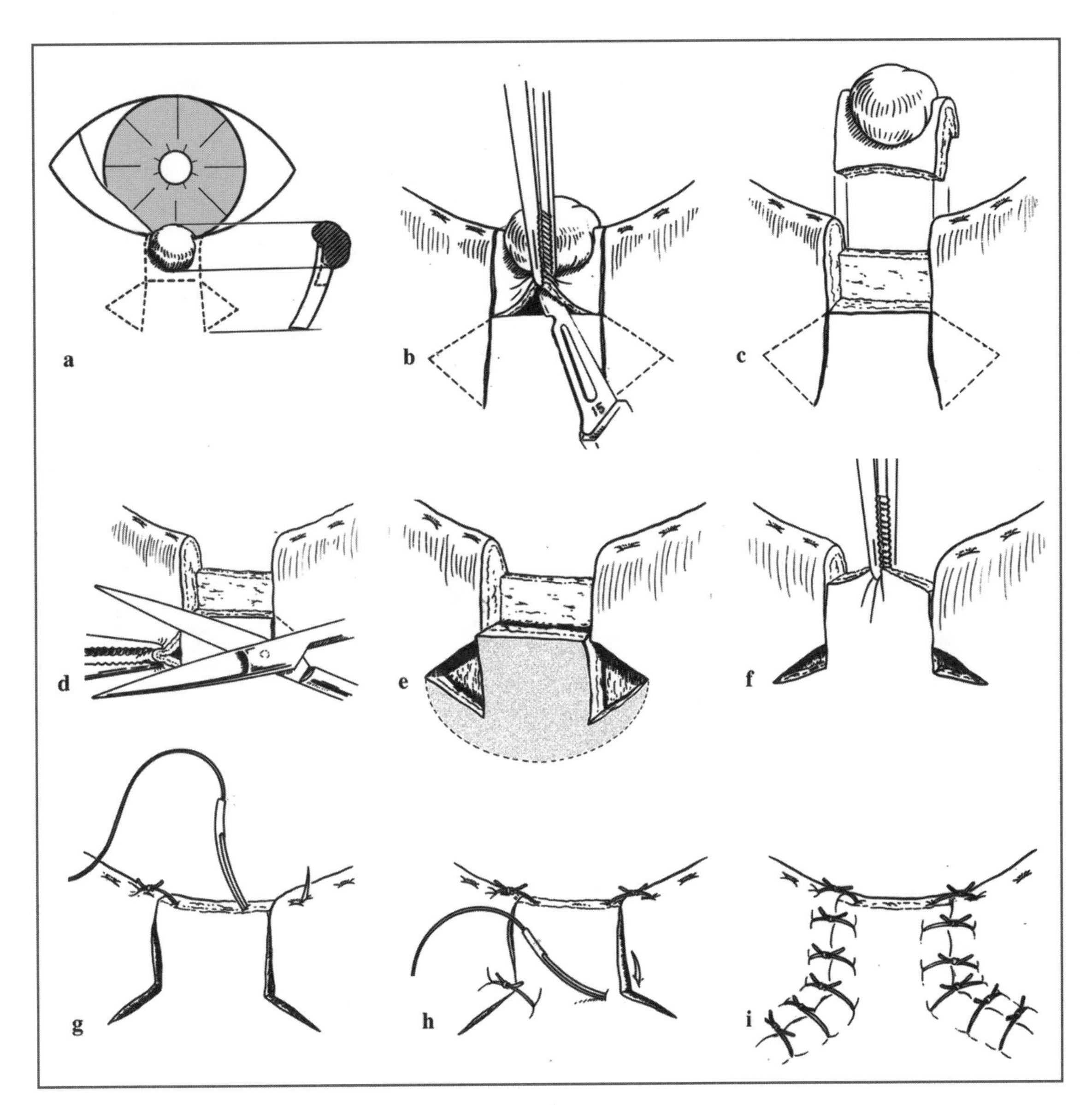

Figure 5-28. Sliding H-flap for large tumor removal.

a. Lower eyelid with large tumor. Lines represent where skin incision will be made. In this case, the skin and edge of the eyelid are involved and the conjunctiva is normal. The normal conjunctiva will not be removed.
b. Undermining tumor starting at base of eyelid and dissecting toward eyelid margin. Normal conjunctiva is left in place.
c. Appearance of eyelid after tumor removal
d. Removing triangular piece of skin with scissors
e. Appearance of eyelid after all tissues removed. Flap has been undermined (shaded).
f. Flap pulled into place.
g. First two sutures placed along edge of lid.
h. Next two sutures are placed at the dogleg.
i. Skin sutures in place. Conjunctiva may be sutured to skin flap with continuous suture (not shown).

b. Modified H-plasty (Fig 5-29). If the entire thickness of the lid must be removed, it may be desirable to transpose upper eyelid conjunctiva to the area of the flap. This will provide additional support and thickness to the skin flap. This will also prevent the edge of the skin flap from contracting. The diseased skin and conjunctiva are removed from the diseased eyelid and a conjunctival flap is prepared from the opposite eyelid. The conjunctival flap is sutured to the conjunctiva in the diseased eyelid with a 6-0 absorbable suture. The skin flap is prepared as before and sutured into place. The conjunctival flap is sutured to the free edge of the skin flap. Then the edges of the eyelids are sutured as a tarsorrhaphy for stabilization as the wounds heal. After two to three weeks, all sutures are removed and the conjunctival flap is trimmed smooth to the eyelids. This technique provides full thickness to the tissues in the area of the lesion.

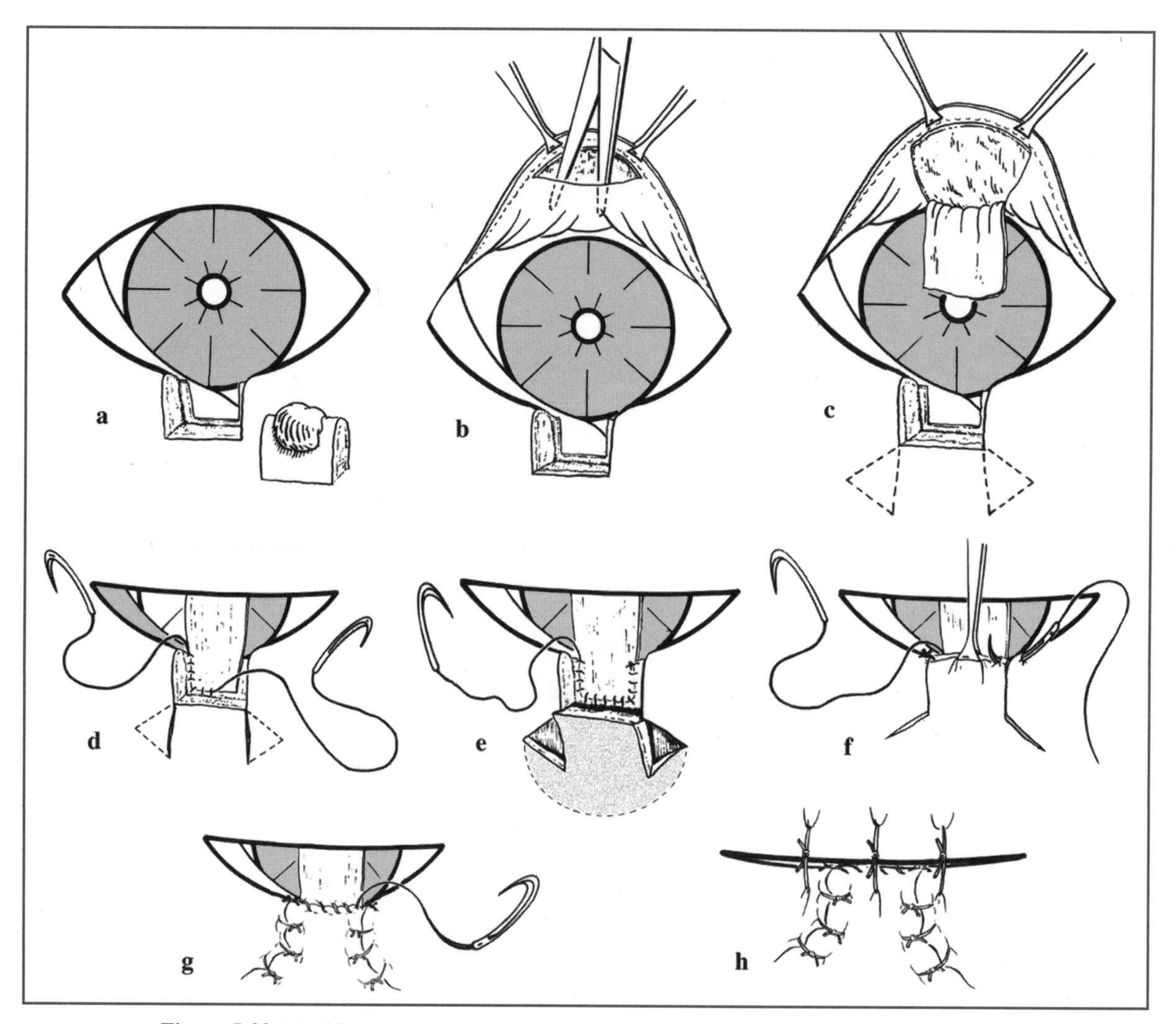

Figure 5-29. Modified H-plasty for full thickness eyelid resection.

a. Appearance of eyelid after tumor removal
b. Undermining conjunctiva from upper lid
c. Conjunctival flap pulled toward defective lower lid
d. Suturing conjunctival flap to conjunctiva of lower lid with double armed suture. Suture started in center of wound.
e. Conjunctival flap sutured to conjunctiva of lower lid with 6-0 absorbable suture. Nasal end of suture is not cut. Remove triangles of skin and pull skin flap into place.
f. Skin flap sutured into place as described in Figure 5-28
g. Suturing conjunctiva along edge of skin flap with continuous 6-0 absorbable suture that was left uncut at the nasal edge of the conjunctival flap
h. Tarsorrhaphy sutures in upper and lower lids

c. Bucket handle technique. Indicated in major full thickness defects. This technique permits a full thickness graft from the opposite eyelid. After the tumor has been removed, the graft is prepared from the opposite eyelid by making an incision 5 mm from and parallel to the eyelid margin. This incision should be at least 2 mm longer than the width of the defect. Full thickness, slightly diverging, incisions are made away from the eyelid margin until a flap has been prepared that will repair the defect. This flap is pulled beneath the intact border of the donor lid and sutured with two-layer closure into the defect. After 14 to 21 days the graft can be cut free at the eyelid margin of the repaired eyelid and the wound in the donor lid repaired.

3. *Comment.* Some eyelids are involved beyond surgical reconstruction, in which case they must be treated by removing the lids and globe.

ENTROPION - Entropion is inversion of the eyelid and eyelashes.

Etiology

1. Inherited - most common cause in dogs, (Table 5-1) and seen as a familial problem. The genetics are unknown. Inheritance also proposed in sheep and Persian cats.
2. Acquired - most common cause in other species
   a. Spastic - as a result of blepharospasm from corneal pain or conjunctivitis (usually unilateral)
   b. Nonspastic - postsurgery or cicatrix (trauma or postinflammatory)

Table 5-1. Conformation changes associated with inherited entropion courtesy of Wyman, Manual of Small Animal Ophthalmology, Churchill Livingston, 1986.

Large orbit	Defective muscle development	Primary lid deformity	Medial entropion
Collie	Chesapeake Bay retriever	Airedale terrier	Boston terrier
Doberman pinscher	Chow chow	Basset hound	Lhasa apso
Golden retriever	Samoyed	Bullmastiff	Pekingese
Great Dane		Cocker spaniel	Miniature pinscher
Irish setter		Curly-coated retriever	Miniature and toy poodle
Rottweiler		Bulldog	Pug
Weimaraner		English setter	Shih Tzu
		German shorthair pointer	
		Great Pyrenees	
		Kerry Blue terrier	
		Labrador retriever	
		Mastiff	
		Newfoundland	
		Old English sheepdog	
		Saint Bernard	
		Shar-pei	
		Springer spaniel	

Incidence

1. Dogs. Very common. The inherited form may occur soon after eyes open or until dog is fully developed. Entropion in any dog that is less than one year of age should be considered inherited entropion until a primary cause can be found. One or both eyes may be involved on first examination with the other developing entropion later. In some dogs, the inciting cause may be ocular irritation, in others spontaneous.
2. Cats - uncommon. Usually acquired after cat fights. Persian cats are predisposed.
3. Horses - uncommon. Generally seen in newborn foals (< 2 weeks of age). Are acquired less in adults.
4. Cattle - very rare.
5. Lambs. Usually seen in the spring after a conjunctivitis outbreak. Therefore, may have high incidence (80%) one year and insignificant the next year. Some ewes may be affected. Inheritance has been proposed. Author has seen small purebred flocks with high annual incidence.
6. Rabbits - usually seen in adults

Signs - Variable depending on the severity of pain and corneal changes

1. Epiphora - caused by interference with punctal function and wicking of tears on the face from lower eyelid hair

2. Prominent third eyelid - indicates degree of pain
3. Eyelid - use minimal eyelid manipulation to avoid stimulating further blepharospasm. Topical anesthetic will reduce blepharospasm, allowing a better evaluation of the eyelids.
   a. Blepharospasm is proportional to the amount of pain
   b. Evaluate degree of entropion when the eyelid is returned to its normal position. The entropion segment will be depigmented and have a waxy appearance. This depigmented zone is the landmark that determines the degree of entropion and in turn the amount of skin to be removed if a skin removal technique is selected for treatment.
   c. Determine if eyelid has developed an entropion memory pattern. This is due to orbicularis oculi muscle fibrosis and a memory pattern that results in the edge of the eyelid flipping over when the muscle contracts to blink the eyelid. After applying topical anesthetic, pull the eyelid away from the eye and then release it:
      1) Chronic entropion will recur immediately or after the first blink, indicating muscle memory pattern
      2) Acute (spastic) entropion will have normal eyelid position and maintain this position for several minutes or until the anesthetic wears off. Spastic entropion can usually be corrected with conservative treatment.
4. Conjunctiva
   a. May or may not have conjunctivitis
   b. Increased lymph follicle development is consistent with chronic entropion
5. Cornea - changes are related to severity of irritant
   a. Pigment - indicates chronic irritation
   b. Vascularization - superficial indicates chronic irritation; stromal occurs with corneal ulceration
   c. Fibroplasia - chronic irritation
   d. Ulceration - the most serious sequelae

Treatment

Choice for treatment is determined by species, age, severity of entropion and presence of corneal ulcers.

1. Repositioning the eyelid. This is often attempted by the owner but is unsuccessful in dogs and cats unless it is spastic and the cause is removed. In foals this may work but if unsuccessful after three to four days recommend injecting with penicillin.
2. Injection of eyelid with subconjunctival aqueous procaine penicillin.
   a. Foals - without corneal ulcers
   b. Rabbits - respond well to injection, except if there is a fracture of the tarsal plate. If injection is unsuccessful, a "V" resection of the fracture area (Fig 5-27) is recommended.
3. Tacking mattress sutures to evert the eyelid. Indicated in neonatal and acute spastic entropion.
   a. Foals (Fig 5-30) - treatment of choice with concurrent corneal ulcers. Sutures should be left in place 7 to 10 days.

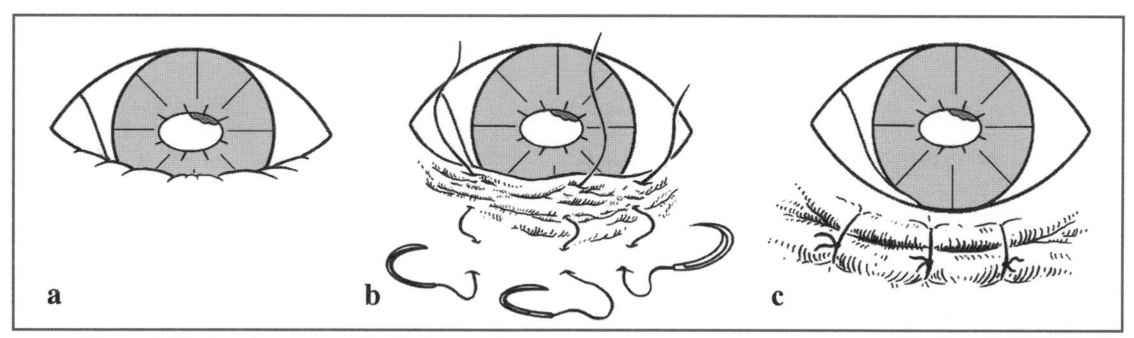

Figure 5-30. Tacking sutures for foal entropion.
a. Appearance of entropion lid
b. Lid after manipulation to correct entropion. Vertical mattress sutures preplaced in lower eyelid.
c. Appearance of lid after sutures have been tied

b. Neonatal entropion in puppies (Shar-pei, chow chow, Akita) (Fig 5-31). A common problem in Shar-pei. Entropion may develop soon after the eyes open and be presented for surgery by 2.5 weeks of age. Puppies at this age can be operated on without anesthesia but the author prefers general anesthesia using a mask and isoflurane. If the sutures remain intact for three weeks, most puppies will outgrow the problem. If it recurs, retacking can be done until the puppy is old enough for permanent surgery (4-6 months of age). If corneal ulcers become a complication, corrective surgery may be necessary sooner. Tacking may be successful on Shar-peis with mild changes as old as six months. Some dogs may need further surgical correction as adults.

c. Adult dogs with acute spastic entropion. Remove sutures after primary cause has been controlled or two to three weeks.

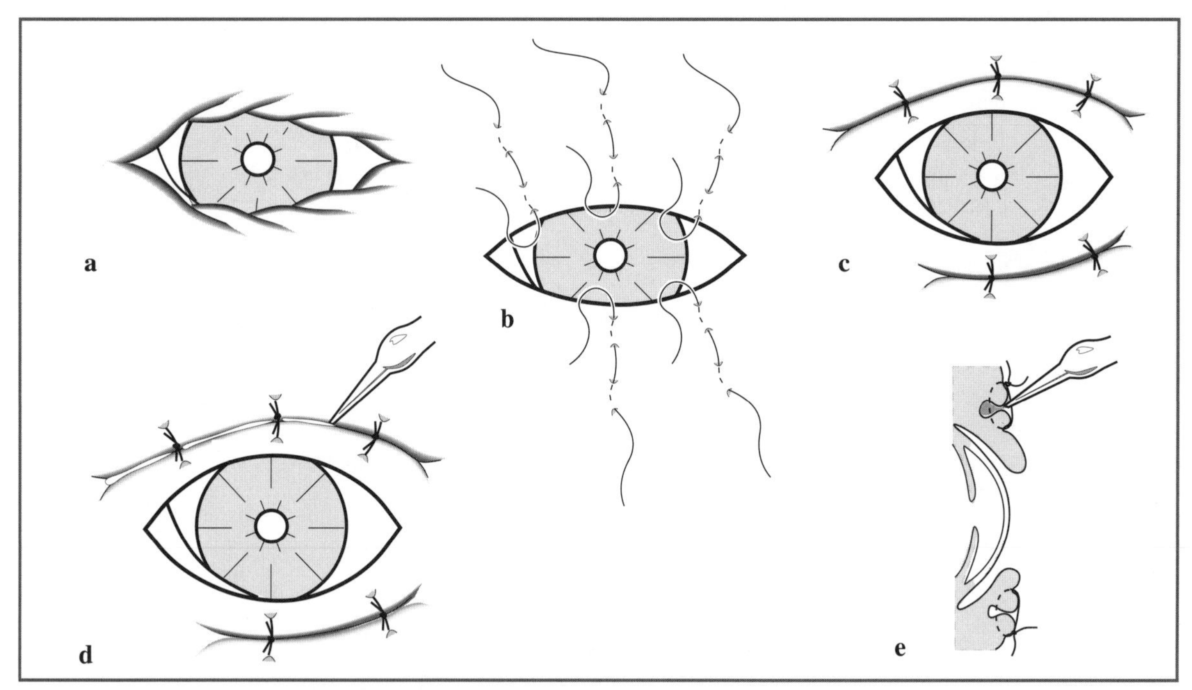

Figure 5-31. Tacking sutures for neonatal entropion in puppies.

a. Appearance of puppy with bilateral entropion
b. Placement of tacking sutures (preplacement as shown in this figure is not necessary)
c. Appearance after sutures are tied
d. Applying "super glue" into furrow created by tacking sutures
e. Cross section of super glue application

4. Medium skin staples - to evert the eyelids
   a. Lambs - the most practical way to treat entropion. Staples are usually allowed to come out on their own.
   b. Dogs - has been used in puppies with normal eyelid skin (chow chow) and adult dogs with acute spastic entropion. ***Do not use in Shar-pei puppies*** because their edematous skin is not strong enough to hold.
5. Surgical correction - many surgical techniques have been described for treating entropion. The simplest procedure is to remove a segment of eyelid skin that matches the shape of the entropion (modified Hotz-Celsus procedure). If there is a corneal ulcer, surgery should be performed as soon as possible. If corneal damage is minimal, a delay of one to two weeks will not cause irreversible damage. In cases with severe conjunctivitis and blepharitis, two to three days of premedication with topical and systemic antibiotics may be beneficial. Postsurgical medication would be determined by any complicating diseases at the time of surgery. Premedication is not generally recommended, but flunixin meglumine will reduce postoperative swelling.

a. The modified Hotz-Celsus procedure is the most popular technique for correcting entropion. Two basic techniques may be used.

The eyelid skin to be removed may be *pinched with a mosquito hemostat* to help delineate the tissue to be removed followed by scissors removal of the crushed portion (Figs 5-32).

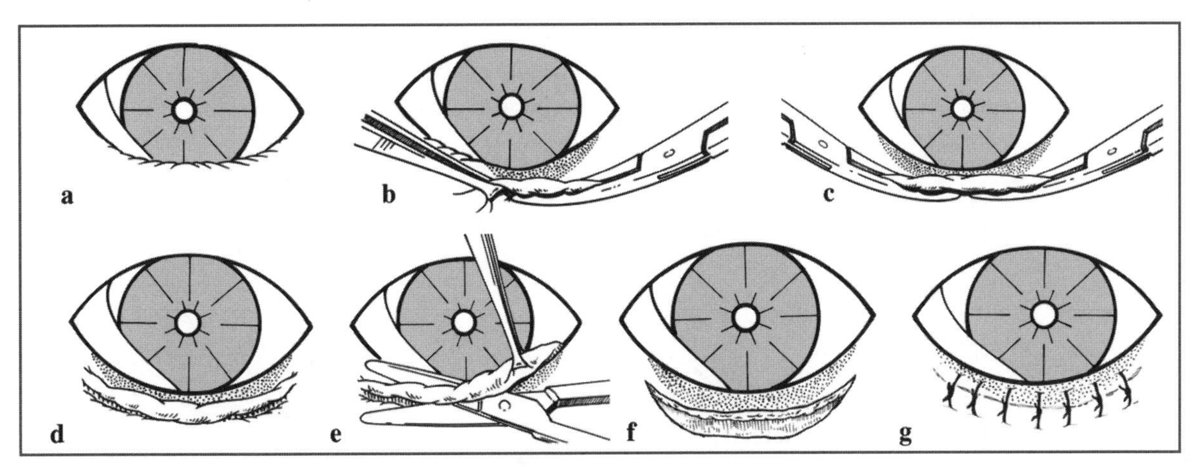

Figure 5-32. Hemostatic crush technique for entropion.

a. Appearance of eye before surgery
b. Grasping skin with curved mosquito hemostatic forceps. Shaded area along edge of the eyelid represents the area of eyelid that was touching the cornea.
c. Positioning second forceps
d. Appearance of eyelid after forceps removed. This incorporates enough skin to bring the eyelid into normal position. The skin that was rolled in is lighter-colored than normal skin.
e. Skin removed with surgical scissors. Be sure to start incision at the temporal canthus.
f. Appearance of wound after skin removal. The orbicularis muscle is not disturbed.
g. Wound sutured with 5-0 or 6-0 suture; 4-0 can be used in large breeds of dogs. Be sure to take a large suture bite so the stitch will not pull out before the wound is healed. The suture should bring the tissues into apposition but not be tight. The eyelid will develop postsurgical edema and sutures that are too tight will pull out.

Alternatively, *freehand scalpel skin incisions* may be used to outline the tissue to be removed. Then the skin within the incisions can be removed with small scissors (Fig 5-33). Scalpel excision is facilitated by using a lid plate (scalpel handle or tongue depressor works fine) to support the eyelid while making the incisions.

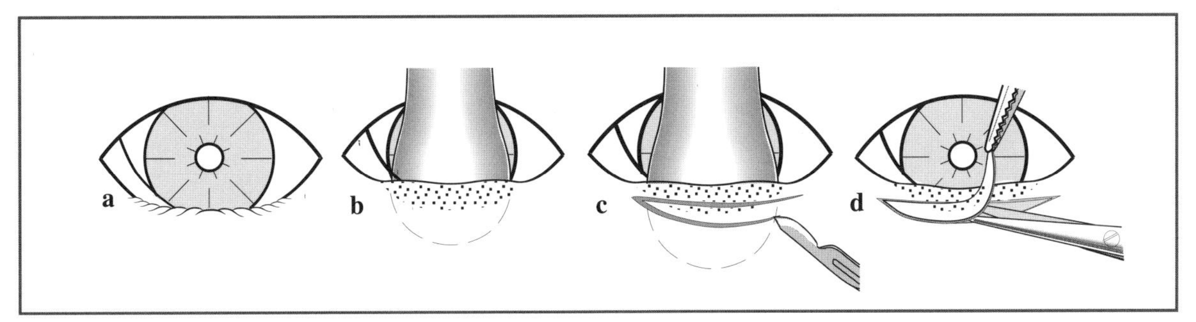

Figure 5-33. Free hand technique for entropion.

a. Appearance of eye before surgery
b. Stabilizing eyelid with lid plate. Shaded area represents eyelid that had turned in.
c. Skin incision same size and shape of tissue that had turned in. First incision should be within 3 to 4 mm from the edge of the eyelid.
d. Skin within incision area dissected free with scissors. The wound is closed in the same manner as in Figure 5-32 f and g.

With either method, ***it is imperative that the incisions be placed properly and tailored to fit the particular case being worked on*** (Figs 5-34 to 5-37). The skin nearest the lid margin should be parallel with the margin and placed just within the zone of eyelid hair growth (i.e. 3 to 4 mm from the lid margin). An incision too far from the margin will reduce the effect the removed skin has on the eyelid edge. An incision too near the margin will make it difficult to properly place the suture and could cause discomfort which would predispose the patient to rub the eye. It is important to entirely remove the skin and subcutaneous layers but it is NOT necessary to deliberately remove the orbicularis oculi muscle. Wound margins should not be beveled. The procedure is completed by closing the defect with simple interrupted sutures of 4-0 to 6-0 sized material, depending on skin thickness. Nonabsorbable sutures are preferred, but absorbable can be used if the owner cannot return for suture removal or if the patient's disposition would necessitate chemical restraint for removal. If the incision is long, two or three sutures dividing the wound will facilitate a smooth closure. Deep suture bites should be taken to close the subcutaneous tissues. Sutures should be

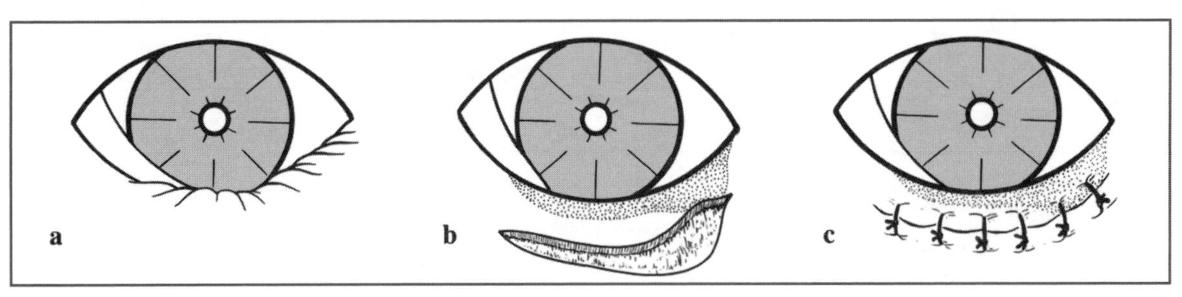

Figure 5-34. Severe entropion at canthus, mild in the center.
a. Before surgery
b. After skin removal
c. After suturing

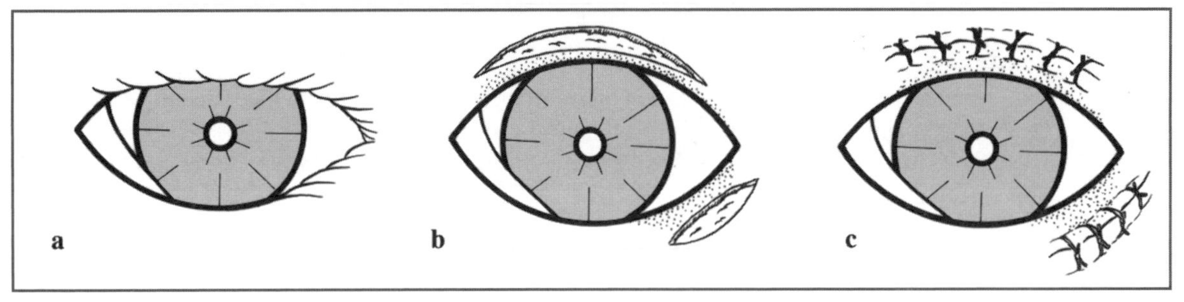

Figure 5-35. Complete entropion upper lid, partial entropion lateral canthus lower lid. This is often seen in the chow chow.
a. Appearance before surgery
b. After skin removal
c. After suturing

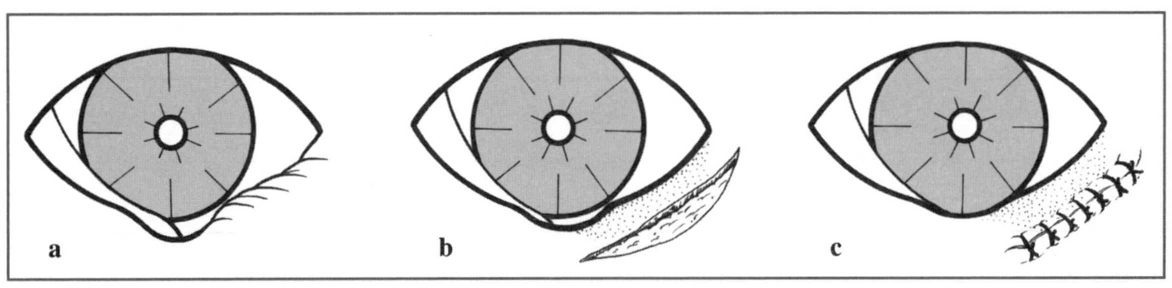

Figure 5-36. Lateral canthus entropion and central ectropion. Typical of St. Bernards.
a. Before surgery
b. After skin removal
c. After suturing

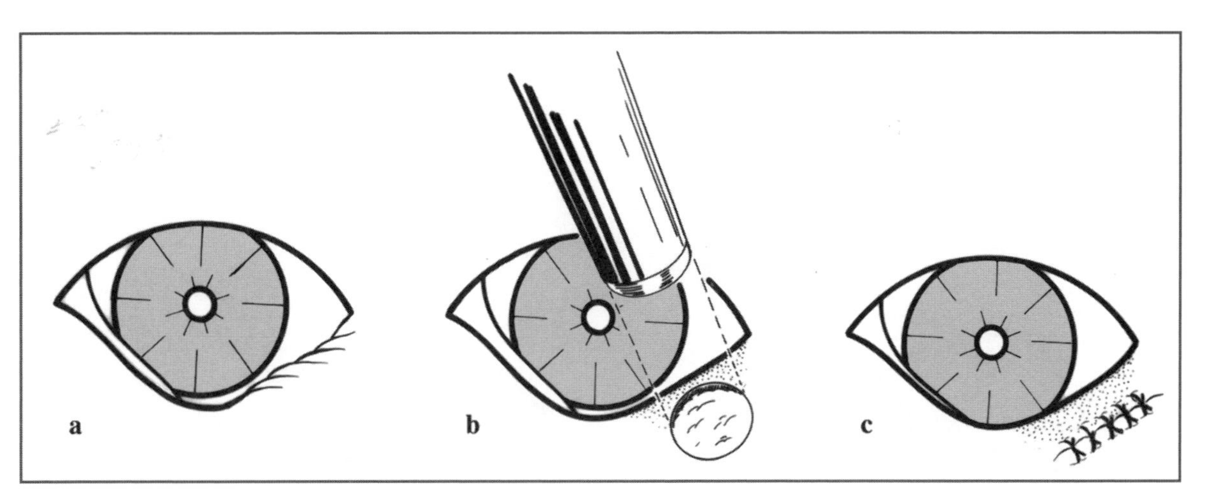

Figure 5-37. Trephine technique for lateral canthus entropion. This procedure works very well in St. Bernards.
a. Appearance before surgery
b. After skin removal with biopsy punch
c. After suturing

placed every 2 to 3 mm and tied to appose the wound margins, but not distort the skin surface. Cut the suture ends close to avoid corneal irritation. The eyelid will swell after manipulation and sutures placed too tightly may cause discomfort. Sutures can be removed in two to three weeks.

b. *Comment*
   1) The animal may appear overcorrected for about three to five days. At seven days the swelling will be gone and the degree of correction can be determined.
   2) If overcorrected, wait 30 days before considering corrective surgery. Some dogs improve with time. One will be more likely to undercorrect than overcorrect. In cases that do not have edema, less tissue needs to be removed. Overcorrection should be avoided.
   3) If a corneal ulcer exists, treat it conservatively. It will improve rapidly as a result of the removal of the irritation. If painful, a collagen shield, extended wear contact or nictitans flap can be used.
   4) Corneal pigment and/or vascularization will improve spontaneously when irritation has been removed.

c. Other techniques

1) Stades correction for upper eyelid trichiasis - entropion. J Am Anim Hosp Assoc 1987;23:603-606. This procedure is very useful in patients with redundant or scarred eyelids (Fig 5-38)

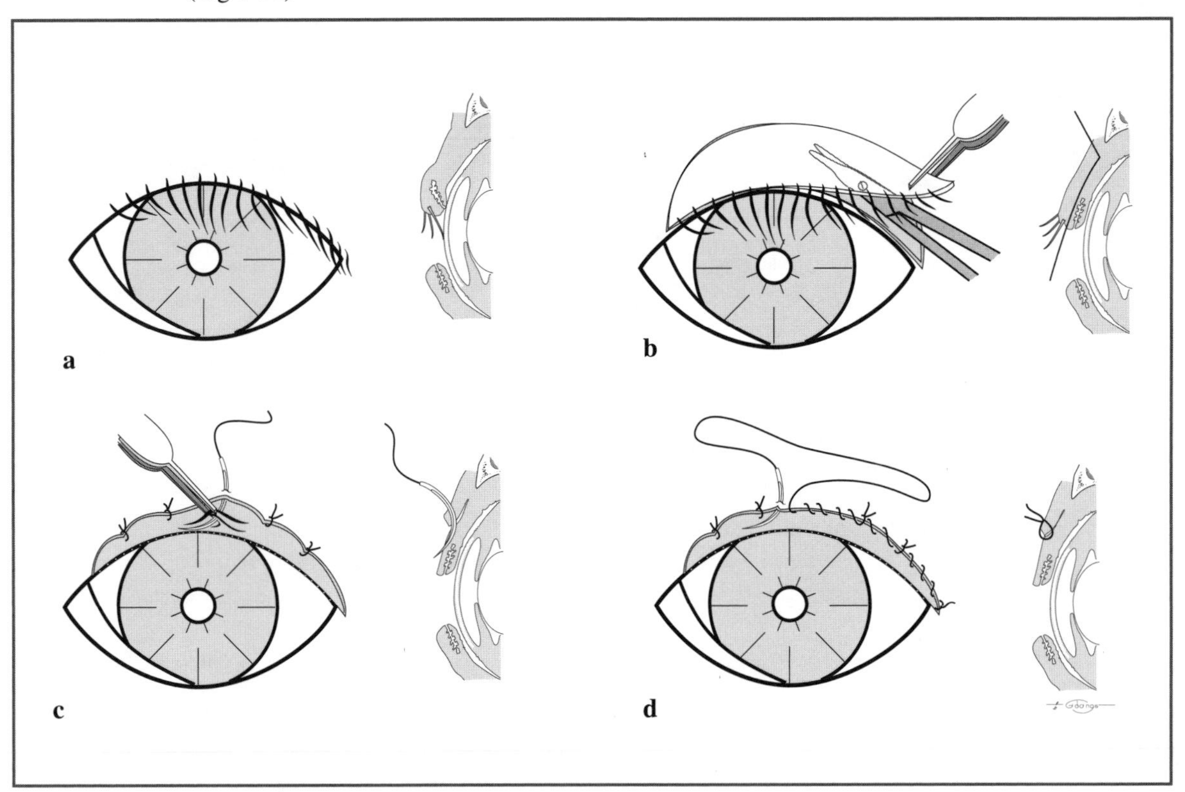

Figure 5-38. Stades correction for upper eyelid trichiasis-entropion.

a. Upper eyelid trichiasis-entropion before surgery
b. First incision made along border of eyelid superior to tarsal gland openings; this includes eyelashes. Second incision extends near dorsal orbital rim. Skin is removed by dissection with blunt-blunt scissors.
c. Superior skin edge anchored near base of tarsal glands with several interrupted sutures.
d. Skin edge oversutured with continuous sutures, allowing margin of the eyelid to heal by granulation.

2) Wyman modified the Hotz-Celsus procedure with a tarsal pedicle for severe lower eyelid entropion in the cat and dog. J Am Anim Hosp Assoc 1988;24:345-349 (Fig 5-39). Multiple pedicles may be necessary in patients with severe entropion.

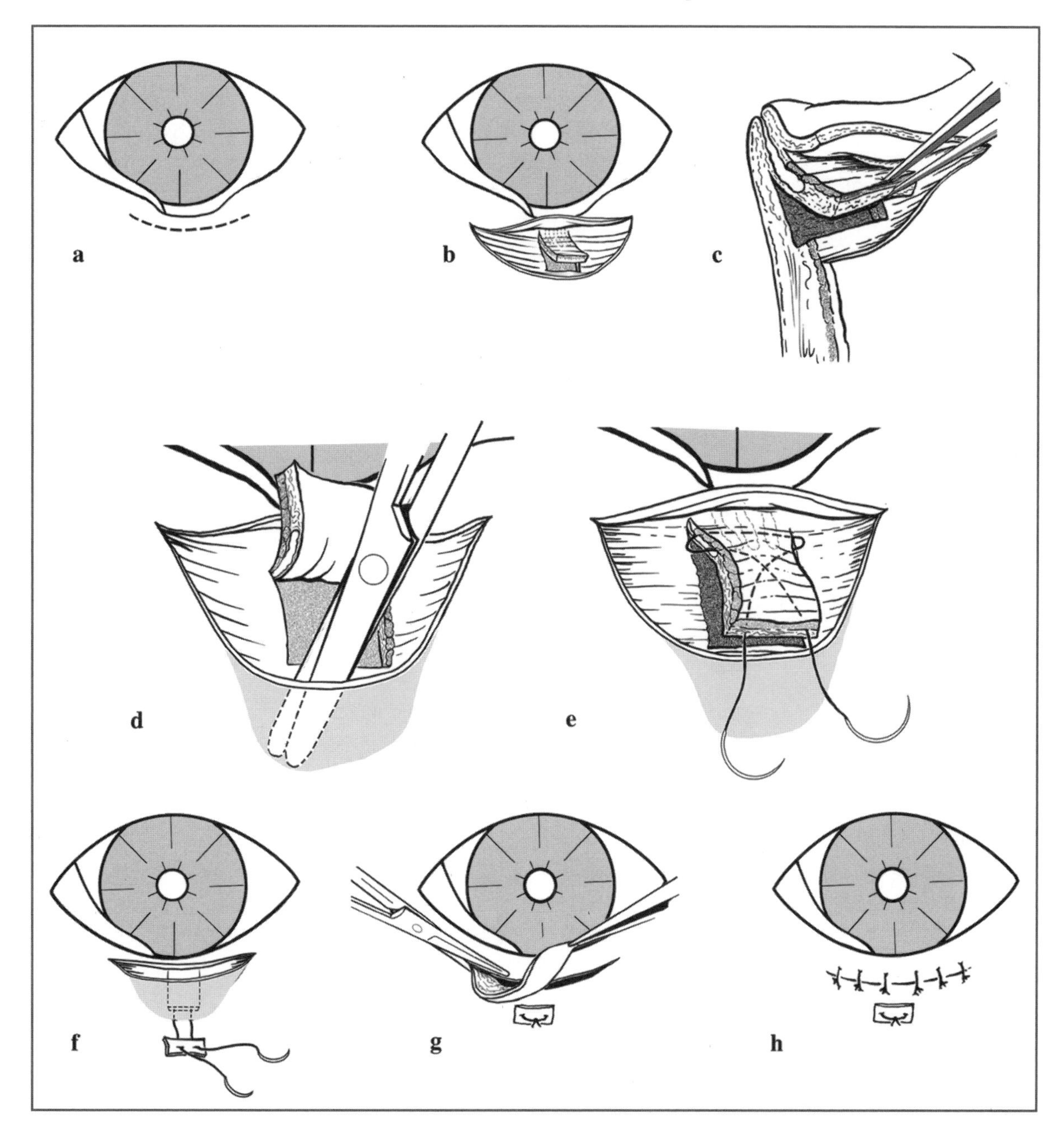

Figure 5-39. Wyman tarsal pedicle technique for entropion.

a. Severe central entropion lower eyelid. Dotted line represents initial incision site
b. Skin elevated along palpebral side of incision. Incision made in orbicularis muscle, and then pedicle flap dissected free to margin of eyelid
c. Cross-section of pedicle flap with base including tarsal glands
d. Subcutaneous pocket created with blunt dissection
e. 5-0 absorbable suture in pedicle flap using Bunnell suture pattern
f. Pedicle drawn into pocket and sutured over stent
g. Excess skin removed from lower side of incision
h. 5-0 nonabsorbable sutures placed in a divergent pattern

ECTROPION

Ectropion is eversion of the eyelid with exposure of the conjunctival surface. It involves the lower lid, is common in dogs, and rare in cats and large animals.

Etiology

1. Conformational - Breeds with loose facial skin and in some breeds considered normal. Hounds, setters, spaniels, retrievers, Saint Bernard, bulldog and boxer.
2. Transient - some hunting dogs will develop physiologic ectropion due to fatigue of the facial muscles. These dogs look normal in the morning and by evening have ectropion. There is nothing surgically or medically that can be done to help these dogs. Ectropion surgery in these dogs may lead to entropion.
3. Paralytic - damage to the branch of the facial nerve supplying the orbicularis muscle or total facial nerve paralysis in patients with large palpebral fissures. Will result in both ectropion and lagophthalmos. Close examination will reveal that the eyelids cannot be closed and tend to stay open, with resultant corneal irritation.
4. Scar tissue after eyelid injury contracting to pull the eyelid down. This would be unilateral.
5. Overcorrection of entropion

Signs

1. The eye is more subject to environmental irritation and frequently has a chronic conjunctivitis.
2. The exposed conjunctiva gives the eye a red appearance.
3. If the puncta are everted, epiphora will occur
4. Paralytic - will have a blinking deficit to the palpebral, corneal and menace reflexes

Treatment

1. Nerve paralysis - if the nerve paralysis is temporary, the condition will be self-correcting. Best to wait a couple of weeks. If the cornea shows progressive deterioration, protecting the eye with a third eyelid flap or a tarsorrhaphy is indicated. If paralysis is permanent, decreasing the palpebral fissure or as a last resort enucleation should be considered.
2. Conformational ectropion
   a. Medical treatment for conjunctivitis
   b. Surgery - seldom recommended
      1) Mild cases - shortening lower eyelid (Fig 5-40)
         a) V-resection at lateral canthus is preferred if there is no eyelid deformity. The edge of the eyelid is notched 3 to 4 mm from the temporal canthus with a mosquito hemostatic forceps. The actual lateral canthus is avoided because the eyelid is half as thick in the canthus as it is where meibomian glands are present in the eyelid. By staying 3 to 4 mm from the canthus, 2 to 3 meibomian glands will remain on the temporal side of the notch.

            The excess length of the eyelid is estimated and the eyelid is notched again to identify the estimated length of the eyelid border that is to be removed. The skin of the lower eyelid is crimped to form a triangle that has sides 2 to 3 times the length of the eyelid edge to be removed. The eyelid is incised with scissors, starting at the notch near the lateral canthus and extending to the crimped area of the skin on the eyelid. The cut edge of the eyelid is grasped with tissue forceps and pulled temporally until the eyelid is tense. The portion of the eyelid that overlaps at the temporal canthus should be removed. If the original estimate of the tissue to be removed was correct, the second notch will be at the point of the overlap.

            The overlapping portion of the eyelid is removed with scissors. The scissors are positioned so that the blade on the conjunctival side of the eyelid extends beyond the lower point of the wound. When the triangular piece of skin is removed in this manner, intact conjunctiva will be present in the lower half of the wound. The wound is sutured in the same manner as previously described for closing an eyelid laceration (Fig 5-25), page 179.

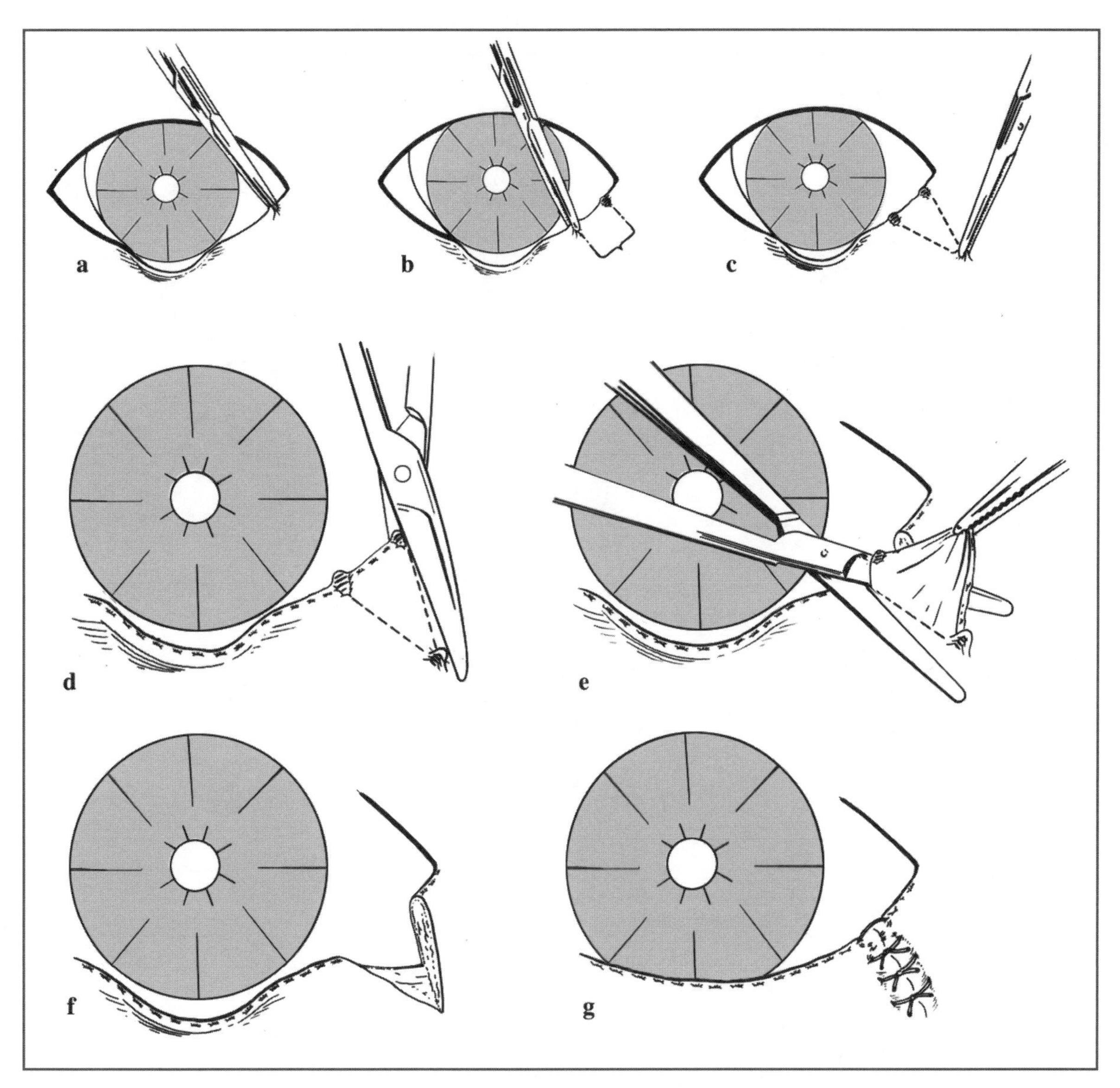

Figure 5-40. Lateral canthus triangle technique for ectropion.

a. Notching the eyelid 3 mm from the lateral canthus with mosquito hemostatic forceps
b. Estimate the excess amount of eyelid and notch the eyelid to indicate the amount of eyelid that should be removed
c. Crimping facial skin to outline triangle of skin to be removed
d. Making first incision from notch at temporal canthus to crimped area on the skin
e. Making second incision with scissors tip extended beyond the lower limit of wound
f. Appearance of eyelid after triangular piece of skin has been removed. Note that the conjunctiva is intact in lower 1/2 of wound.
g. Wound sutured with 6-0 nonabsorbable suture

b) Central eyelid technique for mild ectropion in dogs with damage or deformity of the tarsal plate (Fig 5-41). The technique is basically the same as recommended for the lateral canthus except the palpebral conjunctiva is left intact. Incise the entire thickness of the lid down to the base of the meibomian glands, then complete the triangle by removing only the skin. This leaves the conjunctiva intact. The wound is closed in the previous manner.

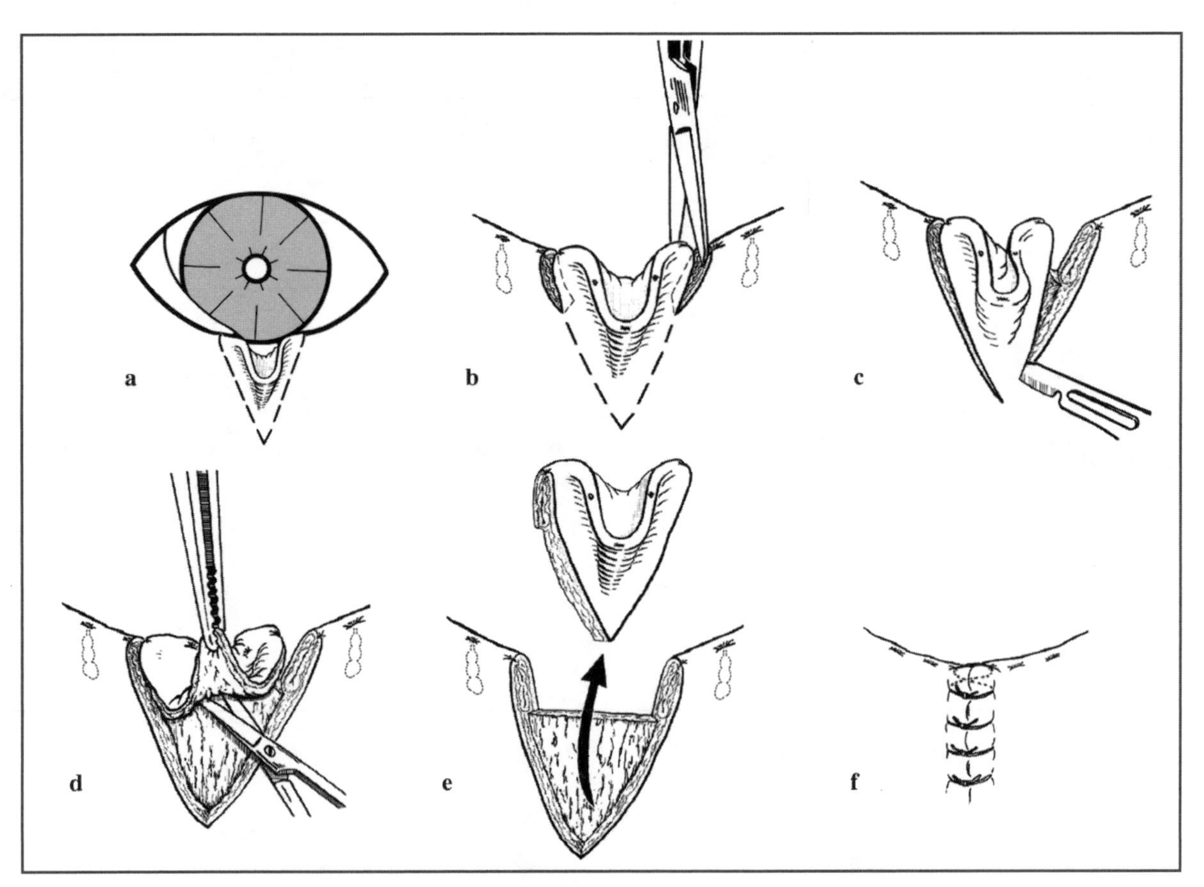

Figure 5-41. Removal of central triangle of skin for ectropion.
a. Eyelid with adhesion pulling lid down
b. Eyelid to be removed incised full thickness through portion of the lid containing meibomian glands
c. Skin only is incised for the remainder of the triangle
d. Triangle of skin being removed from the apex toward the base
e. Wound after the eyelid skin and margin have been removed. The intact conjunctiva is seen.
f. Eyelid wound sutured

2) Moderate to severe ectropion - modified Kuhnt-Szymanowski technique (Fig 5-42). Munger RJ, Carter JD Jr. J Am Anim Hosp Assoc 1984, pp654-656.

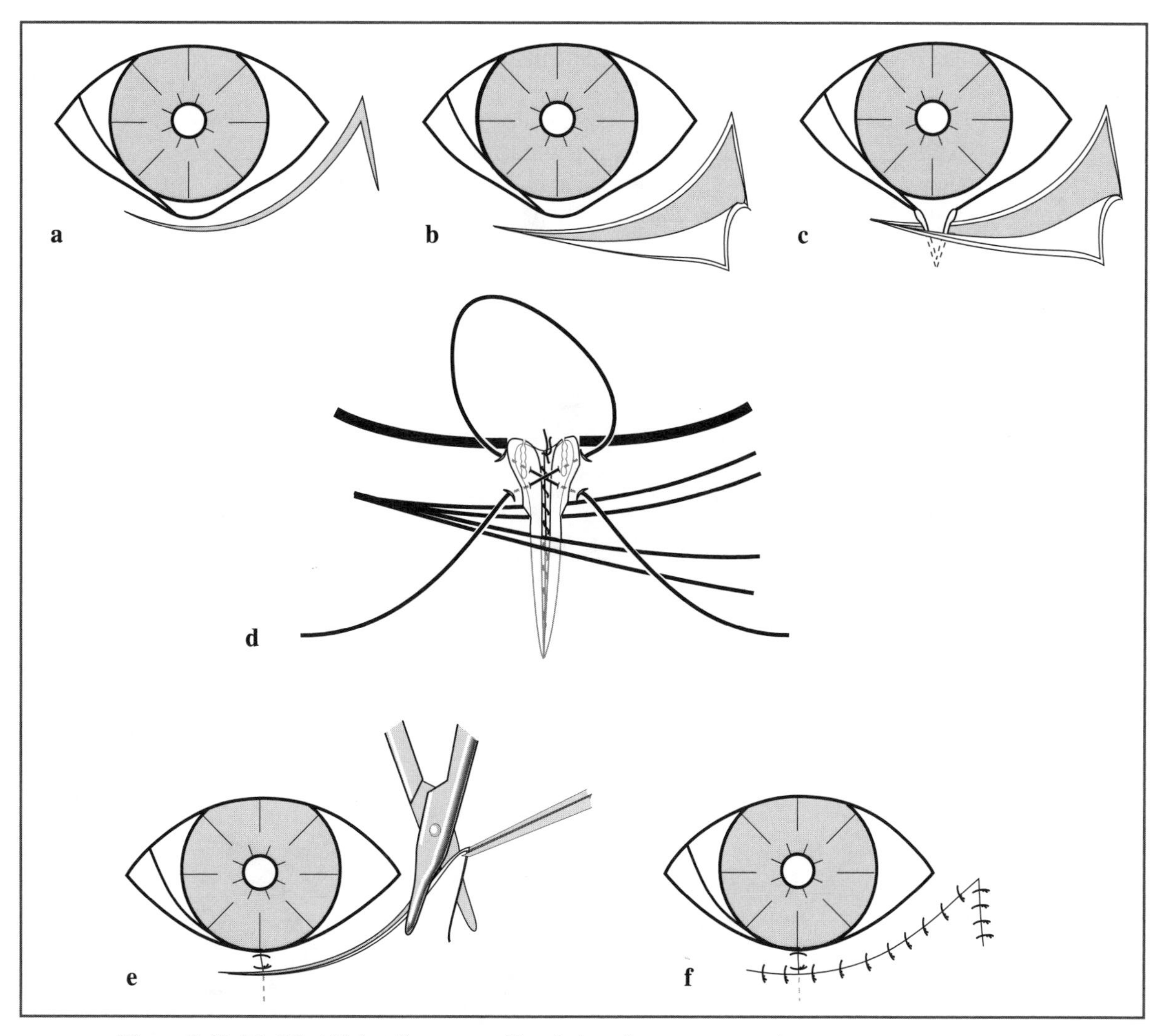

Figure 5-42. Modified Kuhnt-Szymanowski technique for severe ectropion.

a. Initial incision through skin and orbicularis m., 3 mm from and parallel to eyelid margin, extending 1 cm beyond lateral canthus. Second incision extends downward 1 to 5 cm.
b. Skin flap is undermined including orbicularis muscle
c. A triangle of tissue is removed from the lid margin and conjunctiva equal to the excess amount of eyelid
d. The conjunctiva is closed with absorbable suture using a continuous pattern. The eyelid margin is closed with a figure-eight suture.
e. Skin and muscle flap is pulled dorsolaterally and excess tissue excised in a triangle equal to the eyelid and tarsal conjunctiva
f. Final closure with interrupted suture

3. V-Y blepharoplasty for cicatricial ectropion
   a. Indications
      1) Scar tissue contraction from injury
      2) Overcorrection from entropion surgery
   b. Objective - to undermine the scar causing the ectropion and allow the edge of the eyelid to return to normal position
   c. Technique - A V-shaped incision is made that would extend beyond the limits of the ectropion (Fig 5-43). The location of the incisions is determined by a triangle with the base extending beyond the outer limit of the ectropion and the altitude equal to the base. The tip of the incision may nearly be canthus to canthus. The flap of skin is undermined deeply enough to ensure good circulation to the flap. Remove any scar tissue encountered as the flap is elevated. Using 4-0 to 6-0 suture, the wound is sutured from the point of the "V" upward until the flap forces the eyelid back to normal position. From this point, sutures are placed along the sides of the wound to create a "Y" appearance.

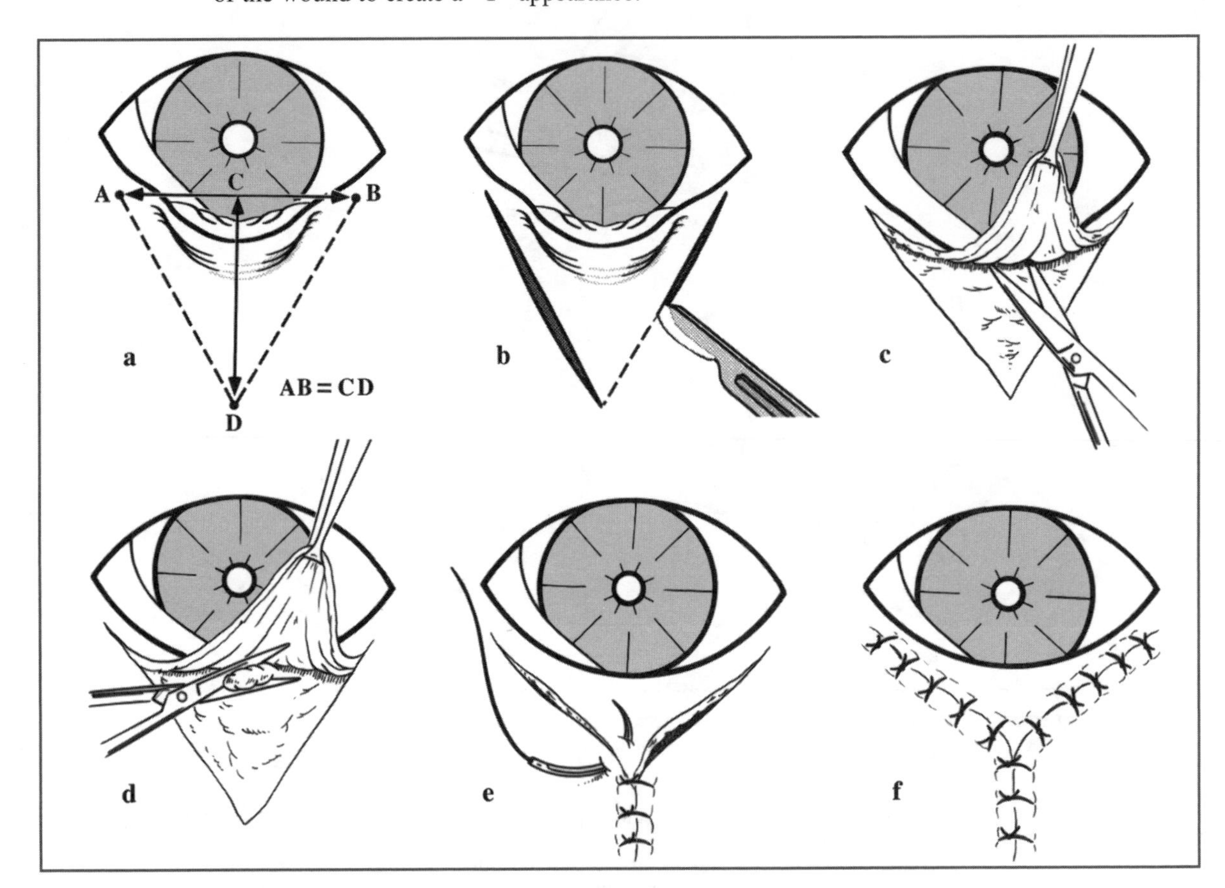

Figure 5-43. V-Y procedure for cicatricial ectropion.
a. Measurements used to determine location of incisions
b. V-shaped incision
c. Flap freed so it can retract upward, allowing edge of eyelid to roll back
d. Subcutaneous scar tissue excised
e. Y-closure to midpoint
f. Y-closure completed

EYELID CONTRACTION

After injury, scar tissue sometimes develops that results in contraction of a lid. Such contraction can be relieved with the Blaskovic canthoplasty to lengthen the eyelid (Fig 5-44).

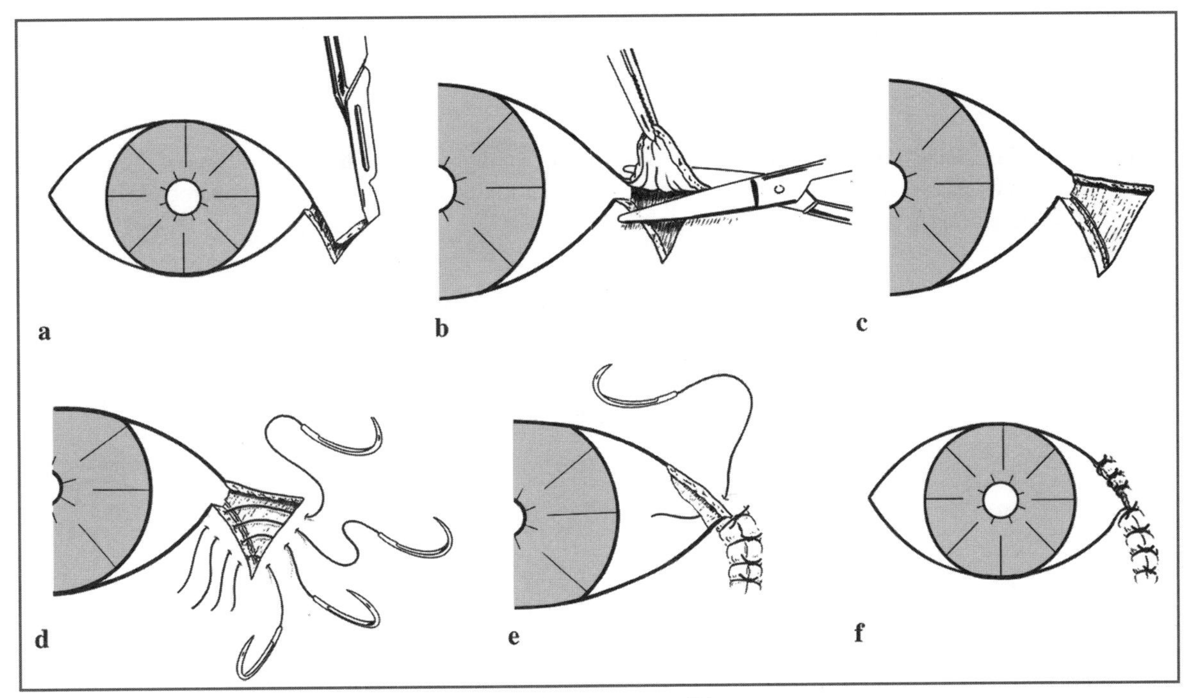

Figure 5-44. Blaskovic canthoplasty to lengthen an eyelid.

a. A "V" incision is made in the skin of the temporal canthus
b. The "V" is undermined and the undermined flap of skin is removed with scissors
c. The conjunctiva is incised along the side of the "V"
d. Sutures are placed in the sides of the triangle. This will add the length of the top of the triangle to the eyelid to be lengthened.
e. Appearance of the eyelid when skin sutures are tied. The conjunctival edge is trimmed and sutured to the skin.
f. Completed surgery

LAGOPHTHALMOS - Failure of the eyelids to meet when they are blinked

Occurrence - most frequent in breeds with marked eye protrusion

Causes

1. Congenital - breed predisposition in brachycephalic dogs with large eyes. May also sleep with the central cornea exposed.
2. Primary nerve dysfunction (facial paralysis)
3. Secondary

SYMBLEPHARON - An adhesion between tarsal and bulbar conjunctiva

SYMBLEPHAROPTERYGIUM - a form of symblepharon in which the palpebral conjunctiva joins the globe with cicatricial band.

These diseases are seen as a complication to infections and superficial neoplasms. Treated by surgically relieving the adhesion. The third eyelid may be involved. Seen most frequently in cats after neonatal herpesvirus conjunctivitis.

PTOSIS (BLEPHAROPTOSIS) - Uncommon. Drooping of the upper eyelid due to paralysis of the levator muscle. Caused by paralysis of CN-III (oculomotor). This is usually a minor problem compared to the loss of the rest of the functions of the CN-III nerve.

DISEASES OF DISTURBED INNERVATION OF THE EYELID

Facial paralysis - results from lesions of the nucleus of the facial nerve up to its termination into the branches that supply the muscles, resulting in a facial paralysis (palsy)

1. Causes
   a. Idiopathic - the most common cause in dogs. Predisposed breeds are boxers, cocker spaniel, English setter, Pembroke corgi
   b. Trauma and surgery
   c. Neoplasia
   d. Otitis media in cats
2. Signs
   a. Normal muscle tone of the muscles of the other side of the face pulls the nose toward the normal side. In dogs the nostril may not be opened as wide on the affected side during inhalation.
   b. The lip on the affected side is flaccid and drooling is common. Some animals will show self-mutilation from chewing on the lip when eating. Horses - trouble picking up hay and moving it back in the mouth.
   c. The eyelids cannot be blinked because of the loss of function of the orbicularis muscle. In small animals the palpebral fissure is slightly larger and in large animals there is slight ptosis. In exophthalmic eyes, exposure keratitis may occur, leading to ulceration. Ulcers in horses are located in lower one-third of the cornea. When the eye is touched, it is sensitive and will be retracted by the extrinsic ocular muscles, but the patient does not blink.
   d. Auricular nerve paralysis results in a lowering of the position of the ear.
   e. Equine - traumatic injury to the peripheral branches affecting nose and lips can occur. This may be permanent or temporary.
3. Treatment
   a. Symptomatic with systemic cortisone for two to four weeks
   b. Keep the eye moist to prevent exposure keratitis and secondary corneal ulcers. Suturing the eyelids or third eyelid flapping may be indicated. Dogs with protruding eyes may have persistent lesions, making eye removal the treatment of choice.
   c. A peripheral conjunctival flap is very effective in controlling the ulcer that frequently occurs in the lower one-third of the cornea just above the lower limbus.
4. Course - allow four to six weeks before considering the disease permanent

Hemifacial spasm - Spasm of the muscles supplied by the facial nerve is usually unilateral and secondary to chronic otitis externa. A rare condition the author has observed in dogs.

1. Causes
   a. Most frequently seen secondary to chronic otitis externa with calcification of the ear canal
   b. Afferent stimulus by demodectic mange of the face
2. Signs - spasm of the muscles innervated by the facial nerve results in:
   a. Pulling of nose to affected side
   b. Elevation of commissure of the lip to give a grinning effect
   c. Constant squint of the eyelids. This may lead to entropion in some dogs.
   d. Spasm of the auricular muscles resulting in an elevated position to the ear. In breeds with erect ears, this will cause the ear to be pulled toward the midline.
3. Differential diagnosis - this lesion results in changes that can be confused with facial paralysis of the opposite side of the face. Thorough examination easily differentiates the diseases.
4. Treatment - none effective. If entropion occurs, may need to do corrective surgery. Alcohol blocking of the auricular palpebral branch of the facial nerve may control the blepharospasm. Do not block the nerve in exophthalmic breeds because of the danger of exposure keratopathy.
5. Course - a permanent change

HORNER'S SYNDROME

Horner's syndrome is paralysis of the sympathetic innervation to the eye and adnexa. Recommended reading—Neer TM. Horner's syndrome: Anatomy, diagnosis and causes. Compend Contin Educ Pract Vet 1984;6:740-747.

1. Neuroanatomy - The sympathetic nervous system maintains the normal muscle tone of the smooth muscles of the periorbita, eyelids (Müller's muscle), third eyelid, and dilator muscle of the iris (Fig 5-45). This tone keeps the eyeball protruded, the palpebral fissure widened, the third eyelid retracted, the normal pupil partially dilated, and vasoconstrictor tone to the cutaneous blood vessels.

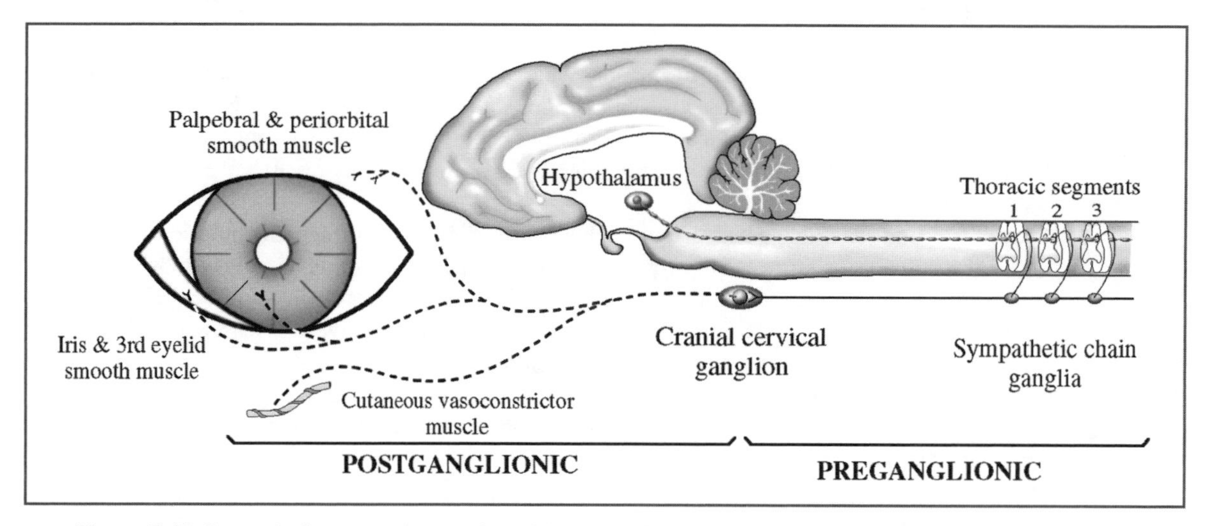

Figure 5-45. Sympathetic nervous innervation of the eye and adnexa
- First order preganglionic nerve fibers originate at the hypothalamus and proceed down the spinal cord (beaded line)
- Second order preganglionic nerve fibers leave at T1 - T3 and extend up the cranial thoracic and cervical sympathetic trunk to the cranial cervical ganglion (solid line)
- Postganglionic nerve fibers disperse from the cranial cervical ganglion to the eye, adnexa and cutaneous blood vessels (dashed line)

2. Etiology - Disruption of sympathetic pathway at any level due to infection, injury or neoplasia. Middle ear disease is probably the most common cause in small animals. Frequently idiopathic - dogs 50%, cats less frequent. Associated neurologic signs may involve facial nerve and/or inner ear.
   a. Preganglionic neurons
      1) First order - brain and spinal cord lesions (uncommon). Usually have additional neurologic changes.
      2) Second order - lesions involving T1-T3, brachial plexus, cranial thoracic sympathetic trunk, and cervical sympathetic trunk. Concurrent neurologic signs if present vary with location of lesion.
   b. Postganglionic neurons - originating at cranial-cervical ganglion. Lesions may involve cavernous sinus, middle ear, guttural pouch in horses, and orbit.
3. Signs - usually unilateral. Severity is variable, ranging from slight miosis to all of the signs listed below.
   a. Miosis of affected eye resulting in anisocoria that is most pronounced in a darkened room.
   b. Enophthalmos - from lack of tone of smooth muscle of periorbita allowing retractor oculi to pull the eye posteriorly
   c. Protrusion third eyelid - caused by enophthalmos and possible lack of smooth muscle tone (cats have definite smooth muscle to third eyelid)
   d. Narrowing of palpebral fissure (squint) - from ptosis of upper eyelid and enophthalmos
   e. Cutaneous peripheral vasodilation - increased skin temperature (especially ear) and sweating of ipsilateral side

f. Species variations
   1) Horses - profuse sweating of face and cranial neck, skin hyperthermia, and prominent ptosis. Moderate myosis and protrusion of the third eyelid.
   2) Cattle, sheep and goats - ptosis and hyperthermia, slight miosis and third eyelid protrusion. Cattle have *decreased* sweating on the surface of the nose.

4. Diagnosis
   a. The presenting signs are sufficient to establish a diagnosis
   b. Localization of the lesion
      1) Good physical and neurologic examination
      2) Possible lab work and radiographs
      3) Pharmacologic testing - to localize lesion
         a) In man a protocol using 4 to 6% cocaine, 1% hydroxyamphetamine and dilute epinephrine has been successful, but this has been unpredictable in animals. This has been modified for animals as follows:

Drug	Central	Preganglionic	Postganglionic
10% phenylephrine	-	-	+
1% hydroxyamphetamine*	+	+	- or poor
6% cocaine*			

* Minimum of two days between hydroxyamphetamine and cocaine.

         b) In animals the most practical test is 10% phenylephrine drops administered in both eyes. In postganglionic Horner's syndrome, the receptor cells are supersensitive and in 20 minutes the affected pupil will dilate more rapidly than the normal eye. In preganglionic Horner's syndrome, the affected pupil will be dilated in 40 minutes.

5. Treatment
   a. Specific - if possible, determine and control the primary cause. As the primary lesion resolves, symptomatic treatment may often be terminated.
   b. Symptomatic treatment
      1) 2.5% phenylephrine (preferred) 2 to 4 times daily PRN
      2) 0.5 to 1.0% epinephrine 2 to 4 times daily PRN. Epinephrine does not penetrate the cornea as effectively and individual variations are greater.

6. Course - most idiopathic cases resolve in eight weeks

IDIOPATHIC NICTITANS PROTRUSION IN CATS

Etiology and signs

1. Cause is unknown and related to an imbalance in the sympathetic innervations to the nictitans (i.e. sympathetic neuritis caused by a slow virus resulting in a decrease in sympathetic tone to third eyelid smooth muscle). It has been referred to as anterior sympathetic cervical ganglionitis.
2. History and/or signs of diarrhea or watery feces
3. May be unilateral initially but usually soon becomes bilateral and symmetrical
4. No other ophthalmic abnormalities are noted
5. Dramatic response to topical epinephrine or phenylephrine
6. Diagnosis is made by ruling out other causes and recognizing the condition. The problem usually lasts two to six weeks, but on occasion the duration may be three months.
7. Other cats in household may develop the disease (suggesting an infectious cause)

Differential diagnosis

1. Systemic disease causing enophthalmia due to debilitation, dehydration, cachexia, etc
2. Ocular pain causing enophthalmia
3. Microphthalmia, phthisis bulbi
4. Horner's syndrome

CHAPTER 6 - THIRD EYELID

ANATOMY AND PHYSIOLOGY

The third eyelid (nictitating membrane, membrana nictitans) is an essential ocular structure for all domestic animals. It is located in the nasal canthus and contains a T-shaped hyaline cartilage giving it rigidity. The base of the cartilage is embedded in a lacrimal gland (gland of the third eyelid, gland nictitans, gland nictitating membrane) (Fig 6-1).

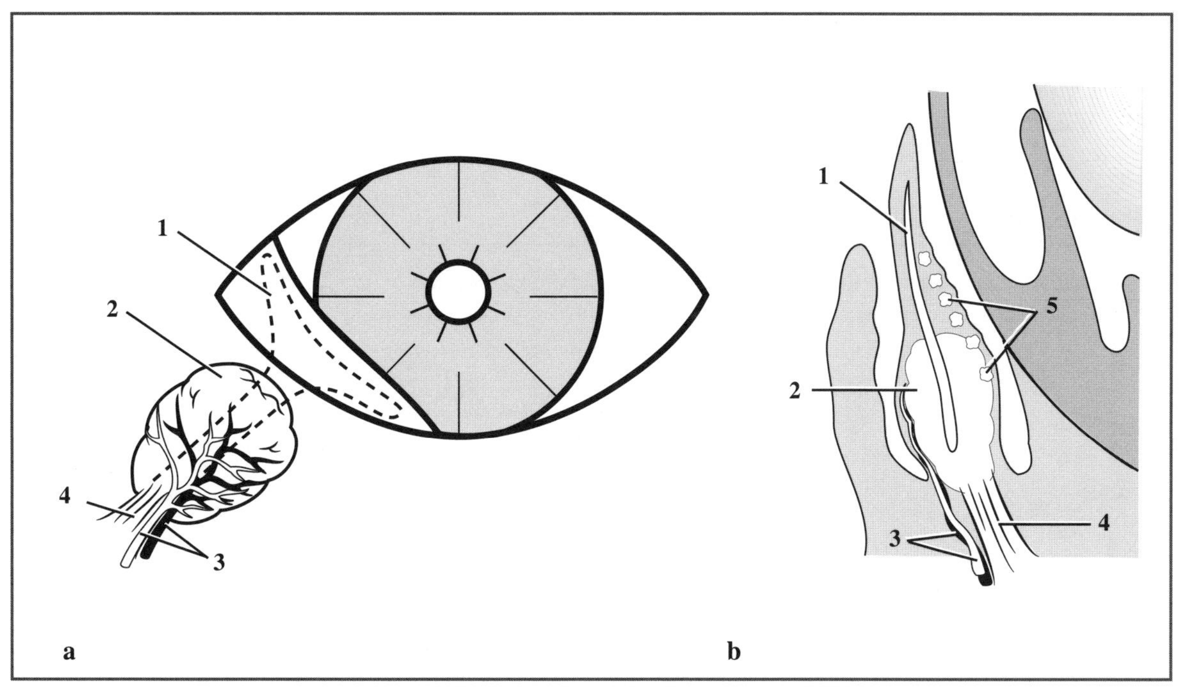

Figure 6-1. Anatomy of third eyelid, dog. 1) Cartilage, 2) Gland, 3) Blood vessel, 4) Connective tissue band to periorbital tissue, 5) Lymph follicles
- a. Cartilage and gland of third eyelid shown schematically and relative location indicated.
- b. Cross section of third eyelid and adjacent structures

FUNCTIONS OF THE THIRD EYELID

Protect the cornea

Reshape the tear film

Lacrimal activity

1. Gland of the third eyelid (gland nictitans)
   - a. It has parasympathetic innervation via the infratrochlear branch of CN-V
   - b. Type of secretion
     - 1) Serous - cat, horse
     - 2) Seromucoid - cattle, dog
     - 3) Mucoid - pig
   - c. Dogs - it produces about 50% (Gelatt 35%) of the tears
2. Harderian gland - cattle, pig, rabbit. A separate lipid-producing gland deeper in the orbit. Phylogenically this was the first lacrimal gland and is still the primary lacrimal gland in many nonmammalian species.

Reticuloendothelial activity - the bulbar surface has a large accumulation of lymph follicles

MOVEMENT

Passive movement - Passive movement is related to retraction of the globe applying pressure on retrobulbar fat, which in turn puts pressure on the gland of the third eyelid and associated cartilage to move the third eyelid over the cornea. By this mechanism, contraction of the retractor oculi forces the third eyelid over the eye.

Active movement

1. Active movement is controlled by smooth muscle fibers attached to the base of the third eyelid and keeping the gland retracted.
2. The cat has striated muscle fibers, originating from the lateral rectus muscle and inserted near the free margin, that provide voluntary control of the third eyelid.
3. Birds. In birds, third eyelid movement is voluntary, moving from dorsal nasal to temporal inferior and is controlled by the pyramidalis muscle.

Stabilization of the gland of the third eyelid

Fibrous attachments between the gland of the third eyelid and periorbital tissues limit the gland's movement and prevent it from prolapsing.

CONGENITAL DISEASES

ENCIRCLING THIRD EYELID

An encircling third eyelid is seldom seen. When present, it may be seen with additional adnexal lesions. Removing the band that dorsally encircles the eyelid is satisfactory treatment.

Beagles and cocker spaniels frequently show an encircling remnant that is pigmented and easily identified during examination. This remnant does not cause any clinical problem.

LACK OF PIGMENTATION

The third eyelid may or may not be pigmented, depending on the hair coat color characteristics of the animal. The lack of pigment may be unilateral or bilateral.

Nonpigmentation results in a reddened appearance to the third lid, which becomes exaggerated with conjunctivitis. Normal pigment in the third eyelid blends with iris and lid color in such a way that most owners are unaware that the third eyelid exists. The pigment is protective. When pigment is missing, the third eyelid may be subject to irritation by the sun and become thickened, precancerous, or develop squamous cell carcinoma.

Dogs - The third eyelid is normally pigmented along the free border. Nonpigment is considered a fault in some breeds (e.g. collies, Shetland sheepdogs). Owners may think a normal eye with a nonpigmented third eyelid has an infection because of the natural redness of the third eyelid, and thus will bring the dog in for examination. Nonpigmented third eyelids are more subject to solar irritation and conjunctival hyperplasia, especially in collies.

Horses - may or may not be pigmented depending on the skin coloring. When nonpigmented, it is subject to solar irritation and has a predisposition for squamous cell carcinoma.

Cattle - often nonpigmented in whitefaced cattle; these are predisposed to squamous cell carcinoma

Cats - usually are nonpigmented but seldom develop pathology because of this. They are less likely to develop solar irritation than the dog and less likely to develop squamous cell carcinoma than large animals.

Treatment - nonpigmentation is not usually treated unless showing solar reaction. Cortisone ophthalmic preparations will help. Tattooing has been used in dogs and horses to arrest irritation, but is more difficult and not as effective as eyelid tattooing. Therefore, seldom recommended. For technique see eyelid tattooing, Chapter 5, page 176 .

DERMOID GROWTHS

Dermoids of the third eyelid are rare except in cattle. In cattle the third eyelid is the most common location of ocular dermoid. These lesions may affect the third eyelid only, or extend out on the globe to include the cornea.

Surgical removal is recommended if the dermoid interferes with normal function or is causing irritation.

ACQUIRED DISEASES

PROTRUSION OF THE THIRD EYELID

The lay term for a prominent third eyelid is haws.

Causes

1. Enophthalmos
   a. Ocular pain
   b. Loss of orbital mass - dehydration, loss of fat
   c. Systemic diseases with increased muscle tone (tetanus, rabies, strychnine poisoning, canine distemper, meningitis)
   d. Neurologic disorders - Horner's syndrome, idiopathic prolapse in cats, generalized dysautonomia
2. Decrease in ocular size - microphthalmos, phthisis bulbi
3. Space-occupying lesion in the orbit - abscess, cyst, hemorrhage, neoplasia
4. Deformity of the orbit - trauma, chronic sinusitis in horses, neoplasia

Treatment

Treat the underlying cause. ***Do not remove the third eyelid for cosmetic reasons.***

EVERSION OF THE CARTILAGE - Eversion of the cartilage is of clinical significance only in the dog.

Causes

1. Inherited - seen most frequently in Weimaraners, Newfoundlands, Chesapeake Bay retrievers, and Saint Bernards. Also reported in bull mastiff, Doberman, German shepherd, German shorthair pointer, Great Dane. Usually occurs before six months of age.
2. Acquired - after injury to the third eyelid or improper suturing of a third eyelid flap (all species).
3. Congenital - author has observed this as a unilateral lesion in one newborn foal.

Signs

1. The cartilage develops an outward curl. This results in scroll appearance to the edge of the third eyelid. The curl may occur anywhere between the narrow portion of the cartilage near the gland or to the free edge of the third eyelid. The tips of the top of the "T" portion of the cartilage may curl, similar to a ram's horn.
2. Secondary changes - conjunctivitis and keratitis may develop, in which case there will be an ocular discharge.
3. There is little physical discomfort unless a secondary conjunctivitis develops or the eversion is due to trauma.
4. In horses, the tip of the "T" may cause a slight irregularity in the surface of the third eyelid. It will not cause any problem, so it should be left alone.

Treatment - using scissors, surgically remove the deformed cartilage from the posterior surface of the third eyelid. Be sure to leave the anterior surface intact (Fig 6-2). ***Do not remove the entire third eyelid.***

1. Technique for removal of deformed cartilage involving the narrow portion of the "T". The third eyelid may be fixed with a chalazion forceps or immobilized with fixation forceps. The conjunctiva is incised over the curled cartilage and then separated free by dissection with delicate blunt scissors (corneal or strabismus). The curled cartilage will protrude through the wound. Next, separate the cartilage from the anterior conjunctiva by blunt dissection until the entire deformed cartilage is free from the conjunctiva. Remove the deformed cartilage and reposition the third eyelid to its normal position. The wound edges should cover the remaining cartilage. If the third eyelid does not lie smoothly, suture the wound with 6-0 or 7-0 absorbable suture. See Figure 6-2 h to k for suturing technique.

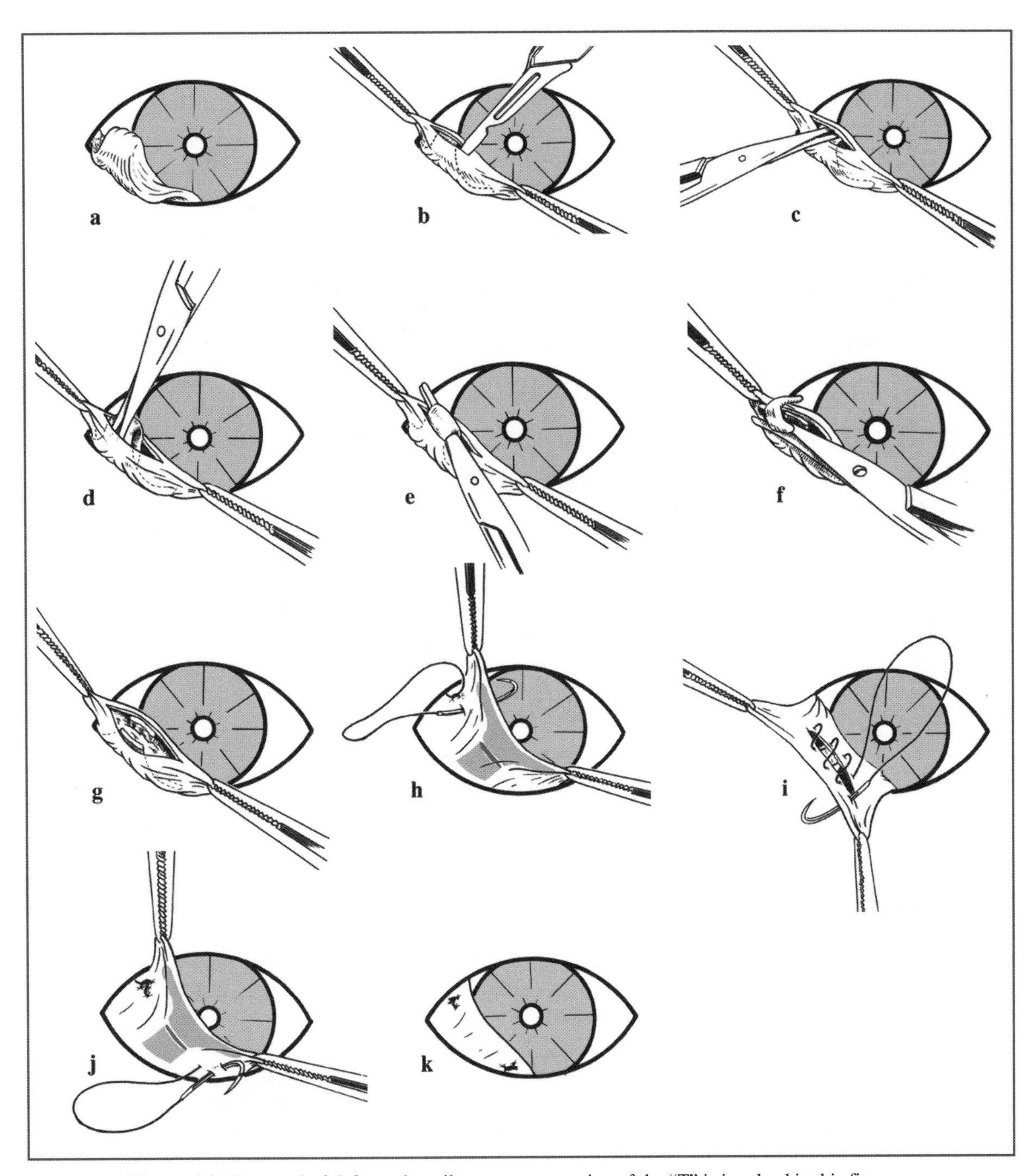

Figure 6-2. Removal of deformed cartilage; narrow portion of the "T" is involved in this figure.

a. Appearance of the everted third eyelid
b. Third eyelid immobilized with forceps exposing the posterior surface. Incising conjunctiva over curl in deformed cartilage.
c. Posterior conjunctiva dissected away with delicate blunt scissors
d. Separating cartilage from conjunctiva near edge of eyelid
e. Scissors introduced beneath cartilage to separate it from the conjunctiva on anterior surface of third lid
f. Removing deformed cartilage
g. Appearance of wound after surgery is complete and third eyelid ready for repositioning
h. If third eyelid does not lay down properly, 6-0 absorbable suture is anchored in the anterior surface of third eyelid and then the suture pulled through to the posterior surface.
i. Wound closed with continuous suture pattern
j. Suture brought back to anterior surface and tied
k. Appearance when surgery is complete

2. When the deformed cartilage involves the "T" at the free edge, the dissection is more difficult and most of the "T" may need removal. This is done similarly to that previously described. The "T" tips can be left in the third eyelid without causing any problems.

FOLLICULAR CONJUNCTIVITIS

Pathogenesis - Lymph follicles are located on the posterior surface of the third eyelid in all domestic animals. The follicles contribute to the tear film and are an essential part of the mechanism of controlling ocular infection. Any chronic irritation or immunologic stimulant will stimulate them to become hyperplastic. If the stimulus persists, new follicles will develop anywhere on the conjunctiva (palpebral, bulbar or anterior aspect of the third eyelid). Increase in the size of the follicles on the posterior aspect of the third eyelid is referred to as folliculitis, folliculosis or follicular hyperplasia. When follicles develop elsewhere on the conjunctiva, it is referred to as follicular conjunctivitis. After the follicles have been stimulated to a certain point, they will sustain themselves even if the initiating cause has disappeared.

Etiology and incidence

1. Dogs - a very common disease
   a. Any prolonged ocular irritation - bacterial conjunctivitis; mechanical (ectropion, entropion, distichiasis)
   b. Any immunologic stimulus - migrating parasites; allergic conjunctivitis (highest incidence in spring and summer)
   c. Tends to be more severe during pollen season
2. Cats - an uncommon disease in cats. When seen often associated with chlamydial conjunctivitis
3. Horses - seen less frequently than in dogs; similar causes to the dog. May be seen with conjunctival *Onchocerca* microfilaria.
4. Sheep, cattle and goats - associated with chlamydial conjunctivitis

Signs

1. Dogs
   a. Persistent mucoid discharge at the medial canthus of the eyes
   b. Picking up the third eyelid and examining the posterior surface will expose hyperplastic follicles. They have a red, roughened appearance. If true follicular conjunctivitis, follicles will be present on all conjunctival surfaces.
   c. Mild cases require cleaning the eyes each morning. As the disease becomes more severe, the discharge must be cleaned several times a day. In severe cases, the eyelids may stick together in the morning until the owner opens and cleans them.
2. Horses
   a. Occasional follicles are seen near the limbus as an incidental finding without other signs.
   b. Severe involvement is rarely seen. When seen, concurrent conjunctivitis will be present.
3. Cats, sheep, cattle and goats - the presence of follicles should cause the examiner to suspect chlamydial conjunctivitis and/or other systemic signs of chlamydial infection.

Treatment

1. Specific - remove initiating cause
2. Symptomatic treatment in dogs. This disease is usually more distressing to the owner than it is to the patient, therefore treatment may be optional.
   a. Mild cases will respond to cortisone-antibiotic ophthalmic medicines. If the case is of short duration, recovery may be complete; if the disease is longstanding, the discharge will generally return when medication is discontinued.

b. Severe cases

1) Removal of follicles from back of third eyelid. Topical anesthesia is usually adequate to treat follicles limited to the bulbar surface of the third eyelid. If all conjunctival surfaces are involved, general anesthetic is recommended.

   a) Technique - grasp the third eyelid with a curved mosquito forceps, parallel to its border, and roll the third eyelid up on the forceps. Then using a gauze sponge, dull blade, or the sharp edge of a copper sulfate crystal, scrape the follicles to rupture as the third eyelid is unrolled.

   b) If a sponge or dull blade is used, mild cauterization of the ruptured follicles with a tincture of iodine swab will reduce regeneration later.

   c) If a copper sulfate crystal is used, scrape the tissues with single strokes, immediately flush liberally with saline solution, and instill a liberal amount of ophthalmic ointment between the cornea and third eyelid before releasing the forceps. Copper sulfate can cause severe corneal damage, therefore do not allow copper sulfate crystals to touch the cornea, and do not scrape the tissues repeatedly.

   d) Aftercare - the eye will be inflamed. Treat with antibiotic/corticosteroid ointment TID as needed. Cyclosporine 1% may reduce recurrence.

2) Removal of follicles from other conjunctiva

   a) Electrocauterization of each follicle is effective but time consuming

   b) Individual removal with scissors

PROLAPSE OF THE GLAND OF THE THIRD EYELID - Prolapse of the gland of the third eyelid is referred to as cherry eye by breeders.

Pathogenesis - The normal gland of the third eyelid has connective tissue bands anchoring it to periorbital tissues. If these bands do not develop properly, postorbital fat can cause the gland to prolapse when the eye is retracted into the orbit by the extrinsic muscles. Any superficial irritation (e.g. conjunctivitis) may act as the stimulus to cause the eye to retract into the orbit. Inflammation and hypertrophy of the gland develop as soon as the gland is prolapsed.

Etiology

1. Dogs
   a. A congenital lack of the connective tissue band to fix the gland to the periorbital tissues. Probably inherited and seen most frequently in beagles, bulldogs, cocker spaniels, Lhasa apsos, and Pekingese
   b. Post-traumatic (wounds to orbit or third eyelid)
2. Cats - inherited problem in Burmese and Persian cats. Littermates have been observed to have corneal dermoids.
3. Horses - posttraumatic

Occurrence - seen frequently in dogs, rarely in cats

Signs - there is often a history of periodic prolapse of the gland before it remains prolapsed (Fig 6-3)

1. The gland protrudes above the free border of the third eyelid, becomes inflamed, and enlarges. After protruding, it becomes red; hence the term "cherry eye".
2. Secondary epiphora and conjunctivitis may occur

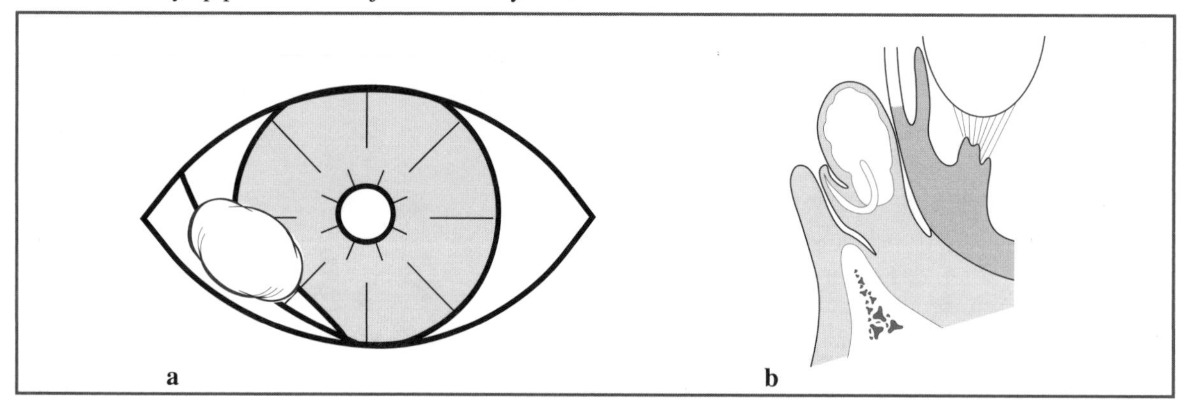

Figure 6-3. Prolapse of the gland of the third eyelid.
a. Frontal view representing the appearance of the patient
b. Cross section view showing the relationship to adjacent tissue

Treatment

1. Do nothing - predisposes the patient to chronic conjunctivitis
2. Remove the gland. This has been a common practice for many years, but cannot be recommended in breeds predisposed to keratoconjunctivitis (bulldog, cocker spaniel, Lhasa apso) or dogs with a Schirmer tear test less than 15 mm in one minute. Therefore owners must be cautioned of this risk if they choose removal, even in breeds that are not at risk.

a. Topical anesthesia is usually adequate - general anesthesia or chemical restraint in hard-to-handle dogs
b. Topical epinephrine or neosynephrine while anesthetizing the conjunctiva will reduce hemorrhage
c. Grasp with forceps and snip off with scissors (Fig 6-4) or electrocautery (Fig 6-5). Some of the cartilage of the third eyelid will be removed with the gland.
d. Reapplication of topical epinephrine and cotton held over the eye for a few minutes will provide adequate hemostasis.

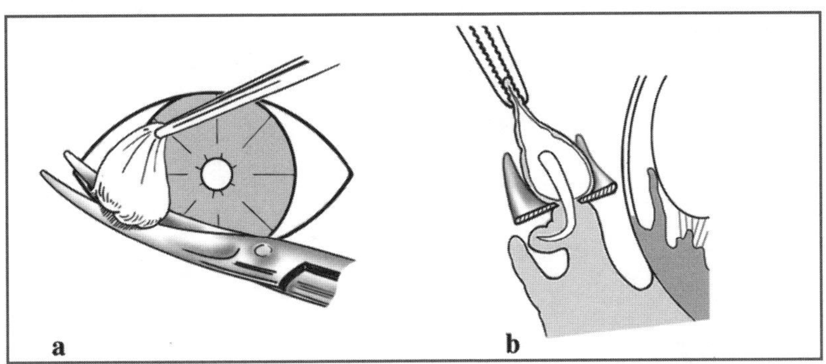

Figure 6-4. Removing prolapsed gland of the third eyelid with scissors.
a. Frontal view
b. Cross section (Tips of scissors seen next to gland)

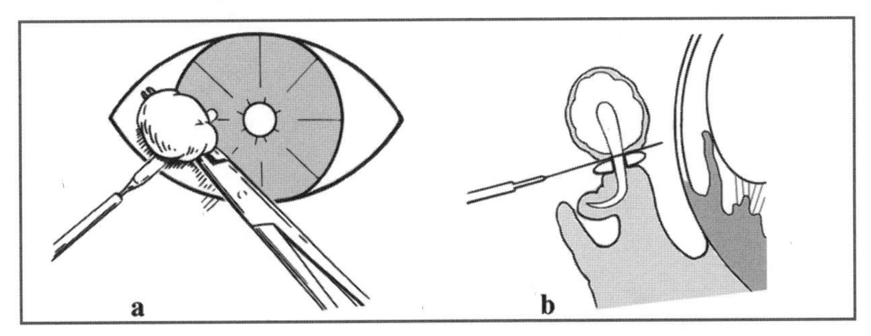

Figure 6-5. Removing prolapsed gland of the third eyelid with mosquito hemostatic forceps and electrocautery. The forceps is placed below the gland and the cautery is used to remove the tissue above the forceps.
a. Frontal view
b. Cross section

3. Reposition the gland
   a. The pocket technique described by Morgan (J Am Anim Hosp Assoc 1993;29:57-59) is effective (Fig 6-6). If the prolapse is long standing, the cartilage may develop a memory for curving. In this case a conjunctival incision in the palpebral side of the third eyelid will expose the cartilage in the area of curvature. Incising the cartilage will facilitate repositioning the gland. Next, after giving general anesthesia, two incisions are made on the posterior surface of the third eyelid, parallel to the free margin, on either side of the prolapsed gland. One incision 2 to 3 mm from the free margin, and the other 6 to 7 mm toward the base of the third eyelid. The length of both incisions is about 1 cm. A pocket is formed with blunt-pointed scissors below the gland, then the gland is returned to its normal position and held in place by suturing the two incisions together with 5-0 or 6-0 absorbable suture using a continuous suture pattern. The knots must be buried to avoid irritating the cornea. If additional support is desired, a second suture layer with an inverting continuous horizontal mattress can be used. Starting and finishing the suture pattern on the anterior surface of the third eyelid (see Fig 6-2, j and k page 211) will eliminate the need for burying the knots.

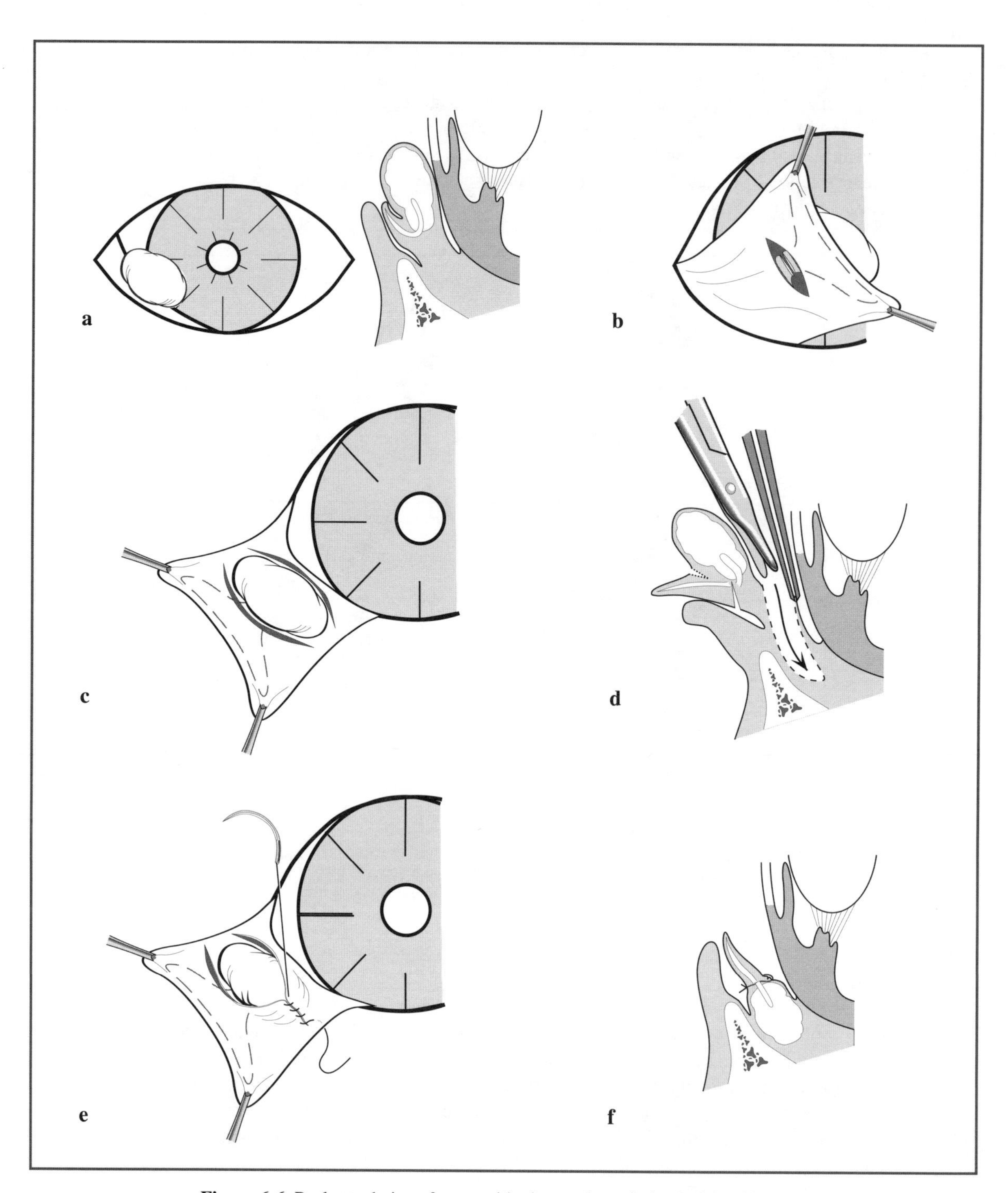

Figure 6-6. Pocket technique for repositioning prolapsed gland of the third eyelid.

a. Frontal and cross-section view
b. If the cartilage is severely curved, the conjunctiva of the palpebral surface can be incised and the cartilage cut in the area of curvature.
c. One cm incisions made above and below the gland
d. Side view showing pocket that the gland will be repositioned into
e. Suturing incisions together to reposition the gland in the pocket. After the continuous pattern is completed, oversew with a Lembert pattern and then bring the suture to the anterior surface of the third eyelid, so it can be tied to the free end as shown in the diagram.
f. Gland repositioned and knots on anterior surface of third eyelid

b. Purse-string technique - described by Moore (Fig 6-7). After general anesthesia, the third eyelid is stabilized with forceps exposing the prolapsed gland on the bulbar surface. Using 5-0 or 6-0 absorbable suture a purse-string suture is placed in the conjunctiva around the gland margins. Next, the conjunctiva over the gland is abraded. The prolapsed gland is returned to normal position with a cotton-tipped applicator and the purse-string pulled tight, the knot tied, and the ends cut short. Aftercare consists of topical antibiotic ophthalmic ointment 5 to 7 days.

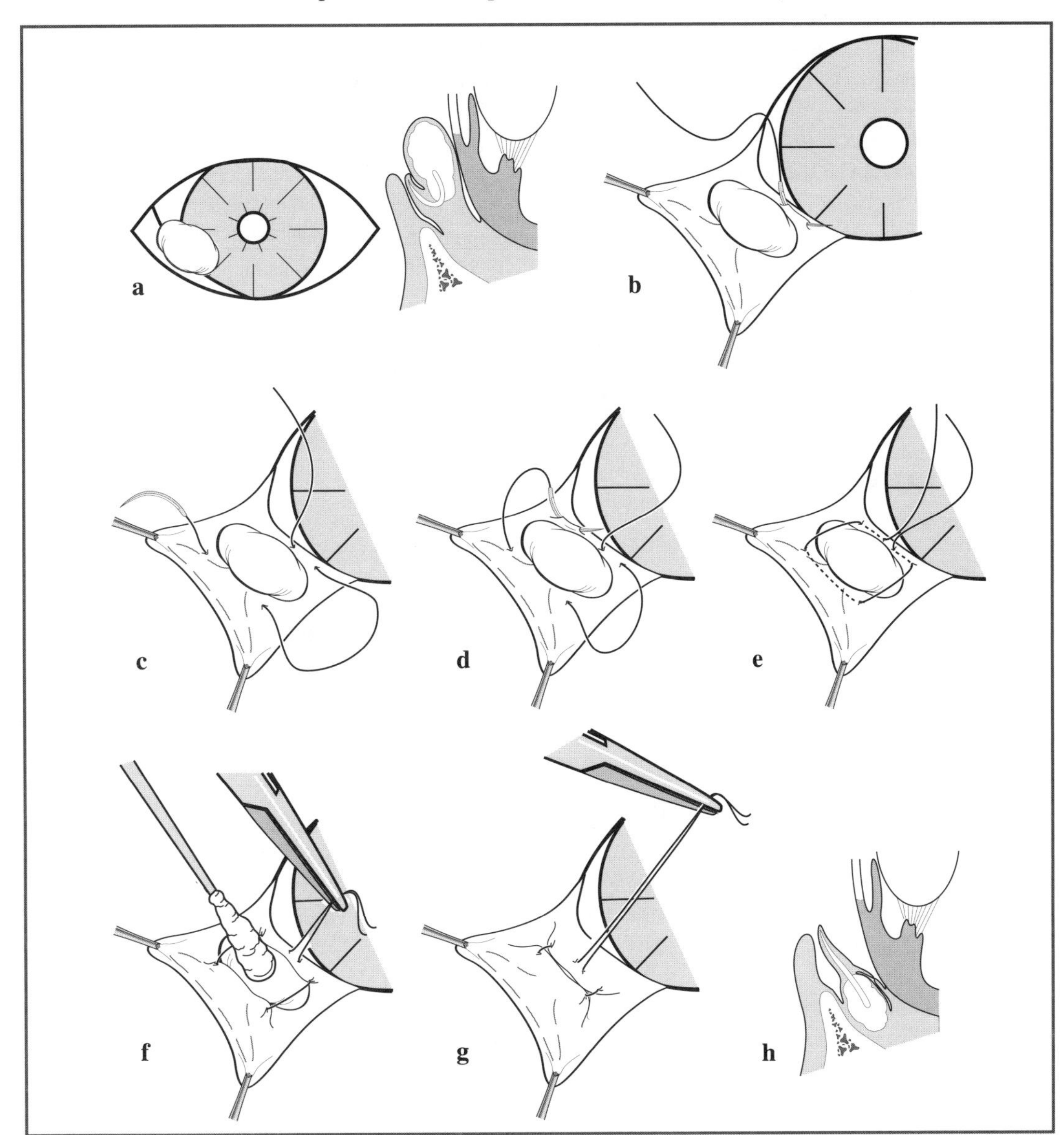

Figure 6-7. Purse-string technique for repositioning prolapsed gland of the third eyelid.
- a. Cross-section appearance of prolapsed gland of the third eyelid.
- b. Third eyelid stabilized with forceps exposing prolapsed gland. First one-half of inferior suture is placed using a 4 mm bite.
- c. Superior suture placed with 8 mm bite
- d. Final position of inferior suture placed with 4 mm bite
- e. Conjunctival surface of gland is ready to be abraded
- f. Gland repositioned with cotton tip applicator as purse-string is drawn tight
- g. Appearance of surface when suture ready for tying the knot. Suture ends cut short.
- h. Cross-section appearance when surgery complete

4. *Comment* After most repositioning surgeries the nictitans mobility is reduced and partial reprolapse is possible. Often the nictitans appears thickened due to poor gland positioning.

CONJUNCTIVAL HYPERPLASIA DUE TO SOLAR IRRITATION

1. Animals with nonpigmented third eyelids may develop chronic solar irritation. This leads to hyperplasia of the exposed conjunctiva of the third eyelid. This thickening is slowly progressive and gives a red, inflamed appearance to the third eyelid. This can be precancerous in horses and cattle. Therefore cytology or biopsy is necessary to establish a positive diagnosis. It generally does not require treatment but, if severe, can be relieved with topical corticosteroid antibiotic ointments.
2. Third eyelid depigmentation and thickening as a result of plasma cell infiltration occurs in dogs with German shepherd pannus. This can occur early in the disease before characteristic corneal changes are obvious.

THIRD EYELID GRANULOMAS

Dogs - Granulomatous thickening will occur in collies and related breeds as part of nodular granulomatous episclerokeratitis before typical lesions occur on the globe (see Chapter 9, page 281).

Horses - Granulomatous nodules may develop on the base of the third eyelid and nasal caruncle as a result of invasion of tissue with *Habronema* larvae. The use of ivermectin has greatly reduced the incidence. The center of the nodule may abscess or undergo a caseous necrosis. Surgical curettage or excision followed by topical antibiotics is effective treatment.

THIRD EYELID CYSTS

The author has seen several dogs with third eyelid cysts associated with the gland of the third eyelid. Surgical removal of the gland and cyst was curative.

NEOPLASIA - presumptive diagnosis should be confirmed by biopsy or cytology.

Dogs - neoplasms are uncommon

1. Histiocytomas are seen concurrently with involvement of the eyelids (see neoplasia eyelids for treatment, Chapter 5, page 180).
2. Adenocarcinoma of the gland of the third eyelid. The gland will enlarge and cause partial prolapse. Unilateral. Remove the affected gland. If there is any chance that the tumor involves the peripheral portion of the gland, it is advisable to remove the entire third eyelid and suture the resulting conjunctival wound.
3. Benign hemangioma is the most common tumor of the third eyelid. These respond favorably to surgical excision. Hemangiomas more commonly involve the bulbar conjunctiva than the third eyelid.

Cats - squamous cell carcinoma is seen occasionally. Surgical removal of the involved part of the third eyelid is adequate if caught early enough. Hyperthermia and cryosurgery can also be used. If extensive, remove the entire third eyelid and suture the palpebral conjunctiva to the bulbar conjunctiva.

Horses - squamous cell carcinoma is more common in animals that lack third eyelid pigment. The method of treatment is at the discretion of the clinician.

1. Small lesions - hyperthermia, cryosurgery or surgical removal. If hyperthermia is used, be careful to avoid excessive treatment that may lead to cartilage necrosis and disfigure the third eyelid. If the third eyelid cartilage is exposed when removing a small portion of the third eyelid, suture the outer and inner conjunctival edges over the exposed cartilage (Fig 6-8). This will speed healing and prevent inflammatory granulation tissue from developing at the site.

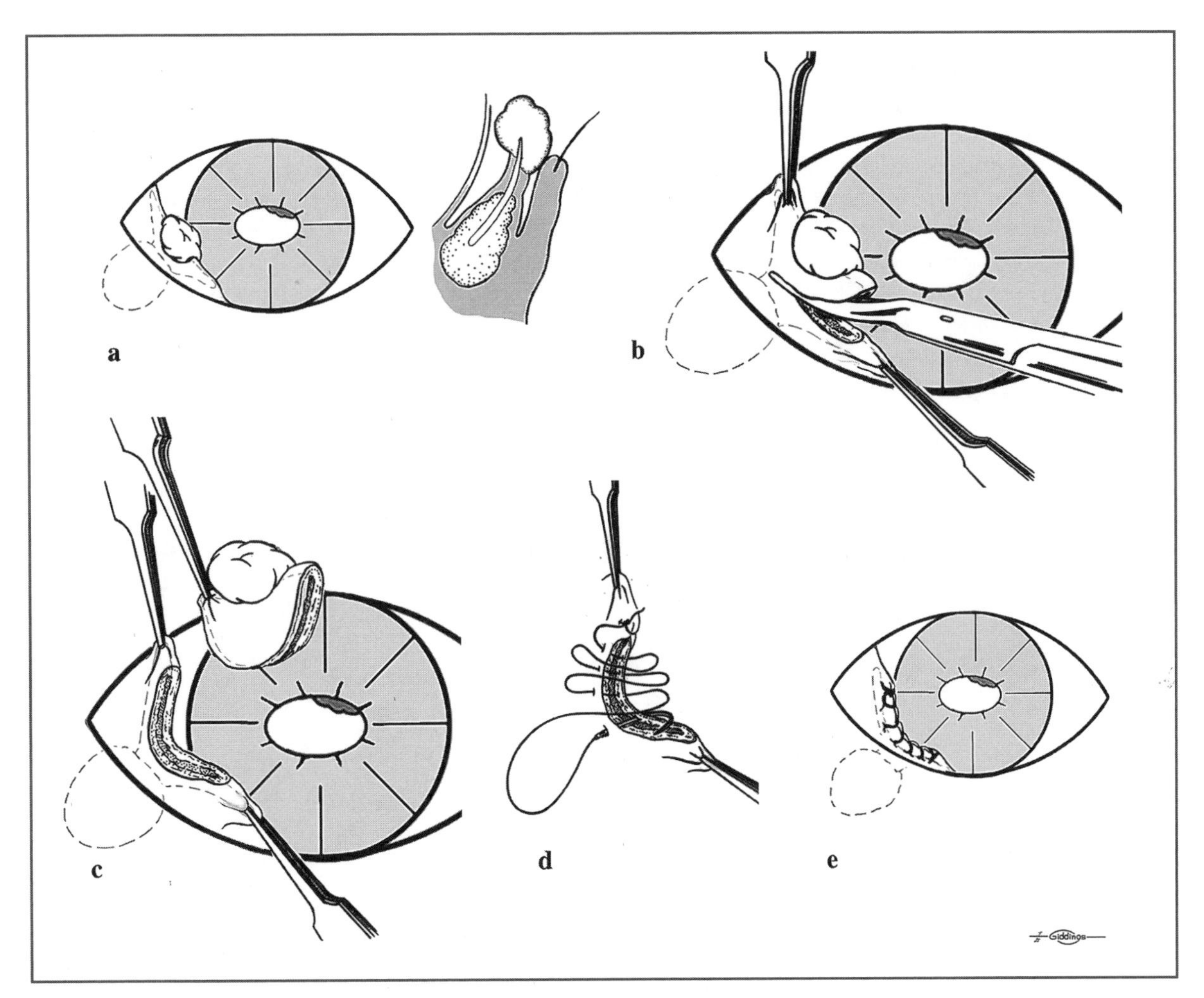

Figure 6-8. Removal of small tumor from the third eyelid.

a. Frontal and cross section diagram of third eyelid with tumor along margin involving the cartilage

b. Fixation forceps placed on third eyelid for stabilization. Affected portion is excised with scissors.

c. Appearance of third eyelid after excision

d. Exterior and inner conjunctival edges sutured together to cover the cut edge of the cartilage

e. Knots are tied on the outer surface of the third eyelid. Absorbable 5-0 or 6-0 suture is satisfactory. Postsurgical medication is not indicated unless there is conjunctivitis, in which case topical antibiotic ointment is satisfactory.

2. Extensive involvement

   a. If the limits of the tumor can be palpated, the author prefers surgical removal of the entire third eyelid (Fig 6-9). Stabilize the ends of the third eyelid with fixation forceps. The ends of the third eyelid are incised from the temporal and nasal attachments with scissors. Next, forceps are attached to the inside and outside conjunctiva at the ends of the incisions. This is to keep the cut edges from retracting. The anterior face of the third eyelid is exposed and the conjunctiva incised near the fornix, joining the first wound. The third eyelid is retracted nasally to expose the posterior surface and the conjunctiva is incised near the base of the third eyelid. Forceps are attached to the cut edges of the bulbar conjunctiva to keep it from retracting. The third eyelid is pulled temporal and the dissection is completed by removing the cartilage and the associated gland of the third eyelid. The conjunctiva is sutured from the center of the wound with 5-0 or 6-0 double armed absorbable suture. If the conjunctival wound is not sutured, postorbital fat will prolapse from the wound and cause a delay in healing for several days.

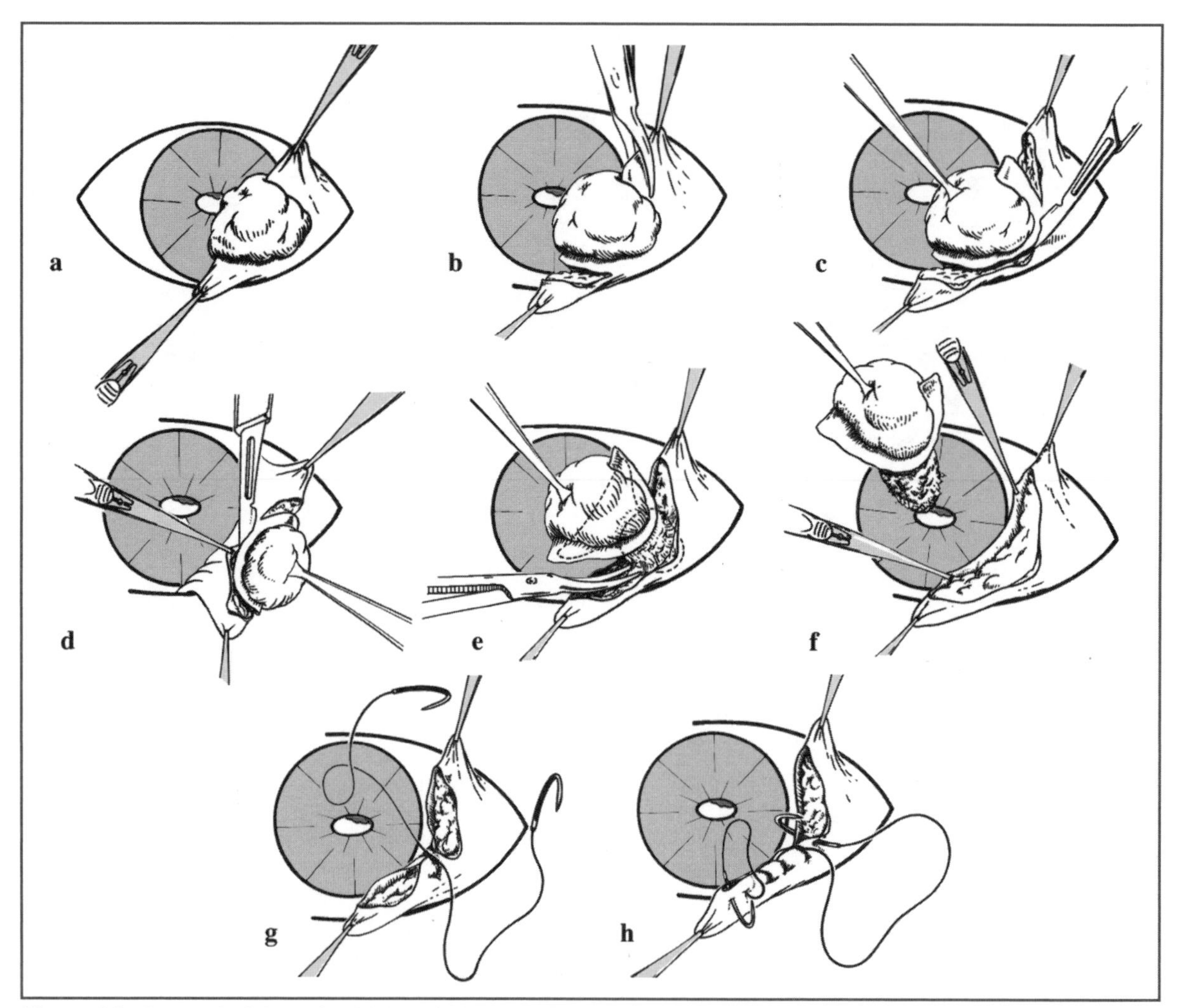

Figure 6-9. Removal of the entire third eyelid because of extensive neoplasia.

a. Stabilizing the third eyelid with forceps at the nasal and temporal limits
b. Incising the nasal attachment of the third eyelid. The temporal side has been incised and fixation forceps are attached to the conjunctiva at the end of the incision.
c. Incising the conjunctiva at the end of the incision
d. The third eyelid has been pulled down, exposing the posterior surface so that the posterior conjunctiva can be incised at the junction between the bulbar conjunctiva and third eyelid conjunctiva.
e. After the conjunctiva has been incised, tension on the third eyelid will pull the gland up into the wound. The third eyelid including the gland of the third eyelid is removed with scissors
f. After the third eyelid and gland have been removed, retrobulbar fat will prolapse into the wound. The free edge of the bulbar conjunctiva is tagged with forceps to facilitate suturing the conjunctiva.
g. Double armed suture is used to close the conjunctival wound. The suture is placed in the center of the wound.
h. The wound is closed by suturing toward the ends of the wound.

b. If the tumor is anchored to the rim of the orbit, or fibrous bands can be palpated extending into the orbit, exenteration of the eye is recommended. If neoplastic tissue is suspected on the orbital rim or adjacent surface, spray freezing the suspicious area with liquid nitrogen is recommended.

Cattle - Squamous cell carcinoma

1. Early lesions - respond well to hyperthermia and cryotherapy
2. Extensive lesions - have a significant incidence of metastasis. Surgical removal with cryotherapy of the surgical area may be considered but exenteration of the eye should be considered.

LACERATIONS

Seen most frequently in small animals as a result of fighting.

Minor lacerations - resulting in a small flap without significant change in appearance of the third eyelid can be removed with scissors after topical anesthesia.

Major lacerations - should be sutured. If there is marked swelling and/or the injury is extensive, two-layer closure of the palpebral and bulbar surfaces is recommended.

Comment - absorbable suture is indicated. Healing is rapid.

CHAPTER 7 - LACRIMAL APPARATUS

ANATOMY AND PHYSIOLOGY

TEAR PRODUCTION

Source of tears - The tears are a composite of the secretions of several glands. The glands involved in tear production vary according to the species (Fig 7-1). The most significant glands are listed below.

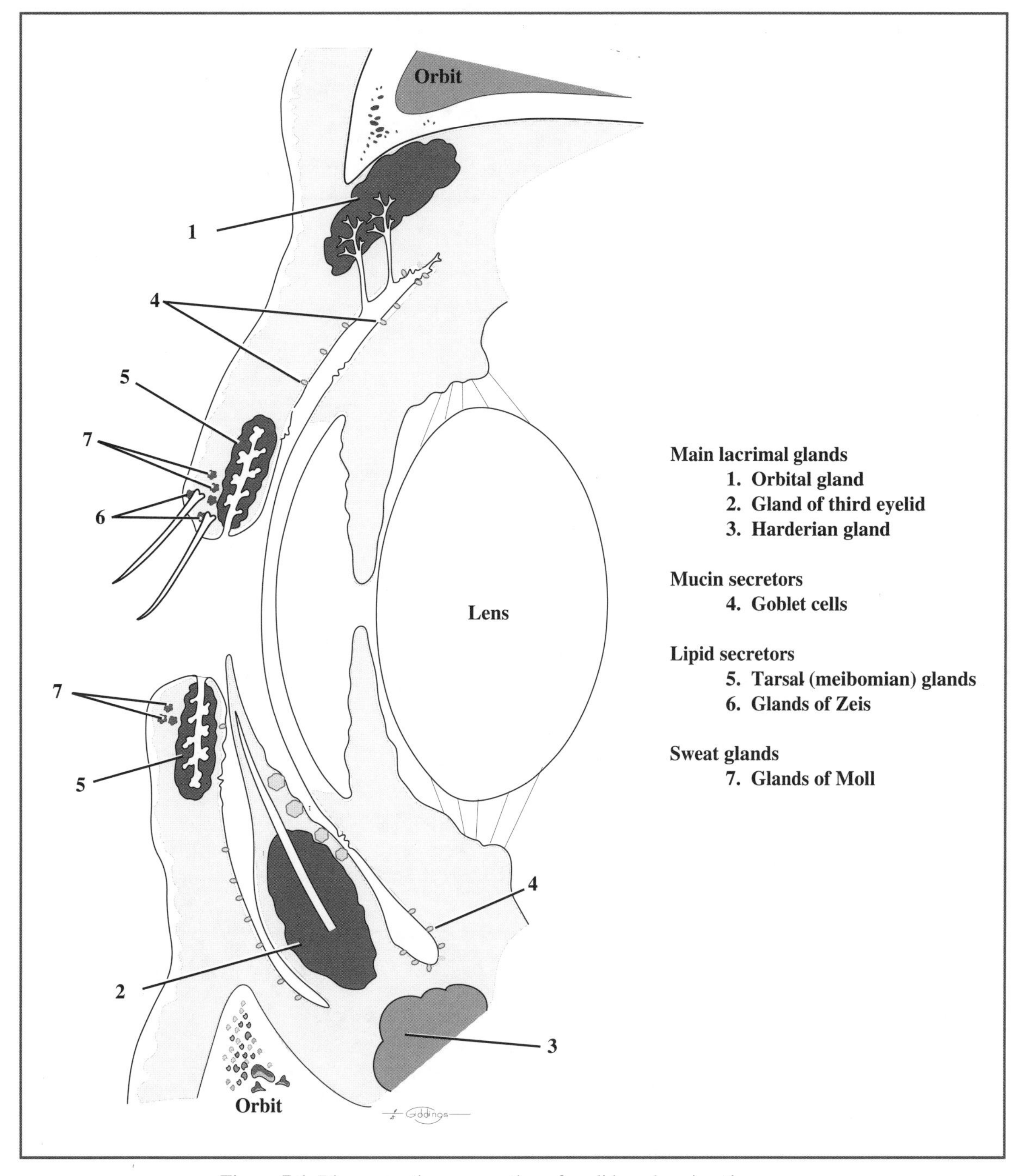

Figure 7-1. Diagrammatic cross-section of eyelids and conjunctiva, showing glands associated with tear production in animals.

1. Orbital lacrimal gland - is a mucoserous gland located in the superior temporal orbit and has several ducts opening into the conjunctiva near the fornix. It is present in all domestic animals and is the primary source of serous tear formation. Phylogenically, this is the most recent lacrimal gland to develop.
2. Gland of the third eyelid - it is closely associated with the cartilage of the third eyelid and is present in all domestic animals. This gland has many small ducts.
3. Harderian gland - not present in domestic animals except for cattle, pigs and rabbits. When present it is located in the base of the third eyelid or in the inferior orbit. It is separate from the gland of the third eyelid. Phylogenically, this was the first lacrimal gland to develop and is still the most important in lower animals, such as snakes and lizards. Primarily a lipid secretor in mammals.
4. Conjunctiva - the goblet cells of the conjunctiva are the primary mucin glands. They are most plentiful in the fornix.
5. Eyelids
   a. Tarsal (meibomian) glands, 30 or more in each eyelid, are the major source for lipid
   b. Glands of Zeis - sebaceous glands at the base of the cilia
   c. Glands of Moll - sweat glands at base of the cilia
6. *Comment.* Removal of either the lacrimal gland or the gland of the third eyelid in normal dogs, does not produce a significant decrease in tears to produce disease. Removal of both glands will result in kerato-conjunctivitis sicca in cats and dogs.

Layers of tears (Fig 7-2)

The tear film is 7 to 9 microns thick and is a complex three-layered film. If it is inadequate or missing, its functions cannot be totally replaced with artificial tears.

1. Outer oil layer - it is primarily from meibomian glands and serves to increase surface tension and retard evaporation
2. Middle serous layer - a composite of secretion of the lacrimal gland and the gland of the third eyelid. It is the major part of the tear layer and is responsible for most of the functions of tears.
3. Deep layer - this is the mucin layer that is the bonding agent between the serous tear and the lipophilic corneal epithelium. It also has the highest concentration of lysozymes and leukocytes.

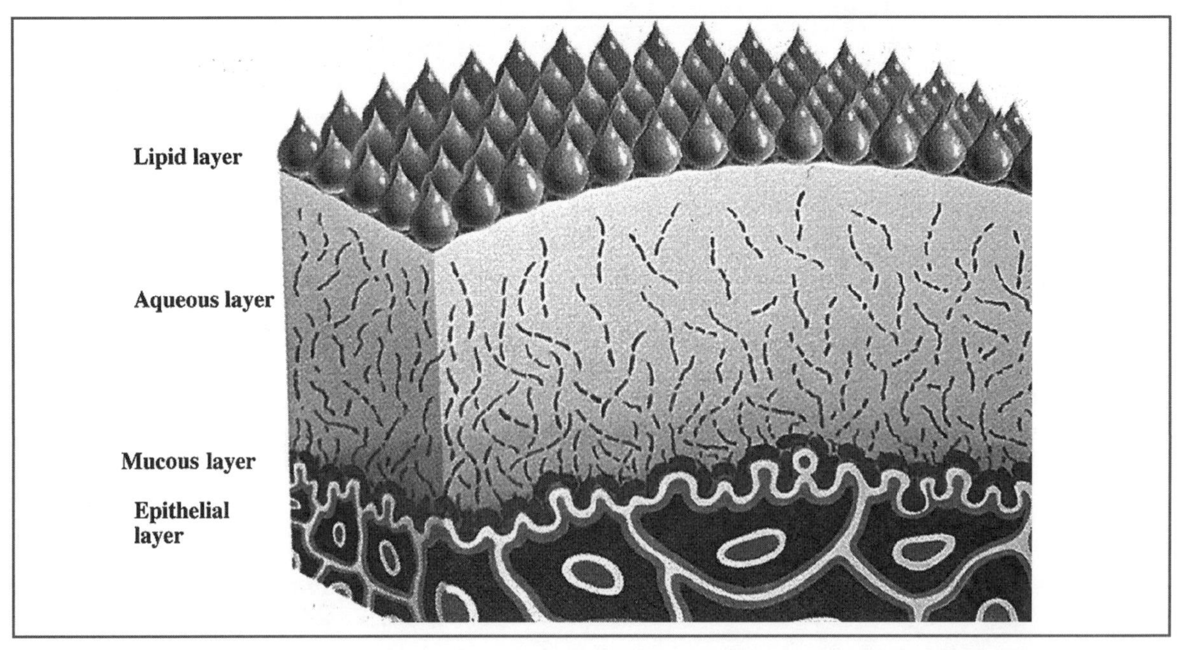

Figure 7-2. Schematic diagram of layers of tears (reproduced by permission from Allergan Labs).

Function - the tears are slightly alkaline

1. Provide antibacterial activity (lysozymes and leukocytes)
2. Maintain the optical activity of the cornea. The tear film is the first refractive surface of the eye and has a refractive index comparable to the cornea.
3. Provide metabolic needs. Oxygen and other needed metabolites are absorbed by the epithelium from the tear film.
4. Remove waste products and debris
5. Provide lubrication for the eyelids

Nerve supply

1. Afferent pathway - trigeminal nerve is the afferent pathway for the reflex arc that stimulates tearing. Loss of this nerve eliminates the stimulus for tearing produced by corneal or conjunctival irritation, glaucoma, uveitis and blepharitis.
2. Efferent pathway for lacrimal flow is via the parasympathetic fibers of the facial nerve nucleus and then to the gland of the third eyelid via the infratrochlear nerve and the orbital lacrimal gland via the lacrimal nerve.
   a. Parasympatholytic drugs (atropine, scopolamine) decrease activity
   b. Pilocarpine stimulates secretion

TEAR FLOW

Tears flow across the eye and by blinking are propelled toward the nasal canthus where they enter the nasal puncta. From there they are carried by the palpebral canaliculi to the lacrimal sac, where they join to form the nasolacrimal duct that ends as the nasal punctum near the mucocutaneous junction of the nostril.

Mucous thread

The fluid portion of the tear flows through the nasolacrimal ducts to the nostrils, but the solids are removed from the eye by means of mucous threads. Mucus collects in the fornix of the lateral canthus and migrates nasally as clear threads in the upper and lower fornices. At the nasal canthus this mucus accumulates and is the "sleeper" that is present in all animal eyes. Ordinarily it is minimal and is easily wiped away. When picked up on a swab at the nasal canthus, it can be lifted from the eye with intact threads pulled out of the upper and lower fornices in a "wishbone" fashion.

NASOLACRIMAL DUCTS AND PUNCTA

Dog - the palpebral puncta are located at the nasal canthus on the inner surface of the eyelids near the opening of the most nasal meibomian glands (Fig 7-3). The lacrimal canaliculi begin at the puncta and pass superficially beneath the conjunctiva to the nasal canthus where they penetrate to the lacrimal fossa of the orbit.

At the fossa, the canaliculi ducts join to form the lacrimal sac. A single nasolacrimal duct leaves the lacrimal sac, goes through the lacrimal foramen emerging on the inner surface of the nasal cavity. The course of the duct in dense bone is usually less than 1 cm (Fig 7-4). From this point, the duct is in soft tissues until it enters the nasal cartilage and then emerges into the nasal cavity as the nasal punctum.

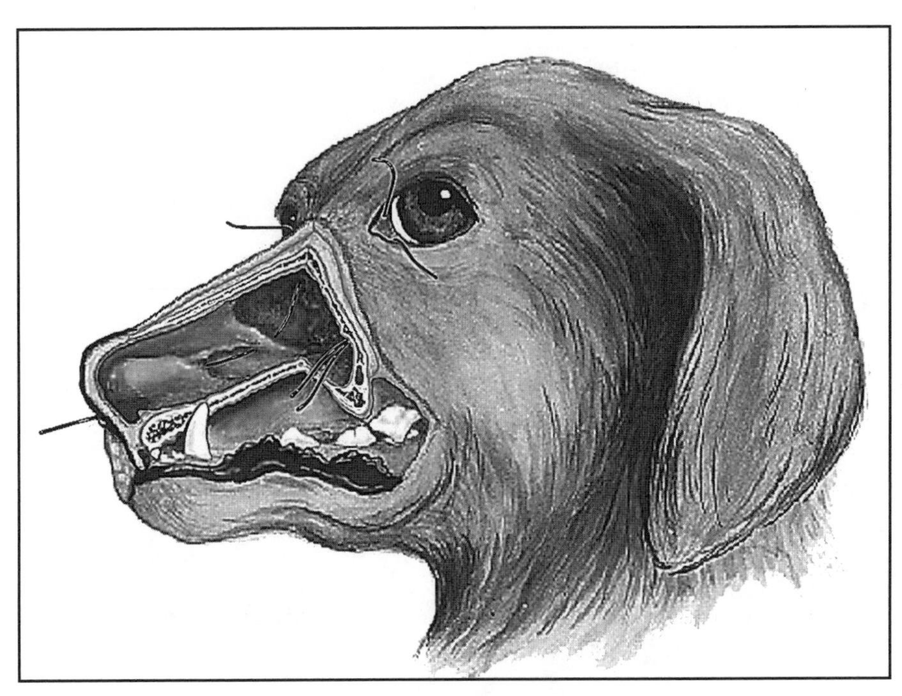

Figure 7-3. Cutaway drawing of the head showing the course of the nasolacrimal duct. Turbinates have been removed.

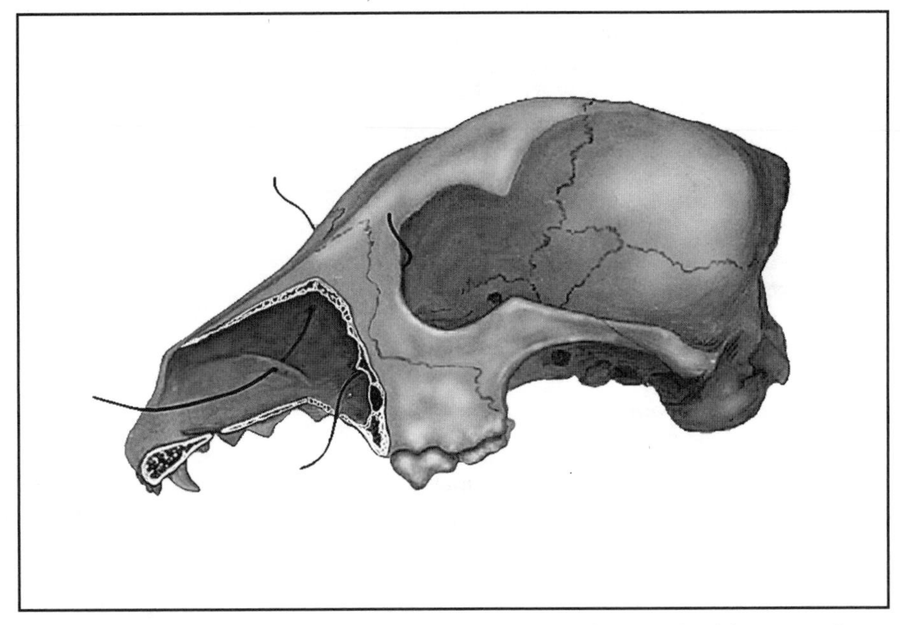

Figure 7-4. Cutaway drawing of skull showing the lacrimal fossa, lacrimal foramen and relative position of the nasolacrimal duct.

The nasal punctum is located about 4-5 mm caudal to the opening of the external nares. It is on the lateral wall about 2 mm above the floor of the nostril (Fig 7-5). An opening in the duct wall is common where the duct crosses over the root of the canine tooth. Tears entering the nasal cavity at this point will flow toward the pharynx if the animal's head is level.

Cat - The ducts and puncta are located similarly to the dog, but due to the size of the external nares, it is difficult to observe the nasal punctum. The palpebral puncta are nearer the margin of the eyelid and are opposite the most nasal meibomian gland.

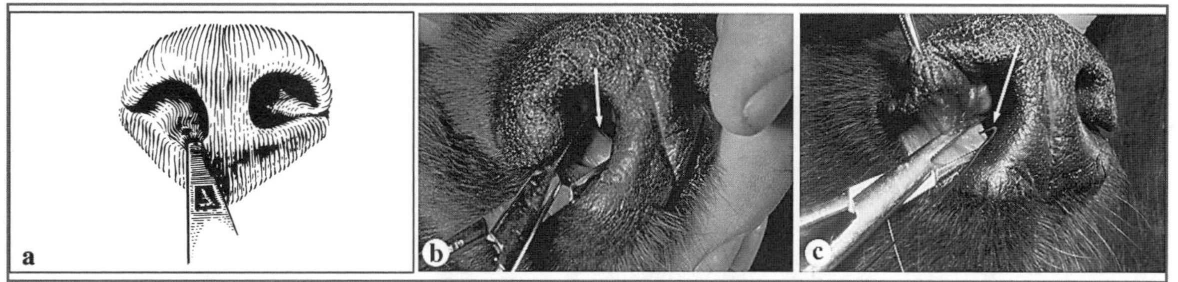

Figure 7-5. Nostril of dog showing location of nasal punctum.
a. Drawing. Nostril opened with forceps showing nasal punctum (arrow).
b. Nasal punctum (arrow) of dog anesthetized and nostril spread with mosquito forceps
c. Monofilament nylon suture coming out nasal punctum (arrow)

Horse - The palpebral puncta are located similarly to the dog. The upper is located near the first tarsal gland (Chapter 1, page 39). The lower punctum is much larger and nearer the canthus. The nasal punctum is easily seen opening inside the nostril on the floor of the nasal cavity near the mucocutaneous junction (Fig 7-6).

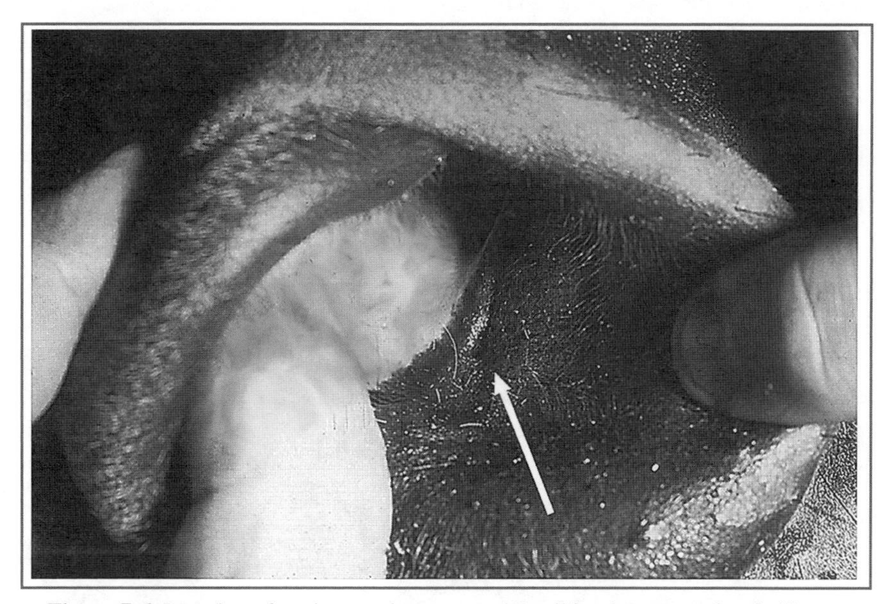

Figure 7-6. Location of equine nasal punctum. Nostril has been spread to facilitate seeing nasal punctum.

Bovine - Cattle are similar to the horse except that the nasal punctum is nearer the lateral side of the nares. The nasal puncta and the osseous nasolacrimal canal are much larger than a horse, literally eliminating the occurrence of dacryocystitis in cattle.

Llama - is similar to cattle, but the nasal punctum is harder to find because the vestibule is smaller.

Rabbit - The rabbit has only a lower eyelid punctum and canaliculus located further from the canthus and further from the eyelid margin. The bony canal is small and makes a bend, thereby restricting catheterization.

CONGENITAL CONDITIONS

PALPEBRAL PUNCTUM (see Chapter 5, page 163)

Imperforate puncta - common in dogs, occasionally llamas

Small puncta - common in dogs, rare in horses

NASOLACRIMAL DUCT - Congenital abnormalities are rarely diagnosed clinically and then only when they cause epiphora

Dog

1. Unilateral anomalous punctum and canaliculus - A six month old German shepherd dog with a history of chronic epiphora was examined. When the upper palpebral punctum was cannulated and flushed, irrigation fluid revealed an anomalous canaliculus with a punctum 5 mm from the nasal canthus.
2. Bilateral bifid distal nasolacrimal canals were identified in a mixed breed dog during retrograde catheterization with monofilament nylon catheters. On catheterization of the dorsal palpebral punctum of the right eye, the catheter was observed coming out the mouth. Oral examination revealed the catheter coming out an opening in the roof of the mouth less than 1 cm behind the first incisor. A catheter passed down the fellow nasolacrimal duct came out an opening behind the other first incisor (Fig 7-7). The nasal puncta were normal in location and patent when the palpebral duct was flushed. Dacryocystorhinography revealed that the accessory ducts left the normal duct before it passed over the root of the canine tooth.

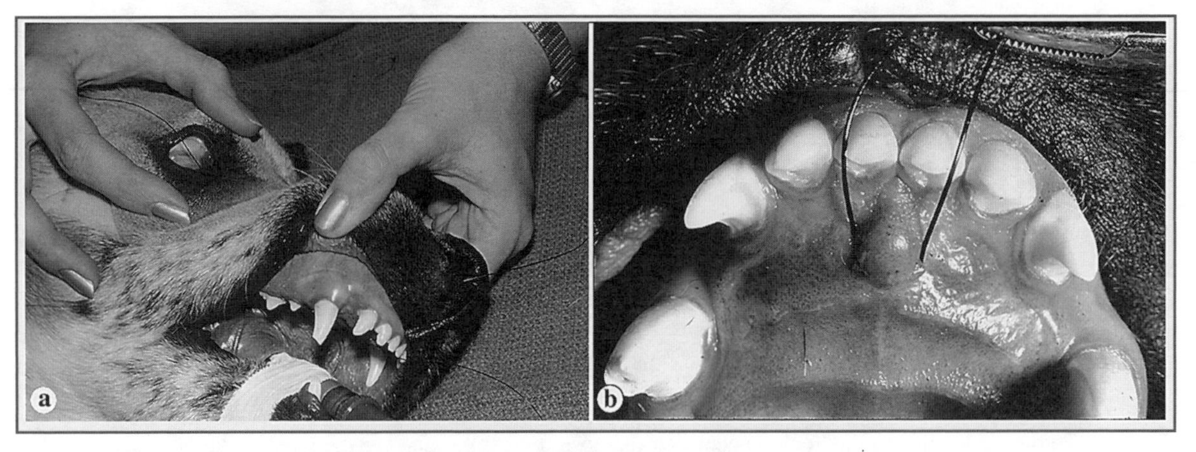

Figure 7-7. Dog with bifid nasolacrimal duct both sides.
a. Size 1 nylon sutures coming out right nostril and behind right incisor
b. Close-up of mouth showing nylon sutures in oral openings of both nasolacrimal ducts

Horse - Unilateral incomplete duplication of the nasolacrimal duct has been seen by the author (Fig 7-8). The dorsal opening of the anomalous duct was beneath a small skin pedicle 4.5 cm inferior to the nasal canthus (Fig 7-8a & b). The inferior opening was in a small pit on the lower lateral margin of the nostril (Fig 7-8c). There was constant moisture at these openings. Dacryocystorhinography revealed that the superior anomalous duct joined the superior nasolacrimal duct at the lacrimal sac and the inferior anomalous duct joined the nasolacrimal duct about 6 cm superior to the nasal punctum.

Another horse was presented with bilateral agenesis of the palpebral puncta and canaliculi replaced by a single lacrimal duct with its punctum located in a cleft between the nasal canthus and the caruncle. There was no epiphora. This was an incidental finding during an ophthalmic examination.

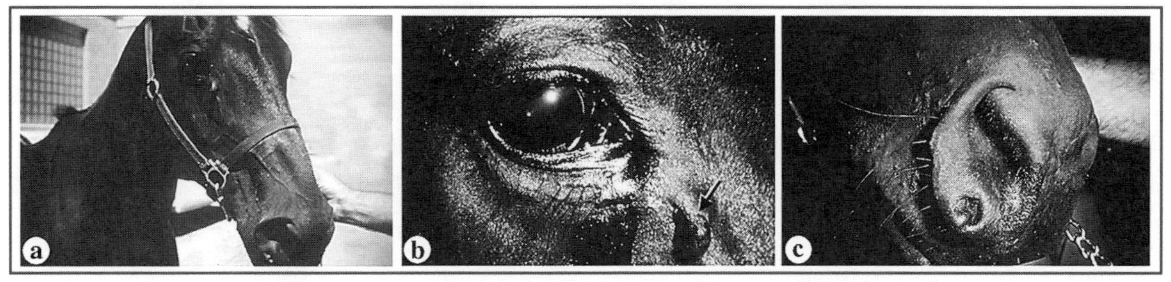

Figure 7-8. Unilateral incomplete duplication nasolacrimal duct in equine.
a. Full face view showing skin pedicle over upper anomalous punctum and nostril deformity with lower anomalous punctum.
b. Close-up of eye and skin pedicle (arrow) obscuring dorsal anomalous punctum
c. Close-up nostril showing nasal deformity with lower anomalous punctum

Bovine - Wyman (J Am Vet Med Assoc 167:145-147, 1975) reported nasolacrimal duct anomaly in 13 brown Swiss calves on a dairy farm. The openings were usually along the proximal 1/3 of the nasolacrimal ducts. Heredity was proposed.

IMPERFORATE NASAL PUNCTUM

Absence of the nasal punctum is the most common congenital abnormality of the nasolacrimal system in horses and is also occasionally observed in llamas. It is rare in other species. The clinical signs are epiphora and excess ocular discharge characteristic of dacryocystitis. On examination the nasal punctum is missing. Catheterization from the palpebral punctum will allow the catheter to be passed to the point of obstruction, which may be at the location where the punctum should be located or 1 to 2 cm short of that location. Treatment is the same as for acquired obstruction and dacryocystitis (Chapter 7, page 242).

ACQUIRED DISEASE

KERATOCONJUNCTIVITIS SICCA

Keratoconjunctivitis sicca (KCS) (dry eye, xerophthalmia) is a chronic disease resulting from inadequate tear production and characterized by ocular discharge and changes in the cornea and conjunctiva. It is common in the dog, less common in the cat, and rare in the horse.

Etiology

1. Primary - congenital lack of lacrimal activity, lack of glands or lack of nervous stimulation
2. Secondary
   a. Autoimmune adenitis - evidence is accumulating that cases previously considered to be idiopathic have an autoimmune adenitis with circulating autoantibodies
   b. During or after systemic diseases - canine distemper, herpes conjunctivitis in kittens and adults, acute hypotensive conditions (shock and Addisonian crisis) or allergy
   c. Chronic ocular infections - leading to secondary dacryoadenitis and atrophy
   d. Trauma to orbital and supraorbital area damaging the lacrimal gland
   e. Lack of normal innervation of the glands - post-traumatic, infections, dysautonomia, or spontaneous from unknown cause. Horses - vestibular disease with facial paralysis, gutteral pouch infection
   f. Toxic - systemic sulfonamides, phenazopyridine and aminosalicylic acid may cause transient or permanent KCS. Pretreatment and periodic Schirmer tear tests are recommended with sulfa therapy. Animals sensitive to sulfas may show toxicity immediately or after chronic therapy. Locoweed poisoning
   g. Topical atropine - temporary hyposecretion can be seen with topical atropine
   h. General anesthesia - temporary hyposecretion is seen in old dogs after surgery. The cause for this is unknown, possibly drug induced from preanesthetics and anesthetic or postsurgical from circulatory disturbance.
   i. Surgical removal of the gland of the third eyelid when there is decreased lacrimal gland activity. Never remove a gland of the third eyelid from a dog with a Schirmer tear test less than 15 mm in one minute or from dogs with a history of KCS in the blood line.
   j. In dogs, loss of conjunctival goblet cells can result in corneal changes as a result of mucin deficiency.
   k. Postradiation
      1) If the lacrimal glands are in the radiation field, a decrease in serous tear production may occur during therapy. Depending on dosage fractionation and total dosage, this may be transient (1-2 months) or permanent.
      2) If the eyelids are in the field, blepharitis may develop. This is characterized by swelling, hyperemia, skin ulceration, hair loss, and tarsal gland necrosis. The skin changes are temporary and new hair growth will be white. The tarsal gland damage is permanent, resulting in an insufficiency of the lipid tear layer and a painful secondary degenerative keratitis.

Incidence in dogs

1. Sex - not significant except in female West Highland white terriers
2. Age - increases with age
3. Neutering - higher in neutered animals, effect not seen until later in life (10 years)
4. Breed predisposition (Appendix IV)
   a. A higher incidence in bulldog, Lhasa apso, and West Highland white terrier
   b. American cocker spaniel - commonly seen because of high relative population. Incidence varies with blood lines.

Clinical signs - The clinical signs are proportional to the degree of hyposecretion and the duration of the disease. KCS can occur concurrently with generalized seborrhea and signs are exaggerated in breeds with prominent eyes and/or lagophthalmos (Fig 7-9).

1. Pain - The patient shows discomfort. Increased blinking, leading to persistent squinting. In the end stage, the cornea keratinizes and pain disappears.
2. Decreased tear film
   a. Mild cases - the eye may appear moist, making the Schirmer tear test necessary for diagnosis
   b. Severe - the eye is distinctly dry
3. Changes in the mucous thread. As the serous tear production decreases, mucous production is increased as a protective mechanism for the eye.
   a. An increase in the size of the mucous thread
   b. Changes from clear to yellow or yellow green
   c. Becomes adherent to the conjunctiva in the fornices
4. Excessive ocular discharge - the eye and eyelids may be covered with a thick discharge which may dry and adhere to the central cornea of the eyelids.
5. Corneal changes (any change characteristic of chronic keratitis may occur)
   a. Ulcers - start out superficially but may deepen and perforate
   b. Opacity - scarring and dehydration
   c. Vascularization - usually superficial
   d. Pigmentation (most severe in breeds with heavily pigmented conjunctiva)
   e. Keratinization (the corneal epithelial response to drying)
6. Conjunctiva - inflamed, thick and may appear dry
7. Nostrils - may be normal or dry. Tears do not provide moisture for the nose. Nasal moisture comes from the nasal mucosa. Therefore, the nose will be normal in uncomplicated KCS, but in neurogenic KCS the stimulation for nasal secretion may be missing and the nostril will become obstructed with debris.

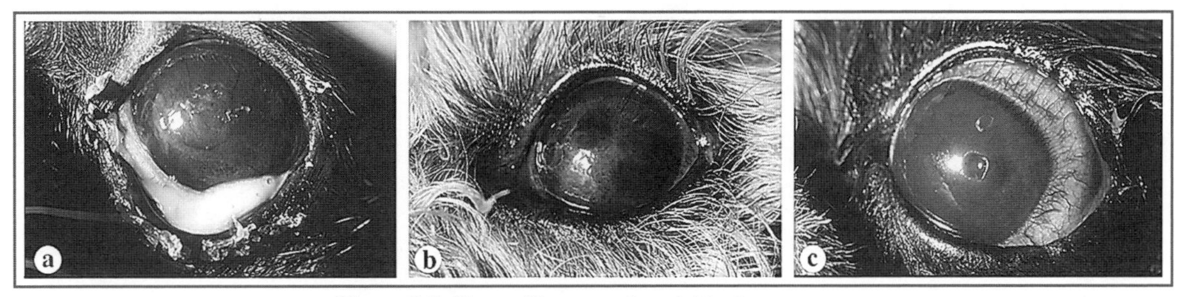

Figure 7-9. Signs of keratoconjunctivitis sicca.
a. Excess mucus
b. Corneal scarring and pigmentation
c. Corneal vascularization and ulceration

Differential diagnosis

1. Infectious conjunctivitis
2. Dacryocystitis
3. Primary corneal disease

Diagnosis

1. Clinical signs
2. Schirmer tear test (STT)
   a. Dogs - most dogs produce 17 to 22 mm in 1 minute
      - Definite keratoconjunctivitis = < 5 mm in 1 min
      - Questionable = 5 to 8 mm in 1 min
      - Satisfactory = 9 mm or more in 1 min
   b. Cats - many cats will have a normally appearing eye with as little as 3 to 5 mm/min
   c. Horses - signs of conjunctivitis will generally develop when tear production drops below 10 mm/min
3. Schirmer tear test with topical anesthetic (STTa) dogs - should be > 5 mm in 1 min

Course

Variable and depends on the etiology. Many cases respond to treatment in less than 60 days.

1. If from systemic disease - most cases recover when the disease is corrected
2. If from trauma or toxicity - many recover unless toxic drug administration was prolonged resulting in irreversible damage to the glands
3. If autoimmune - response to treatment is rapid but may require some degree of permanent treatment
4. If from congenital absence or permanent nerve damage - permanent KCS will result

Treatment

Treat medically first. If it becomes obvious that topical treatment is inadequate, surgery may be recommended.

1. Medical treatment

   GOALS: supplement tear formation, stimulate lacrimal activity, control infection, cleanse the eye, and control corneal changes

   a. Supplement tear formation
      1) Artificial tears (demulcents) - given when the eyes appear dry or the patient starts to squint. Do not use saline solutions unless followed with artificial tears. Saline will wash away the lipid tear layer and result in severe drying soon after.
      2) Ointments (emollients) - lubricate and protect the eye. They are useful at night or during the day when drops cannot be administered as frequently as needed.
      3) Topical viscoelastic preparation for lubrication and protection as frequently as needed (see page 125)
   b. Stimulate lacrimal activity
      1) Topical cyclosporine - 0.2% cyclosporine ophthalmic ointment (Optimmune - Schering Plough) or compounded 1% cyclosporine in oil (see page 98). Cyclosporine is the most effective lacrimator available and in early cases may be the only medication needed. It stimulates tear production and has a beneficial effect on the keratopathy. Initial treatment is BID; if marked improvement, reduce to daily at 30 days and every other day at 60 days. Some dogs may develop blepharitis secondary to 1% drops. Reducing the concentration to 0.5% may eliminate sensitivity. At this time, cyclosporine is the treatment of choice.
      2) Oral pilocarpine - 1 to 4 drops of 1 to 2% ophthalmic pilocarpine solution BID in food. Helps many animals but may cause side effects before effective levels are reached. Begin with one drop in the food BID and gradually increase the dosage until tearing occurs. If toxic signs develop before tearing occurs, discontinue medication. Toxic signs are salivation, anorexia, vomiting, diarrhea and/or colic.
      3) Topical pilocarpine - 1/4% pilocarpine will stimulate functional lacrimal tissue that may be present. Some patients develop a local sensitivity to dilute pilocarpine. Local sensitivity is manifested by severe conjunctival pain and congestion. If this occurs, topical pilocarpine must be discontinued.
   c. Control infection - many cases are bacteriologically sterile but it is wise to do culture and sensitivity studies so that the most effective antibiotics can be used. Use broad spectrum antibiotics until the results are known.
   d. Cleanse the eye - 2.5% and 5% acetylcysteine will remove the mucus and speed healing of ulcers when present. Acetylcysteine may be irritating and can be reduced to 2.5%. If irritation persists, it should be discontinued. When mucous production decreases and ulcers have healed, acetylcysteine should be discontinued. An opened bottle of acetylcysteine will keep six months if tightly capped and refrigerated.

Table 7-1

KERATOCONJUNCTIVITIS SICCA SOLUTION	
1. Antibiotic - to control bacterial infection, if present 2. Acetylcysteine - to provide anticollagenase activity and as a mucolytic agent 3. Pilocarpine - as a lacrimation stimulator 4. Artificial tear - as a qs agent and tear substitute	
Amount used to make 24 ml	**Final concentration in mixture**
1.5 ml 5% gentamicin	0.3%
6 cc - 20% acetylcysteine	5%
1.5 ml 4% pilocarpine ophthalmic	0.25%
Artificial tears qs to 24 ml (about 16 ml)	60% of volume
The mixture is dispensed in a one ounce bottle and will maintain potency at room temperature for two months. Place 2 to 3 ml in a small dropping bottle and instruct the owner to use this as indicated. This bottle may be kept at room temperature and the stock bottle in a refrigerator.	
If the patient has severe KCS, start with hourly treatment and as the owner notices tear productivity returning, reduce the frequency of administration accordingly. Schirmer tear strips can be dispensed to monitor tear production. Advise them to continue medication at a frequency that maintains a test above 6 to 8 mm per minute. KCS solution can be discontinued when cyclosporine can maintain the patient.	

f. Control secondary corneal changes - pigmentation, corneal vascularization, scarring and ulceration
   1) Pigmentary keratitis is the eye's response to chronic irritation. Epithelial pigment will regress quickly as tearing returns. Stromal pigment disappears slowly, if at all.
   2) Corneal vascularization regresses as the tearing returns. If treated early enough in the disease, it will disappear entirely. If ulcers are not present, topical corticosteroids can be used as an adjunct. Care should be exercised in the use of corticosteroids if the animal has a history of recurrent corneal ulceration.
   3) Scarring is seen in chronic cases and will remain. Mild leukoma results from corneal drying; this disappears when tearing returns and should not be confused with scarring.
   4) Ulcers should be treated according to their severity. ***Do not use atropine*** as part of the treatment regimen because it can cause lacrimal shutdown.

   If the eye is sterile, antibiotic is not needed.

Causes of medical treatment failures

1. Lack of tear production (lacrimal gland atrophy or fibrosis)
2. Develop sensitivity to drugs - especially pilocarpine and acetylcysteine, less frequently cyclosporine
3. Owner unable to treat eyes properly
4. Progressive corneal deterioration that may cause blindness if not checked

Surgical treatment - Surgical treatment should not be considered until medical treatment has been unsuccessful after at least 60 days.

1. Transposition of the parotid salivary duct. Lavingnette reported the successful treatment of a case of canine keratoconjunctivitis sicca with parotid duct transposition in 1966. Since then, others have modified this technique. The regional anatomy is illustrated in Fig 7-10.

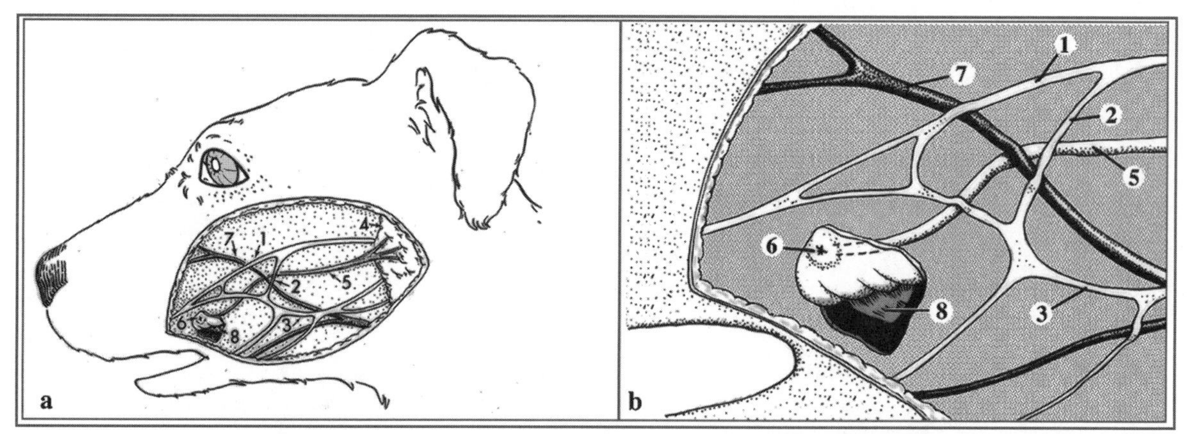

Figure 7-10. Cutaway drawing of the area where the parotid duct enters the mouth. Facial muscles have been omitted to illustrate the essential features. a. Entire face. b. Close-up of area.
1. Dorsal buccal nerve
2. Anastomosis of dorsal buccal and ventral buccal nerves
3. Ventral buccal nerve
4. Parotid salivary gland
5. Parotid duct
6. Papilla of parotid duct
7. Facial vein
8. Upper carnassial tooth

2. The papilla of the parotid duct can be identified above the base of the upper carnassial tooth. Care should be taken to not confuse it with the papilla of the major duct of the zygomatic salivary gland which opens near the gingival border above the last molar. An 0 to 00 monofilament nylon suture, that has had the tip flamed to glaze it, is passed through the parotid duct papilla (Fig 7-11). The suture can be seen moving beneath the skin as it passes down the parotid duct. When the suture cannot be passed any further, cut it so that it protrudes about 1 cm from the papilla. Place a pledget of cotton soaked with 1:50 Betadine solution over the papilla and return the lip to normal position.

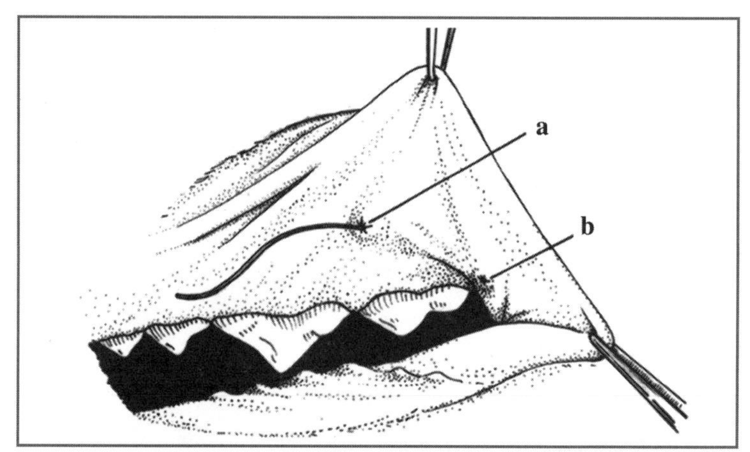

Figure 7-11. Monofilament nylon suture in place in the parotid duct.
a. Suture in duct
b. A papilla of the zygomatic salivary duct seen near the last molar

3. Surgical technique
   a. Open technique (Fig 7-12). The nylon suture in the duct is palpable through the skin over the masseter muscle. Make an incision along the duct through the skin and panniculus muscle layer exposing the duct. Dissect the duct from the masseter muscle and pass a length of 1/8 inch umbilical tape beneath it. Use this to elevate the duct and avoid the possibility of damaging it with forceps. Dissect the duct free posteriorly to the angle of the mandible. Carefully start dissection forward, avoid the facial vein and the anastomotic branches between the buccal nerves. Continue dissection with small blunt scissors beneath the nerve and vein until the scissors tip can be seen in the connective tissue ahead of the vein. Force the tip out, making an opening that exposes the duct. Place another length of umbilical tape around the duct and continue dissection anteriorly to the point where the duct penetrates the orbicularis oris and the oral mucosa. Using a 6 mm biopsy punch or corneal trephine, remove a round plug of mucosa containing the papilla. Center the punch (trephine) over the papilla and cut the mucosa. Take care to avoid cutting the duct. Dissect the plug of mucosa free and pull it into the external facial wound. Suture the oral wound and set aside all instruments used in the mouth. Reglove. Continue dissection of the duct until it is free to the angle of the mandible. A canthotomy may be needed if the eyelid opening is small, but if the animal has a large eyelid opening the duct can be transplanted without canthotomy. Using small blunt scissors (curved corneal, strabismus, or tenotomy scissors), make a tunnel along the surface of the masseter muscle from the angle of the mandible to the lateral canthus. Apply pressure until the scissors tip appears subconjunctivally at the fornix of the lateral canthus. Force the scissors through the conjunctiva, grasp the point with a mosquito hemostatic forceps and then withdraw the scissors and forceps until the forceps appears in the facial wound. Grasp the edge of the mucosal plug (containing the papilla) with the forceps and draw the duct through the tunnel. Suture the mucosal plug to the conjunctiva with four simple interrupted sutures of 6-0 absorbable sutures. Reappose the panniculus muscle with the same suture, close the skin incision and canthotomy with nonabsorbable suture. Remove the nylon suture from the parotid duct. Saliva will usually start flowing through the duct immediately.

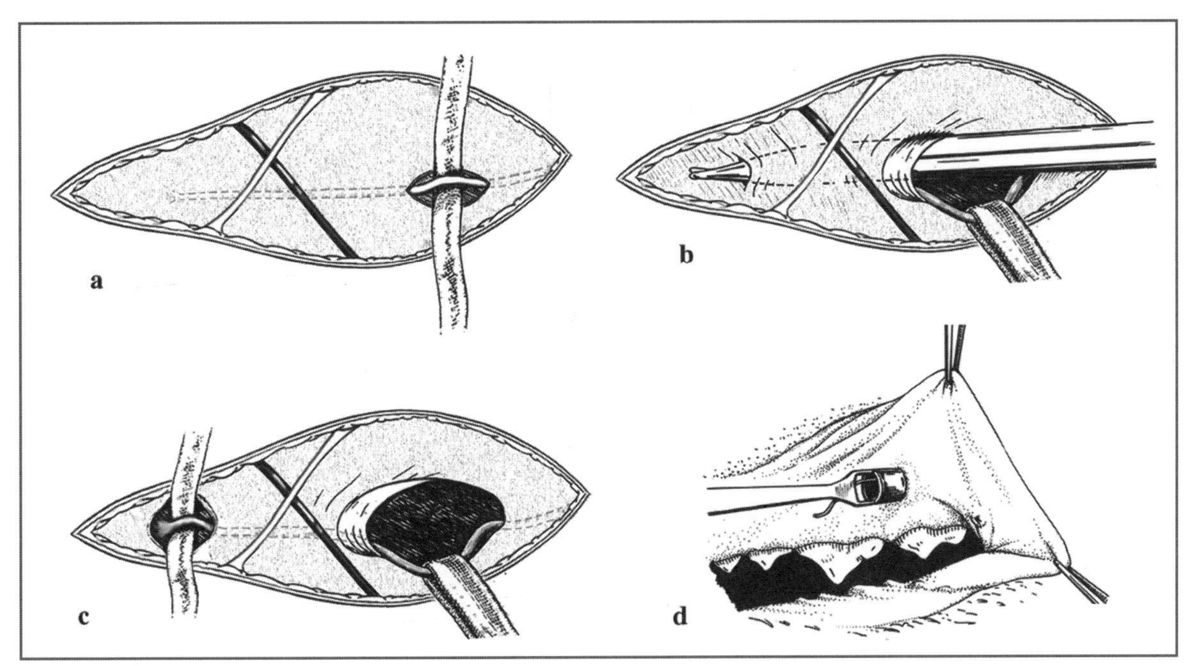

Figure 7-12. Parotid duct transposition, open technique.

a. Umbilical tape passed beneath the parotid duct so the duct can be manipulated without damaging it with forceps.
b. Dissection completed beneath the branches of the buccal nerves and facial vein
c. Parotid duct dissected free to area where papilla opens into mouth
d. Biopsy punch positioned to cut plug of mucosa containing papilla of parotid duct

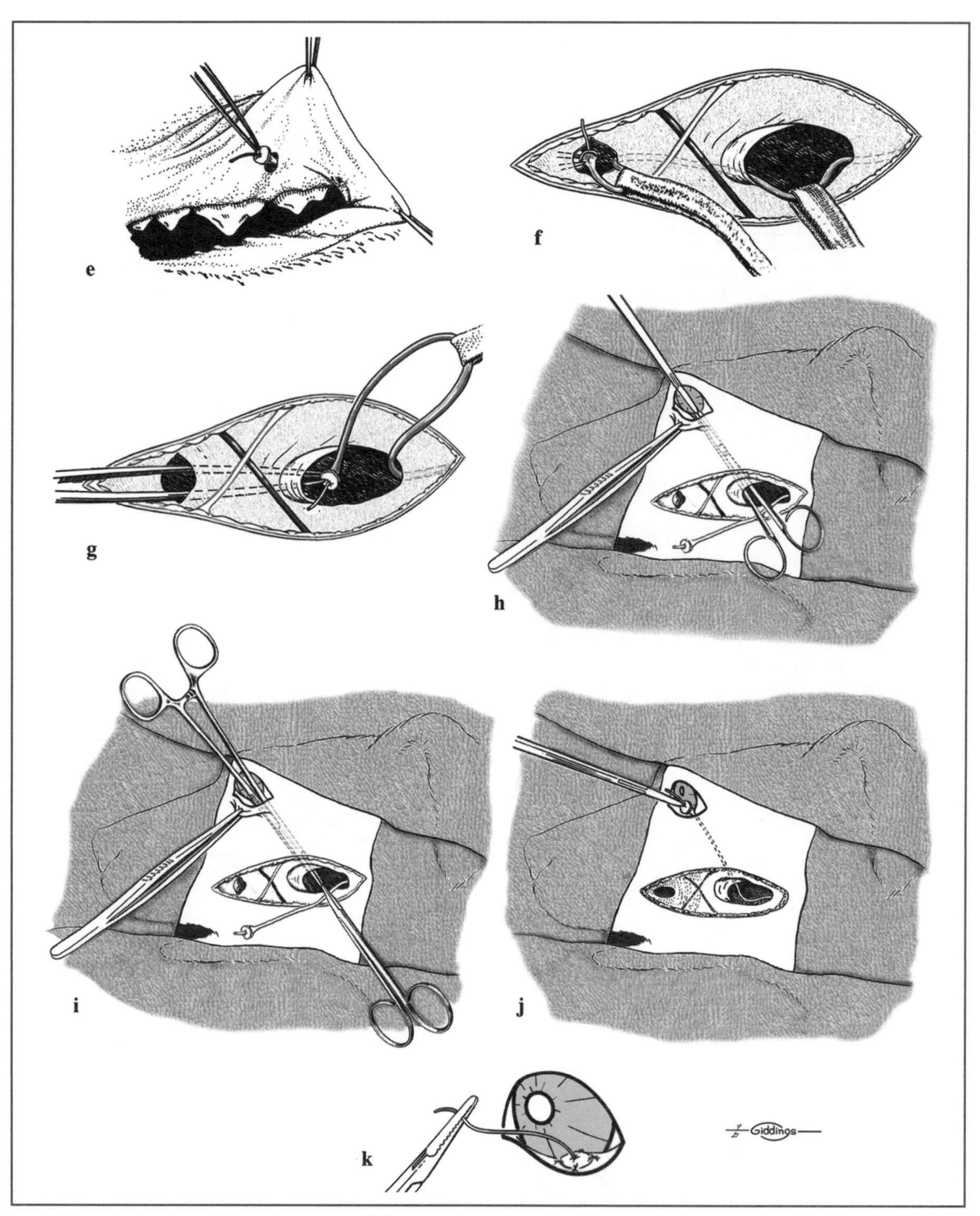

Figure 7-12. Parotid duct transposition, open technique. (continued from page 235)

- e. Plug of mucosa containing parotid papilla and duct dissected from oral mucosa
- f. Mucosal plug with papilla pulled into wound
- g. Mucosal plug with papilla duct forced through tunnel beneath vein and nerve. Parotid duct and papilla are now dissected free to the angle of the mandible.
- h. Tunneling along the fascia of the masseter muscles to the lateral fornix with blunt delicate scissors. The scissors tip penetrates the conjunctiva at the lateral fornix.
- i. Scissors and forceps are rotated 90° and pulled back through the tunnel made in h.
- j. Oral mucous membrane plug with parotid papilla positioned for suturing to the conjunctiva
- k. Mucous membrane plug sutured to the conjunctiva with four simple interrupted absorbable sutures

b. Closed technique. This technique eliminates the need for a facial incision. In this procedure, the initial step is to remove the oral mucosal plug and then, with blunt scissors, dissect the duct free to the angle of the mandible. The duct stretches and is quite easily separated from surrounding tissues. Next, tunnel from the fornix across the masseter muscle with a mosquito hemostatic forceps until the mucosal plug can be grasped with the forceps and transpositioned to the conjunctival sac. This technique eliminates the facial skin incision, but has a greater chance for kinking and damaging the duct.

4. Surgical sequela
   a. Epiphora during eating is the common complaint. This seems to decrease with time. Epiphora is a nuisance, but is far less serious than the untreated disease.
   b. Transposition failure occurs from duct or papilla obstruction
   c. Atrophy or failure of the parotid gland is rare
   d. Saliva does not have the antibacterial qualities of tears. If infection occurs after the transposition, serious corneal damage may result. Saliva exceeds normal tear production and significantly dilutes lysosomes.
   e. Corneal opacity resulting from salivary mineral deposits can occur (Fig 7-13). In some mild cases, this can be controlled by treating the cornea with 1 to 2% EDTA solution (see page 125). In many cases, however, the mineralization remains in spite of treatment. Topical corticosteroid therapy may enhance corneal mineral deposition in some cases and, therefore, may be contraindicated.
   f. Some animals will show severe discomfort from the saliva, which may necessitate surgical replacement of the transposed duct to the mouth.

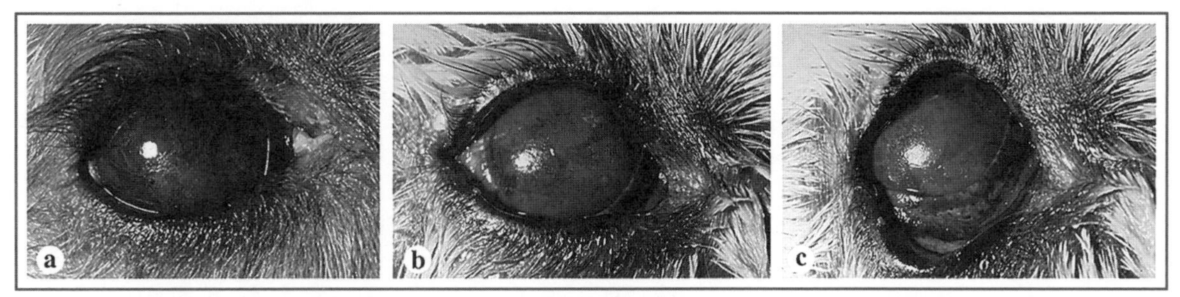

Figure 7-13. Corneal opacity from salivary mineral deposits.
a. Corneal deposit beginning two months postoperative
b. Pigment and corneal opacity
c. Same dog as "b" with eye retropulsed to expose third eyelid. Plaquing also present on third eyelid.

Other methods of treatment

1. Reducing the size of the eyelid opening in dogs with prominent eyes and/or lagophthalmos - success of this procedure is dependent on some lacrimal activity (Fig 5-18 & 19, page 168).
2. Cauterization of the palpebral puncta to prevent tear removal by the nasolacrimal system has been tried. If tearing returns or duct transposition is required, this would then result in epiphora.

EPIPHORA - Epiphora is the abnormal flow of tears over the face.

Etiology

1. Increased tear production (lacrimation)
    a. Hypersecretion from lacrimal gland inflammation
    b. Reflex secretion
        1) Mechanical irritation (foreign bodies, misplaced eyelashes)
        2) Ocular diseases (corneal ulcers, anterior uveitis, glaucoma)
        3) Light and wind
2. Failure of the excretory system
    a. Congenital abnormalities of the nasolacrimal system
    b. Acquired obstruction of the nasolacrimal system. This may be caused by:
        1) Lesions within the nasolacrimal system (inflammatory discharge plugging the duct, foreign bodies, closure of the puncta after conjunctivitis, or calculi)
        2) Lesions in adjacent tissues (tumors, granulomas, osteomyelitis, dental disease, or severe trauma)

Treatment

Since there are multiple causes for epiphora, a routine approach should be followed.

1. First step is to identify and eliminate causes for excess tear production (lacrimation)
2. Second step - evaluate the nasolacrimal system
    a. Nasolacrimal examination
        1) Examine eyelids for punctal size and location
        2) Evaluate conformation of nasal canthus
    b. Test for functional patency with fluorescein applied to the eye
    c. Saline irrigation is necessary to differentiate physiologic obstruction from pathologic obstruction and is the most expedient method in determining patency.

EPIPHORA IN DOGS CAUSED BY NASOLACRIMAL FAILURE

Causes

1. Congenital (see tear staining syndrome, page 246)
    a. Conformation of the nasal canthus interfering with palpebral punctal function
        1) Nasal entropion with or without excess nasal fold
        2) Toy breeds with tight fitting lids and excess hair growing at nasal canthus acting as a wick (poodles, Lhasa apso, Maltese, Yorkshire terrier, and others)
    b. Punctal abnormalities (cocker spaniels)
    c. Severe ectropion
2. Acquired
    a. Eyelid injuries
    b. Dacryocystitis

Examination

1. Evaluate eyelids and conformation of nasal canthus
2. Check functional patency with fluorescein - 30 seconds to 5 minutes
3. Flushing is needed to differentiate passive (functional) obstruction from pathologic obstruction

Nasolacrimal irrigation (Fig 1-44; Chapter 1, page 40)

1. Instill topical anesthesia on the eye three or four times over a period of several minutes. If the patient is tractable, chemical restraint is not needed.
2. Dogs should be positioned with their nose down at a 25 to 30 degree angle so that irrigating fluid will come out the nostril rather than flow toward the pharynx and stimulate coughing.
3. A blunt hypodermic needle or lacrimal cannula is introduced 3 to 5 mm into the superior punctum and saline is injected; if clear fluid passes freely from the nose and lower punctum, no obstruction is present. If there was mucus obstructing the duct, it will precede the clear fluid. If the solution returns out the inferior punctum only, obstruction is present in the nasolacrimal duct. If saline returns only through the superior punctum, there must be obstruction of the upper canaliculus or the inferior canaliculus and nasolacrimal duct. Injection should be tried through the lower canaliculus if the upper is unsuccessful.
4. Frequently, considerable hydrostatic pressure will be required to dislodge a mucous plug from the nasolacrimal canal. If so, digital compression of the inferior punctum at the time of injection of the upper punctum is necessary. Be sure to do aerobic and anaerobic culture and sensitivity.
5. Antibiotic-cortisone ophthalmic solutions should be used TID or QID for several days to hasten healing of the inflamed excretory system. Make changes as indicated by culture results.
6. The patient should be checked and treated for associated conjunctivitis or complicating eyelid and nasal disorders.

Nasolacrimal catheterization - Indicated when irrigation is unsuccessful or dacryocystitis is present. General anesthesia is required.

1. Catheter preparation - Flame the end of 1, 0 or 00 monofilament nylon suture to make a blunt point. The blunt end facilitates passage and reduces damage to the duct. The largest suture that will pass into the osseous lacrimal canal is preferred.
2. Catheterization from the palpebral punctum. Pass the blunt end of the suture into the upper punctum, down the duct, and out through the opening of the external nares.

   If resistance is encountered when the catheter starts through the bony canal, use a smaller catheter. It is not unusual for the catheter to stop at the external nares. When this happens, spread the nares with a mosquito hemostatic forceps, locate the catheter coming out of the punctum, and grasp the end of the catheter with the forceps.

   Occasionally the catheter will exit the lacrimal duct at an opening over the canine tooth and come down the nostril from that point instead of out the nasal punctum. This is satisfactory.

   There is a cul-de-sac in the duct beyond the nasal punctum. In some animals, the catheter may pass beyond the punctum into the cul-de-sac. Should this happen, manipulate the external nares and the catheter until the catheter comes out. If manipulation is not successful, withdraw the catheter and pass it retrograde from the nasal punctum toward the eye.
3. Catheterization from the nasal punctum - Retrograde passage of the catheter is accomplished by spreading the nostril with a mosquito hemostatic forceps and identifying the nasal punctum. The punctum is seen inside the nares near the junction of the lateral wall and the floor. Moisture present in the opening will result in a highlight which facilitates location of the punctum. Stabilizing the catheter with a curved mosquito forceps with the catheter tip about 8 to 10 mm beyond the forceps tip will facilitate starting the catheter into the nasal punctum. The catheter can be advanced 1 to 2 cm at a time with the forceps. The catheter usually will come out the upper punctum. There is a cul-de-sac in the palpebral punctum that the tip may lodge in, but eyelid manipulation frees it immediately.

   About 50% of the dogs have the opening in the lacrimal duct previously described. In many of the dogs, the catheter will enter the nasal cavity at this point and pass into the pharynx. When this occurs, retrograde catheterization will be unsuccessful.
4. Retention tube placement (Fig 7-14) - This is indicated if scar tissue obstruction was encountered during catheterization or if dacryocystitis is present. Polyethylene tubing (PE50 or 90) can be placed over the nylon catheter and then pulled through the nasolacrimal canal and sutured to the skin near the eye and nasal canthus. Preparing the tubing with a tapered tip will facilitate drawing the tubing through the duct. Heating the tubing over a small flame, then applying gentle traction will result in stretching the tubing

and narrowing the diameter. Excess heating or too much traction will cause the tubing to break. Next pass a nylon catheter down the tubing until it lodges in the narrowed area. If the tube is cut at this point, it will fit snugly around the catheter and pull through the nasolacrimal canal without hanging up.

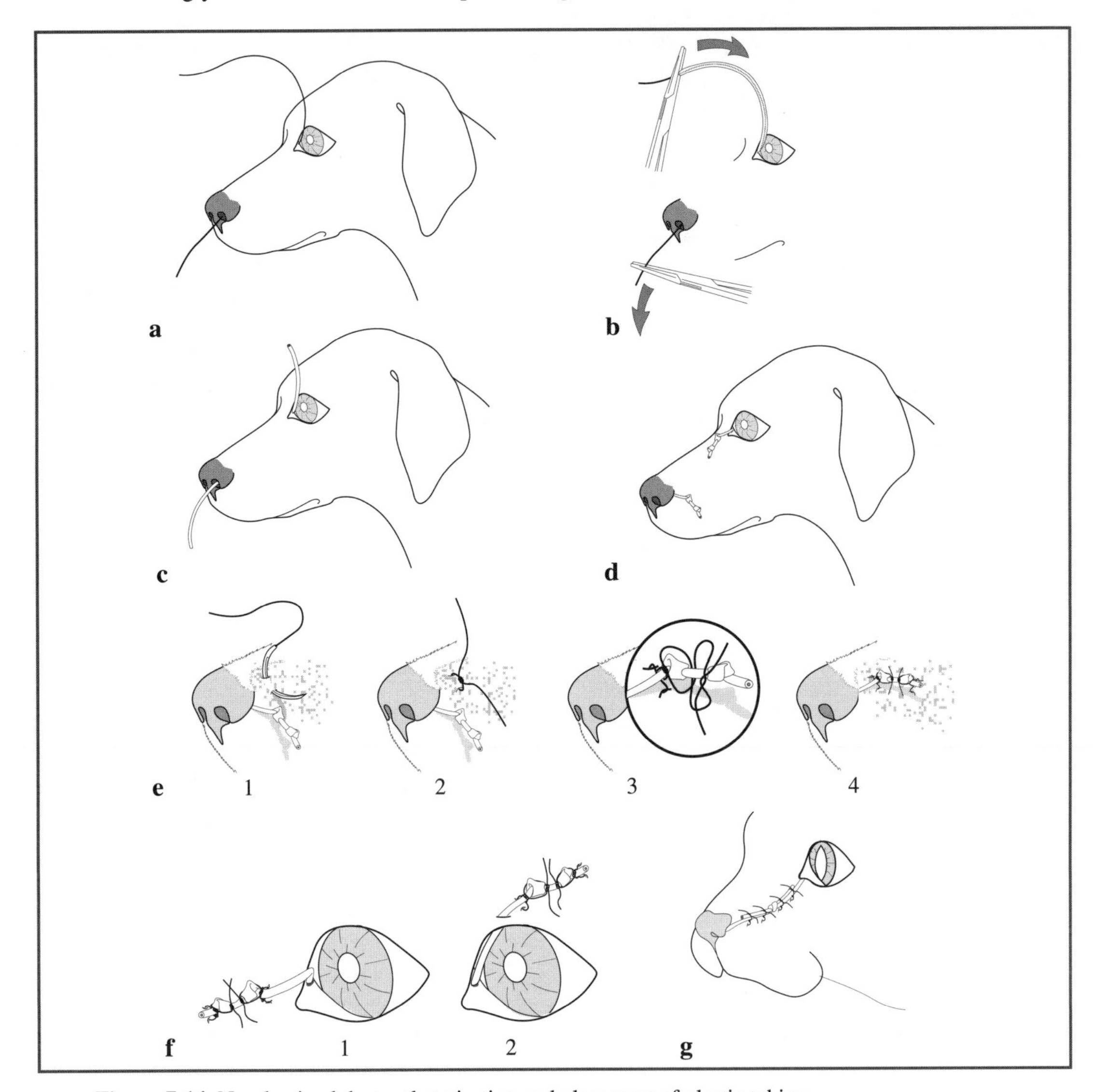

Figure 7-14. Nasolacrimal duct catheterization and placement of plastic tubing.

a. Lateral view of the head showing monofilament nylon suture passed through the upper punctum, lacrimal duct and coming out the nose

b. Lateral view of head with plastic tubing slipped over monofilament catheter. Mosquito forceps are positioned on the catheter so the tubing can be pulled into the upper punctum by applying traction with the forceps near the nose.

c. Lateral view of the head showing plastic tubing pulled through nasolacrimal duct

d. Double knots tied in tubing so suture can stabilize tubing

e. Two-suture technique to anchor tubing at nares
   1. Placing first suture in haired skin above and behind nares
   2. Suture loosely tied in skin
   3. Suture anchored around knot in tubing
   4. Second suture placed in skin and anchored to knot near end of tubing

f. Locations for anchoring tubing near the eye
   1. Bending tubing and anchoring medial to nasal canthus
   2. Suturing above upper eyelid after tubing threaded through upper eyelid trocar

g. In cats, it is simpler to tie the ends of the tubing together and suture the loop of tubing to the facial area

5. *Comment.* Catheterization and retention tube placement is a successful method of treating chronic dacryocystitis and reestablishing patency of the nasolacrimal duct system. The tubing is well tolerated if it comes out the nasal punctum. If it comes out through the imperfection in the duct over the base of the canine tooth, it may cause discomfort manifested by sneezing and/or pawing at the face for the first few hours. Tubing should be left in place four to six weeks if dacryocystitis is present. When placed for correction of a congenital defect, two weeks is often adequate. If dacryocystitis is present, culture and sensitivity should be performed and appropriate antibiotics given for two to three weeks.

EPIPHORA IN CATS DUE TO NASOLACRIMAL FAILURE - Chronic epiphora causes fewer secondary problems in cats than it does in dogs.

Causes

1. Congenital
   a. Atresia puncta - very rare
   b. Conformation - Persian cats. Removal of the gland of the third eyelid usually helps if the Schirmer tear test is greater than 15 mm/min. Use the same technique as described for dogs.
2. Acquired
   a. Post herpesvirus scarring from neonatal conjunctivitis (most common cause)
   b. Dacryocystitis - uncommon

Examination

1. Evaluate eyelid and look for adhesions that would suggest scarring from neonatal herpesvirus
   a. Adhesions between eyelids and third eyelid
   b. Symblepharon
   c. Punctal scarring and/or canaliculus scarring
2. Check functional patency with fluorescein (15 seconds to 1 minute)
3. Flushing ducts

Nasolacrimal irrigation - chemical restraint and a magnifying loupe may be needed

1. Topical anesthesia - 3 to 4 times or several minutes
2. Cats can be positioned with their head level
3. The puncta are smaller than dogs, therefore 25 to 30 gauge needles may be needed
4. It is not unusual for the canaliculus to be obstructed 1 to 3 mm from the punctum after herpesvirus scarring

Nasolacrimal catheterization

1. Catheter preparation - 0 to 00 monofilament nylon is prepared as described for the dog. The technique is the same.
2. Catheterization from the palpebral punctum. If scar tissue does not prevent passage to the osseous lacrimal canal, the catheter will be expected to pass through the rest of the nasolacrimal duct and out the punctum uneventfully.
3. Catheterization from the nasal punctum. The nasal punctum is located similarly to the dog but the nares is not large enough to find it except in large cats.
4. Retention tubing is indicated if scar tissue or dacryocystitis is present. Tubing is positioned similarly to dogs. The preferred method to secure the tubing is to tie the ends together and suture the tubing to the side of the face (Fig 7-14g).
5. *Comment.* Tubing is very well tolerated and should be left in place for the same time frame as described for dogs.

EPIPHORA IN HORSES DUE TO NASOLACRIMAL FAILURE

Causes

1. Congenital
   a. Imperforate nasal punctum is common, usually unilateral
   b. Palpebral punctum abnormality is rare
2. Acquired
   a. Blepharitis from solar irritation
   b. Neoplasia (SCC) nasal canthus
   c. *Habronema* granuloma involving punctum
   d. Lacrimal calculi
   e. Inflammatory stenosis nasolacrimal canal or nasal punctum

Examination

1. Examine eyelids for lesions that would interfere with tear flow
2. Examine floor of nasal cavity for atresia or stenosis of the punctum
3. Checking functional patency of nasolacrimal system with fluorescein is not practical in horses. The nasolacrimal duct has a large fluid capacity resulting in intermittent flow at the nostril.

Nasolacrimal irrigation (Fig 1-44; Chapter 1, page 40) - Nasal punctum irrigation is usually preferred.

1. Nasal punctum irrigation can be accomplished with a curved tip irrigation syringe, teat cannula, plastic tubing or catheters on a 12 cc syringe.
2. Palpebral punctum cannulization requires topical anesthesia and chemical restraint. A 20 or 22 gauge lacrimal needle, IV catheter, feline urinary catheter, or plastic tubing can be used. The lower punctum is larger and usually easiest to cannulate.

Nasolacrimal catheterization

Chemical restraint is required and if atresia of the nasal punctum is present, general anesthesia is recommended.

1. Catheter selection - The largest catheter that will pass through the bony canal is 6 French. Suitable catheters are 4-6 French canine urinary catheters, 5 French feeding tubes or polyethylene tubing (PE90 or 160). Plastic tubing can be prepared with a point (see canine catheterization) to facilitate passage and reduce damage to the duct. The catheter will open scarred portions of the duct system. Most obstructions will occur near the nasal punctum. After the obstruction has been cleared, the catheter can be left in place to keep the duct system open while it heals.
2. Catheterization from the lower punctum - Indicated if the nasal punctum is present and lower nasolacrimal duct obstruction is suspected. Initial catheterization with a 6 French catheter and replacement with an 8 French feeding tube with skin staples or nasolacrimal sutures will reduce the chances of stricture. If possible, a topical antibiotic ophthalmic ointment should be administered BID daily until the catheter is removed at three weeks.
3. Catheterization from palpebral puncta (Fig 7-15). This is indicated with nasal punctum atresia and dacryocystitis. A rigid urinary catheter is preferred. Either punctum can be used.
   a. Punctal atresia with normal duct. The catheter can be passed down the nasolacrimal canal until it is palpated beneath the skin at the mucocutaneous junction. The skin can be incised over the catheter. After forming a new punctum, a six inch segment of tubing can be left in the duct and the end stapled or sutured in the nostril.
   b. Absent or scarred terminal nasolacrimal duct. The catheter can be palpated further up the nostril. It will be necessary to make an incision over the catheter and then hook it out with a muscle hook or grasp it with forceps. These tissues have an abundant blood supply, resulting in marked hemorrhage. The catheter should be secured in the nares.

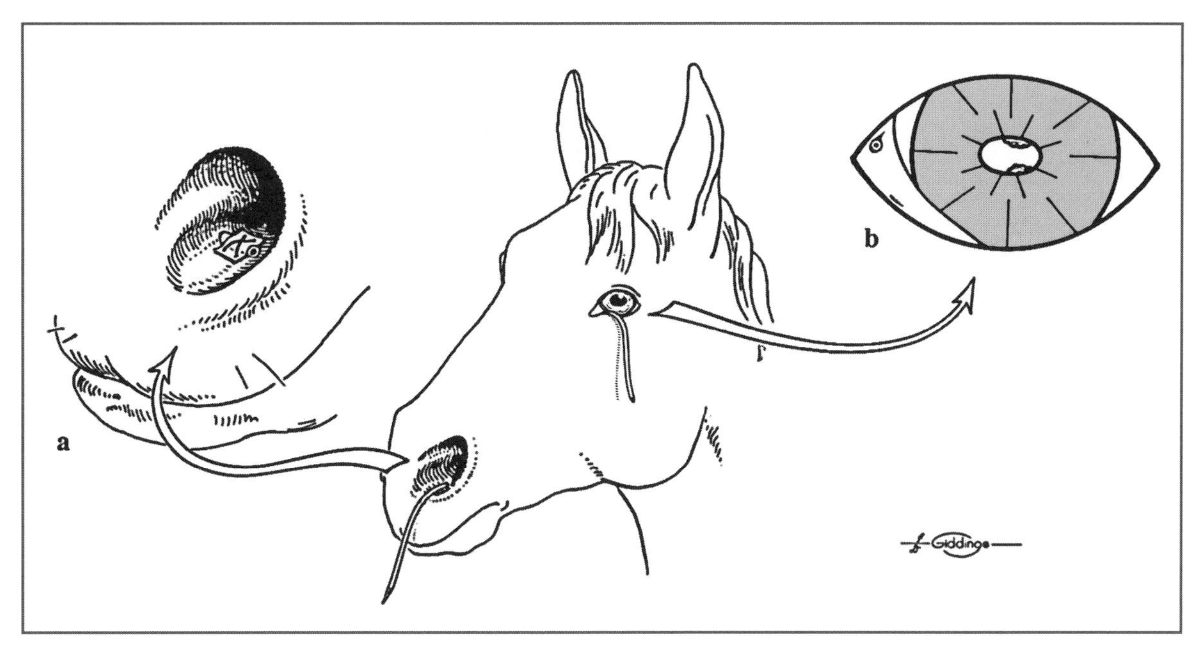

Figure 7-15. Schematic representation of plastic tubing positioned in nasolacrimal canal.
a. Butterfly tape applied over tubing and sutured adjacent to nasal punctum
b. Tubing cut flush to palpebral punctum after secured with butterfly tape

c. Dacryocystitis and inflammatory changes present in the bony canal. After the catheter has been passed, it should be anchored in the nares and then the end coming out the palpebral punctum be cut flush with the eyelid. Systemic antibacterials as indicated by culture and sensitivity should be given for three weeks and the catheter removed in four to six weeks, depending on the patient.

EPIPHORA IN LLAMAS DUE TO NASOLACRIMAL DISEASE

Causes

1. Congenital - atresia of the palpebral punctum, canaliculus or nasal punctum
2. Acquired
   a. Inflammatory obstruction nasolacrimal canal and nasal punctum (dacryocystitis)
   b. Posttraumatic after bone injury

Examination

1. The eyelids can be examined after topical anesthesia. Puncta location is similar to equine.
2. Nasal punctum - chemical restraint is usually needed to examine the nares. The punctum location is similar to the horse and quite large considering the size of the animal.
3. Functional patency with fluorescein is 1 to 3 minutes.

Nasolacrimal irrigation

1. Nasal punctum. After topical anesthesia, the puncta can be cannulated with 20 to 22 gauge lacrimal needle to a depth of 3 to 5 mm and irrigated with saline solution.
2. Nasal punctum. It is located on the floor of the nostril and large enough to be catheterized with size 5 to 8 French catheters.

Nasolacrimal catheterization - The catheterization and retention tubing placement techniques described for dogs are applicable to the llama.

DACRYOCYSTITIS - Dacryocystitis is inflammation of the lacrimal sac and nasolacrimal duct.

Occurrence - seen in dogs, cats, horses, and llamas

Pathogenesis

1. Dogs - usually results from a grass awn(s) migrating from a palpebral punctum to the lacrimal sac where it wedges into the lacrimal foramen or canal. After several weeks, osteomyelitis may develop.
2. Cats - usually associated with osteomyelitis involving the turbinates
3. Horses - may be secondary to congenital atresia (imperforate) nasal punctum. Less frequently, postinflammatory stenosis of the nasal punctum.
4. Llamas - usually involves acquired obstruction of the osseous lacrimal canal similar to dogs.

Clinical signs

1. Thick exudate present at the medial canthus is the characteristic sign. A concurrent, mild conjunctivitis is sometimes seen. The amount of exudate is excessive for the degree of conjunctivitis present. *The exudate at the nasal canthus will frequently have air bubbles in it.*
2. Exudate may flow from the punctum back toward the eye when the eyelid is manipulated in the area of the punctum.
3. Epiphora is present if there is obstruction of the nasolacrimal duct. Horses may show continuous epiphora and purulent discharge may be periodic. Cats, dogs, and llamas have continuous epiphora and purulent discharge.
4. The cornea and anterior uvea are normal.

Differential diagnosis from conjunctivitis

1. Severe conjunctival reaction is present in the conjunctivitis, whereas little or no conjunctival reaction is seen with dacryocystitis
2. Purulent discharge may be seen coming out of the nose in conjunctivitis, whereas there is little or no discharge seen in the nostrils in dacryocystitis.
3. The discharge has a homogeneous appearance in conjunctivitis, whereas there is evidence of normal tears streaking the discharge in dacryocystitis.

Positive diagnosis

1. Diagnosis is established by irrigation of the nasolacrimal duct. Depending on the size of the punctum, use 20, 23, or 25 gauge lacrimal needle. Topical anesthesia is generally adequate, but general anesthesia or sedation may be required in the intractable patient. Irrigation into one punctum will result in thick material coming out of the opposite punctum. In small animals and llamas, if the irrigating material does not reach the nose, there is probably an obstruction where the duct passes through the osseous lacrimal canal. In horses, the obstruction is usually at or near the nasal punctum, rarely it is in the bony canal.
2. Dacryocystorhinography is indicated when the cause of the obstruction is not known. It can be done from the palpebral punctum, nasal punctum, or both if obstruction is complete.
   a. Normograde injection - A small plastic catheter is advanced to about the level of the lacrimal sac, the opposite punctum occluded and then the radiopaque solution is injected, forcing the fluid nasally.
   b. Retrograde injection - Plastic tubing or a small Foley catheter is introduced into the nasal punctum and the procedure repeated.
3. Culture and bacterial sensitivity testing. This is one of the few diseases for which the author does aerobic and anaerobic cultures.

Treatment - same for all species

1. Medical
   a. Irrigation with saline solution to clear the lacrimal duct followed by irrigation with 1:50 Betadine in saline
   b. Topical ophthalmic solution with antibiotic and corticosteroid TID-QID
   c. Depending on culture and sensitivity results, systemic medication may be indicated and should be continued two weeks
   d. *Comment.* If obstruction is recent, medical treatment is quite successful; but if it is chronic, the results of medical treatment alone are usually temporary.
2. Surgical - In dogs, before catheterizing dacryocystitis cases, it is advisable to cannulate the nasal punctum with a lacrimal needle and flush the duct retrograde. This flushing may wash foreign material lodged in the lacrimal sac out through a palpebral punctum. Grass awns migrate from the punctum into the lacrimal sac, where they wedge into the osseous lacrimal canal and cause a dacryocystitis and, unless removed, will continue to cause trouble.
   a. Surgical treatment consists of catheterization and placement of retention tubing the full length of the nasolacrimal ducts. The tubing is left in place for at least three weeks and preferably six.
   b. If the patient and owner will permit, flush the opposite punctum daily for 5 to 7 days or until the discharge is greatly reduced.
   c. Topical antibiotic/corticosteroid ophthalmic solution until the retention tubing is removed
   d. Systemic antibacterial for a minimum of two weeks. If discharge is still present at two weeks or if it returns immediately after discontinuing the antibiotic, assume that an additional grass awn may still be present or osteomyelitis exists. If radiographs were not performed as part of the original examination, they should be taken to evaluate for osteomyelitis. Regardless of the presence or absence of osteomyelitis, reflushing for a persistent foreign body should be considered. This can be performed by trimming the catheter next to the knots used for placing the anchoring sutures. At the nasal end of the catheter, thread a 20 gauge needle into the catheter and attach a 12 or 20 ml syringe. Pull the catheter nasally to a position where the catheter tip that was at the palpebral punctum can be assumed to be in the osseous lacrimal canal. Then vigorously retrograde flush the nasolacrimal duct. If a grass awn is present, it will flush out the palpebral punctum. If in doubt as to where the osseous canal ends, the catheter can be withdrawn in 1 cm increments, followed by flushing. After flushing is complete, a monofilament nylon suture can be passed through the nasal end of the tubing. When it appears at the palpebral punctum, it can be stabilized and the tubing withdrawn nasally. A new tube can be placed over this catheter and sutured in place as previously described. If osteomyelitis is present, antibiotics may be required for several more weeks.

Prognosis - Favorable. Guarded for animals with osteomyelitis.

TEAR STAINING SYNDROME IN DOGS

Tear staining syndrome is a common problem in several toy breeds (especially poodles, hence the term *poodle epiphora*). If the hair color is light, the tears stain where they pass down the face, and this concerns the owner.

Etiology - generally a combination of factors

1. Excess hair growing at the nasal canthus
2. Conformation of the nasal canthus interfering with punctal function
   a. Nasal entropion
   b. Tight fitting eyelids
3. Excess nasal folds

Breeds affected

Poodles, terriers with excess hair at nasal canthus, Lhasa Apso, and other dogs with similar hair characteristics.

Pathogenesis and significance

The disease generally bothers the owner more than it does the dog. Tears contain compounds (porphyrins and catecholamines have been suggested) that react with light and produce a reddish-brown stain to the hair at the medial canthus. This is most noticeable in dogs with light colored haircoats. Black and brown dogs may also have epiphora, but the stain is not apparent. These compounds are also present in saliva and sweat. This will cause staining of the hair around the mouth and the feet. If the dog chews or licks its feet, the discoloration is increased.

In severe cases, a secondary blepharitis and contact dermatitis near the nasal canthus will occur from the constant moisture.

Treatment

1. Do a thorough examination to make sure epiphora is not secondary to some other cause (distichiasis, conjunctivitis, or nasolacrimal obstruction). If a cause for excess tearing can be found, treat it first.
2. Medical treatment - oral broad spectrum antibiotics will tie up the circulating porphyrins. This will reduce, and in some cases stop, the staining.
   a. Tetracycline 25 to 50 mg orally daily. If discontinued, staining recurs in two to three weeks. This will control staining from saliva and interdigital sweating.
   b. Other antibiotics have been reported effective, but I do not have any personal experience with them. Tylosin injection every three to four weeks. Metronidazole 100 mg daily for ten days, then as needed.
3. Surgical treatment (Fig 7-16)
   Removal of part of the gland of the third eyelid. Do not remove this gland unless the Schirmer tear test exceeds 15 mm in one minute. The relationship of the third eyelid to adjacent structures is shown in Fig 7-1.

   The gland is exposed by grasping the cartilage of the third eyelid with two fixation forceps. This is accomplished by pulling the third eyelid out and exposing the inner surface. Grasp the edge of the cartilage with a fixation forceps in the follicle area. The second forceps is placed on the opposite edge of the cartilage. The weight of the forceps will expose the gland. Forceps placed on the free edge of the third eyelid will not put enough tension on the cartilage to expose the gland.

   Epinephrine 0.05 to 0.10 cc of 1:10,000 solution is injected subconjunctivally at the base of the gland. This separates the conjunctiva from the gland capsule, facilitates dissection and reduces hemorrhage. Next, a corneal or strabismus scissors is used to cut the conjunctiva. The conjunctiva is adherent to the gland in the area of the follicles and will have to be cut free. This exposes the gland so it can be grasped at the apex.

The connective tissue band that anchors the apex of the gland to the orbit is cut. The gland is dissected free to its widest point and this portion is removed. This removes about 75% of the gland. The third eyelid is repositioned and 1 to 2% ophthalmic epinephrine solution is placed in the eye to control hemorrhage.

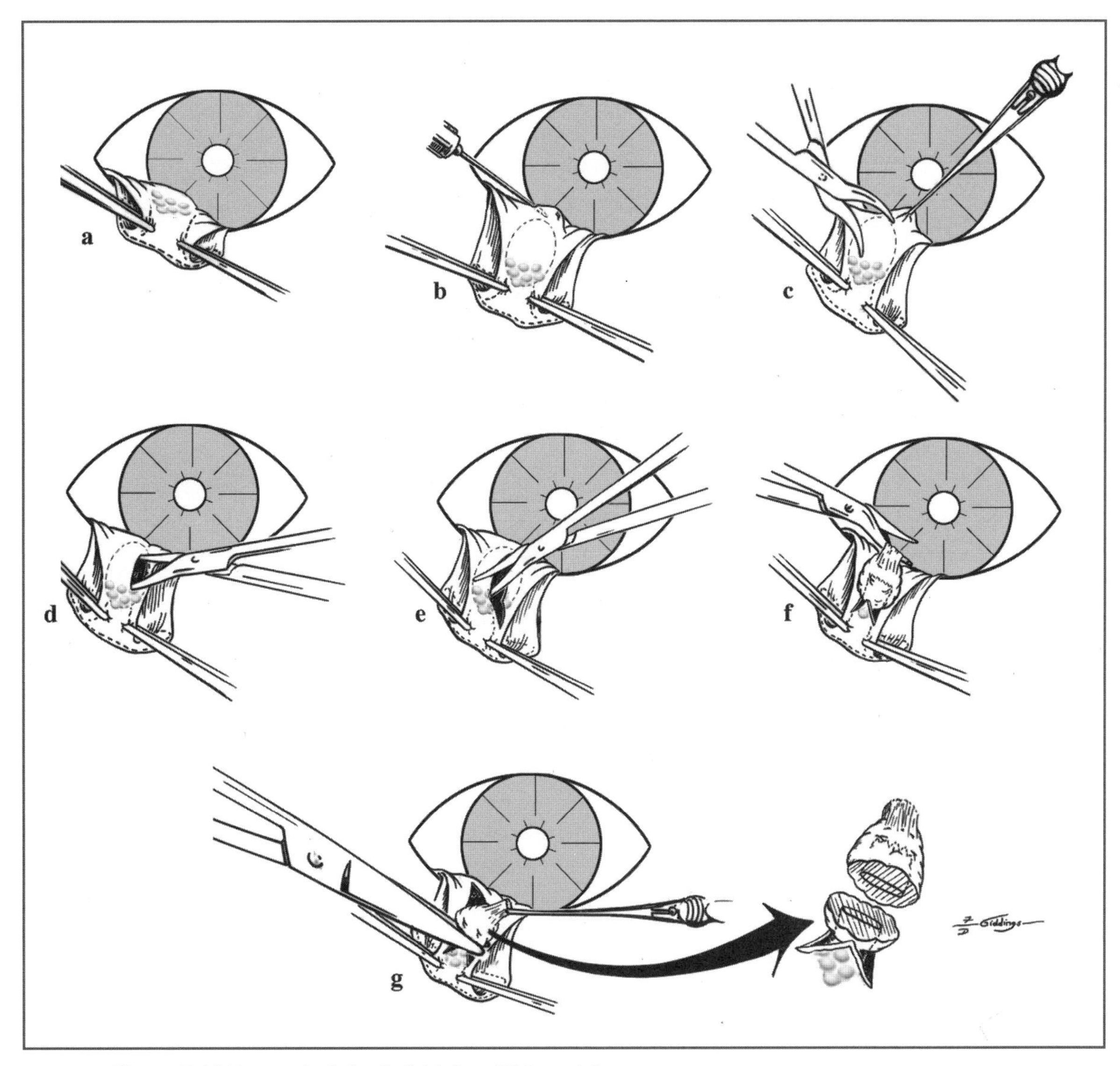

Figure 7-16. Removal of gland of third eyelid for epiphora.

a. Fixation forceps on the edges of the cartilage in the follicle area of the third eyelid
b. Gland of third eyelid exposed by pulling on the forceps. Injecting 1:10,000 epinephrine solution subconjunctivally at the apex of the gland.
c. Cutting the conjunctiva over the gland with corneal scissors
d. Blunt dissection of the conjunctiva from the gland with corneal scissors
e. Cutting the conjunctiva over the base of the gland in the follicle area
f. The connective tissue band anchoring the gland to the periorbital tissue is identified and cut with scissors
g. Removing the gland at its widest point. This removes 75% of the gland.

CHAPTER 8 - CONJUNCTIVA

NORMAL ANATOMY AND PHYSIOLOGY

The conjunctiva is the mucous membrane lining the eyelids (palpebral conjunctiva) and the anterior sclera (bulbar conjunctiva). The palpebral conjunctiva is thick, opaque and red in color. If the lower eyelid is rolled down and the lip elevated, both tissues should have the same appearance.

Bulbar conjunctiva is thin, semitransparent and colorless. The white color of the sclera and Tenon's capsule can be seen deep to the conjunctiva. Blood vessels are present at superficial and deep layers. If the conjunctiva is manipulated with a forceps, these blood vessels will move concurrently. Conjunctival irritation results in congestion of the conjunctival vessels, giving redness (hyperemia) to the conjunctiva. These vessels can be constricted with topical adrenergic drugs (epinephrine and phenylephrine).

The superficial veins of the sclera can be seen beneath the conjunctiva. These vessels do not move when the conjunctiva is manipulated and will not respond to topical adrenergic drugs.

Normal conjunctiva heals rapidly after injury or surgery. Simple lacerations can heal completely in 24 hours.

The conjunctiva should be examined for vascularity, color, edema, surface moisture and abnormal growths. As previously mentioned, it has many small blood vessels that are not easily seen. Irritation will result in congestion of these vessels and redness to the globe. Occasionally a large scleral vein will penetrate the sclera at the limbus and be present in the conjunctiva. This will concern the owner but not have any clinical significance to the patient. Topical anesthetics will cause temporary dilation of conjunctival blood vessels, resulting in increased redness for 20 to 30 minutes.

The conjunctiva is clear except for varying amounts of pigment. The amount of pigment is generally related to the coat color of the patient. White and light colored animals usually have less conjunctival pigment than dark or black animals. Also, the amount of conjunctival pigment increases with age. Pigment is usually most prominent in the temporal part of the globe where the conjunctiva is exposed to environmental irritation at the lateral canthus.

Jaundice will result in a yellow coloration to the conjunctiva and sclera.

Anemia results in a blanched appearance to the globe and paleness to the palpebral conjunctiva.

Hemorrhagic diseases may result in petechial and/or ecchymotic hemorrhages in the conjunctiva. Because of the ease with which the conjunctiva can be examined, it is one of the mucous membrane surfaces to examine in hemorrhagic diseases. Trauma to the eye or choking with a leash can result in gross subconjunctival hemorrhage.

The conjunctiva should always be checked for moisture. Slightly dry appearance may be an early sign of keratoconjunctivitis sicca.

CONGENITAL DISEASES

DERMOID GROWTHS

Ocular dermoids are a form of choristoma (a mass of tissue histologically normal for a part of the body other than the site). Common in the dog, less frequent in horses and cattle, rare in cats.

Tissues involved - Conjunctiva only; conjunctiva and cornea; conjunctiva and eyelids; or if extensive, eyelids, conjunctiva and cornea

Location

Dogs - Usually temporal canthus or limbus
Horses - Temporal limbus or nasal canthus

Appearance

1. Dogs - Typical dermoids have all the characteristics of skin with considerable hair development. The lesion is quite thick and has adipose tissue that is easily identified and separated from normal tissues. These dermoids are easily noticed by the owner and cause surprisingly little discomfort.
2. Horses - Typical dermoids are usually flat and have a rough surface with only a few short hairs visible. There is considerable discomfort when the patient blinks, resulting in epiphora and secondary blepharospasm.

Treatment - Surgical removal

1. If only conjunctiva involved, the conjunctival wound can be left unsutured in small lesions but should be sutured if extensive (Fig 8-1). In large wounds, a "T" closure may be needed (Fig 8-2). Suturing the conjunctival wound will reduce postsurgical healing to two or three days.

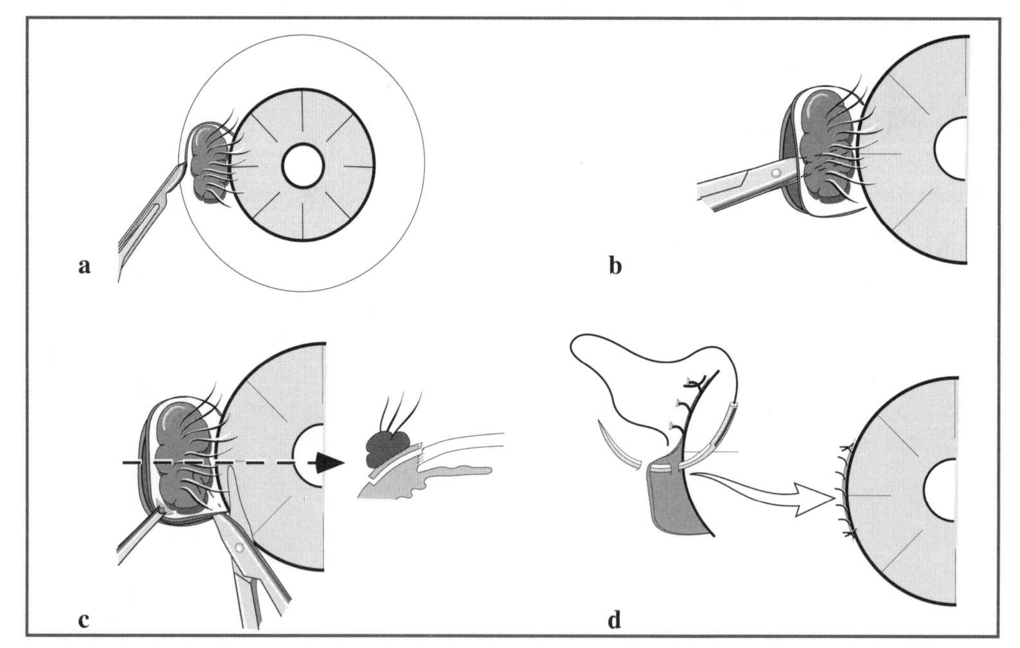

Figure 8-1. Conjunctival dermoid.
a. Incising conjunctiva 1 mm from dermoid
b. Undermining dermoid toward the limbus with a blunt (corneal or strabismus) scissors
c. Dermoid removed from limbus with blunt scissors
d. Closure of conjunctival wound with 6-0 or 7-0 absorbable suture. Suturing results in faster wound healing.

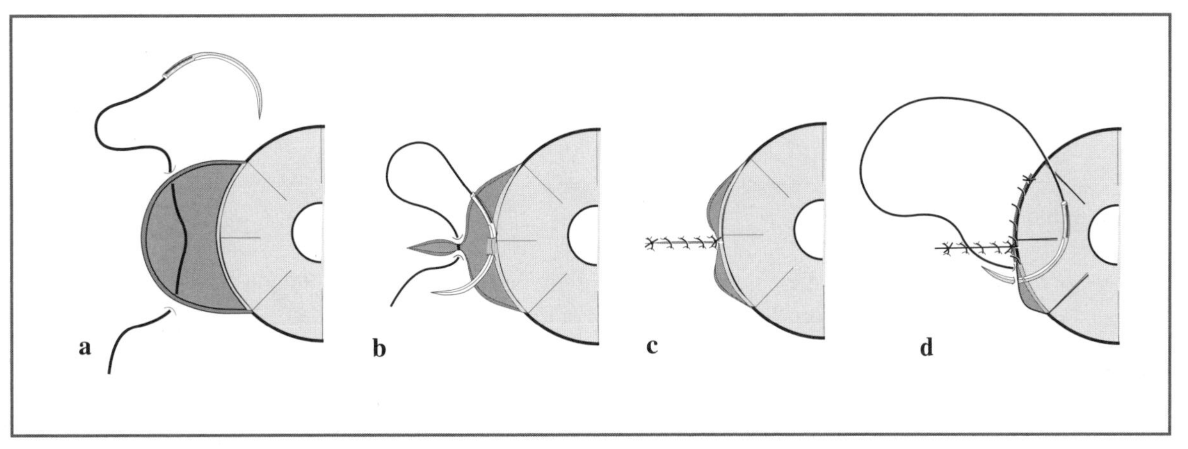

Figure 8-2. "T" closure of large conjunctival wound after dermoid excision.
a. Conjunctival placement of primary closure suture
b. Limbal placement of primary closure suture
c. Primary closure suture tied at limbus, and then continued as continuous suture in conjunctiva
d. Closure of remaining conjunctival wound with continuous suture

2. If conjunctiva and cornea are involved the conjunctival portion should be undermined before starting the superficial keratectomy (Fig 8-3). The surgical ulcer should be treated with topical antibiotics until healed.

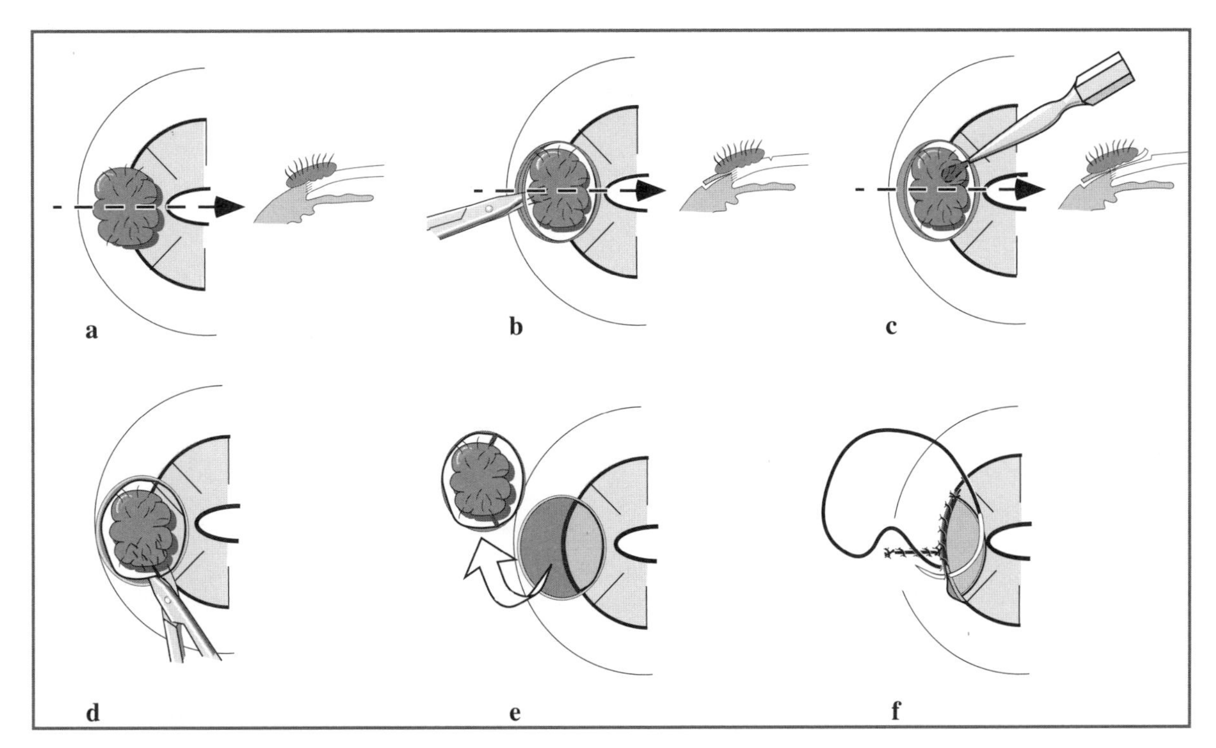

Figure 8-3. Horse with dermoid of conjunctiva and cornea.
a. Frontal and cross-section view
b. Conjunctiva incised and cornea scored 1 mm from lesion before conjunctival portion of dermoid removed with blunt scissors
c. Corneal portion undermined with Martinez corneal dissector to include blood vessels
d. Dermoid removed at limbus with blunt scissors
e. Appearance after dermoid removal (note clear cornea)
f. Conjunctiva sutured to limbus with "T" suture pattern

CONGENITAL CONJUNCTIVAL EXTENSION OVER THE CORNEA

Rarely seen. Occurs along the superior limbus as a thin band of conjunctiva extending 1 to 3 mm out over the cornea. Will remain basically the same throughout the life of the patient without causing clinical problems.

In one case a litter of seven German shorthair pointers were all affected. The breeding was repeated and the litter from that mating was normal.

Observed occasionally in individual animals. This should not be confused with pseudopterygium, which is conjunctival growth out onto the cornea after injury or keratitis.

Pterygium occurs in man and is a conjunctival membrane extending out on the cornea from the nasal limbus. It occurs in adults and is predisposed by actinic radiation. It often recurs after surgical treatment.

ACQUIRED DISEASES

CONJUNCTIVITIS, GENERAL CONSIDERATIONS

Conjunctivitis is inflammation of the conjunctiva. It is the most common eye disease in all species.

Signs - May be acute or chronic, bilateral or unilateral. Acute infections that are not treated may become chronic. Bilateral infections usually indicate infections or systemic disease, whereas unilateral suggests foreign bodies, injury or local infections.

1. Hyperemia. Vascular injection is more severe toward the fornix and the palpebral conjunctiva. Superficial conjunctival blood vessels are small, branch toward the limbus and result in diffuse redness.
2. Papillary hypertrophy. Thickening and increased vascularity (deep red appearance) of the conjunctiva.
3. Chemosis (conjunctival edema). Conjunctival thickening may become so severe that bulbar conjunctiva extends over the cornea and palpebral conjunctiva will extend beyond the edges of the eyelids. The degree of chemosis usually parallels the acuteness of the lesions.
4. Follicles. Normally present on bulbar side of third eyelid, but when present elsewhere indicate chronic conjunctivitis. Will occur with chlamydial infections in cats, sheep and goats.
5. Ocular discharge. Trigeminal innervation controls lacrimal gland secretion and stimulation of goblet cell activity. Discharge usually begins serous and as the disease progresses becomes mucopurulent.
   a. Serous discharge - acute infections (especially viral and chlamydial), allergy, and mechanical irritants
   b. Mucoid - in chronic diseases, especially KCS
   c. Purulent - bacterial infections and foreign bodies that have been causing irritation for several days
6. Pain. May be severe or mild depending on cause. Results in blepharospasm. If chronic may result in spastic entropion.

Etiology - There are many causes for conjunctivitis. Therefore, differentiating primary conjunctivitis (the response of the eye to a local irritant with possible opportune infection) from secondary conjunctivitis due to systemic disease is essential for prescribing appropriate treatment.

1. Physical irritation - probably the most common cause for conjunctivitis in dogs and horses
   a. Wind, dust, solar reaction and weed seeds in all species
   b. Irritating medications applied around or inadvertently to the eye
   c. Overcrowding in corrals or kennels
   d. Eyelid diseases - eyelash problems, tumors (very small eyelid tumors will often result in an unusually severe conjunctival reaction), injuries with eyelid malfunction
2. Infections - May be restricted to the eye or part of a systemic disease. Because of this, all animals with conjunctivitis should be given a thorough physical examination with emphasis on the upper respiratory tract.
   a. Bacterial - Bacteria are present in the conjunctival sacs of most normal animals, therefore their presence does not indicate an infectious process. If an animal has active conjunctivitis and bacteria that can be considered pathogenic are recovered, treatment for these organisms is indicated.
   b. Viral - Systemic and ocular viral agents have been reported in all species.
   c. *Chlamydia* - Important in cats, sheep and goats; not reported in the dog
   d. *Mycoplasma* - Important in cats, sheep and goats
   e. Mycotic - Fungi are present on the conjunctiva of normal animals (Table 8-1).
      Primary mycotic infections are uncommon in domestic animals but when they occur will usually have serious concurrent corneal lesions (see mycotic keratitis, Chapter 10, page 349).
      Frequency of occurrence - equine usually involved, rare in the cat, very rare in dogs and cattle.
   f. Rickettsia - Important in sheep and goats
3. Parasitic - uncommon
   a. *Thelazia sp*
      1) *Thelazia californiensis* - reported in all domestic animals and several wild animals. Seen primarily in Sierra Nevada mountains of California, Oregon and Nevada. Usually cause a mild conjunctivitis and epiphora. Severe cases can cause secondary keratitis.

2) *T. lacrimalis* - reported in horses, primarily in Eastern U.S.
3) Three species in cattle: *T. rhodesi, T. gulosa,* and *T. skrjabini*

b. *Habronema megastoma* - can cause conjunctivitis, eyelid granulomas and lacrimal duct obstruction in horses
c. *Onchocerca cervicalis* - in horses causes conjunctivitis and granulomas
d. Face flies - during the summer a significant cause for conjunctivitis in horses and cattle
e. Mange when observed around the eyes predisposes to conjunctivitis (especially *Demodex* in dogs)

4. Allergic - seen most frequently during pollen seasons and then accompanied by upper respiratory and/or systemic signs. More apt to have pruritus than other forms of conjunctivitis.
   a. Can be associated with type and quality of hay in large animals
   b. Can be serious problem in some hunting dogs
   c. Continual use of topical medications - antibiotics may result in conjunctival sensitivity (neomycin, gentocin). Pilocarpine, tetracaine.
5. Keratoconjunctivitis sicca

Table 8-1. Conjunctival fungal flora of normal bovine, canine, equine, and feline in number of isolates

	Bovine n = 25	**Canine** n = 50	**Equine** n = 43	**Feline** n = 25
Alternaria spp	3	—	6	—
Aspergillus spp	3	—	23	2
Botrytis spp	—	—	1	—
Candida albicans	4	—	1	—
Cladosporium spp	16	3	6	4
Curvularia lunta	5	3	—	—
Drechslera dematioidea	2	—	—	—
Exosporiella fungorum	2	1	—	—
Fusarium spp	4	—	—	1
Geotrichum candidum	—	—	2	—
Gliocladium deliquescens	—	—	5	—
Gliomastic murorum	—	1	—	—
Helminthosporium vellutinum	5	—	1	1
Histoplasma capsulatum	1	—	—	—
Memmoniella echinata	—	—	1	—
Penicillium spp	11	—	19	2
Scopulariopsis spp	6	8	—	1
Torula herbarum	1	—	1	—
Triderma viride	—	—	2	—
Verticillium tenuissimum	—	—	2	—
Yeast	12	1	11	—
Unidentified	20	3	7	1
Total	95	20	88	12

Samuelson DA. Conjunctival fungal flora in horses, cattle, dogs and cats. J Am Vet Med Assoc 1984;184:1240-1242.

Diagnostic procedures

1. Cultures
   a. Bacterial - Culture swabs for bacteria should be made prior to any other diagnostic procedure. Bacterial culturing is not routinely recommended in conjunctivitis patients. It should be considered if the lesion is causing severe changes or if it has been chronic. Chronicity in the presence of continued medication would suggest the development of resistant strains of bacteria. A sterile bacterial culture in a chronic case is reason for reevaluation of the patient; consider the possibility of a viral or noninfectious etiology.
   b. Viral isolation, when available, is helpful in feline conjunctivitis. Viral samples can be taken after topical anesthesia.
   c. Chronic cases should be cultured for fungi.
2. Conjunctival scrapings - Conjunctival cytology gives a rapid evaluation without the one to two day delay associated with culturing. It also evaluates the distribution of organisms and the types of inflammatory cells present. See cytology (Chapter 1, page 36) for collection technique. Several slides should be made for routine staining (e.g. Giemsa, Gram's stain, Diff-Quik) and/or immunofluorescent antibody techniques.
3. Conjunctival stains - Fluorescein will stain ulcerated conjunctiva. This is easiest to see in a dark room using an examining light with a cobalt filter.
4. Schirmer tear test - to diagnose keratoconjunctivitis sicca

Treatment

1. Thorough examination to eliminate physical cause. If secondary to systemic disease, treat the primary disease as well as symptomatic conjunctival treatment
2. Cleanse eye - If there is excessive discharge, thoroughly cleanse eye with an eye wash. Make sure special tests have been completed (culture and Schirmer tear test) before irrigation with an eye wash.
3. Antibacterials - antibiotics or sulfas. The use of broad spectrum agents or mixtures. The drugs are chosen for their effectiveness in the tear film and do not need to penetrate the epithelial barrier. Apply as frequently as needed by the acuteness of the disease. Usually three to four times a day. Hourly in acute conditions.
   a. Neomycin, polymyxin B, bacitracin or gramicidin mixtures. Very effective. These drugs are used only topically and therefore are unlikely to cause systemic drug sensitivity or produce strains that will be resistant to systemic antibiotics.
   b. Chloramphenicol - small animal and equine
   c. Gentocin/tobramycin
   d. Trimethoprim sulfate and polymyxin (Polytrim)
   e. Ofloxacin (Ocuflox)
4. Anti-inflammatory - Corticosteroids are often used in combination with antibiotics to reduce the inflammatory response. In some cases the inflammation appears "quieter" but conjunctivitis lasts longer due to the inhibiting effect on healing. Do not use in those infections where known to be contraindicated (feline herpesvirus or mycoplasma). Acute conjunctivitis from irritants and allergy are definite indications for corticosteroid preparations. Use two to four times daily.
5. Anti-allergy - Corticosteroids topical and/or systemic, depending on severity of case. Topical antihistamines, Cromolyn (mast cell stabilizer) and Ketorolac.
6. If the patient is cooperative, cool compresses may make them more comfortable.

Course and prognosis

Acute conjunctivitis usually responds well to treatment. If it persists more than a week, re-examine and consider cytology and culture/sensitivity testing.

If an animal comes in with a history of treatment for chronic or recurrent conjunctivitis, it is advisable to make cultures before starting the examination, do conjunctival scrapings, and then examine very thoroughly for a maintaining cause.

CONJUNCTIVITIS IN DOGS

Unilateral vs bilateral

1. Unilateral - suspect irritation (foreign bodies, adnexal tumors, injury and eyelid diseases)
2. Bilateral - eyelid diseases, chronic staph infections, secondary to acute systemic viral diseases

Primary vs secondary

1. Primary - usually irritation with secondary infection
2. Secondary to systemic diseases (viral, rickettsia, staphylococcus dermatitis, demodectic mange, leishmaniasis, keratoconjunctivitis sicca)

Bacterial

1. *Staphylococcus* is the most common bacteria present in normal (Table 8-2) and infected eyes (Table 8-3) with *S. aureus* most frequently isolated. Gram negative organisms are less common in normal eyes and their presence in an inflamed eye should be considered significant. Variations in flora may be influenced by geographic location, time of the year, breed, climate, area cultured, and culture technique.
2. Signs - Bacterial conjunctivitis is usually purulent. It may begin acutely and become chronic and it usually has an initiating cause.
   a. Acute from injury or foreign bodies, opportunistic infection after acute viral systemic diseases
   b. Chronic from eyelid diseases (ectropion, entropion, eyelash disease), staph infections or adnexal tumors

Mycotic - Fungal isolates from normal appearing eyes are common (22%, Samuelson - 1984, Table 1) but are much less common in inflamed eyes (4.6%, Gerding, 1988). The most common isolates from normal eyes were *Cladosporium* and *Curvularia.* The author has diagnosed only one case of canine mycotic keratitis.

Viral - usually bilateral and part of systemic diseases

1. Canine distemper begins with an acute serous conjunctivitis. In a few days, secondary bacterial involvement may occur, resulting in purulent discharge. The most successful means of diagnoses are direct and indirect immunofluorescent antibody techniques. Keratoconjunctivitis sicca may occur, which in turn may lead to corneal ulcers.
2. Infectious canine hepatitis - serous discharge may be seen.

Rickettsia - May result in conjunctivitis and subconjunctival hemorrhage

1. Ehrlichiosis
2. Rocky Mountain spotted fever

Parasitic

1. *Thelazia californiensis* seen most frequently in dogs. Remove mechanically after topical anesthesia. Topical weekly administration of an organophosphate miotic may be used for prophylactic treatment.
2. Demodectic mange lesions around the eye predispose to secondary conjunctivitis. Protect the eye with ophthalmic ointment before treating the eyelids with specific medication.
3. Leishmaniasis may cause conjunctivitis and panuveitis

Table 8-2. Frequency of bacteria in the eyes of normal dogs in percentage of eyes sampled

		Staphylococcus			*Streptococcus*				*Coryne-bacterium*	*Bacillus*	*Clostridium*	*Pseudo-monas*	*Neisseria*	*Moraxella*
	No Growth	Total	Epidermidis	Aureus	Total	Nonhem-olytic	Hemolytic alpha	Hemolytic beta						
Bistner[1] N = 70; 140 samples	28	—	46	24	—	0	4	2	75	12	—	x	x	x
Urban[2] N = 150; 300 samples	32*	70	55	45	43	12	34	7	30	6	1	14	26	—
MacDonald[3] N = 100; OS only	22	39	16	23	7	3	3	1	19	29	1	1	2	—
Hacker[4] N = 60; one eye only	12	—	25	31	—	43	5	3	—	18	—	1	—	1

[1]Bistner S. et al. Conjunctival bacteria: Clinical appearance can be deceiving. Mod Vet Pract 1969;Dec 45-47.
[2]Urban M, et al. Conjunctival flora of clinically normal dogs. J Am Vet Med Assoc 1972;161:201-206.
[3]MacDonald P. and Watson A. Microbial flora of normal canine conjunctiva. J Small Anim Pract 1976;17, 809-812.
[4]Hacker D, et al. A comparison of conjunctival techniques in the dog using wet swabs. J Am Anim Hosp Assoc 1979;15:223-225.
[x]All gram - negatiive combined = 7%

*Both eyes were normal in 9% and only 1 eye in 32% of the dogs.

Table 8-3. Frequency of potentially pathogenic bacteria in the eyes of dogs with external ocular diseases expressed in percentage of eyes sampled

		Staphylococcus			*Streptococcus*			*Coryne-bacterium*	*E coli*	*Proteus*	*Bacillus*	*Pseudo-mona*	*Pasteur-sella*	*Kleb-siella*	*Moraxella*
	No Growth	Total	Epidermidis	Aureus	Total	alpha	beta								
Murphy[1] N = 120 animals	32	—	27	68	—	17	19	3	10	11	5	2	—	1	—
Gerding[2] N = 151 eyes	34	39	17	22	32	—	—	4	5	—	2	9	1	—	2

[1]Murphy J, et al. Survey of conjunctival flora in dogs with clinical signs of external eye disease. J Am Vet Med Assoc 1978;172:66-69.
[2]Gerding P, et al. Pathogenic bacteria and fungi associated with external eye diseases in dogs: 131 cases (1981-1986). J Am Vet Med Assoc 1988;193:242-244.

Allergic

1. Acute - may be limited to the conjunctiva or be seen with concurrent upper respiratory signs. Characterized by a serous discharge and considerable chemosis. Conjunctival scraping shows an increase in eosinophils. The owner is often aware that the problem is recurrent after exercising the dog in specific areas.
2. Chronic - discharge may become purulent and have less chemosis
3. Urticaria - eyelids are more severely involved than the conjunctiva. Skin lesions will be present elsewhere over the body. The eyelid and lip lesions are more prone to pruritus and if the dog begins to rub its face, this will produce even greater tissue reaction.

Physical irritation

1. Environmental irritation - wind, dust, smoke, soap or medicines. Sunshine in animals with inadequate protective pigment.
2. Exposure - exophthalmic dogs or in dogs with neurogenic disorders.

Keratoconjunctivitis sicca - All dogs with conjunctivitis should be checked with a Schirmer tear test. The corneal lesions are more serious and treatment is directed toward the corneal change.

CONJUNCTIVITIS IN CATS

Conjunctivitis is a common and perplexing disease in cats. It may occur as a primary conjunctival disease with the same causes as observed in other animals but it occurs most frequently as an acute or chronic ophthalmic manifestation of systemic disease with or without upper respiratory signs. These diseases are:

Pneumonitis (*Chlamydia psittaci cati*)
Feline rhinotracheitis (feline herpesvirus type 1 - FHV-1)
Feline influenza (feline calicivirus) - mild to moderate conjunctivitis, not a significant problem
Reovirus respiratory infection - very mild conjunctivitis; not a significant problem
Mycoplasma infection (*Mycoplasma felis* and *gatea*)

Unfortunately, presenting conjunctival signs of *chlamydia* and feline herpesvirus can be so similar that differential diagnosis is not possible without laboratory assistance and even then the differential diagnosis may not be definite. Mixed infections can occur especially with herpesvirus, *chlamydia* and *mycoplasma.*

Bacterial - The prevalence of conjunctival bacteria in normal cats is much lower than in dogs. Campbell reported an isolation rate of 35%, with *staphylococcus* most frequent (26%) and *mycoplasma* next (5%). Shewen reported a rate of 4% with *staphylococcus* and *streptococcus* equally isolated. Cats with conjunctivitis are less likely to have bacteria isolated than *chlamydia* or feline herpesvirus type 1. When bacteria are isolated they usually occur as a mixed infection with feline herpesvirus 1 or *chlamydia.*

Fungal - Although conjunctival fungi are frequently present in cats with normal appearing eyes (Table 8-1), mycotic conjunctivitis is extremely rare. Deep ocular involvement can occur with blastomycosis and cryptococcosis.

Feline herpesvirus conjunctivitis

1. Pathogenesis. Feline herpesvirus infection begins as a systemic respiratory and conjunctival disease. At that time the oral and nasopharyngeal mucosa are good sites for cytology and culture sampling. Acute cases frequently develop corneal ulcers that begin as punctate lesions, progressing to dendritic and geographic ulcers. If the disease is prolonged, stromal ulcers may develop with perforation as a possibility. Healing begins as virus disappears from the ocular surface. Following the acute phase the virus may localize in the trigeminal ganglion, remaining there as a latent infection to cause ocular relapses the rest of the cat's life. It has been estimated that 80% of the cats become latently infected and 45% of these will react either with asymptomatic virus shedding or recurring clinical signs. By the time cats are one year old, probably 90% of the population will demonstrate FHV-1 titers. Keratitis is secondary to persistent conjunctival infection or reactivated latent infection. Stress (especially environmental) is the major cause to activate latent infections. Virus particles migrate down the trigeminal nerve axons to the corneal and conjunctival epithelium resulting in keratoconjunctivitis. Lacrimal gland involvement will result in decreased tear production.
2. Manifestations vary with age of the patient
    a. Neonatal ophthalmia - conjunctivitis and keratitis (with or without ulcers), KCS, mild respiratory involvement
    b. Neonate to four weeks - bilateral ocular signs, concurrent with severe respiratory involvement
    c. Four weeks to six months - ocular signs concurrent with mild respiratory involvement
    d. Adults - conjunctivitis and/or keratitis with little or no associated respiratory involvement. A common disease with latent carriers, usually unilateral but both eyes can be involved.
3. Signs
    a. Discharge - serous progressing to mucopurulent or purulent several days later
    b. Conjunctival hyperemia with minimal chemosis
    c. Photophobia and blepharospasm
    d. Corneal/conjunctival ulcers
        1) Kittens - diffuse corneal and conjunctival ulcers are common

        2) After six months - corneal ulcers that may be:
            a) Punctate
            b) Dendritic (linear with a branching appearance)
            c) Geographic (covering large area)
            d) Stromal (deep ulcers) - very serious and vision threatened
    e. Keratoconjunctivitis sicca - this may be transient or permanent. Recurrent cases may have reduced tear production as a prodromal sign before conjunctival or corneal changes become evident.
4. Course - variable (two weeks to three months). Many kittens recover completely. Adult cases are usually a relapse from latent trigeminal ganglion infection.
5. Diagnosis - clinical signs are suggestive but often not definitive
    a. Cytology - lymphocytes, neutrophils (chronicity), epithelial giant cells, intranuclear inclusions (rare). Cytology inconclusive.
    b. Serology - serum neutralizing antibody, hemagglutination inhibition, ELISA most sensitive. Recurrent problems may not show a good rising paired titer.
    c. Virus isolation - observe for tissue culture cytopathic effect and the density of virus with virus neutralization or fluorescent antibody tests. Stromal disease cases are difficult to culture.
    d. Indirect immunofluorescence - performed on conjunctival or corneal scrapings and swabs *(best screening test)*. If fluorescein has been used on the eye, place an air dried slide under a light for 12-18 hours to bleach the fluorescein before performing immunofluorescent procedures.
    e. Polymerase chain reaction (PCR) - is more sensitive than either virus isolation or FA. <u>But</u> in clinical situations, FA is still usually the best screening test.
6. Treatment - difficult and relapses due to the latent nature are common. If the host's immune system responds to the virus, the disease will be self-limiting. If immunosuppressed, nothing seems to work well.
    a. Symptomatic
        1) Topical antibiotics - to control secondary bacterial infection
        2) Debridement of corneal ulcers - this is the best way to remove virus infected epithelial cells
    b. Antiviral (see Chapter 2, page 86; also Table 2-5)
        1) Topical treatment - effective only for epithelial virus
            a) Acute infection - idoxuridine appears to be more effective than Vira-A (See page 85).
            b) Chronic infection - Betadine 1:20 to 1:10 in saline QID (is also antibacterial)
            c) Prophylactic - Betadine 1:20 daily or BID in animals with a relapsing history
        2) Systemic treatment for acute infection
            a) Acyclovir sodium (Zovirax), 5 mg/lb BID. Given a minimum of two weeks, maximum of four weeks. It can also be used prophylactically in known carriers who relapse when stressed. Begin treatment 1-2 days prior to an anticipated stressful event (traveling, arrival of grandchildren for vacation, etc.) then continue several days post-stress.
            b) Interferon 3 IU per os daily
            c) Prophylactic - 250-500 mg lysine per os BID.
    c. Anti-inflammatory
        1) Corticosteroids - topical corticosteroids result in delayed ulcer healing and prolonged viral shedding. Some cases that have been started on corticosteroids will relapse when medication is discontinued. Topical steroids can be used when treating severe stromal keratitis if combined with systemic acyclovir and topical antivirals.
        2) Cyclosporine A 1% - may induce recurrence
7. Prognosis - depends on the immunocompetence of the host. In immunosuppressed animals (FeLV/FIV infected), the prognosis is poor.
8. Complications
    a. Kittens - conjunctival and corneal ulcers resulting in adhesions
        1) Punctal occlusion due to palpebral conjunctival adhesions. This is the most common cause for obstructive epiphora in cats.
        2) Palpebral and bulbar conjunctival adhesions that result in interference of third eyelid movement
        3) Conjunctival and corneal adhesions (symblepharon) - if severe may impair vision and/or eyelid movement

b. Adult cats
   1) Fibrovascular keratitis
   2) Permanent keratoconjunctivitis sicca
   3) Corneal sequestration
   4) May have a relationship with eosinophilic keratitis (suspected)

Chlamydial conjunctivitis (*Chlamydia psittaci cati*) - Commonly seen but nationwide incidence is variable. Easily spread between animals in a household. May or may not have a history of recent or current upper respiratory infection.

1. Signs
   a. May be unilateral or bilateral. It is common for the patient with unilateral involvement to develop the lesion in the other eye 5 to 10 days later.
   b. Chemosis - severe at onset and then decreases. It is more severe than expected with herpesvirus.
   c. Hyperemia - not as much as expected with herpesvirus. Slight at first. May become more pronounced later.
   d. Initially serous epiphora. Becomes mucopurulent in several days. Herpesvirus tends to be serous longer.
   e. Blepharospasm - less painful than herpesvirus. A mild squint with slight epiphora may precede overt signs by 12 to 24 hours. Treatment at this stage may resolve the disease in 24 to 48 hours.
   f. Follicle development - may occur on the palpebral and bulbar conjunctiva after several days. *Chlamydia* is the only proven cause for follicle development in the cat, therefore the presence of follicles is of diagnostic value.
2. Diagnosis - cytology (epithelial cytoplasmic inclusion bodies), culture, indirect immunofluorescence (most practical and high degree of accuracy). *Chlamydia* are abundant early in the disease but often cannot be identified after 7-10 days. Organisms may be present in normal appearing animals.
3. Course
   a. If treated, about 3 to 7 days
   b. Untreated, may last months
   c. Short immunity and carriers exist
4. Treatment - if no systemic signs, topical only
   a. Topical
      1) Antibiotics (tetracycline or oxytetracycline are the most specific antibiotics; chloramphenicol, neomycin, gentamicin)
      2) Corticosteroids - beneficial when given concurrently with effective antibiotics, but are contraindicated in mixed infections
      3) Comment - *C. trachomatis* occurs in man and is sensitive to sulfonamides, whereas *C. psittaci* is not. Physicians prescribe sulfonamides commonly for human eye infections and clients often will try to treat their pets with the same products.
   b. Systemic - if respiratory signs are present, systemic doxycycline or azithromycin are indicated.
5. Public health significance - minimal. Human infections with *chlamydia* from cats can occur; especially close contact with children should be avoided.

Mycoplasma conjunctivitis

1. Occurrence - Uncommon as primary infection. When present it is usually seen as a secondary invader with FHV-1, less common with chlamydia.
2. Signs as a primary agent
   a. Unilateral or bilateral - may go to the other eye in a week
   b. Discharge is mucopurulent with pseudomembrane formation on the palpebral conjunctiva
   c. The eye may appear dry, resembling KCS, but tear production is normal.
   d. Mild chemosis and hyperemia
3. Diagnosis - Surface inclusion bodies can occasionally be seen on cytology. Clinical signs are suggestive. A positive diagnosis requires culture.

4. Course
   a. If untreated or improperly treated, the infection will persist about 30 days, then regress spontaneously
   b. If treated properly, the eyes will clear up in five to six days
5. Treatment - Topical is usually adequate.
   a. Erythromycin is most effective; chloramphenicol and tetracycline are also effective
   b. Cortisone is contraindicated because it can precipitate the infection
   c. If penicillin, sulfas, neomycin, or bacitracin are used to treat the eye, there will be a diminution of signs, but the conjunctiva stays red and appears dry. If the treatment is changed to any of the drugs recommended, the eye should clear up quickly.

Neonatal conjunctivitis in kittens - The queen is the most common source of infection and therefore should be examined along with the kittens.

1. Occurrence - kittens one to six weeks of age (usually before four weeks)
2. Etiology - herpesvirus is the most frequent cause in most areas of the US
   a. Herpesvirus - neonatal conjunctival herpesvirus infection from a carrier queen or other household cats. Also occurs after the eyes open. This is responsible for the greatest number of complications.
   b. *Chlamydia* - neonatal conjunctival chlamydial infection from carrier queens or other cats in the household. This usually occurs after the eyes open.
   c. Bacterial - Genital infection of the queen resulting in infection immediately after birth until 10 days. If a kitten develops conjunctivitis before 10 days of age, always examine the queen
3. Signs
   a. If before the eyelids open - the discharge builds up beneath the lids causing them to swell. Discharge may be seen at the nasal canthus before the lids open. There may be delayed opening of the eyelids.
   b. After the eyelids open - the discharge may be serous or purulent depending on the cause. Purulent discharge may cause the eyelids to stick together soon after they open. Corneal ulcers may develop.
   c. Additional signs (if present) depend on the cause - upper respiratory infection, diarrhea, small kittens that are poor-doers and/or death.
4. Differential diagnosis - cytology for IFA and histologic examination, cultures
5. Course - if untreated, corneal changes develop quickly and cause ulcerative keratitis; may lose the eye if the ulcer penetrates.
6. Treatment - never dispense medication without examining the kittens for corneal damage. Examine the queen for vaginitis or respiratory infection. Except for the herpesvirus kittens, there is a rapid response to treatment.
   a. Symptomatic
      1) Open and clean the eyes
      2) Treat with broad spectrum antibiotics (ointments preferred)
      3) ***Do not use medication containing corticosteroids*** because it will interfere with healing of corneal lesions
   b. Specific - if cause is identified, use definitive antibiotics/antivirals
   c. Queen - treat queen with systemic and topical treatment as indicated

CONJUNCTIVITIS IN HORSES

Primary-allergic, irritant or bacterial conjunctivitis is common in horses, especially when stabled in dusty or poorly ventilated environments. Secondary conjunctivitis is usually the result of systemic viral diseases and less frequently bacterial or parasitic.

Bacterial

1. Normal eyes - Bacteria are common in the eyes of normal horses. Mixed isolates of bacteria and/or fungi are often present. Gram positive isolates predominate. *Corynebacterium bacillus, Staphylococcus,* and *Streptococcus*. Gram negative usually represent less than one-fourth with *Neisseria, Moraxella* and *Actinobacter* most frequently isolated. *Pseudomonas is rarely isolated in normal eyes.*
2. Eyes with external eye disease - Mixed infections of bacteria and fungi are observed about 1/3 of the time. The most common bacteria isolated are *Pseudomonas, Enterobacter, Acinetobacter* and *Staphylococcus* (Table 8-4).
    a. When gram negative organisms are present, polymyxin B and gentamicin are good presumptive choices until sensitivity results are available.
    b. When gram positive organisms are present, chloramphenicol, tetracyclines, gentamicin or triple antibiotic combinations are good first choices.
    c. *Moraxella equi* is species specific. Conjunctivitis is the initial sign and may be followed in 5 to 10 days by erosions at the mucocutaneous junction of the eyelid margins and canthal areas.
3. Systemic diseases with secondary conjunctivitis - *Streptococcus equi* (strangles), *Actinobacillus,* and *Rhodococcus equi.*

Table 8-4. Bacterial and fungal isolates from horses with external eye disease (in percentage of eyes sampled)

	Moore[1] n = 38	McLaughlin[2] n = 123
Pseudomonas spp	26	14
Enterobacter group	24	6.5
Acinetobacter spp	16	—
Streptococcus spp	8	44
Staphylococcus spp	13	14
Bacillus spp	—	11
Escherichia coli	—	4
Corynebacterium spp	3	3
Klebsiella spp	10.5	2
Moraxella spp	3	2
Pasteurella spp	3	2
Neisseria spp	—	1
Phycomyces group	5	—
Aspergillus spp	18	2
Penicillium spp	8	—
Fusarium spp	1	1

[1]Moore CP, et al. Bacterial and fungal isolates from equidae with ulcerative keratitis. J Am Vet Med Assoc 1983;182:600-603.
[2]McLaughlin, et al. Pathologic bacteria and fungi associated with extraocular diseases in the horse. J Am Vet Med Assoc 1983;182:241-242.

Fungal - Fungal isolates are common in normal eyes (Table 8-1) but less common in infected eyes (Table 8-4).

1. The most common cause for mycotic keratitis is *Aspergillus spp.* Less common are *Fusarium* and *Phycomycetes*. A mixed infection of *Aspergillus* and gram negative bacteria is devastating.
2. Systemic fungi may have an associated conjunctivitis - histoplasma, sporotrichosis, and rhinosporidium.

Chlamydia has been reported.

Viral - primarily those affecting the upper respiratory tract. They are clinically difficult to differentiate.

1. Adenovirus (usually in immunodeficient foals) - mucopurulent nasal and ocular discharge, chemosis and hyperemia. Intranuclear inclusions occur in conjunctival epithelium.
2. Equine herpesvirus (EHV)
   a. Type 1 - may produce encephalitis with secondary neuropathy with facial paralysis and KCS. Other ocular signs include blindness and nystagmus.
   b. Type 4 (rhinopneumonitis) - Equine abortion virus and respiratory infection. Develop serous conjunctivitis that may turn mucopurulent.
   c. Equine infectious anemia (EIA) - retrovirus that causes conjunctival and retinal hemorrhages
   d. Equine viral arteritis (EVA) - togavirus causing panvasculitis
   e. Influenza type A_2 - mild conjunctivitis and keratoconjunctivitis associated with upper respiratory disease

Rickettsial

Ehrlichiosis (Potomac horse fever) - conjunctival hemorrhage and uveitis

Allergic

Allergic conjunctivitis is characterized by acute chemosis and epiphora, with increased eosinophils in conjunctival scrapings. Seen associated with summer pastures and from hay. Severe chemosis cases develop concurrent lid edema.

Treatment - remove from offending environment. Treat locally with moist heat packs and topical cortico-steroids. Systemic corticosteroids or antihistamines are indicated for severe cases.

Parasitic conjunctivitis

1. Face flies (*M. autumnalis*). Conjunctivitis is common during summer months when face flies are a problem. The eyes should be kept clean and the conjunctivitis treated with antibiotic-corticosteroid combinations. The flies should be controlled as much as possible. Fly screens are beneficial.
2. *Onchocerca cervicalis* microfilaria concentrate in conjunctiva causing granulomatous nodules. These are near the limbus at the temporal canthus, are self-limiting, and when healed leave white scars (vitiligo) that are very noticeable if the conjunctiva is pigmented. These lesions can resemble early squamous cell carcinoma. Therefore, cytology is indicated. See equine conjunctival granuloma, page 270.
3. Habronema produce mild conjunctivitis and nodules near the nasal canthus and along the edges of the eyelids. The nodules may develop caseous necrosis. The palpebral puncta are often involved. Treatment is curettage or surgical excision.
4. *Thelazia sp* - usually asymptomatic or may cause mild conjunctivitis and dacryocystitis. The parasites inhabit the conjunctival sac, nasolacrimal canaliculi and lacrimal ducts.

Solar irritation

Horses with solar blepharitis due to nonpigmented eyelids will develop concurrent conjunctivitis. Fly screens are helpful and eyelid tattooing is recommended.

CONJUNCTIVITIS IN CATTLE

Conjunctivitis in cattle can result from the basic causes previously mentioned but herd outbreaks are frequently associated with infectious bovine keratoconjunctivitis (IBK) or systemic diseases (infectious bovine rhinotracheitis [IBR]; malignant catarrhal fever [MCF]).

Bacteria in normal cattle at slaughter in U.S.

Barber identified bacteria of normal cattle presented for slaughter. Vet Rec 1985;117:234-239.

No growth - 10%
Bacillus sp - 77%
Staphylococcus epidermidis - 69%
Streptococcus faecalis - 45%
Branhamella catarrhalis - 33%
Moraxella bovis - 5%
Corynebacterium bovis - 4%
Escherichia coli, Staphylococcus aureus, and fungi - < 1%

Many bacteria have been isolated from cattle with keratoconjunctivitis with or without the presence of *Moraxella bovis*. Some of these are *Neisseria sp, Achromobacter, Hemophilus, Micrococcus, Pasteurella sp.*

Mycoplasma sp

Several species have been identified that cause mild conjunctivitis with epiphora and hyperemia. Cross infection with *M. bovis* will result in severe lesions. Topical and systemic tetracyclines will shorten the infection.

INFECTIOUS BOVINE KERATOCONJUNCTIVITIS (IBK, PINK-EYE) - Is the most important ocular disease in cattle with an annual financial loss of $150-300 million.

Etiology - A combination of bacterial and environmental factors

1. *Moraxella bovis* is the primary cause
   a. Virulent (piliated) form - is hemolytic and produces dermonecrolysins which combine with enzymes released by inflammatory cells to produce progressive necrosis of the epithelium and then the stroma. This form is usually the cause for summer outbreaks.
   b. Avirulent (nonpiliated) form - is nonhemolytic. This form can be stimulated to the virulent form and is usually identified in winter outbreaks.
2. Mixed infections can occur resulting in more severe signs.

Predisposing factors

1. Ultraviolet light (high altitude)
2. Systemic infections can reduce resistance (e.g. IBR and *Mycoplasma sp*). IBR vaccine administered during an outbreak of IBK will increase the rate and intensity of IBK.
3. Nonpigmented adnexa
4. Environmental - dust, wind, overcrowding, poor nutrition and stress from shipping
5. Large numbers of face flies

Occurrence - All breeds and ages

1. Higher in animals less than four years of age
2. Seen in pasture and dry lot
3. Seasonal - late spring and early summer. Can occur the year around. A regional Holstein herd had a serious problem in its calves continuously for 16 months, until husbandry for the calves was changed.

Transmission - A large number of organisms are shed in ocular and nasal discharges

1. Direct
2. Indirect - flies, aerosol, pasture or feed bunks
3. Carrier animals may be the source for infection when new animals are introduced

Signs - Variable. Some animals with mild changes recover spontaneously without permanent damage. The signs described below indicate all possibilities that occur. Do not expect to see an individual animal go through all stages. The lesions may differ between the eyes of a patient.

1. Conjunctivitis - starts with signs of conjunctivitis (epiphora, hyperemia, photophobia). If treated at this stage, many recover without developing keratitis.
2. Keratitis - develops after two to three days
   a. Corneal edema causing mild leukoma
   b. In one to two days, small foci of dense leukoma develop. These may enlarge until they coalesce forming a central area of dense stromal opacity.
   c. The cornea thickens (2 to 3 times normal thickness) and undergoes stromal necrosis. May develop an appearance of keratoglobus at that time.
   d. Corneal vascularization begins three to six days after interstitial keratitis develops. This is deep vascularization beginning at the limbus and moving centrally in a ring at a maximum of about 1 mm per day.
   e. Ulceration may occur early in the disease (3 to 5 days)
      1) Superficial ulcers result from epithelial necrosis and if limited to the superficial cornea, the eye will usually heal within two weeks of onset
      2) Stromal ulcers occur frequently, resulting in corneal necrosis. This necrotic material may remain on the cornea while granulation tissue is repairing the deep stroma. The necrotic material then sloughs away, exposing nearly healed cornea. In other cases, the necrotic stroma may slough early, leaving a deep ulcer that will fill with granulation tissue or rupture. Granulation tissue is dependent on corneal vascularity and is an essential part of the healing process.
      3) Corneal perforation - may be small with spontaneous healing from granulation tissue or result in massive iris prolapse. After prolapse the iris may seal the corneal wound and the cornea will eventually heal with some vision. Unfortunately, the common sequelae to massive prolapse are:
         a) Panophthalmitis
         b) Phthisis bulbi
         c) Obstruction of the filtration angle leading to glaucoma
   f. Corneal abscesses may develop without epithelial erosion. When this occurs, granulation tissue migrating into the cornea from the limbus will slowly heal the cornea. Extensive scarring is anticipated.
3. Iris changes - anterior uveitis occurs concurrently with keratitis and will be present throughout the disease. The pupil is miotic. The iris is rough, thickened and appears dull in color.

Course - One to six weeks

Morbidity - Varies, may go as high as 60 to 100%

Differential diagnosis

1. Trauma and foreign body conjunctivitis
2. Malignant catarrhal fever
3. Conjunctival form of IBR

Treatment - Frequency of medication is limited by the owner's ability to work with the affected animals. Often single or infrequent treatment is all that is available.

1. Control infection - *M. bovis* responds well to many antibiotics and sulfonamides. The earlier in the disease the treatment is started, the better the results.
    a. Systemic - helps eliminate carriers
        1) Two or three IM injections of long acting oxytetracycline (LA-200), 20 mg/kg, 72 hours apart
        2) Oral or IV sulfadimethazine, 55 mg/kg for one to three days
    b. Topical - TID treatment is desired but often not possible
        1) Fusidic acid (currently not available in US) has prolonged ocular contact time and is very effective
        2) Betadine solution diluted 1:25 to 1:50 in saline can be applied with an atomizer of fine spray
    c. Subconjunctival - gives high tear concentration for 8 to 24 hours
2. Control uveitis - subconjunctival atropine (1 to 2 mg)
3. Control inflammation - the bovine cornea has the greatest regenerative ability of our domestic animals. Because of this, subconjunctival corticosteroids are given to reduce the redness of the eye. If ulcers exist, the corticosteroid will enhance collagenase activity and reduce vascularization, thereby interfering with healing. This cannot be recommended.
4. Ulcer treatment
    a. Ulcer solution prepared with gentamicin is effective (see Table 10-1; Chapter 10, page 320)
    b. Topical or subconjunctival serum
    c. Create a conjunctival wound that provides a continuous source of serum to the tear film for several days.
5. Protect the eye and/or remove from sunlight. If severe corneal damage is present, this is the most important part of treatment.
    a. Suture eyelids together (Fig 4-10 and 4-11; Chapter 4, pages 149 and 150)
    b. Self-adhesive eye patches
    c. Paint eyelids with Tri-dye

Prevention

1. Isolate affected animals
2. Control flies - insecticides and manure removal
3. *M. bovis* bacterins are available. Use three to six weeks before fly season. This will not eliminate the disease but will reduce severity.
4. Provide shade
5. Treat all animals on the premises with single injection of long acting tetracycline

SYSTEMIC DISEASES WITH SECONDARY CONJUNCTIVITIS

Malignant catarrhal fever (MCF)

1. Acute form - develops ocular lesions within the first 24 hours. The eyes are painful and visual impairment is common.
    a. Conjunctivitis and scleritis - chemosis, serous discharge soon becoming mucopurulent
    b. Cornea - begins with limbal edema and cellular infiltration leading to opaque cornea
    c. Anterior chamber - fibrin, hypopyon
    d. Anterior uvea - panuveitis
    e. Retina - vasculitis
2. Chronic form - has variable signs
    a. Mild ocular inflammation
    b. Low grade keratoconjunctivitis
3. Treatment - symptomatic

Infectious bovine rhinotracheitis (IBR)

Herpesvirus infection with multiple syndromes, one of which is conjunctival; others are respiratory, infectious pustular vulvovaginitis (IPV), encephalitis, neonatal viremia and abortion.

1. Signs of ocular form - patients seldom show any discomfort. May be bilateral or unilateral.
   a. Ocular discharge - serous becoming mucopurulent
   b. Conjunctiva - chemosis. Small white plaques that may coalesce, necrose, progressing to conjunctival ulceration
   c. Cornea - usually clear but may develop limbal edema and vascularization. This differs from IBK which starts with central corneal lesions.
2. Diagnosis
   a. Clinical signs and systemic changes are suggestive
   b. Cytology for fluorescent antibody testing is recommended
   c. Serology and virus isolation
3. Treatment - usually not recommended. Permanent damage is unlikely.
   a. Mild cases resolve in 2 weeks
   b. Severe may take one month

CONJUNCTIVITIS IN SHEEP AND GOATS

The most common causes of infectious conjunctivitis in sheep and goats are *Moraxella ovis, Chlamydia psittaci* and *Mycoplasma conjunctivae.*

Bacterial

1. *Moraxella ovis* is the most frequently isolated bacteria in sheep and goats with conjunctivitis. Mixed infections are common.
2. Other bacteria isolated include *Streptococcus spp, Staphylococcus spp, E. coli, Psuedomonas spp, C. pyogenes* and *Bacillus spp.*
3. *Listeria monocytogenes* mixed with *M. ovis* - may cause keratoconjunctivitis with epiphora, hyperemia, chemosis, corneal opacity and photophobia, in addition to neurologic signs

   Treatment - topical antibiotics, especially tetracyclines, for the conjunctivitis.

Viral - infectious bovine rhinotracheitis (IBR) can cause keratoconjunctivitis in goats

Mycoplasma - infectious keratoconjunctivitis

1. Etiology
   a. Sheep and goats
      1) *Mycoplasma conjunctivae* is most commonly isolated. The signs are usually transient and complications are rare.
      2) *Acholeplasma oculusi* may cause mild conjunctivitis with an 8 to 12 day incubation period and a course of 7-10 days.
   b. Goats - additional spp have been reported - *M. agalactiae, M. arghinini, M. mycoides*
2. Signs - young animals are more susceptible and have more severe signs
   a. Sheep - signs vary from lacrimation, blepharospasm, photophobia and mild conjunctivitis, to severe keratoconjunctivitis with purulent discharge. Lambs can develop corneal vascularization with ulceration.
   b. Goats - usually unilateral except in young kids. Signs begin with lacrimation, corneal vascularization and anterior uveitis. Ulcers do not develop. Whitley and Albert reported a young goat that had polyarthritis.
3. Diagnosis - Conjunctival scraping will reveal organism early and later in the disease

4. Treatment
    a. Topical tetracyclines or erythromycin
    b. Systemic long acting oxytetracycline (10-20 mg/kg)

Rickettsia - *Rickettsia conjunctivae (Colesiota conjunctivae)* can be a complication in sheep with kerato-conjunctivitis caused by *M. conjunctivae.*

Chlamydial keratoconjunctivitis

1. Etiology - *Chlamydia psittaci* is highly contagious in sheep and goats.
    a. Conjunctivitis and polyarthritis
    b. Abortion
2. Signs - affects all ages, most common in young animals, signs vary with the strain involved
    a. Bilateral keratoconjunctivitis with blepharospasm; development of lymph follicles; and corneal that include edema, vascularization and ulcers
    b. Anterior uveitis in severe cases
    c. Polyarthritis
3. Diagnosis
    a. Cytology - cytoplasmic inclusion bodies and/or IFA
    b. Serum antibody titer
    c. Culture
4. Treatment - usually self-limiting in 2-3 weeks. Tetracyclines, systemic and oral, depending on signs.

CONJUNCTIVAL HYPERPLASIA CAUSED BY SOLAR IRRITATION

The bulbar conjunctiva in the temporal canthus may thicken and become roughened. Histologically described as solar elastosis. It may reach a stage where it becomes static. In dogs this condition is not of clinical concern. In cattle and horses, these changes should be observed closely to make sure it is not the beginning of squamous cell carcinoma.

CONJUNCTIVAL GRANULOMAS

Dogs - Inflammatory conjunctival granulomas are occasionally seen near the temporal limbus.

1. Etiology - probably post-traumatic or chronic irritation
2. Signs
    a. Single or multiple
    b. Color and appearance
        1) Bright red, smooth, and growing rapidly
        2) Slightly pink to yellow cast and growing slowly
    c. Usually unilateral
3. Differential diagnosis - excisional biopsy may be needed, or response to treatment may be tried
    a. Collie granuloma (nodular granulomatous episclerokeratitis)
    b. Nodular episcleritis
    c. Neoplasia
4. Clinical management
    a. If growing slowly - treat with topical corticosteroid ointment or drops
    b. If growing rapidly - excisional biopsy and treat area with topical antibiotic until pathology report is available. Then, treat accordingly.
5. Post-traumatic granulomas will regress without treatment

Horses - conjunctival granulomas are usually near the lateral limbus and bilateral

1. Etiology - migrating *Onchocerca* larvae, injury or chronic irritation
2. Signs
    a. If from *Onchocerca*, they may initially appear as an elevated smooth red mass, which will contract, flatten and possibly have some roughened areas. If the conjunctiva was pigmented, it will depigment, leaving a white area (vitiligo). As the lesion contracts, fibrous bands will extend in a radial pattern from the limbus. This differentiates it from early squamous cell carcinoma, which will not have the radiating fibrous bands.
    b. If from injury or chronic irritation, granulation will regress quickly when the cause is removed.

CONJUNCTIVAL TUMORS

Conjunctival tumors are most common in the bovine with the horse second. Dogs are next in frequency of occurrence and cats are rarely involved. Impression smears and exfoliative cytology are beneficial in large animals when squamous cell carcinoma is suspected. Tissues removed should always be submitted for histopathologic examination so a definite diagnosis can be made and a proper prognosis rendered.

Dogs

1. Hemangioma - Benign conjunctival hemangiomas are the most common tumor observed in the dog. They may be single or multiple. When grasped with a forceps, the tumor and associated conjunctiva are easily mobile without scleral attachment. They generally do not bother the patient. If injured, they bleed excessively.
   Surgical removal is simple. The tumor is grasped with a forceps and the tumor and adjacent conjunctiva are cut off with scissors. Heat cautery is excellent for controlling hemorrhage. The conjunctival wound is not sutured. The owner should be advised to watch for recurring tumors in either eye.
2. Viral warts - The virus of infectious papillomatosis occasionally involves the eyelid, conjunctiva and/or cornea. Conjunctival lesions grow rapidly, are gray, have a cauliflower appearance. When manipulated, they are very fragile. They may be single or multiple, unilateral or bilateral. A secondary conjunctivitis is usually seen. Oral examination for warts may be negative or show only moderate involvement. Some dogs may never develop oral lesions.
   Surgical removal is the preferred treatment. The tumor and adjacent conjunctiva can be removed with scissors or a knife. The wound will heal without suturing. I have had one patient where a conjunctival wart recurred three weeks after removal of a single conjunctival wart. The second wart was surgically removed and there was no further recurrence. That dog never developed any oral papillomas.
   Cryosurgery and CO_2 laser surgery are less effective. Beware that virus particles may be present in the laser smoke plume.
3. Histiocytoma - Ocular histiocytomas are rapidly growing tumors and may involve the eyelids, conjunctiva and/or cornea. The lesions are usually multiple and affect all adnexal tissues. Lesions may occur on the lips as well. This is not to be confused with inflammatory granulomas, which are slow growing and are not neoplastic. Treatment - see eyelids (Chapter 5, page 181).

Other tumors - Less frequently seen are fibrosarcoma, squamous cell carcinoma, melanoma and malignant melanoma. Malignant tumors of the globe and orbit may extend into the conjunctiva.

Cats - Primary conjunctival tumors are rare. Squamous cell carcinoma near the limbus may involve the cornea and conjunctiva. Early lesions are easily confused with conjunctivitis and secondary keratitis. Exfoliative cytology is the best method of establishing a diagnosis. The eyelids may also be involved. They should be removed surgically and the site treated with radiation (beta), cautery (chemical, electrocautery), and cryosurgery.

Horses

1. Squamous cell carcinoma - most common tumor. Lesions usually start near the limbus with the cornea more extensively involved than the conjunctiva. Occasionally the lesion will be entirely conjunctival or corneal. Early lesions have signs similar to a mild conjunctivitis and/or keratitis. Several months may pass before the appearance of the lesion is diagnostic, therefore, smears or scrapings may be needed to establish an early diagnosis.
   a. Conjunctival lesions - The lesion is removed in the same manner as a conjunctival dermoid (Fig 8-1, page 250). The conjunctiva and the exposed sclera are treated with a strontium ^{90} beta applicator (7500-9500 rads) before suturing the conjunctiva to the limbal sclera (Fig 8-4). If the conjunctival defect is large, closing the conjunctiva is facilitated using a “T” closure (Fig 8-2, page 251). Closing the conjunctival wound will reduce postsurgical healing time to two to three days. This should be followed with topical antibiotics until healing is complete. Lesions involving the cornea will require a superficial keratectomy and resection of the affected conjunctiva as recommended for

dermoids in the same location (Fig 8-3, page 251) followed by beta radiation of the surgical site before suturing the conjunctival wound.

b. Other tumors are uncommon.
   1) Melanocytoma - epibulbar or involving the caruncle. Surgery is adequate if deeper tissues are not involved. Then cryosurgery of the site is recommended.
   2) Small hemangioma/sarcoma limited to bulbar conjunctiva can be successfully treated with surgical removal and beta radiation.
   3) Diffuse hemangiosarcoma/angiosarcoma is slow growing, invades into surrounding tissues and metastasizes to regional lymph nodes. Therefore even with early surgical treatment (including orbital exenteration) the prognosis is guarded. One horse with retrobulbar involvement was successfully treated at CSU with vincristine sulfate therapy and another did not respond.
   4) Mastocytoma near the limbus - surgical removal and beta radiation has been effective

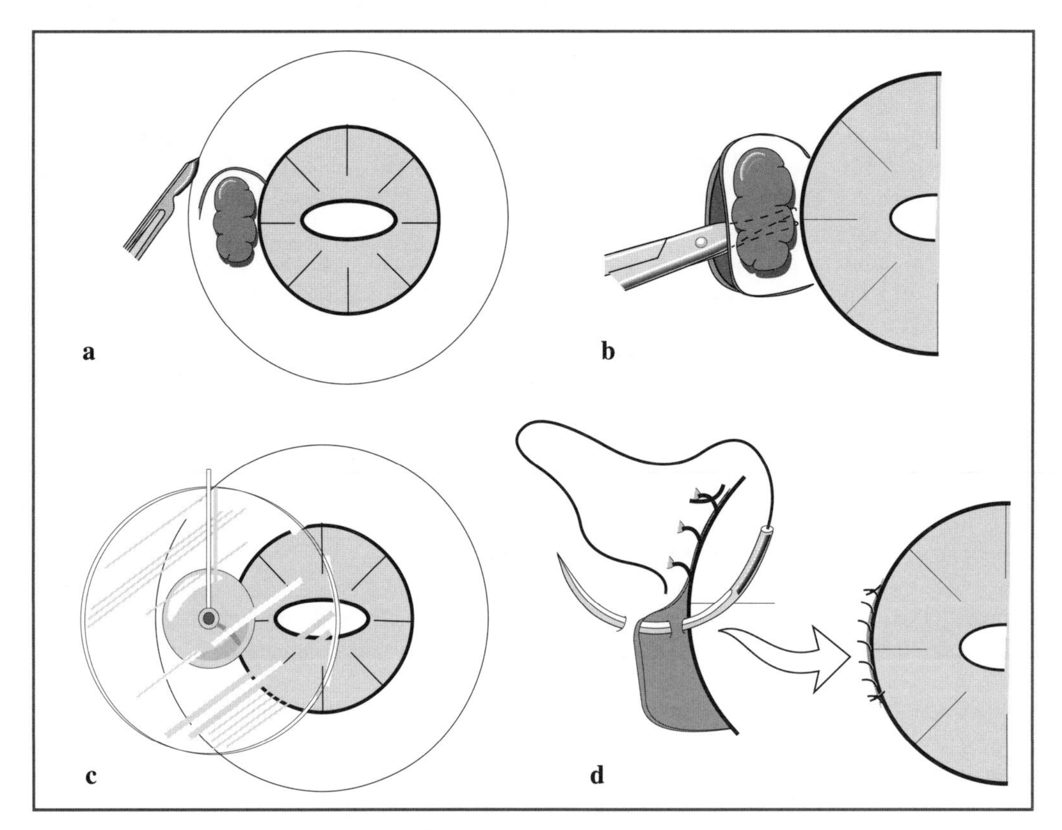

Figure 8-4. Removal of conjunctival-limbal tumor.
a. Incising conjunctiva 3 mm from margin of tumor
b. Tumor undermined and removed from limbus with blunt scissors
c. Surgical site irradiated with a strontium 90 beta applicator before conjunctival wound sutured
d. Conjunctival wound sutured after radiation

Cattle

1. Terminology
   Ocular squamous cell tumors (OSCT) - collective term for benign and malignant tumor
   Ocular squamous cell carcinoma (OSCC) - implies a malignant lesion
2. Etiology - multifactorial
   a. Genetic predisposition
   b. Sunlight (amount and intensity very important)
   c. Viral has been proposed

3. Pathogenesis - tumors develop from the epithelial surfaces of the conjunctiva, cornea and eyelid margins
    a. Predisposing factors - genetic background and age
    b. Globe and third eyelid - hyperplastic plaques progressing to papilloma, then squamous cell carcinoma, or, carcinoma may arise *de novo*
    c. Eyelid margins - keratoma or keratoacanthoma progressing to papilloma, then to squamous cell carcinoma; or carcinoma may arise *de novo*
4. Frequency of occurrence
    a. Predominantly Herefords. Also breeds with similar patterns of perivascular pigmentation (Simmental and Holstein-Friesians)
        1) Seldom seen less than four years of age
        2) Peak age of occurrence - 8 years of age
    b. Sites for malignancy in decreasing order of prevalence
        1) Lateral and medial limbus
        2) Eyelid margins (especially lower)
        3) Third eyelid and caruncle
        4) Nasal canthus
5. Signs - vary with location of lesion
    a. Limbus - grow slowly. Usually starting as whitish hyperplastic plaque progressing to red-colored mass that may become rough and develop necrosis.
    b. Eyelid lesions begin as papillomas or appear as hyperemic areas with mild erosion. As they grow they can be firm, bleed easily when manipulated. They develop a foul odor from necrosis. Extensive lesions may destroy the eyelid and infiltrate the orbit.
6. Course
    a. Lesions of the globe are slow to metastasize
    b. Adnexal lesions metastasize in 15 to 18% of the cases
        1) First to the parotid lymph node
        2) Then to the lateral retropharyngeal node via the tracheal lymphatic ducts to the venous circulation
    c. *In situ* carcinoma will eventually become invasive, encroaching on soft tissue, bone or orbit.
    d. Untreated animals may survive two to five years
    e. Precancerous lesions may undergo spontaneous regression in 30 to 50% of the cases
7. Morbidity
    a. In areas of abundant sunlight, some Hereford herds:
        - 40% of the animals may develop OSCT
        - 10% of the animals may develop OSCC
    b. Condemnation at slaughter
        1) 95% of neoplastic parts condemnations
        2) 54% of neoplastic carcass condemnations
        3) 13% of all bovine carcass condemnations
8. Differential diagnosis
    a. 20% of gross diagnosis of squamous cell tumors are in error
        1) Healed pink-eye
        2) Trauma
        3) Folliculitis of the third eyelid
        4) Fibrosarcoma
        5) Dermoid cysts
        6) Benign keratoacanthomas (wickers) are light brown hornlike crusts along the edge of the eyelid that become coated with lacrimal secretions.
    b. Cytologic diagnosis of smears of lesions (Papanicolaou's stain)
        1) Negative - normal cells
        2) Atypical - cells indicate benign tumor - plaque or papilloma
        3) Suspicious - cells strongly suggest carcinoma
        4) Positive - cells definitely compatible with squamous cell carcinoma

9. Treatment may be one or a combination of:
   a. Surgery - with or without adjunctive therapy
   b. Cryotherapy - excellent for small or superficial lesions; can be combined with surgery on large lesions
   c. Hyperthermia - more time consuming than cryotherapy. Excellent results for small lesions, debulking first is recommended for large lesions. About 90% of the early tumors will resolve with a single treatment.
   d. Immunotherapy - results are variable
      1) Mycobacterium cell wall fraction (Nomagen, Fort Dodge; Regressin-V, Vetrepharm)
      2) Allogenic OSCC extracts
   e. Chemotherapy
      1) Levamisole - has been observed to cause tumor regression and complete recovery
   f. Radiation therapy - expensive and requires special handling; unlike other means of treatment repeated treatment may result in damage to normal tissues
      1) Implants - cesium^{137}, cobalt^{60}, gold^{198}
      2) Surface - strontium^{90}, beta radiation source for surface treatment of thin lesions (1 mm thick) or after surgical removal of lesions on the globe
   g. *Comment*- for best results
      1) Initiate early treatment
      2) Re-examination and retreatment at first signs of recurrence
10. Prevention
   a. Selective breeding
   b. Cull affected animals

INJURIES

1. Lacerations
   a. Causes
      1) Small animals - fighting, cat claws, or bite wounds
      2) All animals - blows to the eye or penetration from foreign bodies or gunshot
   b. Signs
      1) Bloody tears
      2) Blepharospasm with protrusion of the third eyelid
   c. Examination findings and treatment - topical anesthesia or chemical restraint if needed to examine thoroughly
      1) Laceration over the globe - the lacerated conjunctiva will contract, exposing white glistening sclera. The adjacent conjunctiva will be hyperemic and the conjunctival edge swollen, making the wound easy to identify. These wounds heal quickly and need to be sutured only if extensive. Suture with 6-0 or 7-0 absorbable suture.
      2) Laceration near the fornix - penetrating foreign bodies or deep fight wounds are the most common cause. Postorbital fat may be protruding from the wound. X-ray the orbit if the cause is unknown. Clean the wound and remove any protruding fat before suturing the conjunctiva.
      3) Laceration of the palpebral conjunctiva - most of these wounds will heal without sutures
2. Subconjunctival hemorrhage
   a. Causes
      1) Common following trauma to the eye
      2) Less common causes: bleeding disorders, choking on a leash
   b. Source of blood
      1) Hemorrhage beneath the bulbar conjunctiva
      2) Blood migrating anteriorly from retrobulbar hemorrhage
   c. Significance and course - does not cause any harm; examine the eye with an ophthalmoscope to eliminate the possibility of intraocular damage. Will be unattractive until it absorbs in 10 days.
   d. Treatment - if still bleeding, topical epinephrine 1 to 2%. Hemorrhage has stopped by the time most cases are presented; this can be handled as follows:
      1) Will recover without treatment
      2) To hasten recovery, corticosteroids injected into postorbital fat (5 to 10 mg of triamcinolone) may reduce postorbital swelling and speed absorption

SUBCONJUNCTIVAL PROLAPSE OF RETROBULBAR FAT

In cattle, retrobulbar fat can occasionally dissect anteriorly between the conjunctiva and Tenon's capsule. This occurs less frequently in horses and rarely occurs in other species. The lesion is unsightly but does not affect sight.

Etiology - A defect in the orbital septum allows orbital fat to prolapse forward beneath the conjunctiva. May be congenital or acquired.

1. Congenital - Prenatal BVD calves with severe strabismus
2. Acquired
   a. Exaggerated eye movements during examination may result in transient prolapse effect
   b. Space-occupying retrobulbar mass
   c. Obesity in older animals (especially horses)
   d. Post-traumatic

Treatment - Examine thoroughly for signs of exophthalmos and/or retrobulbar mass

1. Not routinely treated because it does not harm vision
2. Excise prolapsed fat; suture conjunctiva to the globe

CHAPTER 9 - SCLERA

NORMAL ANATOMY AND PHYSIOLOGY

The sclera and cornea make up the fibrous tunic of the eye. This tunic is responsible for the size and shape of the eye. The sclera is less extensive in the horse (80% of the globe) than in the dog (85%). The thickest area surrounds the optic nerve. In all animals but the pig, it is thin at the equator and thicker at the limbus. In the pig the equator is slightly thicker than the limbus. The sclera can be divided into three zones: episclera, sclera proper, and inner zone.

The episcleral zone has Tenon's capsule as an outer limit and the sclera as its deep boundary. Tenon's capsule attaches anteriorly near the limbus and can be identified surgically. This zone contains most of the scleral nerves and small blood vessels. The episcleral veins enlarge and are readily visible in glaucoma and anterior uveitis. The deeper scleral veins that drain the anterior uvea can sometimes be seen in the sclera as dark lines. Occasionally, one of these deep vessels penetrates to the surface of the sclera and is readily visible. When this happens, it is an insignificant abnormality and the pet owner should be advised accordingly.

The sclera proper is dense white fibrous connective tissue with many elastic fibers. It has little pigment except in dark-coated pigs where it is richly pigmented. Thinning of the sclera will give it a bluish cast. This is seen near the limbus in chronic glaucoma with enlargement of the globe and near the equator in collie eye syndrome with severe scleral ectasia. The inner layer or lamina fusca is very elastic and may contain pigment. This pigment also contributes to the blue cast seen with scleral thinning.

The opening in the sclera for the optic nerve is called the lamina cribrosa. It is crossed by interlacing fibrous bands that allow the fibers of the optic nerve to penetrate the sclera without causing a weak spot.

The sclera and cornea are both rich in collagen fibers. The arrangement of these fibers is random in the sclera and lamellar in the cornea. This lamellar arrangement in the cornea is one reason why the cornea is clear and the sclera is opaque. There is a transitional zone between these tissues at the limbus. In all species but the horse, the sclera extends anteriorly to the base of the iris 2 to 4 mm, thus obscuring the filtration angle so it cannot be clearly visualized without a goniolens. In the horse, the limbus lies over the filtration angle nasally and temporally, allowing visualization easily through the cornea. Pigment from the inner zone of the sclera may be seen entering the cornea at the limbus.

CONGENITAL ABNORMALITIES

Congenital abnormality of the sclera is often associated with concurrent abnormality in adjacent tissues.

DERMOIDS

Dermoids that involve conjunctiva and cornea may involve Tenon's capsule.

SCLERAL COLOBOMA

A coloboma is a congenital cleft or fissure. In the sclera it is most frequently seen involving or near the optic disk but can occur anywhere in the sclera. The possibility of lesions is enhanced with color dilute genetics. Colobomas near the limbus are rare, but when seen will be dark colored as a result of staphyloma of the ciliary body, which will push back into the globe with minimal pressure. When present near the equator, they may be seen as they bulge the sclera. If present over the retina, they represent a blind spot, therefore size and location will determine the degree of blindness, if any.

Collie eye syndrome - (See Chapter 15, page 433) (collie, Shetland sheepdog, and border collie) - inherited autosomal recessive disease with colobomas typically involving or near the optic disk.

Multiple ocular anomaly in Australian shepherd - Colobomas tend to be near the equator of the globe. This is also autosomal recessive disease.

Charolais cattle - Seen near the posterior pole of the globe. Dominant inheritance.

Rabbits - Colobomas of the sclera occur commonly in microphthalmic rabbit eyes and less frequently in normal size eyes. The optic disk and peripapillary zone are most frequently affected. Recessive inheritance. Coloboma should not be confused with the deep physiologic cup seen in rabbits, especially New Zealand Whites.

SCLERAL ECTASIA (THIN SCLERA)

Occurrence

1. Albino and subalbinotic animals
2. Collie eye syndrome (see Chapter 15, page 433)
3. Australian shepherds with multiple ocular defects
4. Siamese cats
5. Color dilute horses, especially Appaloosas

Cause

1. It can be related to subalbinotic genetics
2. A recessive gene in collies and related breeds.
3. If both subalbinism and collie eye exist, as seen with merles, the changes can be extreme.

Significance

Scleral ectasia in itself does not cause any problems, but it is only one of many ocular changes that can occur in patients with multiple eye defects.

ACQUIRED DISEASE

Episcleritis is inflammation of the superficial sclera. Scleritis involves the deep layers of the sclera. Inflammation of scleral tissues may be restricted to the sclera or occur concurrently with other ocular tissues. In dogs, several syndromes occur that are similar. This has led to confusion in terminology. Whether they are the same disease with multiple manifestations or separate diseases is yet to be determined. These diseases have specific features and respond to different specific clinical treatments. Therefore they will be presented according to clinical appearance and response to treatment.

DIFFUSE EPISCLERITIS

Etiology - The specific etiology is generally unknown but it is a hypersensitivity reaction in the outer layers of the sclera that occurs in animals one year and older.

Occurrence - This is the most common form of scleral disease

Signs - It usually begins in the exposed episclera of the temporal canthus. Lesions have gradual onset, becoming progressively more severe. Severe and longstanding cases may become generalized, affecting all of the anterior episclera. Lesions may be unilateral or bilateral.

1. Episcleral blood vessels are engorged and the overlying conjunctiva is congested and red. Topical epinephrine or phenylephrine will differentiate between conjunctival and episcleral congestion.
2. The cornea adjacent to episcleral lesions develops leukoma and may show neovascularization at the limbus. In longstanding lesions, the entire cornea may develop leukoma and corneal vascularization can extend to central cornea.
3. Tonometer determinations of intraocular pressure reveal a soft eye
4. The iris is normal in color and pupil size
5. Aqueous centesis is normal
6. Ocular discharge - Episcleritis does not cause an ocular discharge. If there is a concurrent conjunctivitis, ocular discharge may be present.
7. No pain

Differential diagnosis - Diffuse episcleritis must be differentiated from other causes of the red eye.

1. Conjunctivitis. Conjunctivitis has a history of acute onset, ocular discharge (serous or purulent), congestion of superficial blood vessels (that are very responsive to topical epinephrine or neosynephrine), and physical discomfort with moderate to severe blepharospasm. Uncomplicated conjunctivitis does not have any corneal change and intraocular pressure is normal.
2. Anterior uveitis
    a. Differences. Anterior uveitis usually has a more rapid onset, increased ocular discharge (epiphora), blepharospasm secondary to intraocular pain, generalized perilimbal vascular flush, abnormal anterior chamber contents, and iris changes (swelling, dull color, sluggish miotic pupil).
    b. Similarities. Both will have superficial and episcleral vascular injection, corneal edema (peripheral edema with episcleritis and more generalized edema with anterior uveitis), corneal vascularization (episcleritis will have perilimbal vascularization while uveitis will begin with limbal vascularization and become generalized more rapidly). Both diseases have a soft eye.
3. Glaucoma
    a. Differences. Glaucoma can have sudden or chronic onset, ocular discharge (epiphora), blepharospasm secondary to intraocular pain, dilated pupil and increased intraocular pressure
    b. Similarities. Both may have superficial and episcleral vascular injection, corneal changes (corneal edema is generalized in acute glaucoma but in chronic glaucoma it may be limbal similar to episcleritis), limbal vascularization (generalized limbal vascularization with glaucoma; perilesional with episcleritis).

Treatment - Anti-inflammatory and immunosuppressives

1. Topical - May be adequate early in the disease or used with systemic treatment
   a. Topical 1% prednisolone acetate three or four times a day may be effective in early cases with minimal corneal changes. As the lesion improves, gradually reduce frequency of administration. In early cases, treatment can usually be discontinued after one to two months.
   b. Cyclosporine BID - The author has not found this to be very effective when used as the only treatment. Synergistic with topical corticosteroids.
2. Systemic -Indicated in longstanding and severe cases, or when topical treatment has not resulted in marked improvement in a week
   a. Oral prednisolone at anti-inflammatory levels (see page 94). After the lesion has disappeared, discontinue oral prednisone but continue with topical medication for as long as needed.
   b. Imuran (azathioprine) (see page 98) can be given in cases that are nonresponsive to corticosteroid therapy or in patients that are developing undesirable side effects due to systemic corticosteroids. Imuran is probably most effective when combined with topical and systemic prednisolone.
3. Subconjunctival injection. Subconjunctival injection of repository (depot) corticosteroids every one to four months can be used if lesions require long term treatment or oral corticosteroids are causing undesirable side effects.

Prognosis and course - Prognosis depends on the duration of the lesion and initial presenting signs

1. With treatment
   a. Early lesions without degenerative secondary changes
      1) The prognosis is favorable
      2) Course - Most appear normal in one month and do not require further treatment when medication is discontinued.
      3) Recurrence - In about 1/4 of the patients may recur and again respond well to treatment
   b. Persistent cases - This is uncommon and should be given a guarded prognosis because of possible degenerative complications that can lead to blindness
      1) Corneal lipid (cholesterol) deposits leading to interference with vision
      2) Limbal corneal ulceration
      3) Anterior uveitis
      4) Necrotizing scleritis with secondary glaucoma
   c. Longstanding cases - Longstanding cases of episcleritis with corneal degeneration and/or anterior uveitis should be given a guarded prognosis until response to treatment can be determined. There is a high probability of poor response to treatment and the development of persistent corneal lesions
2. Prognosis and course without treatment - The prognosis is guarded to unfavorable without treatment. Some mild cases may be self-limiting and resolve spontaneously. Other animals may be presented with a history that suggests the disease is recurring with more severe involvement with each recurrence. Persistent cases, when untreated, will eventually develop uveitis, scleritis and eventually obstructive glaucoma. If presented after these complications develop, it may require histologic examination of the eye to differentiate the eye with secondary glaucoma from intraocular neoplasia.

NODULAR (PROLIFERATIVE) SCLERITIS

Nodular episcleritis is characterized by firm swelling within the sclera with or without concurrent diffuse episcleritis.

Signs

1. Firm swelling in the sclera near the limbus. Initially the margin may be indistinct. As the lesion enlarges, it extends along the limbus resulting in a "bean-shaped" appearance. In some cases, a nodule may develop within two or three weeks. The nodules produce smooth elevation in the sclera. The conjunctiva remains smooth and can be easily moved over the nodule. The nodule is immobile and a definite structure within the superficial sclera.

2. Corneal changes. A vascular reaction and leukoma develop in adjacent cornea. Chronic cases may develop cholesterol deposits that have a potential of spontaneous recovery if the animal responds well to treatment.

Differential diagnosis of nodular scleritis

1. Collie granuloma (nodular granulomatous episclerokeratitis - NGE) with bulbar lesions
   a. Differences
      1) Animals with ocular collie granuloma have concurrent lesions on the third eyelid
      2) Location - Collie granuloma lesions may be corneal, scleral or involve both equally
      3) Vascularization - Conjunctival and episcleral blood vessels are normal
      4) Conjunctiva - The conjunctiva is involved and securely attached to the lesion
      5) Cornea - The cornea adjacent to the lesion will have a narrow band of edema but will not have neovascularization
      6) Intraocular pressure is normal
   b. Similarities
      1) Both lesions are immobile
      2) Filtration angle is normal
2. Ocular nodular fasciitis
   a. Differences
      1) Location - The lesion is located between the conjunctiva and the episclera. Thereby, forceps manipulations will reveal the conjunctiva is movable over the lesion and the fasciitis nodule is movable over the sclera.
      2) Cornea - Ocular nodular fasciitis does not have visible corneal involvement
      3) Vascular changes - There is minimal conjunctival and episcleral blood vessel injection
   b. Similarities - Both are smooth, elevated perilimbal masses on or in the sclera. The filtration angle is normal in both diseases.
3. Ciliary body tumors with scleral infiltration - Ciliary body tumors can erode through the sclera, resulting in a weakened sclera that will bulge over the area of scleral disease. If pressure is applied to the area, it can be easily depressed because of the loss of scleral rigidity. Obstructive secondary glaucoma is a common complication to intraocular tumors. This may be the result of tumor invading the filtration angle or producing iris bombé which in turn results in obstruction. Ultrasound will reveal anterior uveal changes with tumors.

Treatment

The treatment is the same as diffuse episcleritis and is more likely to require concurrent immunosuppressive therapy (azathioprine).

Prognosis and course

Guarded because more likely to develop complications than diffuse episcleritis.

NECROTIZING SCLERITIS

Necrotizing scleritis is a rare complication of diffuse and nodular scleritis that may result in sclerouveitis and secondary glaucoma.

Signs

1. It is characterized by thinning of the sclera resulting in dark patches as a result of being able to visualize the deeper uveal pigment
2. Severe corneal lipid degeneration
3. Limbal corneoscleral erosions (ulcers) may occur

4. Anterior uveitis
5. Obstructive glaucoma - Nearly always occurs.

Treatment - Usually unsuccessful

1. Systemic prednisolone and azathioprine
2. If corneoscleral erosion develops - Permanent peripheral conjunctival flap is indicated
3. Glaucoma - Enucleation

OCULAR NODULAR FASCIITIS

Ocular nodular fasciitis is a benign nodular lesion of connective tissue. It has been reported occurring in sclera, cornea, and/or third eyelid. The author has seen it as a scleral lesion.

Occurrence

1. Dogs - Uncommon. No specific age incidence; range in our cases - 1 to 13 years
2. Cats - Rare. One case at CSU.

History - May grow rapidly up to 6 x 10 mm in three weeks or grow slowly over several months

Signs

1. Location
   a. Usually located on the episclera near the limbus. May involve adjacent cornea.
   b. Less frequently near equator of the globe between sclera and extrinsic ocular muscles
   c. Third eyelid involvement has been reported, but not observed at CSU
2. Examination findings
   a. A firm pink mass that when grasped with forceps may be movable or moderately anchored to the sclera
   b. If near the limbus, the lesion may extend slightly into the superficial stroma of the cornea
   c. The conjunctiva will be freely movable over the nodule. This differentiates fasciitis from collie granuloma

Treatment

1. Does not respond to topical medication or intralesional injection with corticosteroids
2. Surgical removal - Excellent results
   a. Episcleral masses near the limbus are usually well encapsulated and easily dissected from the conjunctiva and sclera. The conjunctiva is incised and reflected from the nodule before scleral dissection. After removal of the nodule, the conjunctival wound is sutured with 6-0 to 8-0 absorbable suture.

      Nodules near the equator of the globe tend to infiltrate the sclera and are more difficult to remove. Do not worry about leaving part of the tissue because it does not tend to recur if not completely excised. If there is belief that the nodule is neoplastic rather than fasciitis, beta radiation of the surgical site with 9,000 rads may be performed before the conjunctiva is sutured.
   b. Corneal involvement. Superficial keratectomy of the lesion. Beta radiation to the surgical site will reduce postsurgical corneal vascularization without delaying healing.

Prognosis - Favorable, does not recur

NODULAR GRANULOMATOUS EPISCLEROKERATITIS (NGE - COLLIE GRANULOMA)

Collie granuloma is a fleshy appearing lesion that occurs at the temporal limbus and/or on the third eyelid of young to middle aged collies. Less frequently seen in Shetland sheepdogs, border collies and Australian sheepdogs, rarely other breeds.

Etiology - Not known

Histopathology indicates an immune-mediated inflammatory response. Some authors suggest these lesions may be a variation of either nodular fasciitis or episcleritis. I believe they are similar but distinctly separate diseases.

Signs

1. Ocular lesions
   a. Usually involve conjunctiva and superficial sclera, and extend into the superficial layers of the adjacent cornea
   b. When manipulated with a forceps, the conjunctiva cannot be moved separately and the lesion is fixed firmly to the sclera.
   c. Occasionally lesions may be entirely corneal. Advanced lesions may cover the entire cornea.
   d. Rates of development - May be rapid (3-5 mm in less than a month) or gradual (taking several months)
2. Third eyelid lesions - They are characterized by granulomatous thickening near the free margins of the third eyelid. In rare instances, only third eyelid lesions may be present. They are always present if bulbar lesions occur.
3. Some dogs may have concurrent lesions of the eyelids that are more suggestive of discoid lupus.

Treatment - Systemic treatment with Imuran is most effective

1. Local treatment
   a. Topical corticosteroids - Minimal value
   b. Subconjunctival and/or intralesional - Temporary response
   c. Surgical removal followed by topical corticosteroids successful in some cases, but most return
   d. Surgical removal and immediate beta radiation of the surgical site (7500 rads) followed by topical corticosteroids. Quite effective.
2. Systemic treatment
   a. Systemic corticosteroids - Little or no value
   b. Imuran (azathioprine) - .66 to 1 mg/lb daily until lesion regresses. Regression usually takes place in less than 10 days. Current treatment with topical 1% prednisolone is beneficial. Reduce oral medication gradually over several months to as little as 0.5 mg/lb every 7 to 10 days. After four to five months, attempt withdrawal of oral medication and continue topical prednisolone. Most dogs will require low level maintenance.

Precaution - Imuran has hepatotoxic qualities and a liver profile should be checked before starting treatment, then monitored periodically during treatment. Long term use may result in blood dyscrasias. Therefore, periodic CBC and platelet count monitoring is indicated.

SCLERAL TUMORS

Primary tumors of the sclera - Are uncommon except for epibulbar melanoma in dogs and cats

Extension through the sclera from other tissues - Is more common

1. Dogs - Anterior uveal tumors may erode through the sclera and give the appearance of a large scleral tumor. In some cases they weaken the sclera to a point where the tumor prolapses through the sclera (scleral staphyloma). Hemangiosarcomas and malignant melanomas are most likely to occur.
2. Cats - Rare
3. Horses - Extension of squamous cell carcinomas from the conjunctiva and cornea is most likely. Intraocular melanomas eroding the sclera can cause glaucoma and multiple scleral staphylomas
4. Cattle - Invasion of ocular squamous cell carcinoma

Epibulbar melanomas - Epibulbar melanomas have been observed in dogs and cats and are usually benign melanocytomas

1. Dogs
   a. Signs
      1) Scleral lesions - May be restricted to a small scleral nodule or a diffuse subconjunctival lesion with minimal elevation
      2) Limbal lesions - May be seen in young dogs, some less than one year of age, suggesting they were present at birth and were not noticed until later or have just started to grow. See corneal melanomas (Chapter 10, page 312). Others may extend equally into the cornea and sclera with minimal thickening of the tissues.
   b. Treatment
      1) If small and stationary, treatment may not be necessary. The owner should watch closely. Some may start to grow fairly rapidly after remaining stationary for years.
      2) If significant corneal involvement or start to grow
         a) Sectional superficial keratectomy (Fig 10-9; Chapter 10, page 296) and debulking of the scleral portion followed by cryotherapy has been very satisfactory for the author. Suturing the conjunctiva at the limbus is optional.
         b) Surgical resection of the entire affected cornea and sclera replaced with a corneoscleral graft has been successful
   c. Prognosis - The tumors are usually benign. The author had a case with rapidly growing corneal malignant melanoma that metastasized resulting in death of the patient.
2. Cats - Usually seen in cats over eight years of age and restricted to the sclera

TRAUMA

Episcleral hemorrhage - Can be differentiated from subconjunctival hemorrhage by close examination. In episcleral hemorrhage, conjunctival nerves can be seen superficial to the hemorrhage. In conjunctival hemorrhage, conjunctival nerves cannot be identified in the area of the hemorrhage.

Laceration

1. Equine - Severe blows to the eye may result in laceration of the sclera about 1 to 2 mm from the limbus. This is apparently a weak area only in the equine eye, because similar injury to other species does not cause this tear. The ciliary body, iris and/or lens may prolapse through this wound. The extent of internal hemorrhage and retinal detachment determines if the eye will be visual after repair. The lesion is repaired by replacing the prolapsed tissues and suturing the sclera with 6-0 absorbable suture. All the basic principles described for intraocular surgery involving corneal lacerations should be followed. Severe injuries may be followed by phthisis bulbi.
2. Small animals - Most scleral lacerations occur after fights with other animals or auto accidents. The extent of internal eye injury determines the prognosis. The wound is repaired and the eye allowed two to four weeks to recover before the outcome can be determined. An owner will usually prefer a blind eye to removal of the eye. Severe injuries may lead to phthisis bulbi. Signs of phthisis may begin in two weeks and be obvious by four weeks after injury.

SCLERAL STAPHYLOMA

Scleral staphyloma is prolapse of the uvea through the sclera. It is rare and occurs after trauma or erosion of the sclera by ciliary body tumors. Generally the lesion causing the staphyloma is so serious that the eye is blind and the presence of the staphyloma is not significant.

CHAPTER 10 - CORNEA

ANATOMY AND PHYSIOLOGY

ANATOMY

Gross

1. Size of the cornea (relative area of the globe) - roughly 20% in most domestic animals. Nocturnal animals have larger relative corneas than diurnal animals. Some strictly nocturnal animals have as much as 35% of the globe area represented by cornea.

Man	17%
Dog	17%
Horse	14%
Cat	30%

2. Thickness - In man, the cornea has basically uniform thickness but in domestic animals it is slightly thinner toward the center. These differences are not clinically significant.
   a. Dog - averages .62 mm (females thinner than males)
   b. Cat - about .56 mm
   c. Horse - about 0.6 mm at center and about 1 mm at periphery
   d. Bovine - about 0.8 mm
   e. Sheep - about 0.8 mm
   f. Pig - about 1 mm
   g. Fish, amphibians and birds (except nocturnal) - thin center and much thicker at periphery
3. Location of cornea to central axis of the globe. Cornea is central in herbivore. Located nasal to central axis in animals with binocular vision.
4. Shape and diameter
   a. Nearly circular
      1) Cat - nearly circular, horizotal diameter 17 mm, vertical 16 mm
      2) Dog - nearly circular, except it extends slightly outward at the dorsotemporal limbus, horizontal diameter 13-17 mm, vertical 23-27 mm
   b. Oval in grazing animals with oval pupils
      1) Horse - slightly pear-shaped with smaller end lateral, horizontal diameter 28-34 mm, vertical 23-27 mm
      2) Bovine - slightly pear-shaped with smaller end lateral
      3) Sheep - slightly pear-shaped with smaller end lateral
      4) Camelids - oval
      5) Pig - oval
5. Refraction - the cornea is the main refractive structure of the eye (70% of the total refraction of canine eye)
   a. Man - 48 D
   b. Dog - 43 D

Microscopic (Fig 10-1)

1. Layers of the canine cornea: anterior epithelium, stroma, Descemet's membrane, endothelium (posterior epithelium) (Fig 10-1a)
   a. Epithelium (Fig 10-1b) - Several cell layers thick (5 to 7 in cats, dogs, rabbits and birds; and up to 20 in large animals). It is continuous with the conjunctiva. There are stratified squamous cells at the surface with columnar cells at the basement membrane, which is securely attached to the stroma. Normal epithelium is constantly desquamating at the surface with a cell half-life of about 36 to 48 hours. It is completely replaced every six to eight days. The epithelium can be abraded quite easily, especially in horses. Drying of the cornea will result in transient epithelial damage and if prolonged, will cause ulceration. Eyes of anesthetized animals that have been preanesthetized with atropine or that will remain open during surgery should be protected with an ocular lubricant.

Pigment is normally restricted to the limbus in all species, with the exception of calves and sheep, in which case some pigment may occur throughout the epithelium. Epithelium does not contain any collagen. The basal epithelial cells are attached to the basement membrane by hemidesmosomes which in turn anchor the basement membrane and stroma together.

b. Stroma (substantia propria) - 90% of the cornea. Collagen fibers are formed by keratocytes (modified fibroblasts) and represent nearly all of the solid matter of the cornea. They are arranged in a laminated pattern allowing light to pass through without internal reflection, thereby giving the cornea transparency. Collagen fibril turnover is very slow (half-life about 180 days), taking nearly two years for normal replacement. This accounts for the slow rate of scar disappearance in corneal injuries. Flattened keratocytes are located in the interfibrillar spaces. The stromal fibers are so densely packed that the cornea is devoid of blood vessels except for small capillary loops at the limbus. The matrix surrounding the collagen fibers is composed of glycosaminoglycans. The most anterior stroma has a thin (1 to 2 microns) cell-free zone that corresponds to Bowman's (anterior limiting) membrane in primates. Distinct anterior limiting membranes occur in birds and to a lesser degree in the bovine (Fig 10-1c).

c. Descemet's membrane (posterior limiting membrane, elastic membrane) (Fig 10-1b). An elastic membrane composed of atypical collagen. It is an exaggerated basement membrane for the endothelium. If damaged, it will be dependent on the endothelium for regeneration. There are three layers at the limbus. The anterior fibers join the sclera, the middle attach to the ciliary muscle, and the posterior pass to the iris to form the pectinate ligaments of the iridocorneal angle.

d. Endothelium (posterior epithelium or mesenchymal epithelium) (Fig 10-1d). It lines the posterior surface of the cornea, is one cell layer thick, composed of polygonal-shaped cells, and regenerates

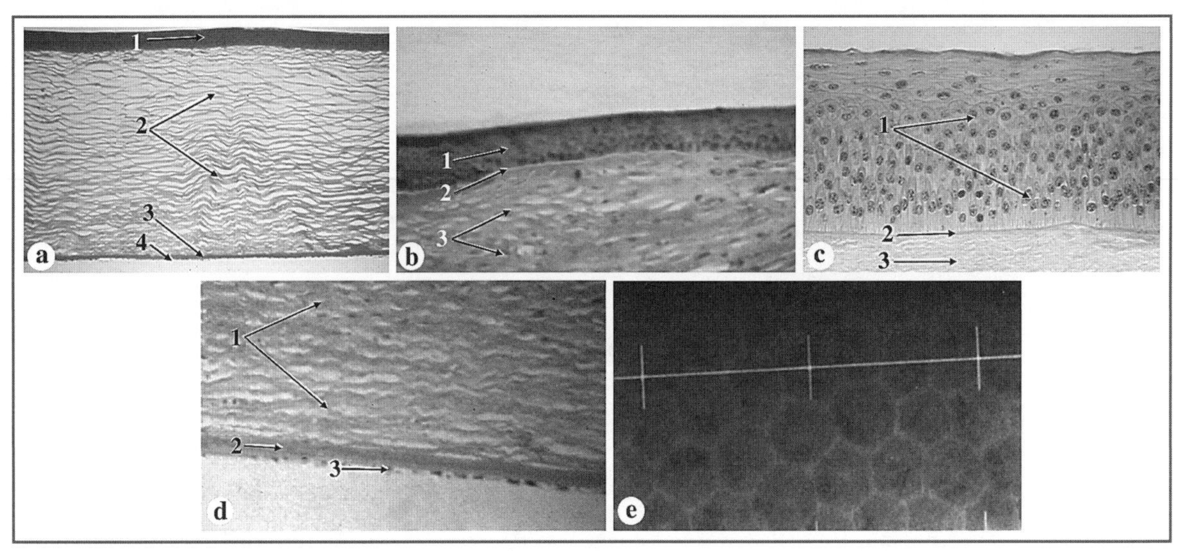

Figure 10-1. Microscopic anatomy of the cornea.

a. Cross-section of canine cornea
   1) Epithelium
   2) Stroma
   3) Descemet's membrane
   4) Endothelium

b. High power magnification of superficial canine cornea
   1) Epithelium
   2) Basement membrane
   3) Stroma

c. High power magnification of superficial bovine cornea
   1) Epithelium
   2) Bowman's membrane
   3) Stroma

d. High power magnification of deep canine cornea
   1) Stroma
   2) Descmet's membrane
   3) Endothelium

e. Specular microscopy of young adult canine corneal endothelium, demonstrating normal hexagonal arrangement of cells. Modified from Gelatt: Canine ophthalmology, Philadelphia, Lea & Febiger, 1991.

more slowly without mitosis than anterior epithelium. The endothelial cell count for dogs and cats is 2,700-2,800/mm^2 and decreases with age. When this count drops below a critical level, corneal edema results. The regenerative capability varies with species and age. Cats have minimal regeneration and young dogs good regeneration.

Endothelium is the most sensitive layer to mechanical irritation. Rubbing during intraocular surgery, anterior synechia, or adhering fibrin clots after anterior uveitis can cause permanent endothelial damage.

2. Nerve supply (sensory only) - trigeminal > ophthalmic branch > ciliary ganglion > cornea (Fig 10-2). The cornea is abundantly supplied with nonmyelinated nerve fibers entering at the limbus at two layers. The superficial layer is near the basement membrane of the epithelium and the sensory nerve endings penetrate into the epithelium, making it one of the most sensitive tissues of the body. The deep layer is above Descemet's membrane. Superficial fibers are sensitive to touch and deep fibers are sensitive to intraocular pressure. Corneal epithelial metabolism and mitotic rate are related to normal sensory innervation.

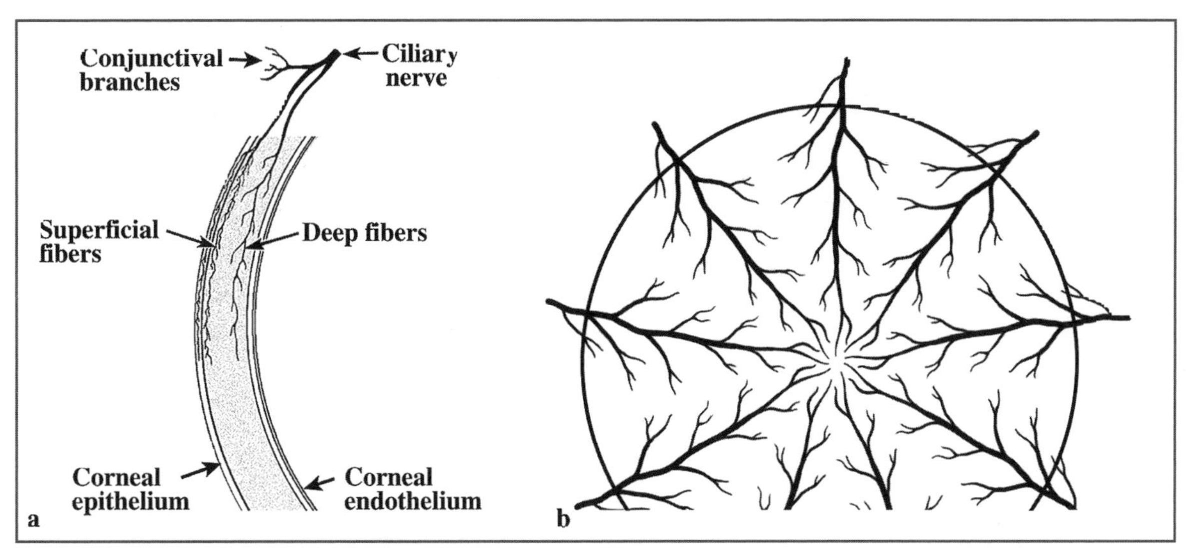

Figure 10-2. Diagram of sensory nerves entering the cornea Modified from Prince: Anatomy and histology of the eye and orbit in domestic animals. Springfield, Charles C. Thomas, 1960.
a. Nerves divide into superficial and deep fibers
b. Radial arrangement of entering nerves

PHYSIOLOGY

Metabolism

Many of the metabolic functions of the cornea are unknown. The normal cornea is 81% water, 18% collagen, 0.04% lipid. The epithelium and endothelium are high in lipid (4.3% dry weight) when compared to the stroma. The epithelium and endothelium have greater metabolic activity than the stroma and carry an aerobic metabolism. Stromal metabolism is anaerobic. The cornea can utilize oxygen from the tear film (dissolved from air), limbal capillaries, and aqueous. The tear film is the major source of O_2.

Permeability

The normal cornea acts as a semipermeable membrane with water freely moving through it. Drugs penetrate the cornea primarily by differential solubility (Fig 2-1; Chapter 2, page 63).

Transparency

1. The collagen fibers of the cornea have uniform diameter and a lamellar arrangement (Fig 10-3). They cross the cornea from limbus to limbus in an orderly fashion. Proteoglycans and other components of

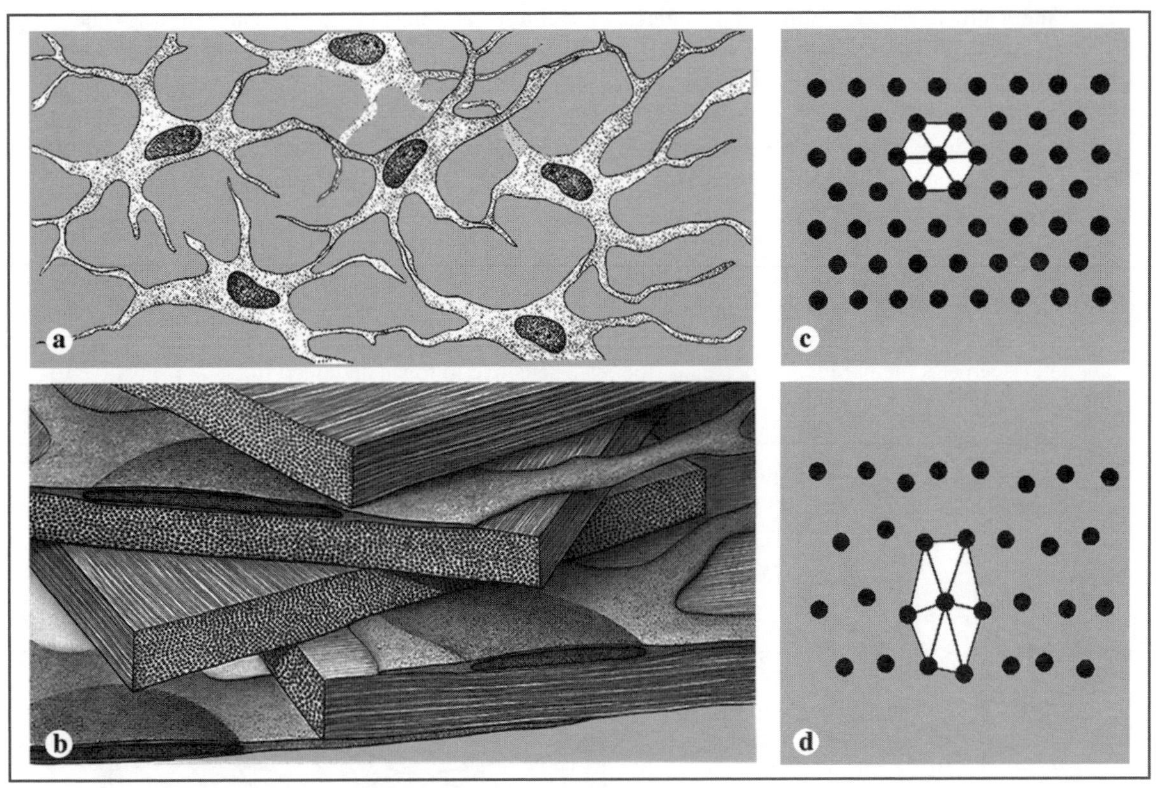

Figure 10-3. Arrangement of collagen fibers.

a. Fibroblasts. This diagram shows six fibroblasts lying between the stromal lamellae. The cells are thin and flat with long processes that contact fibroblast processes of other cells lying in the same plane. These cells were believed to form a true syncytium, but electron microscopy has disproved this idea. There is almost always a 200Å. wide intercellular space that separates the cells. Unlike fibroblasts elsewhere, these cells occasionally join each other at a macula occludens.

b. Lamellae. The cornea is composed of a very orderly, dense, fibrous connective tissue. Its collagen, which is a very stable protein having a half-life estimated at 100 days, forms many lamellae. The collagen fibrils within a lamella are parallel to each other and run the full length of the cornea. Successive lamellae run across the cornea at an angle to each other. Three fibroblasts are seen between the lamellae.

c. Diagram to show the theoretical orientation of the corneal collagen fibrils. Each of the fibrils is separated from its fellows by an equal distance. Maurice has explained the transparency of the cornea on the basis of this very exact equidistant separation. As a result of this arrangement, the stromal lamellae form a three-dimensional array of diffraction gratings. Scattered rays of light passing through such a system interact with each other in an organized way, resulting in the elimination of scattered light by destructive interference. The mucoproteins, glycoproteins and other components of the ground substance are responsible for maintaining the proper position of the fibrils.

d. Orientation of the collagen fibrils in an opaque cornea. The diagram shows disturbance of the orderly positions of the fibrils. Because of this disarrangement, scattered light is not eliminated by destructive interference and the cornea becomes hazy. Fluid in the ground substance also produces clouding of the cornea by disturbing the interfibrillar distance. From Hogan MJ, et al: Histology of the human eye, Philadelphia, WB Saunders, 1971.

the ground substance are responsible for maintaining the proper position of the fibrils. This arrangement of collagen fibers results in the cornea being transparent. The collagen fibers in the sclera have variable diameters and are arranged at random. This results in the white appearance of the sclera.

2. If the arrangement of corneal collagen fibers is changed, it appears cloudy or becomes white (e.g. thickening from edema, thinning from drying out, disruption by trauma, or replacement with scar tissue).
3. Transparency is dependent on the degree of hydration of the cornea and controlled by the epithelium and endothelium. The normal cornea contains much less water than it is capable of imbibing and any increase in water content will reduce its transparency. This state of containing less water than it is capable of imbibing is called deturgescence.
4. Deturgescence is dependent on:
   a. Barrier function of the intercellular junctions of the epithelium and endothelium

b. Na-K ATPase metabolic pump which carries water from the stroma to the aqueous

5. Loss of epithelium can result in a two-fold increase in corneal thickness; loss of endothelium can result in a five-fold increase in corneal thickness.

CORNEAL HEALING

Species differences in corneal reaction and healing

The horse shows the most severe reaction to irritation or injury; the bovine reacts the least. In a horse with severe corneal involvement, we expect to see severe edema, marked leukoma, slow healing and marked scar formation. In the bovine, the cornea is highly regenerative with minimal amount of scarring. The reactivity to irritation is:

1. Horse - most sensitive, slowest healing
2. Dog - develops considerable vascularity
3. Cat - severe ulcers may heal with minimal scarring
4. Bovine - least sensitive, fastest healing, also the thickest cornea of domestic animals, which may have some benefit
5. Sheep, goats, llamas - heal similar to cattle

Healing of epithelial wound (Fig 10-4) - Superficial wounds involving only the epithelium heal quickly. Mild edema occurs and healing is a two-stage procedure.

1. Cell migration - Epithelial cells begin to migrate into the defect within one hour regardless of the wound size. Basal cells touching the wound stretch out in a pseudopodial manner to cover as much as nine times the area of a normal cell. Then the next cell slides over it in a leap-frog fashion and so on. If the cornea is damaged near the limbus, conjunctival epithelium will migrate onto the cornea.
2. Cell mitosis - Mitosis in the basal layer of the epithelium is inhibited for several hours after injury and begins in 24 hours. Superficial wounds may be closed by cell migration before mitosis begins. The larger the wound, the longer the period of mitotic inhibition. Regeneration of the basement membrane is much slower and therefore new epithelium is loosely attached and very sensitive to new injuries.
3. It may take six to eight weeks before epithelium is firmly attached after a corneal ulcer or chronic epithelial erosion.

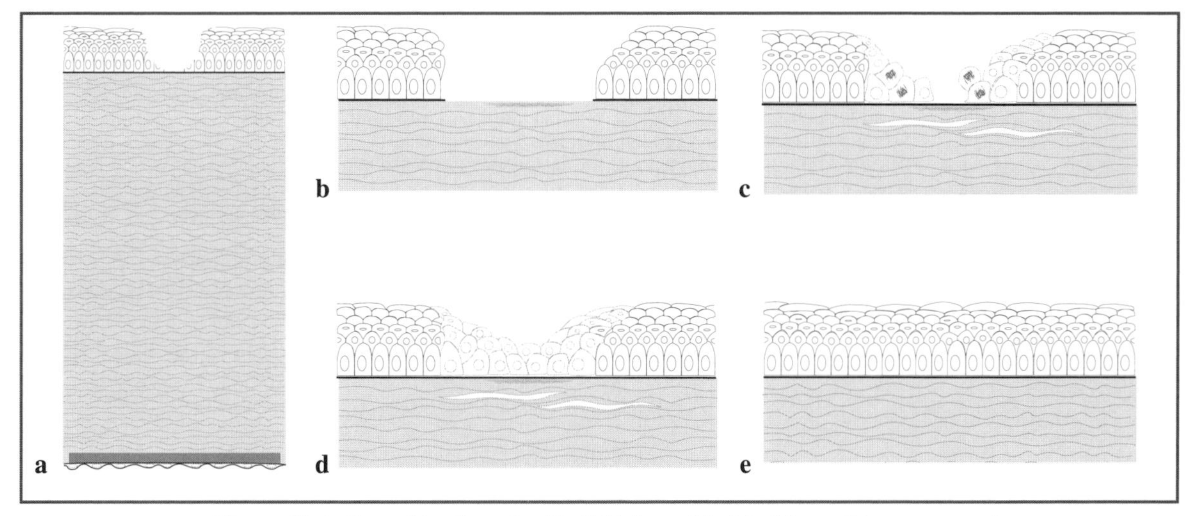

Figure 10-4. Corneal healing of epithelial injury. Modified from slides courtesy of Dr. Milton Wyman and The Ohio State University.

a. Schematic cross-section of cornea with epithelial injury
b. Enlarged area of epithelial injury
c. Migration of epithelial cells begins immediately after injury
d. Migration covers injury and ceases
e. Mitosis responsible for regeneration of epithelial thickness

Healing of superficial stromal injury (Fig 10-5)

1. The stroma becomes edematous (cloudy) and the cells become pyknotic or swell and burst. This provides an opening for neovascularization to invade the lesion if healing is delayed.
2. In 24 hours leukocytes from the tear film and limbal vascular arcade involve the base of the lesion as a result of a polypeptide chemotactic response.
3. If infection occurs, there will be an accumulation of mucopurulent discharge and exudate within the ulcer and its margins.
4. If infection did not occur or is controlled by the animal's own defenses or clinical antibiotics, intrinsic corneal hydrolases (e.g. collagenase) will establish a demarcation between normal and necrotic tissues. The necrotic tissue sloughs and epithelium fills the crater.
5. Fibroblasts arise from stromal keratocytes and histiocytes to fill the crater of the defect as the epithelium thins to its original thickness.
6. Vascularization begins at the limbus in three to six days and progresses toward the injury at a rate of about 1 mm per day. If the injury epithelializes before the blood vessels reach it, they may regress without developing granulation tissue that will fill the defect, leaving a permanent indentation. An ulcer that persists more than 7 to 10 days will usually have a halo of blood vessels surrounding it.

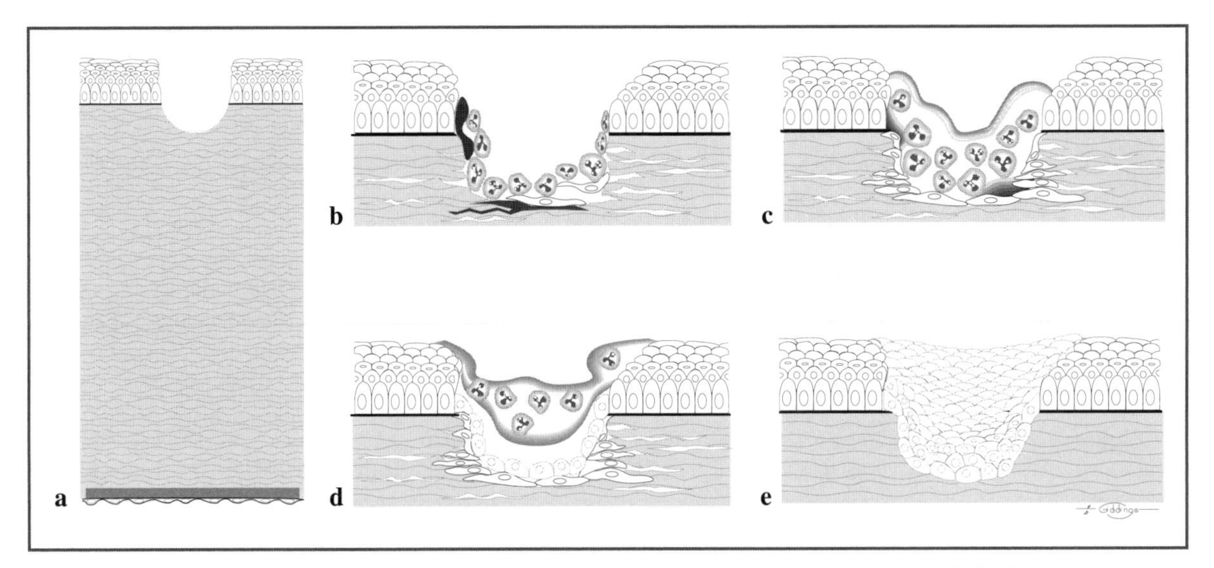

Figure 10-5. Healing of superficial corneal stromal injury or ulcer with controlled infection. Modified from slides courtesy of Dr. Milton Wyman and The Ohio State University.

a. Schematic cross-section of superficial stromal injury
b. Within 24 hours, leukocytes line the lesion and fibrocyte activation occurs
c. Fibrocytes line the lesion
d. Corneal hydrolases establish demarcation between normal and necrotic tissues, which slough from the lesion and epithelial cells line the defect
e. Epithelium fills the lesion and will thin as fibroplasia re-establishes normal stromal thickness

Healing of deep stromal injury (Fig 10-6)

Epithelial migration and fibroblastic stimulation is the same as with superficial stromal injury but will be inadequate to heal the injury. In this case, vascularization and the accompanying fibroplasia (granulation tissue) fill the defect. After healing is complete vascularization regresses spontaneously. In places where the stromal lamella are disorganized, the invading fibroblasts and regenerating keratocytes are not laid down in parallel rows and scarring results. The more rapidly an ulcer heals, the less the scar.

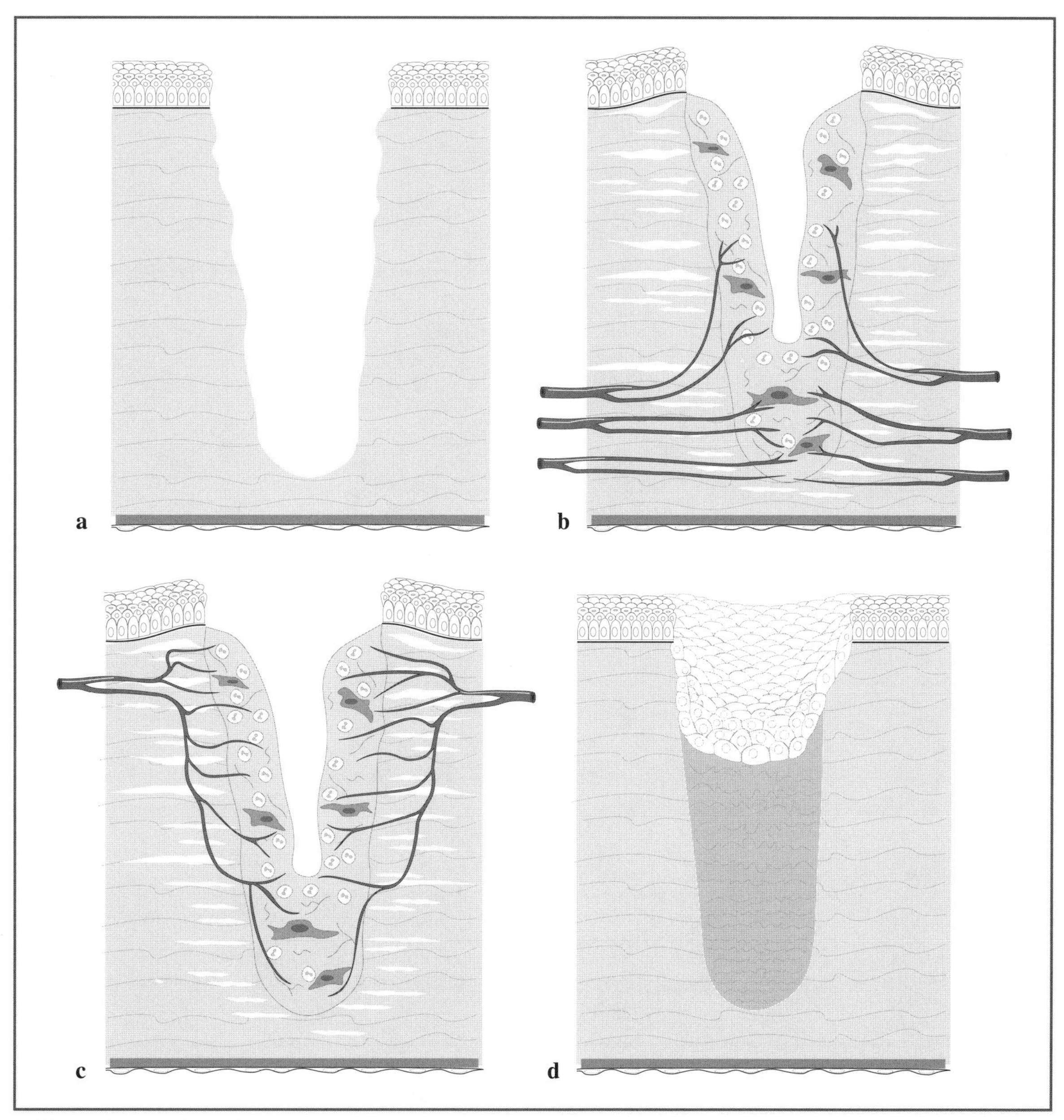

Figure 10-6. Healing of the deep corneal stromal injury or ulcer with controlled infection and collagenase activity. Modified from slides courtesy of Dr. Milton Wyman and The Ohio State University.

a. Schematic cross-section of deep stromal ulcer
b. Ulcer near the limbus - Deep vascularization and fibrostimulation leading to granulation begin to fill the wound
c. Central ulcer - Superficial vascularization migrates to the lesion to provoke the granulation tissue to fill the wound
d. After healing is complete, vascularization regresses, the invading fibroblasts and regenerating keratocytes are not laid down in parallel rows, and scarring results

Sequelae to excess collagenase activity (Fig 10-7)

If the rate of collagen destruction exceeds formation, the ulcer will enlarge and possibly perforate. There are several lysosomal hydrolases involved (glycosidases, collagenases, 5-nucleotidases, and oxidases), of which collagenase is the most prominent proteinase. These all have the ability to digest the proteinaceous matrix of the cornea and result in a "melting" ulcer.

1. Descemetocele
2. Perforation

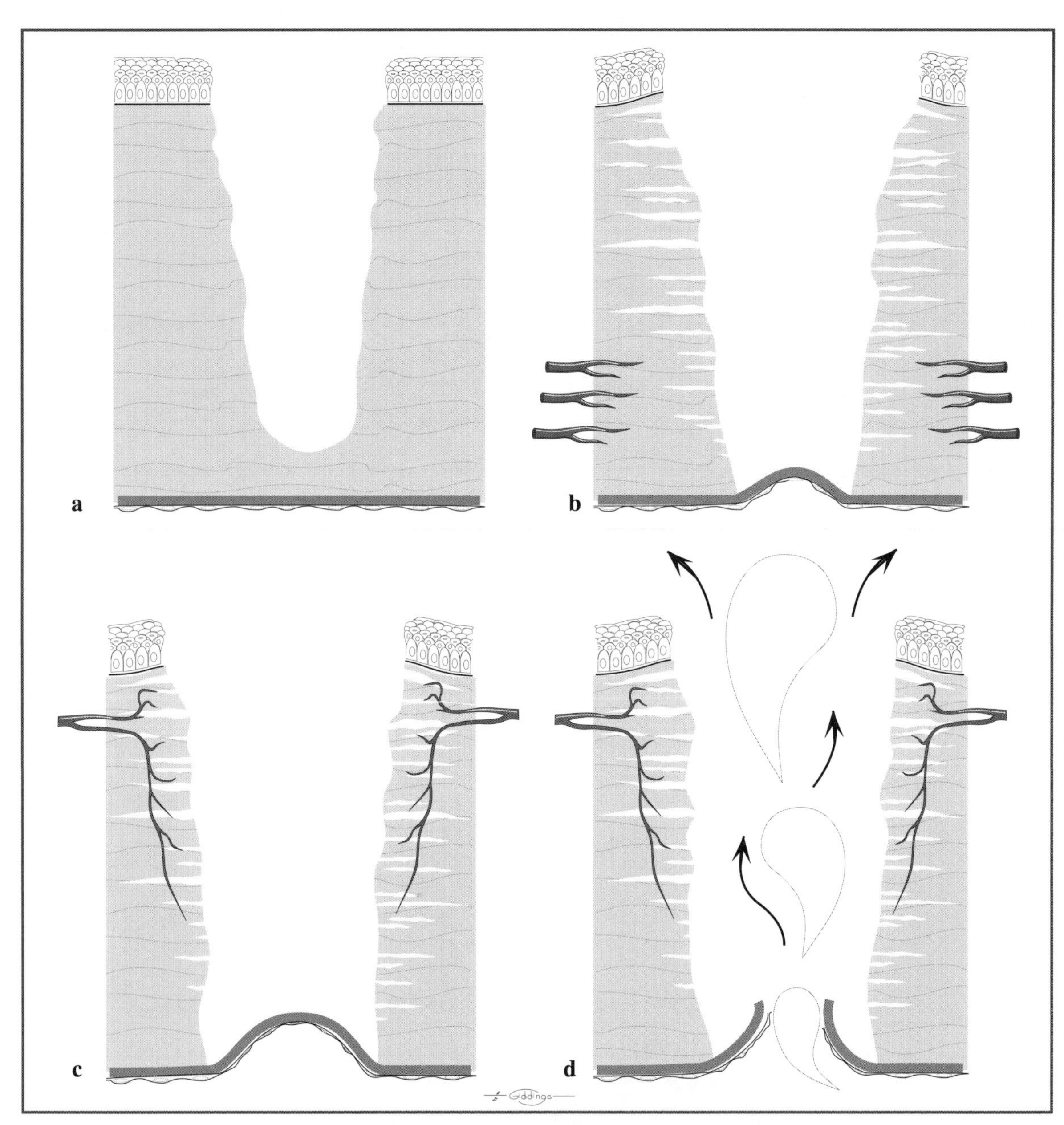

Figure 10-7. Sequelae to excess collagenase activity, which causes descemetocele and perforation. Modified from slides courtesy of Dr. Milton Wyman and The Ohio State University.

a. Schematic cross-section of deep corneal ulcer or laceration
b. Excess protease activity resulting in limbal descemetocele. Note deep vascularization.
c. Excess protease activity resulting in central descemetocele. Note superficial vascularization.
d. Descemetocele ruptures and aqueous escapes

DRUGS USED TO IMPROVE CORNEAL WOUND HEALING

Collagenase inhibition

1. Corneal collagenase production
   a. Normal epithelium produces a minimal amount of collagenase. This is involved with the normal turnover of the corneal cells and does not significantly penetrate the stroma. If the cornea is injured, the epithelial cells that are dividing rapidly produce an increased amount of collagenase. If the outer glycoprotein layer is disrupted, collagenase will break down the collagen fibers of the stroma. In the absence of a serious injury, the glycoprotein layer immediately beneath the epithelium prevents collagenase from penetrating into the stroma.
   b. Budding endothelial cells that are a part of the corneal vascularization after injury produce collagenase
   c. Leukocytes present in an inflammatory reaction are active in collagenase production
   d. Some bacteria and fungi produce large amounts of collagenase or other proteinases that will denature collagen
   e. Summary of collagenase production - If the cornea is superficially scratched, it will heal without cell mitosis and thereby without increased collagenase activity. In severe wounds, there will be increased collagenase production beginning about five days after injury. This will break down the injured cornea and allow healing to take place. In some corneal lesions, especially alkali burns, collagenase activity may result in excess destruction of the cornea, and thereby result in an ulceration that continues to increase in size rather than heal. Collagenase-producing bacteria or fungi may cause a lesion to spread rapidly.
2. Collagenase potentiators - Corticosteroids will increase the activity of collagenase by 14 times. Therefore, they are contraindicated in a collagenase producing cornea.
3. Collagenase inhibitors (see page 123)
   a. Chelating agents (EDTA), tetracycline
   b. Cysteine (acetylcysteine)
   c. Penicillamine
   d. Iodine preparations
   e. Alpha macroglobulins (blood/serum)
   f. Antiplasmin agents
4. If collagenase activity is controlled, corticosteriods will improve healing by inhibition of leukocyte infiltration and angiogenesis, immunosuppression

NSAIDS - Inhibition of prostaglandin synthesis and indirect inhibition of angiogenesis, inhibition of PMN degranulation

Retinoids - Maintenance of normal corneal epithelial growth and proliferation

Cyclosporine - Immunosuppression, inhibition of PMN activation

Sodium hyaluronate (viscoelastics) - Tear film substitute, stabilization of epithelial surface

Fibronectin - Promotion of cell adhesion and migration

Aprotinin - Inhibition of plasmin leading to protection of fibronectin and laminin

Epidermal growth factor - Stimulation of epithelial cell proliferation and angiogenesis. Very expensive but is present in fresh serum

Polysulphated glucosaminoglycan - Promotion of cell adhesion by inhibiting plasmin and plasminogen activators

CHARACTERISTICS OF CORNEAL DISEASE

Loss of transparency

Various degrees of opacity are described: nebula (very faint change that can be seen with oblique illumination), macula (appears as a light gray spot in natural light), leukoma (any dense white spot). Leukoma is the degree of opacity that is of clinical importance. Adherent leukoma is a white spot that occurs in the cornea from an anterior synechia.

1. Leukoma
   a. Edema of the cornea (hydration) that may result from:
      1) Interstitial keratitis
      2) Anterior uveitis
      3) Glaucoma
      4) Corneal ulcers
      5) Endothelial dystrophy or degeneration
   b. Cellular infiltration
      1) Leukocyte
      2) Cicatricial
   c. Metabolic infiltrates - lipid and cholesterol deposits; calcium deposits
2. Pigmentation - Corneal pigmentation may be:
   a. Superficial as the result of migration of pigment cells from the limbus and perilimbal bulbar conjunctiva. It is the cornea's response to chronic irritation.
   b. Iris pigment that may become trapped in the cornea after corneal injury
   c. Congenital pigment deposits in the stroma
   d. Ruptured anterior uveal pigment epithelial cysts adhering to the corneal endothelium
   e. Silver nitrate trapped in the cornea after cauterization
3. Foreign bodies

Corneal vascularization - Vascularization occurs at the level (depth) of the irritation **(Fig 10-8).**

1. Superficial vascularization - It has a tree-like branching appearance and indicates chronicity. Pannus, blood vessels going to granulation tissue.
2. Deep (interstitial) vascularization - After stromal injuries, surgical incisions, and interstitial keratitis. It appears as a deep red halo near the limbus and is characterized by small parallel vessels.

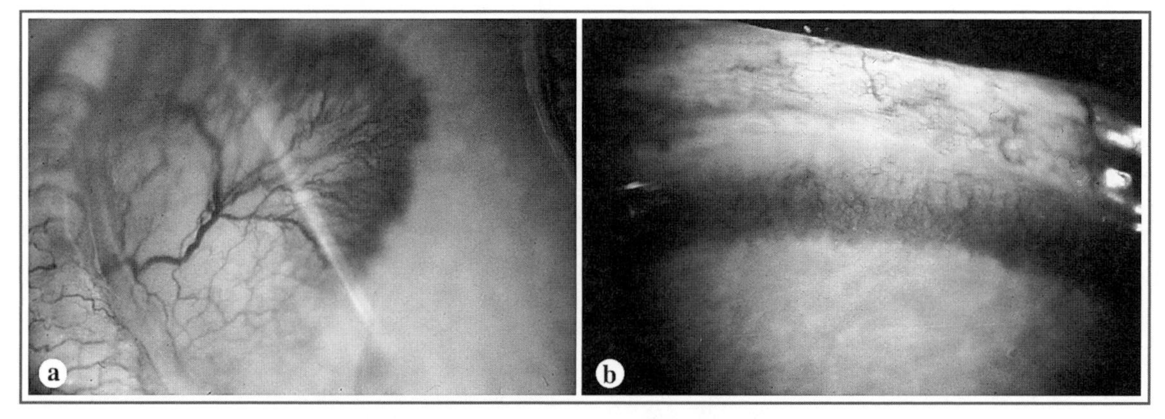

Figure 10-8. Characteristics of corneal vascularization.
a. Tree-like branching characteristic of superficial vascularization
b. Small parallel blood vessels characteristic of deep vascularization

Circumcorneal injection - Dilated vessels close to the limbus and diminishing toward the periphery.

Cellular debris and protein clots (keratic precipitates) deposited on the endothelium from the aqueous humor - These occur with interstitial keratitis and iritis. Hypopyon results if severe.

Change in corneal contour

1. Edema
2. Proliferative masses - dermoid, tumor, staphyloma, descemetocele
3. Loss of tissue - ulceration, laceration, perforation

SUBJECTIVE SIGNS OF CORNEAL DISEASE

1. Pain - does not occur with all forms of keratitis, but when present it will result in:
    a. Photophobia
    b. Blepharospasm
    c. Epiphora
2. Loss of vision if cornea is severely diseased

CONGENITAL

DERMOID GROWTHS (CHORISTOMA) - Most common congenital corneal lesion. Seen most frequently in bovine, dog and horse. An inherited disease in Burmese cats.

Appearance - Two types are encountered:

1. Thick mass with long hair growing from it. In this case, usually has a thick layer of deep fat that can be distinctly separated from cornea. This lesion typically causes mild irritation and in some cases none. This is typical of the bovine and dog.
2. Thin elevated mass with short hairs. Usually pigmented. This lesion is quite discomforting because the patient can close the eyelids over it, resulting in secondary irritation to the lids. Typical of the equine. If severe blepharospasm is present, the lesion may be difficult to examine until topical anesthetic is used. This is typical of horses.

Location - Most are near the temporal limbus. May involve conjunctiva and sclera as well.

Treatment

1. Surgical removal (Fig 10-9). Be sure to remove all of it because hair follicles will regenerate if not completely removed. I have never encountered one that went so deep into the stroma or sclera that it prohibited complete removal. The keratectomy is started in clear cornea and dissected toward the limbus. If the dermoid involves cornea and conjunctiva, the conjunctival portion of the lesion is undermined before starting on the superficial keratectomy (Fig 8-3; Chapter 8, page 251).
2. The corneal wound is treated the same as a fresh corneal ulcer.

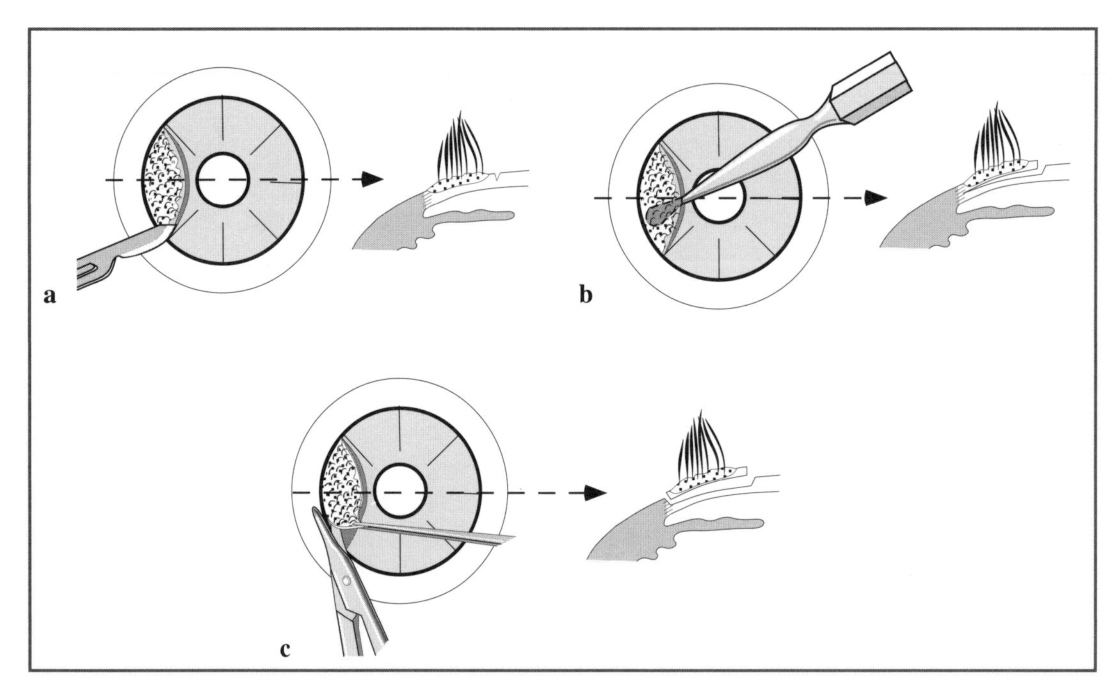

Figure 10-9. Sectional superficial keratectomy for corneal dermoid.
a. Cornea is incised to the depth of the dermoid
b. Dermoid undermined to the limbus with Martinez corneal separator (shown above). Corneal scissors, #15 Bard Parker blade, or #64 Beaver blade are also satisfactory.
c. Limbal incision completed with corneal scissors

CORNEAL COLOBOMA WITH STAPHYLOMA

Uncommon. We have had one case in the dog. The lesion was near the limbus with a circular corneal defect about 4 mm in diameter. Slit lamp examination revealed complete absence of corneal stroma, resulting in a staphyloma of the base of the iris covered by epithelium and Descemet's membrane. The eye was normal in all other aspects. The dog was six months old and not showing any untoward signs; because of this, the owner elected to observe the animal rather than have the lesion surgically removed. The danger of perforation exists. Replacement of the staphyloma and a corneal transplant to fill the defect would be the treatment of choice.

TRANSIENT SUBEPITHELIAL DYSTROPHY IN PUPPIES

Subepithelial opacities in puppies are sometimes observed when the eyes are opened. These are usually faint opacities and are easily missed on a routine examination. If severe, they may be thick enough to cause surface irregularities. Easily seen with transillumination and an Optivisor. No breed predisposition. May occur as an individual problem or affect the entire litter.

We have seen this in a litter of coonhounds (4 of 8) and a litter of salukies (6 of 7) that were severely affected. The white subepithelial plaques regressed without treatment. All of the coonhounds had normal appearing corneas by six months. The salukies were more severe and at six months, four were clear and two had small areas of opacity that were clear by one year. The fundus was clearly seen and vision was assumed normal in all puppies.

CORNEAL LIPID INCLUSION CYSTS - Lipid inclusion cysts may be congenital misplacement of sebaceous cells or acquired after trauma.

1. Congenital. The author observed one dog that was presented at four months of age with a cyst that the owner had been aware of since purchase (six weeks of age). It was growing slowly but not bothering the dog. After removal, histopathology revealed a small lipid-containing inclusion extending into the superficial stroma.
2. Acquired
    a. Occurs occasionally in adult dogs presented with a history of previous ocular injury.
        1) The lesions can be removed by superficial keratectomy. Good prognosis.
        2) If the cyst should spontaneously rupture into the corneal stroma, it will cause a granulomatous reaction with marked vascularization. Surgical removal of the granuloma will give excellent results.
    b. Rare in horses. Same clinical appearances as dogs and responds well to surgical removal.

CORNEAL DYSTROPHY - These are uncommon, therefore difficult to determine inheritance.

The term *corneal dystrophy* is frequently used to describe any corneal degeneration. This should be avoided. In ophthalmic terminology, corneal dystrophy has been defined as "hereditary primary alteration or degeneration of the cornea that affects either of the limiting membranes and/or the stroma, occurs bilaterally and usually begins at an early age; is not accompanied by an inflammatory phenomenon or by vascularization; may be slowly progressive or stationary; and in general is not associated with metabolic disorders or other systemic anomalies."

Endothelial dystrophy

1. Endothelial dystrophy secondary to persistent pupillary membrane adhering to the cornea (see iris, Chapter 12, page 364). The strands of iris adhering to the cornea may disappear before maturity but will result in a permanent area of leukoma. First described in the basenji and observed occasionally in other breeds. Inheritance is proposed for the basenji. No treatment. Mild cases will have adequate vision with some clearing of the cornea with maturity. Severe cases with multiple lesions can cause the eye to be blind.

2. Endothelial dystrophy leading to corneal edema in domestic cats has been observed by the author. One occurrence was a nine month old queen that had affected kittens. The owner had noticed the queen's corneas had been cloudy since six weeks of age. Examination revealed a central corneal edema with a ground glass appearance. The lesions became progressively worse, leading to blindness. In another instance, central stationary corneal edema was diagnosed in a male and female farm cat who were related.

Stromal dystrophy

1. Cats
   Hereditary corneal dystrophy in the manx cat (Bistner, Aguirre and Shively) begins as an anterior stromal edema progressing to marked epithelial edema. There are no opacities located within the cornea. The endothelium is normal but alterations in Descemet's membrane are seen. The lesion causes loss of the eye. The mode of inheritance is not known.
2. Dogs - Stromal lesions vary in appearance and location.
   a. American cocker spaniel posterior polymorphous dystrophy - Occurs in American cocker spaniels and is characterized by multiple irregularly shaped opacities present at Descemet's membrane. The condition is present at birth and nonprogressive. Dominant or incomplete dominant inheritance is proposed.
   b. Airedale terrier - sex linked, central anterior stromal lipid deposit, begins 4 to 12 months of age, decreased vision by four years
   c. English toy spaniel - familial inheritance is proposed, circular paracentral stromal crystalline opacity
   d. Samoyed - inheritance suspected, develops six months to seven years, central stromal dystrophy with donut-shaped appearance, usually bilateral
   e. Siberian husky - recessive with variable penetrance, usually shows up between five months to two years, may be as late as eight years, bilateral, lipid, stromal donut appearance (Fig 10-10)
   f. Other breeds - Alaskan malamute, beagle, golden retriever, greyhound, Afghan, pointer, Shetland sheepdog, and whippet

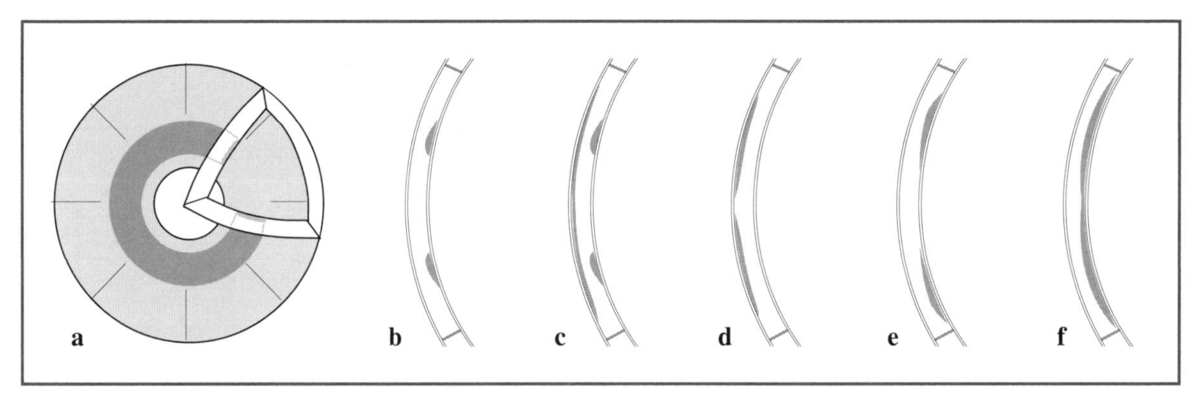

Figure 10-10. Drawing of Siberian husky crystalline corneal dystrophy, demonstrating five commonly occurring patterns.
a. Crystals in pre-Descemet's stroma results in a gray ring and clear central and peripheral cornea
b-f. Slit view of common patterns
b. Pattern represented in "a" above
c. Gray, homogeneous, smudgy deposits within the anterior stroma and crystals in the posterior stroma, with clear stroma between
d. Gray-brown, homogeneous deposits in the anterior stroma, with the remainder of the stroma clear
e. Gray homogeneous deposits involving the posterior two-thirds of the stroma
f. Gray-brown, homogeneous deposits involving the entire stromal thickness. Modified and adapted from MacMillan AD, Waring GO III, Spangler WL, Roth AM: Crystalline corneal opacities in the Siberian husky. J Am Vet Med Assoc 175:829, 1979.

Subepithelial dystrophy - Has been observed in several breeds - bearded collies, bichon frise, rough collie, Lhasa apso, mastiff, miniature pinscher, miniature poodle, weimaraner, Cavalier King Charles spaniel

Metabolic storage diseases (uncommon)

1. Etiology
   a. Dogs with mucopolysaccharidosis type I and VI
   b. Cats with mucopolysaccharidosis type II and VI and gangliosidosis Gm1 and Gm2
2. Signs
   a. Bilateral diffuse hazy corneas. Animals may exhibit blepharospasm.
   b. Skeletal and neurologic signs of the primary disease
3. Diagnosis
   a. Ophthalmic and clinical signs
   b. Diagnostic tests

ACQUIRED DISEASES

Keratitis can be characterized as:

1. Superficial with vascularization (e.g. pannus, pigmentary keratitis, granulation tissue, chronic infectious keratitis, and neoplasms)
2. Superficial without vascularization (e.g. punctate keratitis, metabolic infiltrates, corneal degenerations, healed injuries with scarring)
3. Interstitial (deep) keratitis
4. Ulcerative keratitis
5. Keratoconjunctivitis

GERMAN SHEPHERD PANNUS (ÜBERREITER'S SYNDROME, CHRONIC SUPERFICIAL KERATITIS)

Pannus is defined as subepithelial vascularization and infiltration of granulation tissue into the cornea, extending into the superficial layers of the stroma.

German shepherd pannus is typically blood vessels, lymphocytes, plasma cells, and melanocytes advancing from the temporal limbus and invading the superficial stroma, resulting in a pigmented subepithelial bed of granulation tissue.

Etiology - Unknown. Believed to be an immune-mediated disease with breed predisposition and aggravated by ultraviolet radiation.

1. Breed predisposition
   a. Seen primarily in German shepherds and shepherd crosses (90% or more of the cases) and dogs of similar ancestry
   b. Other breeds
      - Belgian Tervuren, has greater predisposition than German shepherd
      - Border collie
      - Greyhound
      - Siberian husky
      - Australian shepherd dog
2. Ultraviolet radiation (elevation) - Risk factor for dogs at 5,000 to 7,000 feet elevation is 2.87 times greater than for dogs at 3,000 to 5,000 feet, and 7.5 times greater for dogs at over 7,000 feet than those at 3,000 to 5,000 feet.
3. Sex factors - Intact females less frequently affected

Age of onset - Lesions can occur as early as nine months of age and as old as 10 years. Most cases present to CSU between three and six years.

Course and symptoms - Bilateral

1. Begins near the temporal limbus. Lesions next appear at the nasal limbus, then grow toward each other. The last area to be involved is the cornea near the dorsal limbus. When a case is seen early, one eye is usually more advanced than another. In time, the lesion will completely cover both corneas and produce blindness.
2. Small foci of edema are present in the clear cornea adjacent to the pannus lesion
3. When a lesion is covered with pigment, the owners may not be aware of the problem until the animal begins to show signs of blindness. Unpigmented lesions have a fleshy appearance.
4. The disease may have an acute onset, becoming noticeable in two to three weeks, or be chronic, taking months to develop.

5. Longstanding lesions characteristically develop lipid corneal degeneration (cholesterol deposits) that may eventually become severe enough to interfere with vision even though the pannus lesion is controlled by topical treatment.
6. The third eyelid may depigment and become thickened along the margin with an infiltration of plasma cells.

Treatment - Provides temporary arrest and must be continued for life. Response to treatment is related to environment. Much more difficult to control at higher elevations (above 5,000 feet). The course and recommended treatment used at CSU are:

1. Early cases - topical medication
   a. Corticosteroids
      1) More potent preparations preferred. Dexamethasone 0.1%, prednisolone acetate 1%, or prednisolone phosphate 1%
      2) Topical corticosteroid treatment four to six times daily until improvement, then two to four times daily depending on response
      3) Ointments or drops. May use in combination with antibiotics. For routine treatment, prefer preparations without antibiotics.
   b. Cyclosporine - Cyclosporine 1% in corn oil is beneficial on vascular lesions and moderately effective on reducing epithelial pigment. Start with BID treatment and reduce as patient improves.
   c. Combination - Cyclosporine BID combined with topical corticosteroids QID. Has a synergistic response. As the patient improves, corticosteroid may be reduced to BID and cyclosporine to daily. This may be most helpful in animals with systemic sensitivity to QID topical corticosteroids.
2. Moderately advanced cases or lesions where topical treatment is becoming ineffective (see page 93).
   a. Subconjunctival injection with repository corticosteroids
      1) Depo-Medrol - 8 to 12 mg/eye. Be careful—permanent deposits of the Depo carrier may result.
      2) Betamethasone - 3 mg per eye
      3) Triamcinolone - 5 to 10 mg/eye
   b. Follow with topical treatment, as before
   c. Expect improvement in seven days. This may be effective one to six months depending on the patient.
   d. Some animals will develop transient polydipsia and polyuria for three to five days after injection
3. Animals with advanced lesions that have minimal scarring or lesions that progress in spite of corticosteroid and cyclosporine treatment
   a. Beta radiation and concurrent subconjunctival cortisone injection
      1) Thick lesions - 7500 rads per application site
      2) Thin lesions - 4500 to 6000 rads per application site

      The applicator is placed so that the entire lesion and adjacent limbus are covered. When using small applicators, multiple applications are needed. Areas of clear cornea and normal limbus are not treated. This is followed by topical treatment as previously prescribed.
   b. The eye will improve in a week and be maximum in 30 days. This treatment is especially useful in eyes with corneal pigmentation. Usually 60 to 70% of the pigment will have disappeared in 30 days. The lesion may not regress as expected if areas have been missed with the applicator or if the lesion exceeds 1 mm thick. In this case, repeat subconjunctival cortisone and wait 30 more days. If the results are not satisfactory by that time, beta therapy may be repeated at one-half the original dosage.
4. Advanced lesions causing blindness with severe scarring, severe cholesterol deposits and/or pigment deposits in the stroma.
   a. Superficial keratectomy (Fig 10-11). A #15 Bard Parker blade is used to start the keratectomy. It is important to dissect deeply enough to remove all blood vessels. When the dissection is deep enough to see clear cornea, the cornea separates easily with a #64 Beaver blade, Martinez corneal dissector or fine pointed corneal scissors. Remove the cornea to the limbus. Any adjacent pigmented conjunctiva should be removed for 3 to 5 mm from the limbus.

b. Beta treatment - 6000 to 7500 rads per site to the entire limbus postsurgically to prevent postsurgical neovascularization.
c. Antibiotic ophthalmic ointment until re-epithelialization (9 to 12 days). An antibiotic corticosteroid ointment can be used if the patient is closely observed. After healing is complete, topical medication is continued. If there is some vascularization associated with healing, subconjunctival cortisone can be used after re-epithelialization.
d. Surgery can be repeated two to three times. The cornea becomes progressively thinner with each keratectomy and eventually will reach the point where it can no longer regenerate.

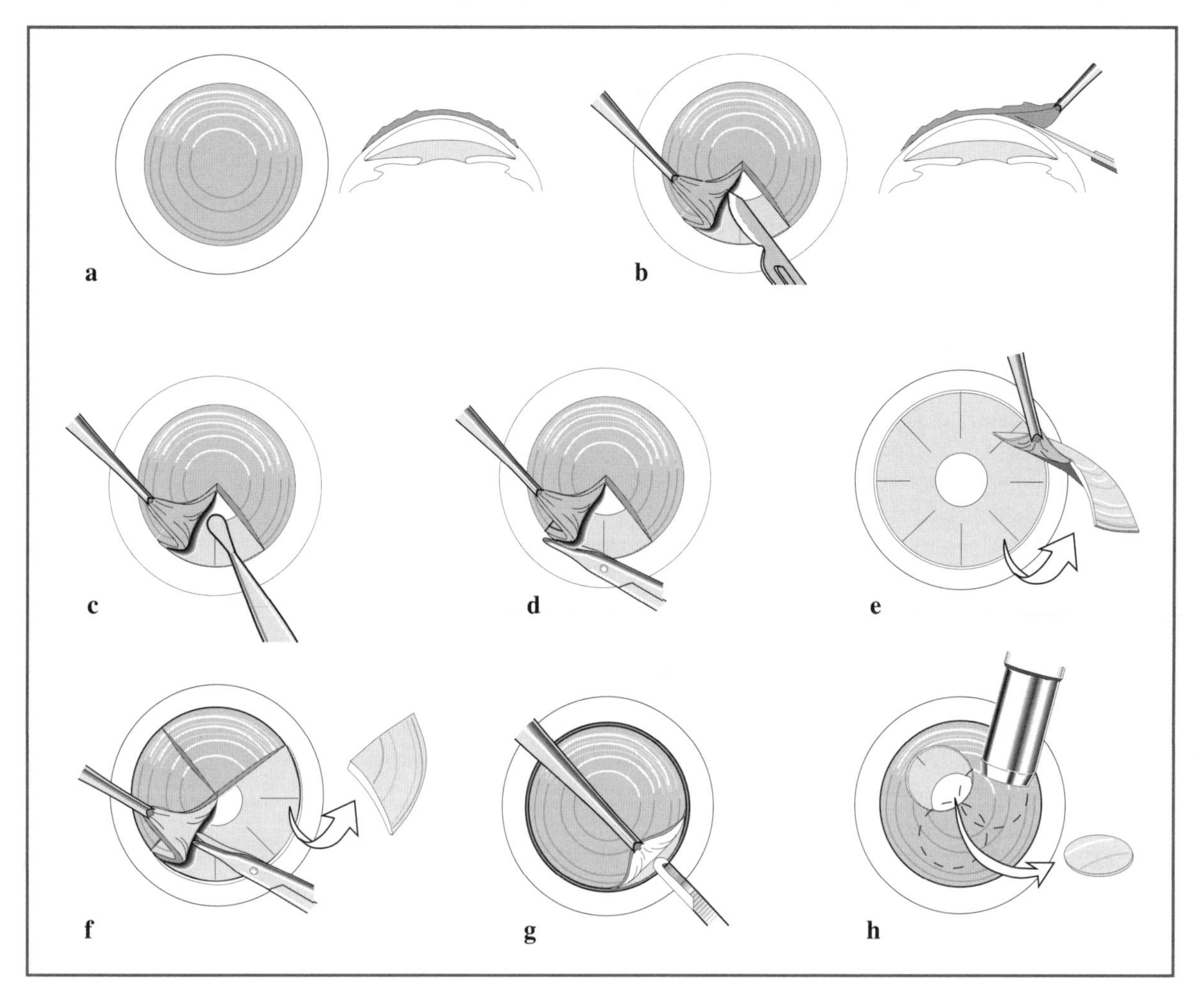

Figure 10-11. Superficial keratectomy for German shepherd pannus. Several methods are shown. The choice is the preference of the surgeon.

a. Frontal and cross-section view of advanced German shepherd pannus. Note the thickness of the lesion.
b. Superficial keratectomy with a #15 Bard-Parker blade or #64 Beaver blade. An incision is started into the lesion at a 45° angle until clear cornea is seen. As soon as the proper depth is reached, the lesion is removed by directing the blade along the lamellar plane of the cornea.
c. Dissecting along lamellar plane with Martinez separator
d. The lesion is dissected free at the limbus with corneal scissors
e. After the lesion has been removed the cornea is smoothed, making sure all blood vessels have been removed from the cornea. The cornea is clear at this time but will turn cloudy in a few days.
f. After dividing cornea into quadrants with incisions, the cornea is separated along lamellar planes with blunt dissection by forcing the closed scissors forward, then opening them and repeating the procedure.
g. A perilimbal incision is made in the conjunctiva about 0.5 mm from the limbus. The dissected cornea is removed from the limbus toward the center.
h. Scoring the cornea with a large corneal trephine followed by keratectomy. All affected cornea is removed.

Prognosis

Depends on geographic location. More favorable at low elevation. Lesions will recur if treatment is stopped, but at lower elevations some can be treated as infrequently as two or three times a week. In the intermountain area can usually keep an animal visual for three to five years. Owners may choose to discontinue treatment on animals that do not respond well to treatment. Most dogs adapt well to blindness and are very content if they are confined to a yard.

Complications

1. Superficial corneal degenerations - These are due to the chronic nature of this disease.
   a. Subepithelial and anterior stromal cholesterol opacities. One year after onset, subepithelial opacities often occur. These generally occur in the area of the original lesion and have a tendency to progress to form a central band. This band may be incomplete or quite distinct. In other cases there may be focal areas of opacity. Cholesterol deposits can be expected to become static or even regress when treated with topical cyclosporine.
   b. Superficial cystic degeneration - Epithelial cysts have been observed in eyes after superficial keratectomy, beta radiation, and in some patients that have received only topical corticosteroids. The lesions are usually small (1 to 2 mm) inclusion cysts containing clear fluid. They occasionally coalesce.

      After prolonged treatment, subepithelial cysts may develop in the superficial stroma that lead to bullous keratopathy. In these animals, the cornea undergoes severe degeneration from a combination of factors that deplete the regenerative ability of the cornea. These are: several years of continuous corticosteroid therapy, repeated superficial keratectomy, and/or repeated beta radiation.
2. Corneal ulceration or injury. Prolonged corticosteroid therapy lowers the regenerative ability of the cornea. If the cornea is scratched or suffers a deep corneal penetration, corticosteroid therapy should be stopped immediately and not started again until the cornea has healed. Delayed healing is common.
3. Infection. In man, continuous cortisone therapy predisposes the eye to infection, especially fungal. We have not observed this in pannus patients. Occasionally acute bacterial infections occur that respond to preparations containing antibiotics.

PANNUS AS A RESULT OF CHRONIC IRRITATION OR INFECTION

Chronic infection or irritation may result in a lesion similar to German shepherd pannus. When this occurs, the cause should be determined and if infection exists, culture and sensitivity should be used to select the most appropriate antibiotic. If infection is present, the infection is treated first and then the pannus lesion, in the same manner as described for German shepherd pannus. These dogs do not show the tendency toward recurrence that is seen with German shepherd pannus. If the eye is infected and blind, a superficial keratectomy must not be done until infection is controlled.

FELINE EOSINOPHILIC KERATITIS

Etiology - This has been proposed to be a corneal manifestation of the same processes seen with eosinophilic dermatitis. More recently feline herpesvirus has been identified in some of these cases.

Clinical signs

1. Superficial vascular lesions with moderate leukoma resembling German shepherd pannus develop near the limbus. These slowly progress centrally. If not treated, lesions can eventually cover the entire cornea. This may take more than a year.
2. White elevated plaques develop, becoming larger as the lesion progresses. On first impression, these plaques are suggestive of mycotic keratitis.
3. Some lesions may be very thin with a fine vascular network and minimal leukoma.
4. Usually bilateral. Little or no discomfort. Minimal ocular discharge.

Positive diagnosis

1. Clinical signs are adequate for presumptive diagnosis
2. Corneal scraping is diagnostic. Eosinophils and mast cells will be seen. Degenerating eosinophils may rupture, resulting in many free eosinophilic granules seen on the slide.

Treatment

1. Some early lesions respond to topical corticosteroids - This is not usually effective enough to justify as initial treatment but may be effective for long term prevention of recurrence or supplemental to reduced megestrol acetate (Ovaban) treatment.
2. Oral Ovaban - Initial treatment 5 mg daily is usually adequate; refractory lesions may require 10 mg. Lesions usually regress rapidly with marked improvement in five to seven days. To determine maintenance, the dosage is reduced to 2.5 to 5 mg every 7 to 10 days. Treatment can be discontinued in some animals. Before using Ovaban, the owner should be advised of adverse reactions (see Chapter 2, page 95).
3. Subconjunctival depot corticosteroids may be needed if not showing adequate response to Ovaban.

GRANULATION TISSUE AFTER DEEP ULCERS

Granulation tissue is a necessary step in the healing process of severe corneal diseases. It is to be encouraged until it has served its purpose, after which it should be retarded or removed if it does not spontaneously regress. An excellent example is the change that occurs in many prolapsed eyes after replacement. Ulceration is followed by interstitial keratitis and granulation tissue. Later the cornea spontaneously clears from the limbus inward.

Treatment - If the granulation tissue becomes exuberant and persists, it must be destroyed. This can be done in several ways.

1. Mild granulation
    a. Topical corticosteroids or subconjunctival at source of blood supply work well for mild granulation
    b. Beta radiation followed by topical corticosteroids is indicated for those dogs that would be prone to delayed corneal healing if the lesion was surgically removed
    c. Electrocauterization of the feeding blood vessels at the limbus. This has not worked very well for me (can be done with deep topical anesthesia)
    d. Cryotherapy at the limbus to destroy blood vessels (can be done with topical anesthesia)
2. Severe granulation responds very well to beta radiation and subconjunctival corticosteroid. Alternate treatments are:
    a. Strong cauterizing agents - trichloracetic acid, phenol (not recommended)
    b. Surgical removal

    After either of these two methods, treat as an ulcer

PIGMENTARY KERATITIS

The deposition of pigment in the cornea is a response to irritation. It may be superficial or deep.

Etiology

1. Trichiasis or distichiasis
2. Protruding eyes - more subject to environmental irritation
3. Entropion, excess nasal folds
4. Any chronic keratoconjunctivitis, especially keratoconjunctivitis sicca
5. German shepherd pannus
6. After corneal injuries (this may be superficial or deep)
7. Congenital predisposition - some blood lines of Pekingese and pugs will show this in a high percent of pups as early as six to seven months of age. The author has observed it in pugs less than three months of age

Occurrence - Most common in protruding eye breeds - Boston terrier, Pekingese and pug

Significance - Pigment that becomes deposited in the stroma is permanent and should be removed surgically if it interferes with sight. If sight is adequate and close examination reveals the lesion has become static, it is best not to do surgery. Superficial pigment will slough if the irritation is stopped.

Treatment of superficial pigment

1. Remove irritating cause
2. Treat with topical corticosteroids. Should see marked improvement in 30 days.
3. If not removed in 30 days, treat with beta application
4. In extreme cases where the cause has been removed but the eye does not clear, superficial keratectomy will be beneficial. Treat postsurgically the same as described for pannus keratectomy. ***Do not do a superficial keratectomy in dogs with protruding eyes.***
5. In dogs with protruding eyes, consider nasal and/or temporal canthoplasty

Prognosis

1. Good if cause can be removed
2. If cause cannot be removed, continue topical treatment with corticosteroids and possibly antibiotics. This can be arrested with treatment but not cured.

CORNEAL DEGENERATION AND METABOLIC INFILTRATES

Several forms of noninflammatory corneal degenerations occur that result in corneal edema or stromal deposits.

Acquired corneal degeneration can occur from chronic keratitis, or metabolic disease, after corneal surgery or spontaneously from unknown causes. These lesions are usually permanent and are generally progressive.

The etiology and pathogenesis of corneal degeneration in many patients may remain obscure or unknown.

Endothelial degeneration

1. Endothelial degeneration in dogs - Endothelial dystrophy allows overhydration of the cornea with thickening. Topical treatment with 5% NaCl ophthalmic ointment QID may have transitory value. It is usually progressive and leads to blindness. If severe, it can cause keratoconus and eventually bullous keratopathy. Corneal transplants have been helpful if the cornea is still avascular. After corneal vascularization, their benefit is questionable.
   a. Breed predisposition in Boston terrier (usually female), poodle, chow, Chihuahua and Pomeranian as the result of a gradual spontaneous endothelial degeneration beginning about 8 years or older. Will eventually lead to blindness.
   b. Senile spontaneous endothelial degeneration in dogs - Old dogs may develop complete opacity from corneal edema in one to six weeks without any other change in the eye. A 1 to 2 mm ring of normal cornea may be present at the limbus. Does not respond to treatment.
   c. After corneal surgery - Corneal perforations and incisions can sometimes cause permanent endothelial damage. This is a possible complication to limbal incisions for lens removal. Usually the edema is limited to the area of the injury and the rest of the cornea will remain clear.
2. Endothelial degeneration in cats - Corneal edema from permanent endothelial damage after uveitis can occur. Results in severe corneal thickening and irreversible damage.
3. Endothelial degeneration in horses
   a. Corneal opacity is sometimes seen in horses that do not show any signs of anterior uveitis. These animals respond to cortisone, thus suggesting endothelial damage resulting from corneal sensitization.
   b. Anterior uveitis with severe corneal involvement can sometimes result in permanent endothelial damage. In some cases this is severe enough to result in bullous keratopathy. Topical 5% sodium chloride ophthalmic ointment is definitely beneficial.
4. Endothelial degeneration in cattle - Cattle wormed with phenothiazine may develop corneal edema as a sunlight photosensitivity. This may last two to three months if they remain outdoors, or clear in a weekend if kept indoors.
5. Striate keratopathy - Occurs most frequently in dogs and horses with chronic glaucoma and results from breaks in Descemet's membrane. They may be single or branching. When examined with magnification, a stria appears as two white parallel lines. During periods of high pressure there will be edema near the stria. If the pressure drops or returns to normal, the edema will disappear and only the stria remain.

   Striate keratopathy that is not glaucoma related can occur in horses. In these cases the striae may vary from a single line to a wide irregular pattern.

Stromal lipid keratopathies (calcium cholesterol and lipid substrates) - These can occur at any depth of the cornea but are usually superficial and slow growing.

1. Cause - The cause may be a primary corneal dystrophy or secondary degeneration from corneal or systemic disease. In either case, deposits of lipid metabolites (cholesterol) build up in the cornea, primarily beneath the basement membrane. These deposits are dynamic and close observation over an extended period of time will reveal subtle changes in their appearance. Degenerations are classified as:
   a. Secondary degeneration to chronic corneal disease. Frequently in dogs. Rarely in cats.
      1) German shepherd pannus - Subepithelial deposits will occur frequently after six months to three years. Usually slowly progressive and tend to form a central ring. Repeated observations will often reveal that the areas of opacity are not stationary but constantly shifting.
      2) After superficial keratectomy for dermoids, tumors or granulomas. These lesions develop an arc that outlines the periphery of the lesions and are usually static.
      3) After ulcers. This is not common and should not be confused with scar tissue.
      4) After episcleritis. In this case, the lesions tend to be near the limbus and may clear up completely if the episcleritis does not recur.
   b. Secondary to diseases affecting lipid metabolism. This is uncommon but a serum lipid profile may be considered in diseases with hyperlipoproteinemia or hypercholesterolemia. Some hypothyroid animals with high serum lipids develop a cloudy cornea from lipid infiltration that will disappear if the serum levels of lipid return to normal.

      High cholesterol levels, especially if greater than 1000 mg/dl, result in cholesterol deposits. This infiltration begins near the limbus in a circular fashion and will proceed toward the center of the cornea. These deposits can be so thick that they make the corneal surface appear irregular. These lesions are reversible only when the serum cholesterol level returns to normal early in the disease. If advanced, the lesion is not reversible. Corneal vascularization occurs in advanced lesions.
   c. Spontaneous from unknown causes - May occur in animals of any age. Usually begin centrally but can occur near the limbus. In the younger dogs (< 8 yrs), may be slowly progressive and then stop. Some cases disappear. Others, especially older dogs (> 8 yrs), are progressive and may eventually interfere with sight.
2. Signs - variable
   a. Appearance - may begin as a faint haze, crystalline ground glass or amorphous white appearance
   b. Shape - varies with the cause, breed and duration of lesion
      1) Generalized haziness
      2) Axial opacity that gradually grows (e.g. spontaneous)
      3) Faint crescent or arc that eventually develops in a ring (e.g. immune-mediated disease)
      4) Limbal arc that grows toward the center of the cornea (e.g. hypothyroidism)
   c. Vascularization - develops in longstanding lesions
3. Treatment
   a. Restrict dietary fat if lipid metabolism is abnormal
   b. If an immune disease is suspected, topical cyclosporine 1%
   c. 1 to 2% EDTA (see page 125). One drop QID is effective in some cases
   d. If loss of vision - superficial keratectomy
   e. If secondary to systemic disease (hypothyroidism) - treat primary disease

Epithelial calcification (band keratopathy) - Band keratopathy refers to subepithelial deposition of calcium

1. Causes
   a. Chronic keratitis (common cause)
   b. Hypercalcemia (hyperparathyroidism, hyperadrenocorticism)
2. Signs - a rough gritty corneal deposit
   a. A gray-white superficial corneal opacity that usually follows the palpebral fissure
   b. Plaques may slough leaving craters
   c. Uveitis may be present
3. Treatment
   a. Surgical removal and treat with 1 to 2% EDTA solution
   b. Treat initiating ocular diseases

Epithelial cystic degeneration

1. Signs - Small epithelial cysts may occur in animals with chronic corneal disease. These may be singular or multiple. If multiple, they may coalesce to form bullae. Can occur as a complication to German shepherd pannus, chronic keratitis with corneal vascularization, or after the healing of ulcers or lacerations. These cysts are located in abnormal epithelium overlying damaged superficial stroma.
2. Treatment - may or may not be indicated. If from pannus or chronic keratitis, the cornea in the area may be severely damaged and opaque. In this case the cyst may be the least problem. If after a laceration or ulcer, the adjacent cornea is normal and the cyst should be removed.
   a. Surgical removal is the most satisfactory. Make sure surrounding epithelium is removed until it is normal and the stromal surface is smooth so the normal epithelium regenerates. If there is severe stromal damage in the area, cyst formation will recur.
   b. Extended wear contact lenses are sometimes helpful after removing the cysts.

Bullous keratopathy - Seen most frequently in dogs and horses. The development of bullae (vesicles) within the corneal stroma. May be the result of severe stromal damage or secondary to extreme stromal hydration from endothelial damage.

1. If from severe disease - bullae can occur anywhere in the stroma and the prognosis is unfavorable. Treatment would be directed at protecting the eye to allow as much spontaneous healing as possible.
2. If from endothelial damage - the bullae are in the superficial stroma and the treatment and prognosis depend on whether the endothelial damage is reversible. If reversible - favorable. If not reversible - unfavorable.

   Transient endothelial damage is usually seen with uveitis whereas fibrin adhered to the corneal endothelium may cause additional mechanical irritation. Fluid is imbibed by the stroma faster than it can escape from the epithelium, resulting in a bullae that is similar to blister beneath the skin. If the bulla is ruptured, the epithelium will reattach if the cornea can be dehydrated. Dehydration depends on healing of the endothelium and dehydrating the cornea with 5% sodium chloride ophthalmic ointment.

SUPERFICIAL PUNCTATE KERATITIS

Punctate keratitis is characterized by punctate ulcers, epithelial and subepithelial opacities (corneal dystrophy), and varying signs of pain.

Etiology

This is a chronic superficial keratitis of unknown cause that probably has multiple etiologies resulting in similar clinical changes. An autoimmune corneal epithelial disorder may be a common factor. Some proposed causes are listed.

1. Dogs
    a. Abnormal tear film - Dice: Corneal dystrophy in Shetland sheepdog. Trans Am Coll Vet Ophthalmol 1984;241-242.
    b. Herpesvirus keratitis - Keller et al: Experimentally produced canine herpetic keratitis. Gaines Vet Symposium 1972;23-26. Herpesvirus has never been recovered from clinical punctate keratitis in dogs.
2. Horses - Equine herpesvirus I (EHV-I) has been isolated from corneal epithelium in horses with punctate keratitis. But herpesvirus ***has not been demonstrated*** in any horses seen with punctate keratitis at CSU.

Breed predisposition in dogs

1. Shetland sheepdog - abnormal tear film. A genetic factor has been proposed, therefore breeding affected animals should be discouraged.
2. Dachshunds - especially longhaired and wirehaired. Punctate keratitis with extensive vascularization.
3. Breeds predisposed to German shepherd pannus.

Clinical signs - There is enough variation in the clinical signs to justify discussing them separately.

1. Tear film abnormality - seen most frequently in Shetland sheepdogs and occasionally poodles and other breeds
    a. Age of onset - six months to six years (usually two to four years)
    b. Signs - bilateral and associated with a premature breakup of the tear film. Dice divides Shetland sheepdogs into two groups: asymptomatic (those with only corneal dystrophy) and symptomatic (those with corneal dystrophy, blepharospasm and corneal ulcers).
        1) Asymptomatic - multifocal 1 to 3 mm central superficial circular or ringshaped lesions. In time, these may develop throughout the cornea.
            a) No blepharospasm
            b) Normal Schirmer tear test
            c) Tear film breakup time 6 to 10 seconds (normal controls 10 to 15 seconds)
        2) Symptomatic - usually in older dogs
            a) Blepharospasm
            b) Schirmer tear test is reduced
            c) Tear film breakup time four to six seconds
            d) Fluorescein staining may identify small punctate ulcers that precede new cholesterol deposits and some of the rings may contain superficial slit-like epithelial erosions
            e) Some rings have sealed central facets
            f) Corneal vascularization is minimal
            g) If untreated, the entire cornea may be involved, resulting in blindness
2. Punctate keratitis with extensive vascularization is characteristic but not limited to dachshunds. It may be unilateral or bilateral and is painful.

a. Initial changes - Punctate ulcers are present with marked discomfort. These are evidenced by punctate areas of corneal edema and positive fluorescein staining. Blepharospasm, epiphora, conjunctival hyperemia and superficial corneal neovascularization will be seen. Bacterial cultures will be negative.
b. Established cases - Corneal vascularization is prominent. Ulcers may coalesce, resulting in larger ulcers with new punctate lesions developing in previously unaffected areas. The appearance of the cornea at this stage must be differentiated from German shepherd pannus.
c. Advanced cases - The entire cornea may vascularize, resulting in visual impairment. Fluorescein staining may be diffuse or linear patterns. Pain is still an outstanding feature.
d. Differential diagnosis - is not a problem except in breeds predisposed to German shepherd pannus
   1) German shepherd pannus is not painful, has gradual onset, normal conjunctival blood vessels and is negative to fluorescein stain
   2) Vascularizing punctate keratitis is painful, has epiphora, injected conjunctival blood vessels and will be positive to fluorescein stain

3. Punctate keratitis in horses - Unilateral or bilateral
   a. Moderate keratitis with edema, superficial vascularization, and pain with lacrimation and photophobia
   b. Multiple superficial punctate white opacities. Some may be positive to fluorescein and others pitted and fluorescein negative
   c. In two to three weeks, some focal areas of granulation may develop
   d. Viral culture may identify EHV-I. The author has not identified EHV-I virus but the cases may have been too chronic to shed virus when presented.
   e. Punctate keratitis can also result from multiple small plant fiber foreign bodies embedded in the superficial cornea. These are very painful and may require 5-10 power magnification to be clearly seen. In these cases superficial keratectomy of the affected cornea will result in rapid healing.

Treatment

1. Cyclosporine 1% BID. Improvement is anticipated in one week and a marked response in three to four weeks. After the lesion is in remission, cyclosporine may be reduced or eventually replaced with corticosteroid preparations. If the animal relapses, cyclosporine would again be indicated. If a dog has German shepherd pannus, a combination of cyclosporine and corticosteroid therapy is probably indicated after the ulcers heal.
2. Treatment without cyclosporine - variable response
   a. Topical antibiotics QID until ulcer heals
   b. After ulcer heals, topical antibiotic/steroid combinations. Shetland sheepdogs will sometimes respond quickly to corticosteroids including ulcers, but have a variable response on long term therapy.
   c. Sodium chloride 5% ophthalmic ointment or drops are always indicated for ulcers that do not heal in 7 to 10 days
   d. Horses - Topical antivirals will usually be helpful but recurrence is frequent (in man a nonspecific beneficial response has been seen in chronic ulcers that were ***not*** caused by herpesvirus, therefore improvement seen in horses may be a nonspecific response).

Prognosis - Lifelong treatment usually needed in dogs

1. Shelty punctate keratitis - favorable if treatment started before severe dystrophy develops. Guarded if advanced corneal dystrophy.
b. Canine vascularizing punctate keratitis - favorable if owner continues treatment
c. Horses - recurrence has been reduced by cyclosporine treatment

FOCAL SUPERFICIAL NECROSIS (Corneal sequestration, cornea nigrum)

Occurrence - considered a feline disease

1. Cats - can occur in any breed but seen most frequently in Persian, Siamese, Burmese and Himalayan
2. Dogs - very rare. The author has seen corneal sequestration in dogs with hypertension and concurrent glaucoma with buphthalmos. A multiple neuropathy dog with facial and trigeminal paralysis developed a corneal sequestrum when treated with 1% epinephrine.
3. Guinea pig - author had one case after a corneal ulcer

Etiology - Although the cause is unknown, several events are consistent

1. There is always a history of signs of chronic corneal irritation or ulcers. In cats, this is frequently a complication of feline herpesvirus keratitis.
2. Animals with corneal sequestration have a dark brown discoloration to the dried mucus around the eyes and the hair at the nasal canthus. When a Schirmer tear strip is removed, the strip will have a "tea" stain from the tears
3. Lastly, this staining compound combines with the degenerating collagen to form a dark brown plaque

Clinical signs

1. Blepharospasm and epiphora with brown staining of the hair at the nasal canthus and eyelid margins
2. Accumulation of dried dark brown mucus on the eyelids and nasal canthus
3. Corneal changes
   a. Usually begin in central cornea. Early lesions may be firm and tan. Soon the lesion becomes dark brown with fluorescein staining around the perimeter.
   b. Depth involvement is variable
      1) Superficial lesions that appear elevated with distinct margins that are separating from the stroma
      2) Deep lesions with well attached margins. These lesions usually do not penetrate beyond midstroma, but they can extend to Descemet's membrane
   c. Moderate corneal vascularization

Differential diagnosis

Pigmentary keratitis will be negative to fluorescein around the periphery and lack the firmness of a sequestrum.

Treatment

1. Determine and remove the source of irritation
2. Conservative treatment - small superficial lesions may be self-limiting and slough in several weeks. Topical treatment with antibiotics or if herpesvirus is suspected, treatment with antivirals is indicated.
3. Surgical treatment is indicated if the eye is painful, the lesion is deep, or if there is no change after two to four weeks of conservative treatment
   a. Small superficial lesions with free edges can sometimes be dissected free after topical anesthesia
   b. Deep lesions require general anesthesia and a superficial keratectomy. Be cautious to not penetrate Descemet's membrane when deep involvement occurs. Lesions up to one-half corneal depth can be protected with indirect support, such as a third eyelid flap. A conjunctival flap or sliding corneoscleral graft (Fig 10-26) should be considered when the keratectomy exceeds one-half thickness.
   c. After surgery, the cornea should be treated as a fresh ulcer. If herpesvirus is suspected, specific antiviral agents (oral acyclovir, 5 mg/lb BID, and topical idoxuridine, 4-6 times daily) or 0.5% povidone-iodine QID should be administered until healing is complete.

Prognosis

The owner should be advised recurrence is possible, especially when herpesvirus is suspected. In these cases, prophylactic treatment with 0.5% Betadine in saline may be indicated.

If the brown staining characteristic of the tears persists, recurrence is likely. If the tears remain clear, the prognosis is favorable. The author has observed antibiotic/weak corticosteroid drops (Gentocin durafilm; Anaprime) will suppress the dark tear formation, but increases the risk of herpesvirus keratoconjunctivitis relapse.

NEOPLASIA

Corneal neoplasia is most common in the bovine, fairly common in horses, and uncommon in cats and dogs. Corneal tumors in all species are characterized by the adjacent corneal tissue remaining clear without a transition zone between healthy cornea and the lesion. If a corneal growth is from an inflammatory process, the adjacent cornea is edematous, opaque and usually shows vascularity.

Dogs

1. Occurrence - uncommon
2. General considerations - In the dog, neoplasms usually occur at the limbus and extend out onto the cornea. If small, excisional biopsy followed with specific treatment according to cell type is recommended. If extensive, biopsy to determine best treatment.
3. Cell types seen
    a. Squamous cell carcinoma - uncommon
    b. Melanoma (nevus) and malignant melanoma - congenital corneal melanosis (melanomas) may remain static until the animal reaches maturity and then start to grow. Primary melanomas and malignant melanomas can originate at the limbus. As the tumor extends into the cornea, it is often preceded by a cholesterol band. In some cases the tumor grows rapidly, resulting in a black spongy corneal mass with minimal scleral involvement. Remove surgically (Fig 10-9, page 296), treat surgical site with beta radiation or cryotherapy and check for malignancy. If malignant and recurs, remove the eye. Some lesions are amelanotic. Prognosis - guarded to unfavorable. See Chapter 9, page 284, for epibulbar melanomas of the cornea and sclera.
    c. Histiocytomas - usually will have concurrent lesions on the eyelid, conjunctiva and/or lip. The corneal lesion cannot be diagnosed by its clinical appearance because it looks the same as corneal lymphosarcoma and collie granuloma. Diagnosis is established with biopsy and treatment is with Cytoxan (see eyelids, Chapter 5, page 181).
    d. Corneal lymphosarcoma - rare, when seen usually has concurrent skin lesions. Diagnose by biopsy, very unfavorable prognosis. Consult with an oncologist regarding treatment.
    e. Fibrosarcoma - very rare. One case at CSU - had to remove the eye
    f. Hemangioma/hemangiosarcoma - surgical removal and beta radiation. If the lesion recurs, consider chemotherapy with vincristine or remove the eye. Hemangiomas have a favorable prognosis, hemangiosarcomas guarded to unfavorable.
    g. Viral papillomatosis - this is probably the most common corneal tumor seen in young dogs. May be limited to the cornea or have lesions of the adnexa and/or mouth. Corneal warts appear similar to beginning oral papillomas. Are quite irritating. Respond very well to surgical excision and/or cryosurgery. Author has had one case recur and it required a second surgical removal.

Cats

Corneal tumors are uncommon. Epibulbar melanomas can occur similar to dogs. Squamous cell carcinoma will usually involve conjunctiva and/or eyelids.

Horses

1. Squamous cell carcinoma is the most common corneal tumor in the horse. It is seen most frequently in animals with reduced pigmentation such as white, pinto, albino and other color dilute animals.

   If diagnosed early, they can be treated successfully. If allowed to become extensive, they may invade the orbit. Early lesions are easily confused with infectious keratitis. May appear as thin lesions or thick and fleshy. These lesions are easily confused with chronic keratitis and require impression smears or biopsy for diagnosis.

   a. Small lesions - Small lesions involving only the cornea should be removed surgically as soon as possible (Fig 10-9, page 296) and the surgical site treated with radiation, hyperthermia, or cryotherapy to prevent recurrence.
      1) Radiation - Treating the surgical area with a strontium ^{90} beta radiation source is effective. A surface dosage of 9000 rads per each application site of the applicator is recommended. Superficial lesions, less than 0.5 mm thick, can be treated without surgery.
      2) Hyperthermia - Is effective but the probe temperature must be watched carefully. Temperatures exceeding 51°C may cause corneal necrosis and scarring.
      3) Cryotherapy - Spraying is preferred to a probe, because probes may distort the cornea during freezing and mechanically damage endothelium or Descemet's membrane.
   b. Circumscribed lesions involving conjunctiva and cornea should be removed in the manner described for removal of dermoids involving the limbus (Fig 8-1; Chapter 8, page 250) The surgical site should be irradiated before the conjunctival wound is closed.
   c. Extensive lesions
      1) Surgical removal and irradiation. If all visible tumor is removed, beta radiation is very effective. If surgical removal is incomplete, beta radiation is usually effective if the remaining tumor is less than 0.5 mm thick. If thicker, implanting a radiation source in the eyelid directly above the lesion is recommended. It may be necessary to suture the eyelids together to position the radiation source over the affected cornea and sclera. The needles are left in place until the lesion can be exposed to 6000 to 9000 rads.

         If the lesion was nearly removed surgically, the reaction to radiation is minimal. If severe infiltration into the tissues is present after surgery, marked necrosis will occur after irradiation and it will take 20 to 30 days before the eye appears to be responding well. If the lesion has extended beyond the point where the eye can be saved, it should be removed.
      2) Radiation only can be used if surgery is not considered.
      3) Eye removal may be the best treatment. Primary SCC of globe is slow to metastasize, therefore enucleation has a favorable prognosis.
2. Other tumors are uncommon
   a. Corneal mast cell tumors appear like caseated material in the cornea. They grow rapidly and respond well to surgical excision and surface irradiation.
   b. Angiosarcomas - Same treatment as small animals. Guarded to unfavorable prognosis.
   c. Melanomas (corneal or epibulbar) - remove or debulk and follow with cryotherapy. Favorable prognosis.

Bovine

1. Squamous cell carcinoma - see conjunctiva (Chapter 8, page 272)
2. Young animals with viral papillomatosis can occasionally develop ocular papillomas that heal spontaneously

INTERSTITIAL KERATITIS (Deep keratitis)

Etiology

As a response to:

1. Systemic disease - canine distemper, leptospirosis in horses, pink-eye in cattle
2. Superficial infections invading deeper corneal structures
3. Deep corneal ulcers and stromal abscesses
4. Traumatic injuries
5. Secondary to anterior uveitis
6. Secondary to chronic glaucoma

Characteristics - Interstitial keratitis is the involvement of all layers of the cornea and is characterized by:

1. Marked leukoma - In horses, the edema reaction is so severe that jelly-like ripples may be seen at the epithelial surface of the cornea. Bullae may result from this severe edema.
2. Deep vascularization
3. An associated iritis
4. May or may not have hypopyon
5. Ciliary injection

Treatment - Because a secondary uveitis is present, the treatment is the same as recommended for uveitis.

1. Topical atropine
    a. To dilate pupil, thereby reducing the chance for synechia
    b. Reduce pain by relieving the ciliary spasm seen with the anterior uveitis
2. Corticosteroids - systemic and topical (do not use if ulceration is present)
3. Antibiotics (broad spectrum antibiotics if infection is suspected) - Continue all treatment until the cornea starts to clear. Then continue only the cortisone.

Sequela - corneal scarring

CORNEAL SCARRING

The fibroplasia that occurs with stromal injury or chronic corneal disease does not lay down collagen fibers in a lamellar arrangement and consequently corneal opacity results. The more rapidly cornea heals, the less the scarring. This opacity decreases in time, but severe scarring is unsightly and may interfere with vision. The affect on vision depends on location and degree of opacification, which in turn determines how it may be treated:

1. Central opacity affecting vision can be treated with central corneal transplant. See Parshall corneoscleral transposition, page 338.
2. Small scar not affecting vision can be treated cosmetically with corneal tattoo or fitted with a colored extended wear contact lens.
3. Blind eye with severe scarring can be tattooed, fitted with an extended wear contact lens, or a rigid scleral sheet (prosthesis).

Tattooing for corneal scarring

The owner should be advised that corneal tattooing is permanent and that scars will very gradually improve with time. Therefore, in the eye that is visual except for the scar, the vision after tattooing will not improve, whereas if the scar is not tattooed, vision gradually improves over the next few years.

1. Chemicals
   a. Tattooing agent - 2% platinum (IV) chloride aqueous solution. Powder and solution forms are available (Aldrich Chemical CO or Sigma Chemical Co) for preparing the 2% solution. If the powder contacts humid air for any period of time, it will solidify, but it will go back into solution when water is added. It is, therefore, suggested that 1 gm powder be divided into 100 mg units and repackaged in airtight vials. These vials can be used to make 5 ml of 2% solution.
   b. Precipitating agent - 2% hydrazine in water. Hydrazine anhydrous (Sigma Chemical Co) is diluted to 2% in distilled water. 0.5 ml of hydrazine q.s. to 25 ml with distilled water is suggested. Hydrazine is stable when refrigerated; therefore, keep refrigerated when not in use. It crystallizes at 0°C and will return to solution as the temperature rises. ***Caution: Hydrazine is explosive and has been identified as being a carcinogen!*** Therefore, it should be handled cautiously. We have not observed any problems in animals that have had their corneas tattooed.
2. Filter paper method of pretesting solutions - solutions should be shaken before using. Place 3 to 4 drops of 2% platinic chloride on filter paper. After the platinic chloride soaks into the paper, a slight yellow stain will be noted. Add 1 to 2 drops of 2% hydrazine to the same area. Black precipitation will begin in 30 seconds and be complete in 5 minutes. If this test does not work, it is possible that the platinic chloride or hydrazine have become contaminated or are inactive, and fresh solutions should be prepared.
3. Test tattooing of cadaver cornea - remove a cadaver eye and keep it moist until the test is performed. The test technique is as follows:
   a. Scrape epithelium from central cornea
   b. Apply 2% platinic chloride to abraded cornea with a cotton applicator until the cornea takes on a yellow-brown cast. This should take 1 to 2 minutes. Use a new cotton applicator whenever additional platinic chloride is needed. This will avoid contamination of the dispensing bottle.
   c. With a new cotton applicator, apply 2% hydrazine to the pretreated area. Continue to work hydrazine into the cornea until change is prominent. The time for color change in the cornea is similar to the filter paper test. It begins in 30 seconds to 1 minute and is complete in 5 to 7 minutes.

4. Tattoo technique
   a. General anesthesia is needed
   b. Stabilize the eyelids with a retractor, and the globe with forceps placed at the limbus
   c. Remove corneal epithelium from the scarred area. Rubbing the area with a scalpel blade is satisfactory.
   d. Platinic chloride 2% is applied to the corneal abrasion using a cotton applicator. The platinic chloride is applied and pressed into the tissues for a period of 2 or 3 minutes. Care is taken to avoid allowing any tears to come across the abraded cornea at this time. Tears into this area will dilute the platinic chloride and wash it away, interfering with tissue absorption. The cornea takes on a yellow stain after it has been saturated with platinic chloride.
   e. Hydrazine 2% is applied next with a new cotton applicator. Continue to apply hydrazine until a deep black color develops within the cornea. Note that the corneal stroma will have absorbed platinic chloride and hydrazine, which will result in precipitation of black stain 1 or 2 mm into subepithelial clear stroma beyond the limit of the epithelial abrasion.
   f. If the scarred area is not adequately tattooed, the procedure can be repeated.
   g. After tattooing is complete, the cornea and conjunctival sac should be thoroughly irrigated with saline to wash away any excess chemicals.
5. *Comment:* corneas that have been tattooed heal in the same fashion as any other noninfected superficial corneal abrasion; therefore, they should be treated with antibiotics to prevent reinfection and topical atropine to control secondary pain due to sympathetic uveitis.

Colored extended wear contact lenses (Cutting Edge) - can be used to improve the appearance of a visual or nonvisual eye. They have been used most extensively in show horses. Following topical anesthesia, the colored contact lens is placed on the cornea. Continuous wear is not recommended. Owners should be advised that a horse with an irregular corneal surface is predisposed to losing the lens.

Corneoscleral shell (prosthesis) - a 1-2 mm thick rigid prosthesis can be fabricated that fits the cornea and sclera precisely. Normal iris and scleral features are painted on the prosthesis. These can be prepared by an ocularist from a casting made from the eye as described in Chapter 17, page 487 for phthisis bulbi. This prosthesis is recommended only for the blind eye. Topical anesthesia is needed for placement and removal. They are indicated for short term (daily) use because they do not permit normal corneal oxygenation from the atmosphere and therefore would be damaging to the cornea with extended wear.

INFECTIOUS CANINE HEPATITIS (ICH) OCULAR CHANGES ("BLUE EYE")

An acute reaction may occur in dogs recovering from natural infection with street virus or after vaccination with canine adenovirus I (CAV-I). In naturally occurring hepatitis, the reaction can occur in about 20% of the recovering cases. It is routinely mild and clears up spontaneously. I have seen only one clinical case where there was some permanent corneal damage. The reaction is much more severe when observed from CAV-I vaccine and is much more likely to have complications. Canine adenovirus II (CAV-II) will protect against hepatitis and has a remote chance, if any, to cause an ocular reaction.

Pathogenesis

1. After vaccination with canine adenovirus I (CAV-I) or during natural infection, there is a viremia with virus localization in the iris and corneal endothelium
2. This will be followed by primary iridocyclitis that generally resolves without clinical evidence or sequela. This uveitis is often unnoticed.
3. In some cases virus persists in the anterior uvea and cornea. Local antibody production occurs that reacts with the cell-associated viral antigen and initiates a focal hypersensitivity of the Arthus type. Increased vascular permeability allows diffusion of serum antibodies into the anterior uvea, aqueous and cornea making the reaction more severe. This can occur from 7 to 28 days after vaccination. Most occur by 14 days.

Clinical signs - Usually occurs in one eye but both may be involved. If both are involved, they are usually affected to different degrees. Usually the owner is unaware of the reaction until it has been present for 12 to 24 hours.

1. Initial - a ciliary flush to the bulbar conjunctiva
2. By 8 to 12 hours - flush increases to mild chemosis and photophobia develops. Close examination reveals anterior uveitis with iris edema and aqueous flare
3. By 18 hours - severe anterior uveitis, intense ciliary flush, marked chemosis, blepharospasm and photophobia. The eye is hypotonic.
4. By 24 hours - corneal edema resulting in "blue cornea". Clumps of coagulated protein may be present in the anterior chamber and pupil. The fundus often cannot be visualized.
5. Course - without treatment, 21 to 28 days.

Treatment - Treat like any other uveitis and interstitial keratitis

1. Topical atropine to relieve pain and dilate pupil
2. Systemic corticosteroids to stop the hypersensitivity reaction. Continue for at least two weeks.
3. Antibiotics are not needed unless secondary infection develops.

Complications

1. Endothelial damage
2. Chronic anterior uveitis
3. Glaucoma

Comment

Infectious canine hepatitis ocular reactions to CAV-I vaccine are serious enough in breeds prone to glaucoma to warrant delaying hepatitis immunization until 6 to 12 months of age. Reaction to CAV-II vaccine is so rare that the author does not hesitate recommending vaccination to any breed in accordance with the manufacturer's recommendations.

ULCERATIVE KERATITIS (GENERAL CONSIDERATIONS)

Causes

1. Mechanical
   a. Abrasions - clippers while grooming dogs with prominent eyes; can be self-inflicted from rubbing at the head; ropes and whips in horses
   b. Eyelash diseases
   c. Foreign bodies
   d. Exposure due to prolapsed eyes, eyelid paralysis, or general anesthesia
   e. Entropion
2. Chemical
   a. Soap/detergents
   b. Acids/alkalies
   c. Insect repellents
3. Infectious
   a. Local - most require a break in the epithelium
      1) Bacterial - *Moraxella, Strep, Staph, Pseudomonas, E. coli*
      2) Mycotic (primarily equine) - *Aspergillus, Fusarium, Alternaria, Mucor*
   b. Systemic diseases
      1) Viral - feline herpesvirus; equine herpesvirus I has been proposed
      2) *Chlamydia* and *mycoplasma* - sheep and goats
4. Metabolic
   a. Keratoconjunctivitis sicca
   b. Endothelial disease leading to bullae formation and epithelial erosion
   c. Hypoandrogenism (neutering or senile) may be a contributing factor in indolent ulcers
5. Neurotropic - failure of sensory innervation ophthalmic branch of CN V
6. Immune mediated punctate keratitis

Signs

1. Pain - manifested by blepharospasm. The cornea is very sensitive and ulcers are painful. In addition, secondary uveitis produces ciliary muscle spasm, resulting in intraocular pain (photophobia).
2. Epiphora - serous or purulent discharges may occur
3. Conjunctivitis - the degree is usually proportional to the severity of the ulcers
4. Corneal changes
   a. Loss of transparency - When the epithelium is disrupted, the stroma imbibes fluid and the cornea becomes cloudy. The more severe the damage, the greater the opacity. Deep ulcers will become clear when Descemet's membrane becomes exposed. Descemet's membrane does not imbibe fluid and therefore remains clear. Therefore, clearing in the center of an ulcer is an unfavorable sign because it indicates exposure of Descemet's membrane.

      The cornea in some superficial ulcers remains quite clear. This is because the outer glycoprotein layer of the stroma is not disturbed and therefore the cornea does not take on much fluid.
   b. Vascularization - The natural response to corneal damage is vascularization. It begins three to six days after injury or ulceration and progresses in from the limbus at a rate of approximately 1 mm per day.
   c. Change in contour - deep ulcers are easily seen. Superficial are often hard to distinguish without staining.
      1) Superficial ulcers with only epithelial erosion appear smooth. As the ulcer becomes deeper, excavation of the stroma will be obvious.
      2) Rapid collagenase breakdown (melting ulcer) is indicated by the ulcer being filled with white gelatinous debris. This is an unfavorable sign and warrants immediate intensive treatment.
      3) The extent of corneal edema surrounding the ulcer will correlate with the degree of compromise of endothelial integrity. Severely damaged endothelium will allow fluorescein to pass into the anterior chamber resulting in a green tint to the aqueous.

        4) Slit lamp examination facilitates determination of ulcer depth and the degree of edema in adjacent cornea
5. Anterior chamber and iris changes do not become obvious unless stromal involvement is present.
    a. Anterior uveitis results with stromal involvement
    b. ± aqueous flare
    c. ± hypopyon

Diagnosis - Diagnosis is based on clinical examination and fluorescein staining.

Management of corneal ulcers - ***Three basic steps must be considered in the management of all corneal ulcers.*** These are:

1. Determine the initiating cause
2. Appropriate medical treatment
3. Protect and/or support the cornea

Determine cause

1. Thorough examination to identify and remove any physical cause, including fluorescein staining.
    a. Schirmer tear test
    b. Fluorescein staining
2. If refractory or progressing rapidly:
    a. Cultures - conjunctival sac and ulcer (this is done before fluorescein staining)
    b. Cytology - from the ulcer

Medical management

1. Topical medical treatment - usually adequate for most ulcers that occur in healthy cornea.
    a. Control infection - Frequency of medication depends on severity and etiology of the ulcer. Hourly with melting ulcers, QID for less severe.
        1) Bacterial - may need to do cultures to determine best drugs. Try a broad spectrum antibiotic initially (e.g. gentamicin or neomycin-polymyxin-bacitracin mixtures). Culture and sensitivity results will determine the most appropriate antibiotic.
        2) Viral - herpes ulcers in cats can be treated with idoxuridine if acute or dilute Betadine if chronic
        3) Mycotic - require frequent treatment (every 1 to 2 hrs), therefore medicine delivery systems are usually recommended.
        4) Chlamydia - tetracyclines drug of choice
    b. Relieve pain with a cycloplegic - Atropine three or four times daily, then may reduce to BID after several days
    c. Anticollagenase for stromal ulcers showing rapid collagen breakdown or more than five days duration (see page 123)
        1) Topical - acetylcysteine is very effective
        2) Topical immunoglobulins (alpha macroglobulins) - fresh or immune serum (tetanus antitoxin)
        The ulcer healing capability of fresh blood has been observed for over 100 years. Physicians were treating corneal ulcers with fresh blood drawn from their patients in the late 1800's. Similar treatment was also being used by ranchers. Calves with ulcers were roped and held down while a knife incision was made along the inside of the upper eyelid. Then salt would be sprinkled on the eye and the animal released.
    d. Ulcer solution contains the topical medications beneficial for ulcer treatment (Table 10-1)
    e. Anti-inflammatory agents
        1) Corticosteroids are contraindicated in infectious ulcers or any ulcer showing collagen breakdown. They can be used with caution in ulcers associated with immune responses.
        2) Antiprostaglandin preparations can be used topically in ulcers with collagenase activity

Table 10-1. Ulcer solution

ULCER SOLUTION CONTAINS

1. Antibiotic - to control bacterial infection*
2. Acetylcysteine - to provide anticollagenase activity and speed ulcer healing
3. Atropine sulfate - to relieve ciliary spasm and intraocular pain
4. Artificial tear - as a qs agent and contact-prolonging carrier

INGREDIENTS (to make 24 ml)

Amount used	Final concentration in drop
1.25 ml chloramphenicol succinate or,*	1%
1.5 ml 5% gentamicin	0.3%
1.8 ml 4% tobramycin	0.3%
6 ml 20% acetylcysteine**	5%
6 ml 1% atropine ophthalmic solution ***	0.25%
Artificial tears to qs to 24 ml	31% of volume

Chloramphenicol is present in proprietary ophthalmic preparations at concentrations of 5 to 10 mg/ml, gentamicin 3 mg/ml, and tobramycin 3mg/ml. Acetylcysteine should be 5% concentration. Irritation has occurred with concentrations that were over 5%. Atropine should be at least 0.25% to produce desired results. Artificial tear is the qs agent and the concentration is dependent on amount of other preparations.

An opened bottle of acetylcysteine will keep six months if tightly capped and refrigerated. This mixture will keep its potency at room temperature for two months. We dispense a 5 cc ophthalmic dropper bottle and show the owner how to fill the dropper bottle. We instruct them to keep this bottle at room temperature and the stock bottle in the refrigerator.

The frequency of administration will vary as to the owner's capability in medicating the eye. We generally recommend hourly treatment the first day, every two hours the second, and decrease the frequency until the animal is being treated three to six times a day. Patients are re-examined in five days. We have been pleased with the rate of ulcer healing using this mixture.

* Chloramphenicol, gentamicin and tobramycin are reasonable presumptive choices. When culture results are available, the most appropriate antibiotic should be chosen. Fortified antibiotic concentrations are indicated in severely infected ulcers. Refer to Table 2-4, page 83 for antibiotic concentrations recommended to prepare fortified ophthalmic solutions.

** Mucosil 20%, Dey Laboratories Inc, Napa, CA 94558 or Dallas, TX 75238-8880, (214)349-7275; or a local distributor (In Colorado, Stuarts Drug and Surgical, Denver, CO 800-833-4112).

*** Atropine can result in decreased gut motility in horses and should be used cautiously after mydriasis occurs.

2. Subconjunctival injection used most frequently in horses. Can be used to supplement topical treatment or in place of it when routine topical treatment is not possible.
   a. Indications
      1) Rapidly developing deep ulcers
      2) Patients that can only be treated every few days
      3) Refractory ulcers that have not responded to routine topical treatment
   b. Drugs injected
      1) Antibiotics (see Table 2-4; Chapter 2, page 83) - gentamicin, chloramphenicol, or tobramycin are most frequently used
      2) Mydriatic/cycloplegics - atropine (1 mg), or atropine (1 mg) and phenylephrine (5 mg) mixture
      3) Fresh or immune serum - equine tetanus antitoxin can be used in all species (small animals 0.3 ml, large animals 0.3 to 0.75 ml)

4) *Comment* - Antibiotic and antitoxin can be mixed in the same syringe

3. Systemic medications
   a. Anti-inflammatory drugs to reduce secondary uveitis
      1) ***Systemic corticosteroids will not interfere with ulcer healing***
      2) Systemic antiprostaglandins are very beneficial in horses with severe pain and ocular inflammation
   b. Antimicrobial drugs
      1) Antibiotics usually have no effect on corneal ulcers
      2) Acyclovir in acute feline herpesvirus ulcers
      3) Systemic antifungals may be helpful in horses with severe mycotic ulcers

Protect and/or support the cornea

Protection is a necessary and important step when treating rapidly developing, deep or refractory ulcers. Protection alone will heal many ulcers. In man, the first step is to bandage the eye and thus protect the cornea. Selection of specific method is determined by the characteristics of the ulcer.

1. Indirect means of support - Generally indicated for the treatment of epithelial or superficial stromal ulcers where protection is the main goal. These are simple procedures that can be performed with minimal instruments and anesthesia.
   a. Third eyelid flap
   b. Temporary tarsorrhaphy
   c. Extended wear contact lens
   d. Collagen shield
   e. Bandage or hood
2. Direct forms of support - should be considered in rapidly developing ulcers more than 1/3 depth of stroma or chronic ulcers more than 1/2 thickness.
   a. Conjunctival flaps
      1) Limbal-based flaps provide immediate blood supply and support. The blood supply provides continuous anticollagenase activity.
      2) Free grafts give support but DO NOT provide blood supply
   b. Suturing - useful on small deep ulcers
   c. Corneoscleral transposition - maintains visual cornea
   d. Corneal transplant - primarily a bandage. Cornea will usually become opaque.
   e. Adhesives - give temporary support but may slough before ulcer heals. If too thick, may result in a foreign body reaction.
3. In horses, fly screens or protective hoods are good protection. All horses with adnexal and corneal problems should be fed on the ground rather than using hay feeders.

REFRACTORY SUPERFICIAL ULCERS, GENERAL

Refractory ulcers are ulcers that do not heal in 7 to 10 days with normal treatment. If allowed to continue, they may become undermined. When this happens, they will not heal without surgical and medical treatment. They have some form of maintaining cause that must be corrected before they will respond to medical treatment. See punctate keratitis.

Causes

1. Dogs - Most are the result of mechanical cause. Diseases for special consideration are:
    a. Misplaced eyelashes are a most common cause for refractory canine ulcers
    b. KCS
    c. Basement membrane disease
    d. Senile lack of regenerative ability (especially neutered animals)
    e. Chronic corneal edema due to endothelial disease
2. Cats
    a. Chronic herpesvirus ulcers
    b. Basement membrane disease
3. Equine - Chronic ulcers less frequent than small animals
    a. Foreign bodies adherent to palpebral conjunctiva
    b. Corneal erosion from persistent corneal edema after periodic ophthalmia
    c. Basement membrane disease
    d. Treatment with corticosteroids. Occasionally patients are presented with superficial ulcers of two or three weeks duration with a history of topical corticosteroid therapy. When this is stopped, the ulcer heals within a week with minimal topical treatment.
4. Bovine - Refractory ulcers are uncommon in the bovine because of the great corneal regenerative ability. Most are the result of mechanical irritation from adnexal foreign bodies.

Examination and diagnostic procedures

1. Remove mechanical cause and most will then heal spontaneously
2. If no obvious cause, it may be well to:
    a. Do culture and sensitivity
        1) Bacterial
        2) Chlamydia
        3) Mycoplasma
        4) Feline herpesvirus
    b. Make corneal impression smears and scrapings for cytology and FA testing.
    c. Be sure to measure tear production

Treatment

1. Control infection with topical medication
    a. If bacterial, specific antibiotics. Start out with broad spectrum and as soon as culture results are available, switch to most effective agent. This can be combined in ulcer solution.
    b. Feline herpesvirus. Topical and systemic antivirals; if chronic or for prophylaxis, dilute Betadine 1:20 to 1:10 drops.
2. Nonspecific response to topical Idoxuridine (IDU) has been reported of value for some chronic sterile ulcers in man. The mechanism for this is unknown. This may account for the benefit reported in some ulcers in animals.
3. Subconjunctival injection with antibiotics and tetanus antitoxin. This can be repeated in three to five days.

4. Agents that promote healing
    a. Topical 5% NaCl ointment or drops TID to QID until ulcer is healed, and continue for 30 to 60 days
    b. Hormone replacement - see corneal erosion
    c. Good nutrition and vitamins
    d. Consider eye protection - small animals: third eyelid flap, extended wear contact lens or collagen shield; large animals: contact lens or collagen shield

BASEMENT MEMBRANE DISEASE (CORNEAL EROSION, INDOLENT ULCER, BOXER ULCER)

Incidence - common

1. Species - seen primarily in dogs, less frequently in cats and horses
2. Canine breed predisposition - usually seen in dogs six years or older (boxer, Samoyed, dachshund, miniature poodle, Welsh corgi, wire hair fox terrier
3. Sex - no proven sex predisposition. The author feels neutered animals of either sex are predisposed.

Etiology - It is associated with degeneration in the basal epithelial cells and their basement membrane leading to delayed healing following epithelial injury.

1. Studies of human chronic corneal ulcers revealed that frequently the tears had a high plasmin activity (Salonen et al 1987). Plasmin, a proteinase, interferes with fibronectin, a glycoprotein that anchors regenerating epithelial cells to the basement membrane. Fibronectin is very susceptible to proteinases. Therefore, mild proteolytic activity will neutralize surface fibronectin and detach epithelial cells from their substratum. Plasmin is derived from plasminogen, a proenzyme present in large quantities in body fluids.
2. Increased proteolytic activity of the tear film is present in most dogs with erosion and returns to normal when the erosion heals (Willeford, Miller and Abrams, 1997).
3. Chronic corneal edema from corneal endothelial degeneration can be a predisposing cause leading to corneal bullae that rupture and become recurrent erosions.

Signs - may be unilateral or bilateral

1. Mild pain - evidenced by mild epiphora and blepharospasm
2. Corneal transparency - the cornea remains clear except in the area of the ulcer, which can take on mild leukoma. This indicates the ulcer is superficial.
3. Minimal corneal vascularization - some ulcers do not cause any vascularization. Others only minimal reaction. It may take months before vascularization will lead to granulation tissue and healing.
4. Fluorescein stain - reveals epithelial undermining

Treatment

Examine the eye thoroughly to determine the cause of the initial epithelial defect that preceded the corneal erosion and if possible, control the initiating cause along with symptomatic treatment of the erosion. Symptomatic treatment objectives are:
- Surgical treatment of ulcer (epithelial debridement)
- Appropriate medical management
- Corneal protection (if necessary)

1. Surgical treatment
    a. Remove the undermined epithelium (Fig 10-12). Topical anesthesia is usually adequate but in some cases chemical restraint may be necessary. A cotton swab soaked in dilute Betadine 0.5% in PSS is excellent to debride the epithelium. Diseased epithelium rubs off without effort. Therefore, the debrided area will be larger than the original erosion. Healthy epithelium cannot be rubbed away unless the cornea is allowed to dry out or an epithelial toxic agent has contacted the cornea.

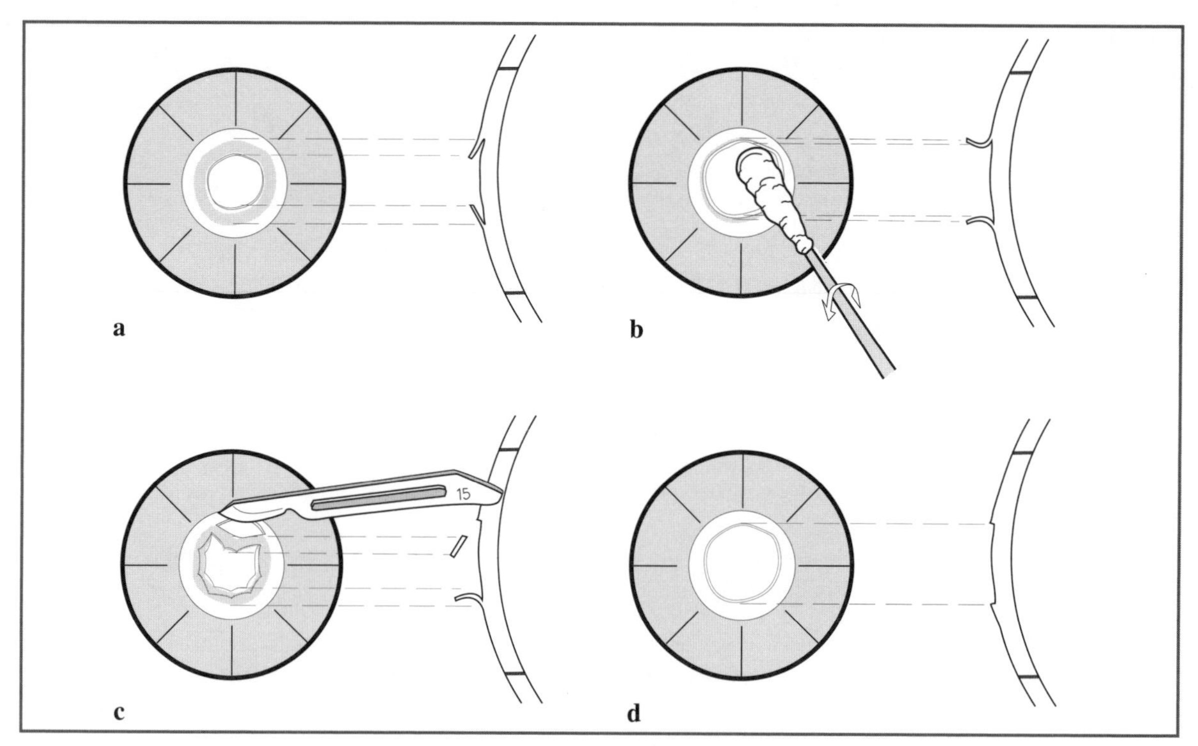

Figure 10-12. Debridement of undermined corneal ulcer (erosion).
a. Frontal and cross-section view of ulcer showing undermined zone
b. Cotton swab soaked with dilute Betadine being used to rub loosened epithelium back to where it is securely attached
c. Cutting loosened epithelium from cornea with a sharp blade
d. Appearance of ulcer after debridement

b. Prepare the ulcer surface for epithelial regrowth
   1) Superficial keratotomy - to provide anchoring sites for the regenerating epithelium
      a) Multiple punctate keratotomy (Fig 10-13) using a 20 gauge needle. The needle is pressed against cornea causing superficial penetrations (1/4 to 1/3 thickness). These multiple punctures are spaced 0.5 to 1.0 mm over the lesion.
      b) Multiple linear keratotomy (Fig 10-14) - using a #15 Bard Parker blade or the sharp edge of a 20 or 22 gauge needle with the tip bent at a 90° angle. Multiple scratches are made 0.5 to 1 mm apart in a crosshatching pattern.

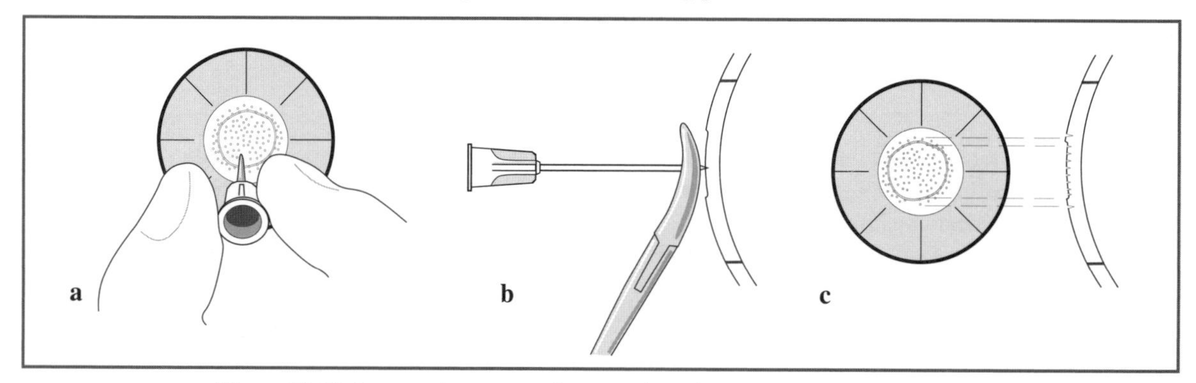

Figure 10-13. Punctate keratotomy for corneal erosion.
a. Multiple punctate perforations with the surgeon holding a 20 gauge needle. Keratotomy depth is 1/4 to 1/3 corneal thickness and 0.5 to 0.1 mm apart
b. Punctate keratotomy performed with 20 gauge needle held with mosquito forceps
c. Appearance of cornea after punctate keratotomy

2) In rare situations, the superficial layers of the ulcerated cornea are damaged to the extent that regenerating epithelium cannot reattach. When this occurs, superficial keratectomy to the depth of normal stroma may be necessary.

2. Medical treatment
   a. Antiprotease drugs (see page 123 for details) - 2-4 times daily
      1) Acetylcysteine 5% - indicated if stromal involvement is present

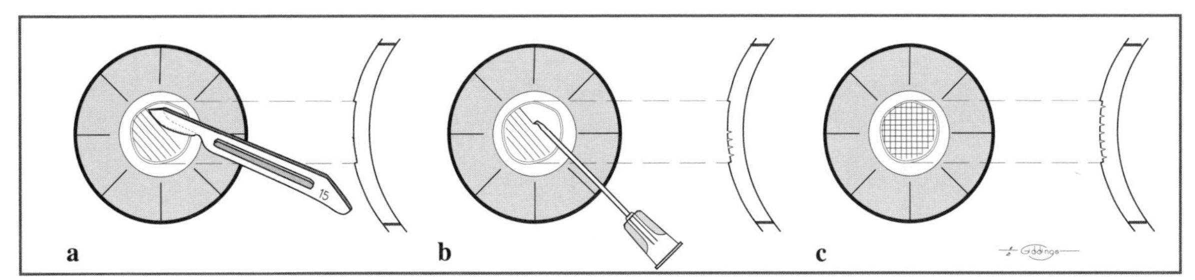

Figure 10-14. Multiple linear keratotomy for corneal erosion.
a. Crosshatching with #15 Bard-Parker blade
b. Crosshatching with a 22 gauge needle with the tip at a 90° angle
c. Appearance of ulcer after crosshatching

      2) Polysulfated glycosaminoglycan (Adequan) 5% solution - has been reported to be 70-80% effective. (See page 123)
      3) Fresh serum - has epithelial growth factors as well as antiprotease activity.
   b. Antibiotics - 2-4 times daily. Optional as prophylactic treatment to prevent infection.
   c. 5% sodium chloride ophthalmic ointment or solution QID to reduce edema and enhance epithelial reattachment. This should be continued for one to two months after the erosion heals.
   d. Experimental
      1) Topical epidermal growth factor 100 μg/ml QID has been studied and found effective (price is prohibitive).
      2) Topical fibronectin has been shown to be beneficial
      3) Topical aprotinin is helpful in man; benefit in animals is questionable. See page 123.
   e. If the patient has been neutered, the author feels replacement hormones have been beneficial, especially to prevent recurrence. Depending on the size of the dog, 1 to 4 mg diethylstilbestrol initially with 1 mg every 5 to 10 days for maintenance. This can be used in males or females. Testosterone will assist healing in old males with testicular atrophy. Intact females with a history of irregular heat periods or anestrus with hypothyroidism can benefit from short term estrogen therapy.

3. Corneal support or protection - Epithelial debridement, keratotomy and medical treatment will be successful in most cases. If the erosion is not healing after 7 to 10 days, or if undermining is recurring, repeat previous treatment and consider some form of corneal support or protection.
   a. Collagen shield (Soft Shield®, Oasis). Although it may not be necessary, the author automatically places a shield after surgical treatment. This breaks the corneal pain cycle, thus reducing blepharospasm and any tendency for the dog to rub the eye.
   b. Extended wear contact lenses (Cutting Edge, Diamond Springs, CA) can be placed for two to four weeks. They protect the new epithelium until it is firmly attached to the cornea. A temporary tarsorrhaphy suture may be needed to retain the contact.
   c. Third eyelid flap - should be left in place a minimum of two weeks
   d. Surgical adhesive - application of a thin layer to the erosion site has been recommended. Be careful to not use excess adhesive because it may result in a foreign body reaction
   e. Conjunctival flaps may be necessary in refractory erosion cases secondary to corneal edema from endothelial degeneration.

Prognosis - Recurrence rate is about 50%, less frequent with hormone replacement

Favorable unless:
1. Deep ulceration secondary to infection becomes a complication
2. The patient has corneal endothelial degeneration resulting in severe corneal edema

SUPERFICIAL STROMAL ULCERS (Less than 1/3 thickness)

Superficial stromal ulcers will usually heal quickly after initiating cause has been identified and sound medical treatment started.

If proper topical medical treatment cannot be provided in horses, subconjunctival injections of antibiotic and atropine every two to three days or a medication delivery tube may be necessary.

If there are predisposing factors for delayed healing (prominent eye, reduced tear production, neurogenic diseases), indirect protection and support with a third eyelid flap or temporary tarsorrhaphy is indicated.

Tarsorrhaphy or third eyelid flaps are usually left in place two weeks.

Reasons to take flaps or tarsorrhaphy down before two weeks:

1. If obvious improvement is not noticed in five days (decreased blepharospasm, relief of enophthalmos, reduction of ocular discharge)
2. Development of acute pain, bloody discharge, or recurrence of purulent discharge

DEEP ULCERS

Deep ulcers are dangerous since perforation will result in prolapse of the iris. The most important features of treating deep ulcers are to provide mechanical support to the weakened cornea and stop further corneal destruction with sound medical management.

Causes

1. Deep injuries that become infected
2. Bacterial infections with highly destructive capability (*Pseudomonas, Staph, and E. coli*)
3. Mycotic infections in horses
4. Protruding eyes - Pekingese and related breeds are very subject to deep central ulcers
5. Corticosteroid therapy on collagenase-producing corneas
6. Cattle with severe pink-eye ulcers
7. Feline herpetic ulcers with stromal involvement
8. Canine distemper with ulcers complicated by decreased tearing

Treatment of large ulcers without immediate danger of rupture (chronic ulcers less than 1/2 depth with peripheral corneal vascularization)

1. Support cornea
   a. Small animals - suture third eyelid
   b. Large animals - suture eyelids.
   c. Leave protective tarsorrhaphies up to 7 to 14 days, depending on the diameter and depth of the ulcer. It is difficult to leave a flap up or the eyelids sutured together when one is worried about the cornea undergoing further deterioration. As long as healing appears to be progressing satisfactorily, it should be left alone.
2. Favorable signs that would go along with proper healing
   a. Clear ocular discharge
   b. Holding the eyelids open exposing the sutured-up third eyelid
   c. The contour of the affected eye will be the same as the healthy eye
3. Unfavorable signs that would warrant taking out the third eyelid sutures to examine the eye
   a. Hemorrhage appearing in the discharge or discharge showing increase in pus
   b. Evidence of acute pain
   c. Holding the eyelids tightly together when they were previously open
   d. The eye contour is flat or severely enophthalmic

Small, deep ulcer with danger of perforation - These are usually central in dogs with prominent eyes.

1. Suture the edges of ulcer together with absorbable suture (Fig 10-15). Use horizontal mattress sutures that are placed the depth of the ulcer. Preplace the sutures and then draw tight slowly. Allow the cornea to stretch and aqueous to pass out the filtration angle. This may take three to five minutes. DO NOT RUSH IT. Ulcers up to 5 mm in diameter can be closed in this fashion. The cornea will be flattened and distorted but is self-correcting in the next few days.
   a. Third eyelid flap or tarsorrhaphy if cornea was weakened with severe edema or collagenase activity
   b. In horses, subconjunctival injection with tetanus antitoxin and antibiotic
   c. Ulcer solution topically
   d. If possible, leave sutures in place 14 days. Then remove the sutures from the third eyelid and allow corneal sutures to come out spontaneously. If the third eyelid flap starts to come down earlier, remove the sutures holding it. The corneal sutures can be removed when granulation tissue fills between the edges of the ulcer.

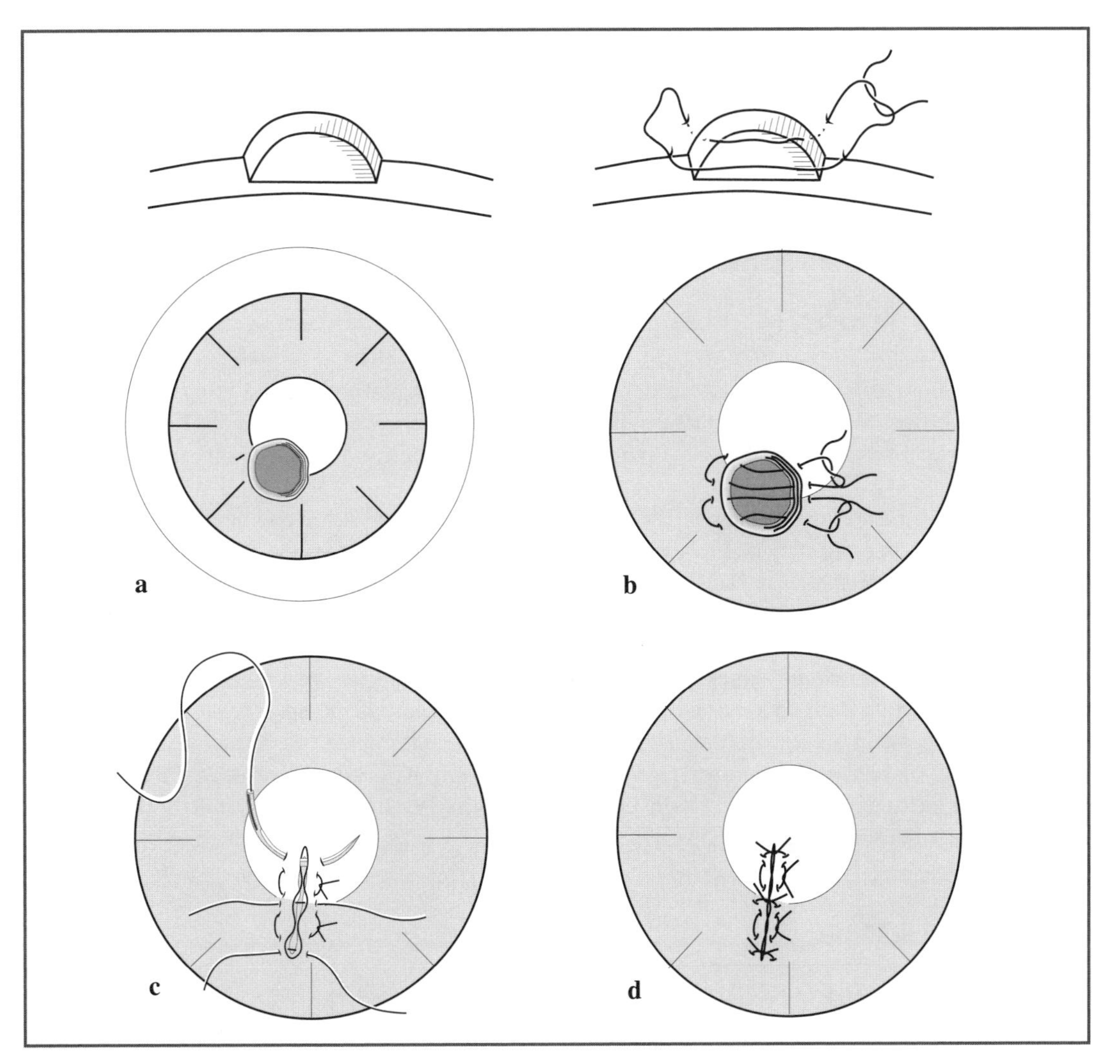

Figure 10-15. Suturing small deep ulcer.
   a. Frontal and cross-section diagrams of ulcer
   b. Two horizontal mattress sutures placed in ulcer. Small ulcers can be closed with one horizontal suture.
   c. Horizontal sutures are slowly drawn tight. If the epithelial edges do not appose satisfactorily, simple interrupted sutures can be placed between the mattress sutures for additional support.
   d. Appearance after all sutures are tied. The cornea is flattened at this time but will return to normal shape in several days.

2. Pedicle conjunctival flap
    a. Will provide blood supply and is the safest procedure if there is any question of the healing ability of the cornea
    b. Further support is usually not needed
    c. Topical medication with ulcer solution advisable for next 7 to 10 days
    d. Flap can be removed after six weeks
3. Free conjunctival graft - Is suitable if cornea is healthy and vascularization is approaching the ulcer
4. Corneal adhesives - maintain support for about seven days, then corneal vascularization is necessary for final healing

Treatment of large deep ulcers with potential to perforate

1. Preferred treatment direct support
    a. Conjunctival flap
    b. Supporting keratoplasty
        1) Lamellar corneal transplant
        2) Corneoscleral transposition
2. If direct repair is not possible, then a third eyelid flap or tarsorrhaphy can be used, but a ***guarded*** prognosis should be given.
    a. Cattle (food animals) have very regenerative corneas, therefore third eyelid-eyelid combination flaps are usually adequate to maintain a visual cornea
    b. Cats have a very strong Descemet's membrane. If the cornea was healthy before the ulcer developed, they have a reasonable chance to heal with indirect support.

CONJUNCTIVAL FLAPS

The most common means of supporting the deep corneal ulcers and perforation and bringing blood supply directly to the cornea. Follow-up treatment is directed more toward systemic antibiotics because the flap will provide direct blood supply to the tissues. Frequency of topical medication can be reduced.

Conjunctival flaps should involve the conjunctiva only. Conjunctiva is elastic and nearly transparent. If deep tissues, such as Tenon's capsule, are included with the conjunctiva, it reduces the elasticity of the flap, making it more difficult to position. Thick flaps are not transparent, therefore will interfere with sight. If there is severe corneal degeneration the entire flap may be left permanently. In this case, a thin flap is transparent enough to permit some vision. Thin flaps are difficult to dissect until the surgeon has gained some experience handling the conjunctiva. Some surgeons prefer a subconjunctival injection of a small amount of PSS to help separate the conjunctiva from underlying tissues. Absorbable sutures, 7-0 to 8-0, are recommended for small animals and 6-0 to 7-0 in horses. Suture patterns may be simple interrupted or continuous. If a continuous pattern is used, 2 or 3 anchoring sutures are recommended first. After transposition, the deep conjunctival surface will adhere to any area where corneal epithelium is missing. It will not adhere to cornea with intact epithelium. Most flaps have served their purpose in four to six weeks and the nonadhering stalk can be removed.

Peripheral flap (Fig 10-16)

An incision is made through the conjunctiva at the limbus. The conjunctiva is liberally undermined from Tenon's capsule with fine blunt scissors (corneal or strabismus). If tags of Tenon's capsule are adherent to the flap, they are trimmed free. A suture is placed at each end of the flap and it is anchored to the sclera at the limbus. Flaps that are perpendicular to the motion of the eyelid will adhere to the ulcer quickly and require minimal suturing to the cornea. Flaps that are not perpendicular require suturing along the edge of the ulcer.

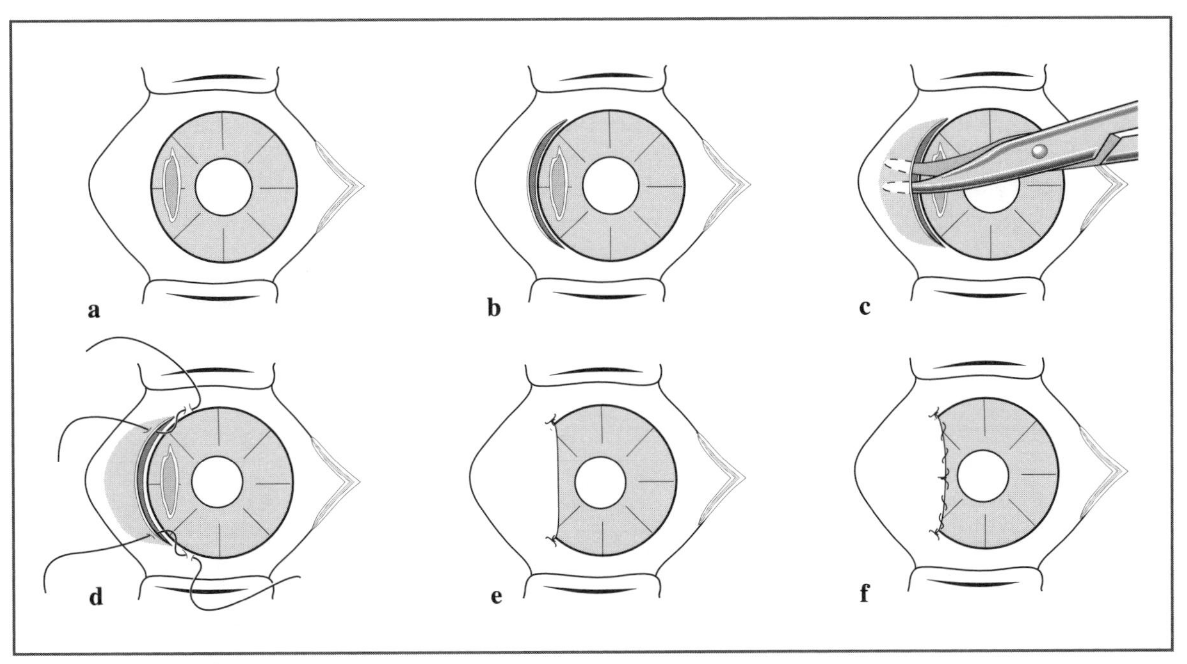

Figure 10-16.1. Peripheral conjunctival flap for corneal lesion near limbus.

a. Appearance of peripheral ulcer.
b. A perilimbal conjunctival incision is made adjacent to the wound
c. Undermining the conjunctiva with blunt scissors
d. Sutures are placed in the sclera at the limbus and along the edge of the undermined conjunctiva
e. Sutures tied at the limbus
f. Appearance of flap if margins sutured to cornea

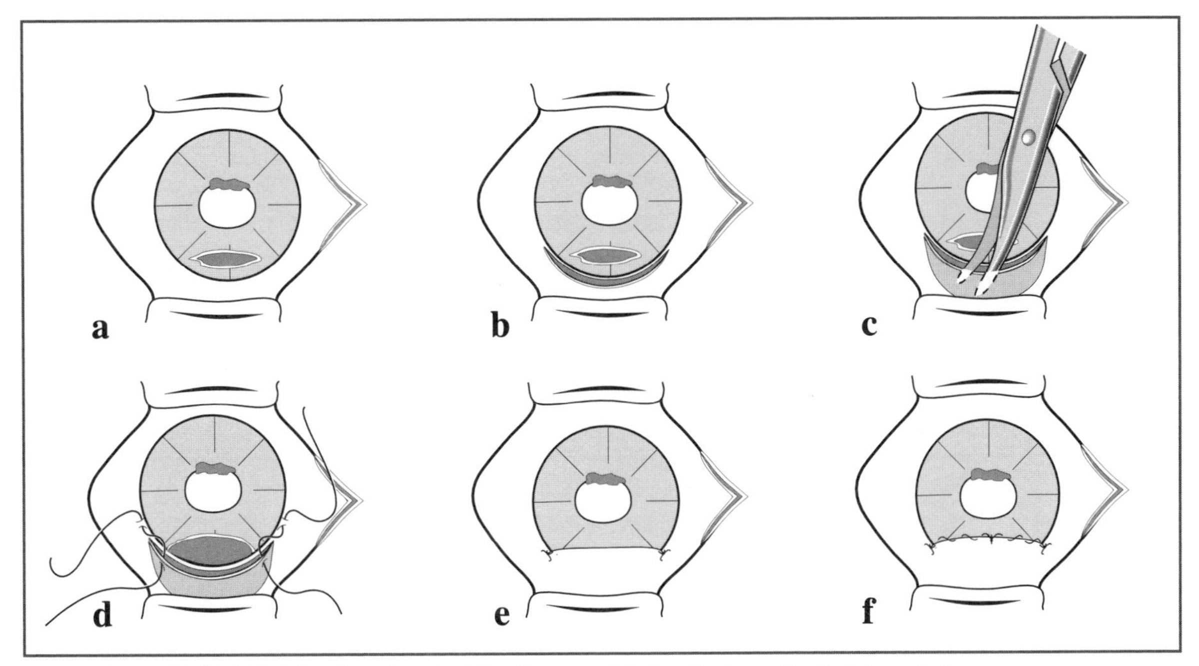

Figure 10-16.2. Peripheral conjunctival flap for corneal lesion due to equine facial paralysis.

a. Appearance of peripheral ulcer.
b. A perilimbal conjunctival incision is made adjacent to the wound
c. Undermining the conjunctiva with blunt scissors
d. Sutures are placed in the sclera at the limbus and along the edge of the undermined conjunctiva
e. Sutures tied at the limbus
f. Appearance of flap if margins sutured to cornea

Advancement flap (Fig 10-17)

A small incision is made through the conjunctiva at the limbus and a subconjunctival pocket is made with small blunt scissors to the desired depth. The limbal incision is extended and side incisions are made perpendicular to the limbus. This results in the base of the flap being wider than the apex. The graft is extended down to cover the ulcer. If there is tension on the graft, further undermining is indicated. Next the graft is sutured to the rim of the ulcer with absorbable suture. A simple interrupted or continuous pattern may be used. This type of flap does the best job of preserving the conjunctival blood supply.

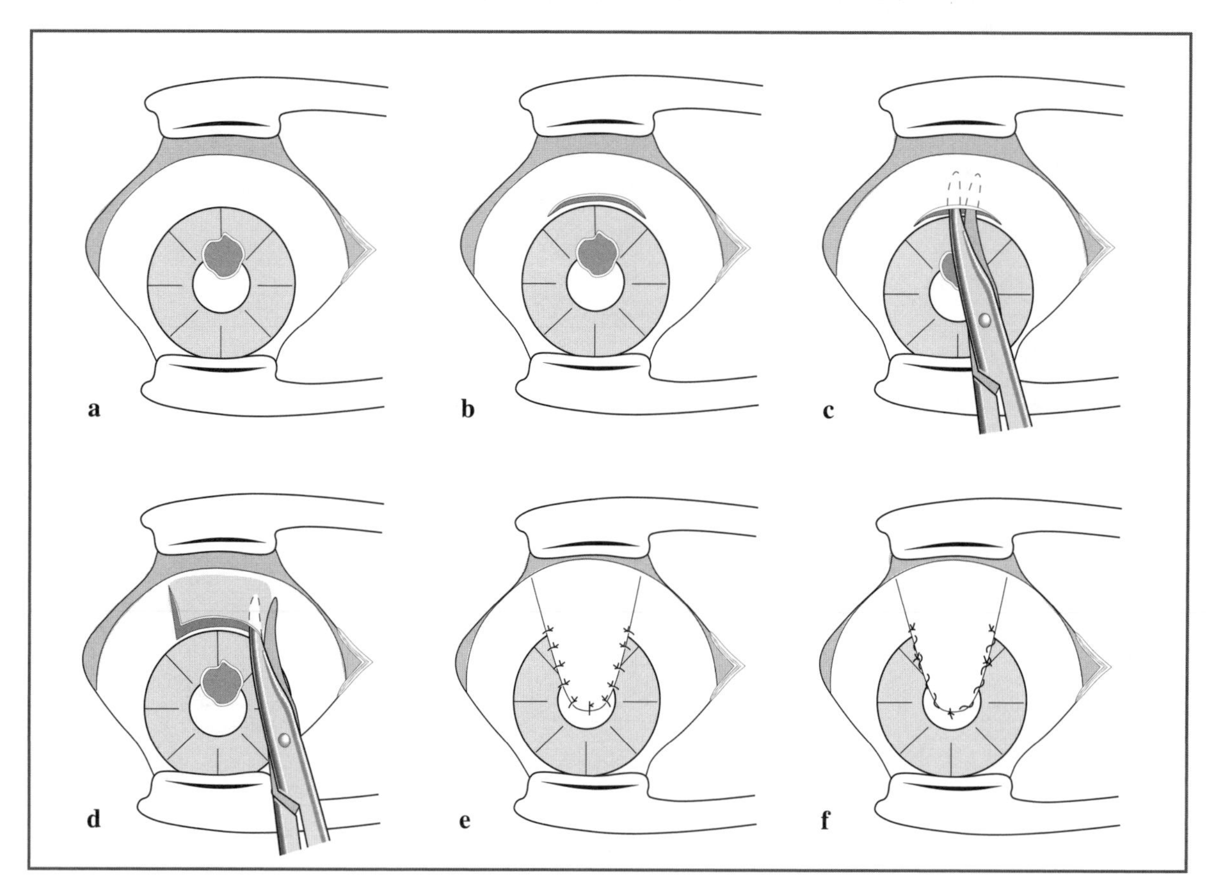

Figure 10-17. Advancement (pedicle) conjunctival flap.

a. Appearance of corneal ulcer
b. Conjunctival incision near the limbus has been extended to anticipated width for the flap
c. Subconjunctival pocket made with blunt scissors (corneal, strabismus). Care should be taken to stay above Tenon's capsule.
d. Incisions are made in the conjunctiva perpendicular to the limbus
e. Conjunctival flap extended over ulcer and sutured with absorbable suture using an interrupted suture pattern. Suture size depends on species and degree of corneal edema: small animals 8-0 healthy cornea, 7-0 marked edema; large animals 7-0 healthy cornea, 6-0 marked corneal edema.
f. Conjunctival flap sutured with continuous pattern is faster but presents greater risk of flap dehiscence. Several anchor sutures are recommended.

Rotation flap (Fig 10-18)

Rotation flaps allow greater length to the flap but may have temporary limitation of blood supply because of more disruption of the conjunctival blood supply. The length of the limbal incision determines the length of the flap. The width is determined by the location of the second incision which is parallel to the limbus. The wider the base, the better the conjunctival circulation. This is an excellent flap for central ulcers. Ideally the incision should be made so the flap is perpendicular to eyelid motion. Again, the flap is sutured to the rim of the ulcer with continuous or interrupted absorbable suture.

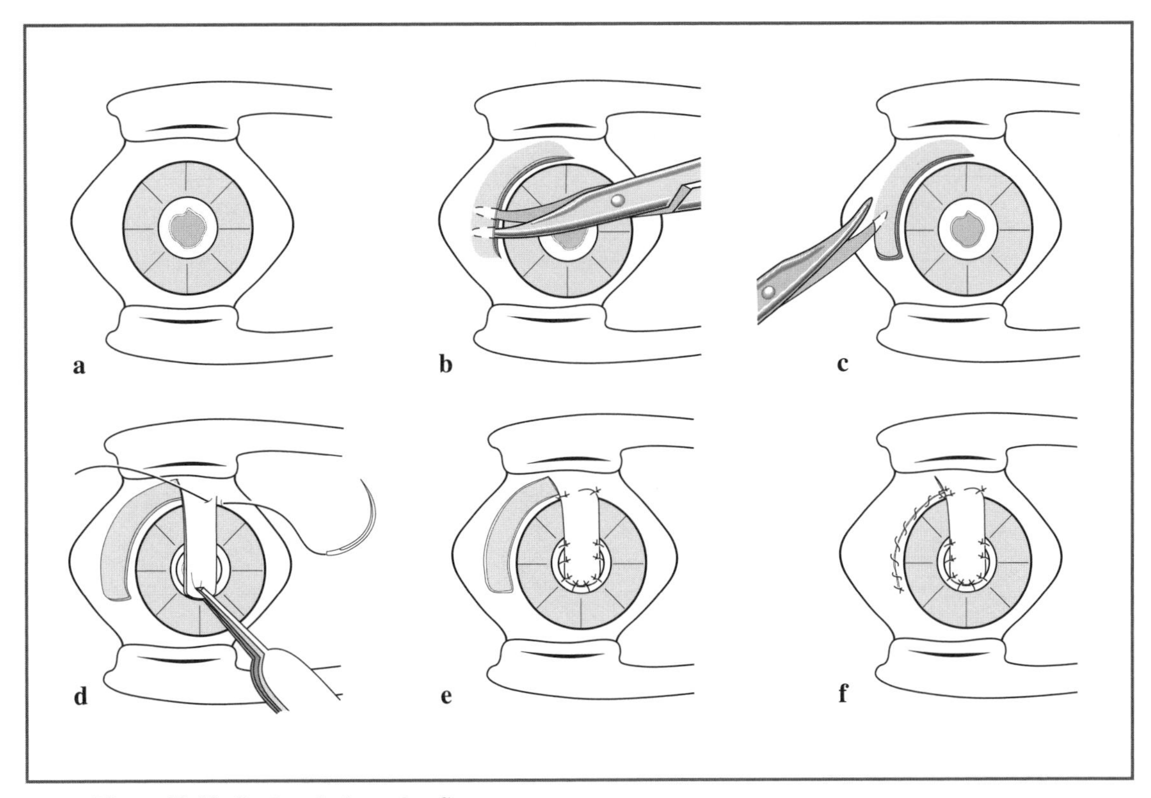

Figure 10-18. Conjunctival rotation flap.

a. Central corneal ulcer
b. A small conjunctival incision is made near the limbus and is extended as the conjunctiva is undermined with blunt scissors. The length of the limbal incision determines the length of the flap. If possible, the incisions should be made so that when the flap is rotated, it will be perpendicular to eyelid motion.
c. The undermined conjunctiva is cut to form the rotation flap
d. The conjunctival flap is rotated over the ulcer and a fixation suture placed before trimming the edge to fit the ulcer
e. After trimming, the flap is sutured to the ulcer edge and anchor sutures are recommended where the flap crosses the limbus
f. Suturing the conjunctival donor site is optional.

Central bridge flap (Fig 10-19)

An incision is made at the limbus and it is undermined in the same manner as a peripheral flap. A second incision is made in the undermined conjunctiva parallel to the limbal incision, thus forming a conjunctival bridge. The distance between the incisions determines the width of the bridge. The bridge can be pulled into place and held there with four interrupted sutures at the limbus. One must ensure that the flap crosses the eye vertically. When the flap is vertical, blinking of the eyes will not cause the flap to shift its location and the conjunctiva will heal to the ulcer in three to five days without suturing. If the bridge is not as secure as desired at the point of corneal injury, it can be sutured directly to the cornea with continuous or interrupted sutures.

The flap is left in place until healing is complete, then the flap is cut free at the limbus. It will adhere to the area of the central injury. It is trimmed free there. Any material that is left on the cornea will regress spontaneously in a few weeks.

When a wide bridge flap is prepared, closure of the conjunctival donor site with a 6-0 to 7-0 absorbable suture is suggested.

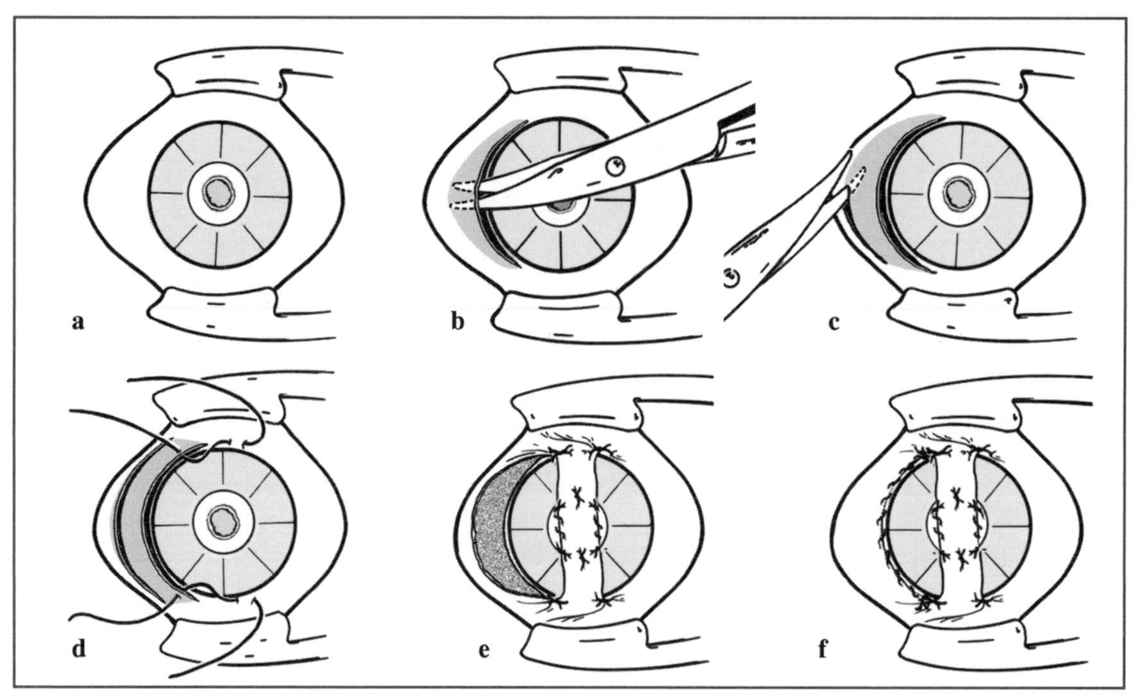

Figure 10-19. Central bridge flap for central corneal lesion.
- a. Central corneal ulcer
- b. A perilimbal conjunctival incision is made along the temporal or nasal limbus. The conjunctiva is then undermined with scissors.
- c. Making parallel incision in undermined conjunctiva
- d. Preplacing sutures in the sclera and edge of the conjunctival flap
- e. Final appearance of flap after all sutures have been placed and tied
- f. Suturing conjunctival donor site is optional

Central tongue flap (Fig 10-20)

This is a modification of a bridge flap with one end dissected free. It allows greater mobility and requires less dissection. The conjunctiva is undermined as described for the bridge flap but the flap is cut free at one end. The flap is stretched across the cornea and a subconjunctival tunnel is made at the limbus. The end of the flap is pulled through it. The flap is sutured in place at the tunnel and at the opposite limbus. It may be secured along the sides as previously described.

This flap is easier to perform but does not have as much blood supply as a bridge flap.

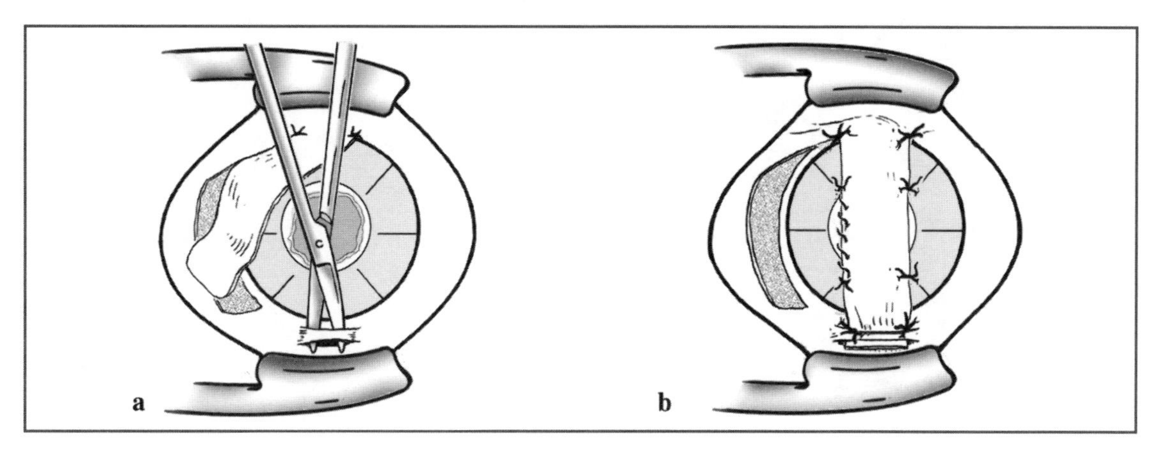

Figure 10-20. Central conjunctival tongue flap.

a. The flap was prepared the same as for a bridge flap but then cut free at one end. A subconjunctival tunnel is made at the limbus with scissors.

b. Tongue flap drawn through the tunnel and sutured in place. The flap is shown sutured to the cornea to prevent shifting. For illustrative purposes, one side has been sutured with a continuous pattern and the other with interrupted sutures.

Total conjunctival flap (Fig 10-21)

A conjunctival incision is made near to and around the limbus. The flap is undermined back a distance of one-half to two-thirds of the diameter of the cornea. The flap can be sutured in place by two methods: 1) purse-string suture (unfortunately sutures often pull out before the cornea has healed), and 2) horizontal interrupted mattress sutures, closing the wound in a linear fashion. This is a better suturing technique.

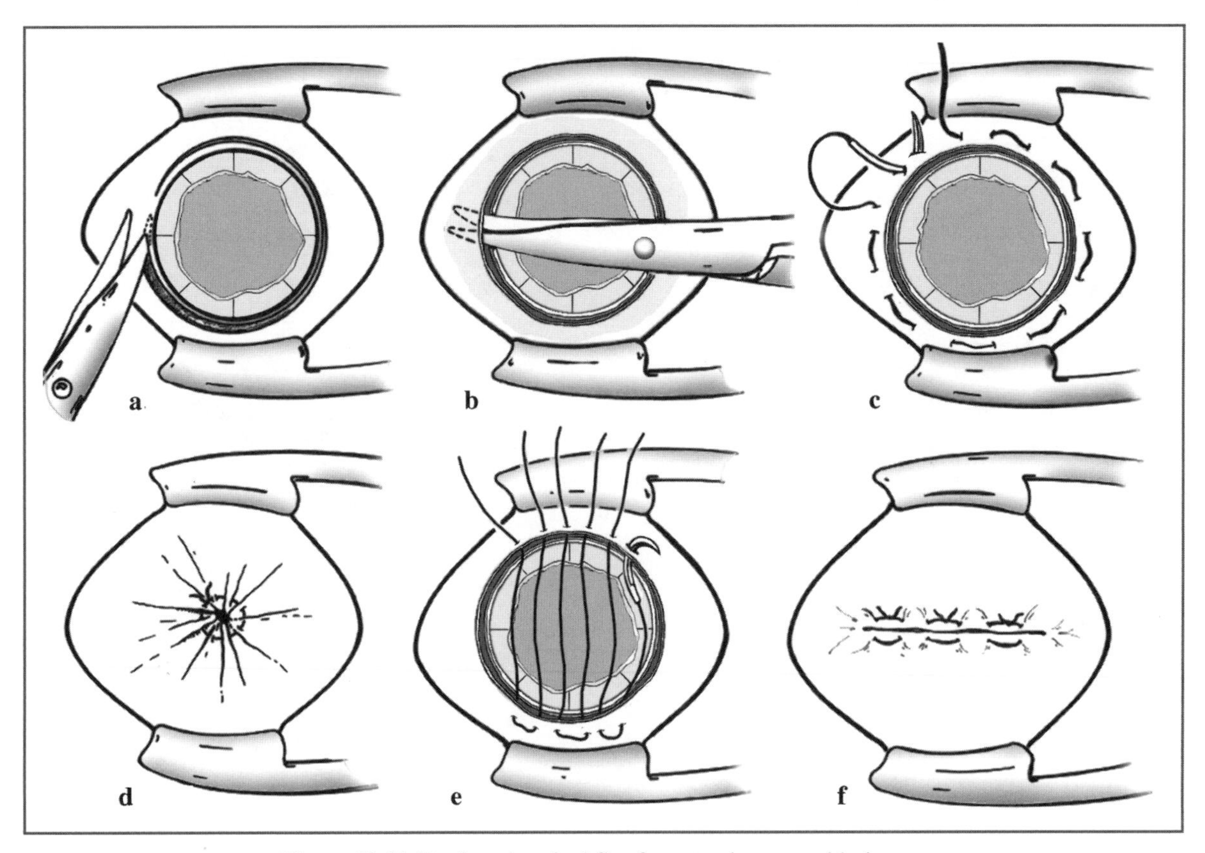

Figure 10-21. Total conjunctival flap for extensive corneal lesion.
a. Completing perilimbal conjunctival incision
b. Undermining the conjunctiva
c. Preplacing purse-string suture
d. Appearance after suture has been tied
e. Preplaced mattress sutures
f. Appearance after mattress sutures have been tied

Palpebral-conjunctival pedicle flap (Fig 10-22)

Recommended for perforating ulcers but can be used on any deep ulcer. The upper eyelid is everted with forceps or sutures. The conjunctiva is incised at the fornix and dissected free to the base of the tarsal glands. The flap is then sutured to the cornea with an absorbable suture. A temporary tarsorrhaphy may be indicated if eyelid motion appears to be a problem.

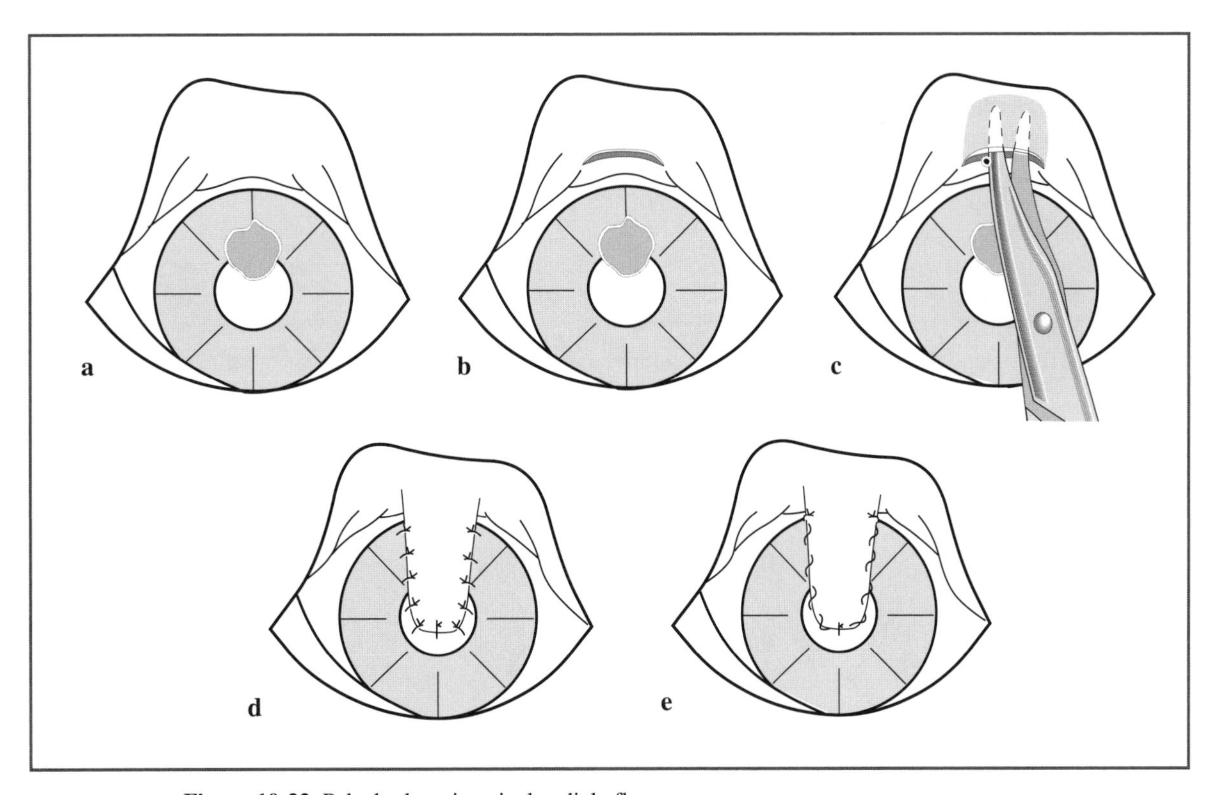

Figure 10-22. Palpebral-conjunctival pedicle flap.

a. Corneal ulcer with upper eyelid everted
b. The upper eyelid is everted and a conjunctival incision is made near the limbus
c. The conjunctiva is dissected free to the base of the tarsal glands
d. Perpendicular incisions free the graft and it is sutured to the cornea with interrupted sutures. A temporary tarsorrhaphy will stabilize the flap.
e. Flap may be sutured with continuous sutures

SUPPORTIVE KERATOPLASTY

Conjunctival graft
Corneal transplant
Corneoscleral transposition

Conjunctival graft (Fig 10-23)

1. Conjunctival grafts from the globe or anterior surface of the third eyelid can be used to support corneal ulcers. Although it does not have blood supply, it will usually remain viable and gradually be replaced by regenerating cornea.
2. Indications are stromal ulcers where a third eyelid flap or temporary tarsorrhaphy might not be adequate but the blood supply of a conjunctival flap is not needed.
3. Contraindications - septic and melting ulcers
4. Technique - A conjunctival graft slightly larger than the lesion is cut from the donor site and anchored to the cornea with stay sutures. It is then sutured with 7-0 absorbable sutures to the ulcer edge with a continuous suture pattern.
5. The graft is supported with a third eyelid or temporary tarsorrhaphy for four to six weeks

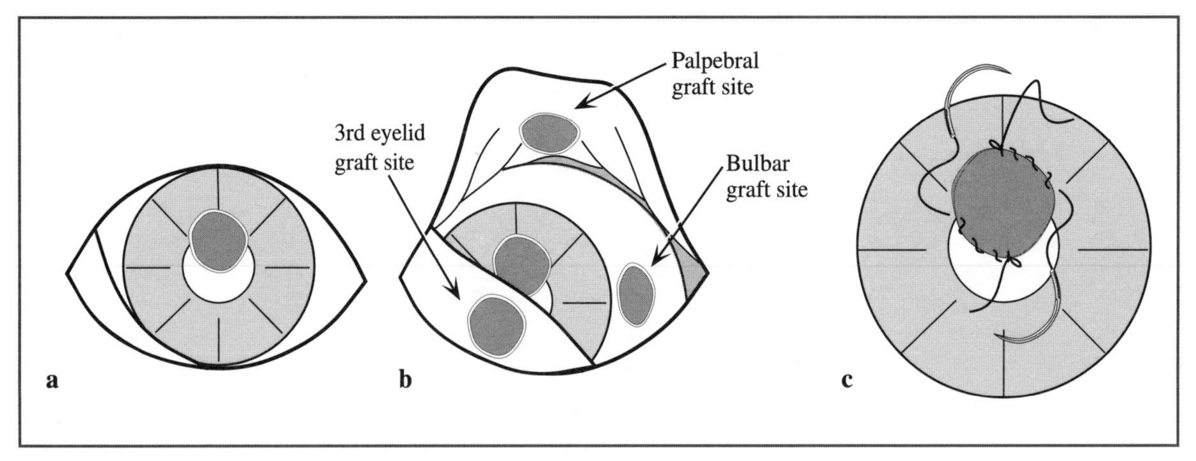

Figure 10-23. Conjunctival graft to support corneal ulcer.
a. Corneal ulcer
b. Donor sites for conjunctival graft
c. Continuous double suture technique

Corneal transplants - Seldom recommended in veterinary medicine. Successful corneal transplants require proper surgical instruments, surgical microscope and microsurgical techniques. Graft rejection is a problem, especially if the cornea is vascularized. Rejection is characterized by the graft becoming opaque and/or vascularized. The author has experienced the greatest success in the cat, moderate success in dogs, and universal rejection in horses.

Grafts may be fresh or preserved.

Lamellar transplants would be indicated in deep ulcers (Fig 10-24) and full thickness in perforating ulcers (Fig 10-28). The donor tissue contracts after removal, therefore the donor grafts should be larger than the recipient site. One-half millimeter larger for recipient sites up to 5 mm, and 1 mm larger for recipient sites larger than 5 mm is recommended.

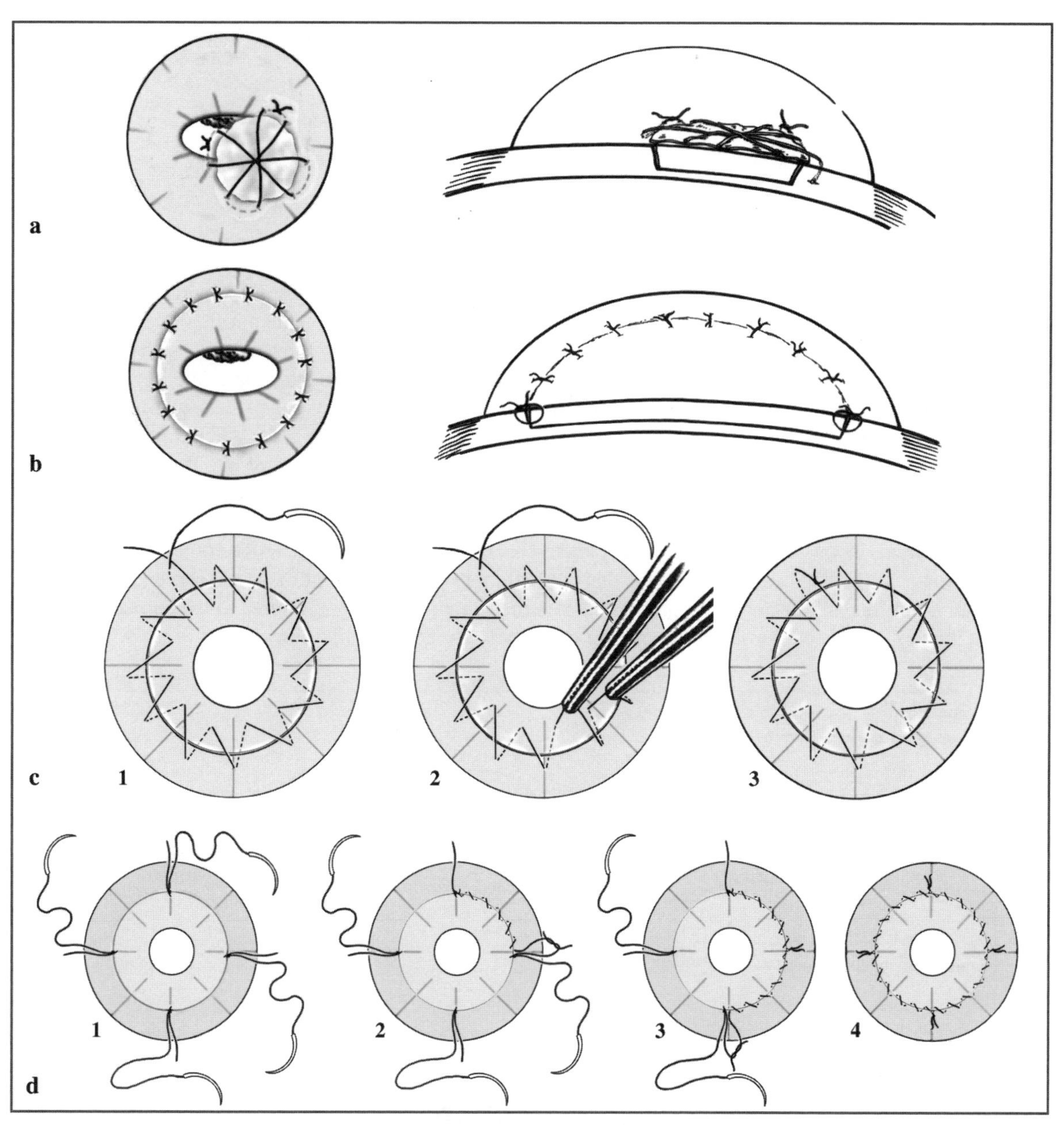

Figure 10-24. Lamellar corneal transplants for large deep ulcer. Several suturing patterns can be used. Nylon (8-0 to 9-0) or PDS suture produces minimal tissue reaction. If severe corneal edema is present, 7-0 suture may be necessary. Some suturing patterns are:

a. Transplant held in place with eggshell membrane and figure-8 sutures in recipient cornea. 6-0 or 7-0 suture is used. If desired, the membrane can be sutured directly to the cornea.

b. Large transplant held in place with simple interrupted sutures. An eggshell membrane can be sutured over this for additional support.

c. Continuous suture pattern.
   1. Placement of equally spaced suture bites
   2. The suture should be carefully tightened to assure equal tension throughout the incision
   3. Suture tied

d. Combination of four interrupted sutures and running sutures.
   1. Four interrupted sutures with a needle and a long end
   2. Running suture from 12 to 3 o'clock being tied to long end of 3 o'clock interrupted suture
   3. Running suture from 3 to 6 o'clock being tied (the surgeon may prefer to place the 6 to 9 o'clock running suture before the 3 to 6 o'clock suture)
   4. Final running suture from 9 to 12 o'clock tied and suture ends cut

Lamellar corneoscleral transposition (Parshall CJ, J Am Anim Hosp Assoc, May/June 1973;9:270-277) **(Fig 10-25)**

Dr. Parshall developed the lamellar corneoscleral transposition technique for animals.

1. Advantages over other forms of keratoplasty
   a. Does not require a donor
   b. Autograft, therefore no rejection problems; higher chances for clear cornea after surgery
2. Disadvantage - The eye must have an area of clear cornea as large as the ulcer
3. Technique - An area of healthy cornea is selected for lamellar transposition by marking it with parallel incisions from the outer edges of the ulcer to the limbus. Next the donor cornea is elevated with a corneal separator or Beaver blade. The cornea is separated at the depth of the ulcer. The separation is extended to the limbus between the parallel incisions. The corneal flap is cut free along the incisions with scissors. A conjunctival flap is prepared by making incisions perpendicular to the limbus outward from where the original corneal incisions touched the limbus. Next one tunnels between the incisions with scissors. The conjunctival and corneal flaps are still attached to the globe at the limbus. This attachment is cut with scissors. Now the cornea and conjunctiva can be moved into the corneal defect. The edges of the cornea are trimmed to match the wound. The transpositioned cornea is sutured to the recipient cornea with 8-0 to 9-0 nylon suture. This will result in minimal scarring. Absorbable sutures can be used. If the conjunctival flap is not under excess tension, it is sutured to the cornea with continuous suturing. If the flap has excess tension that may interfere with healing of the transpositioned cornea, the flap is cut free at the scleral attachment and then the conjunctival flap is sutured to the cornea and sclera at the limbus. If nonabsorbable sutures are used, they are removed after three weeks.

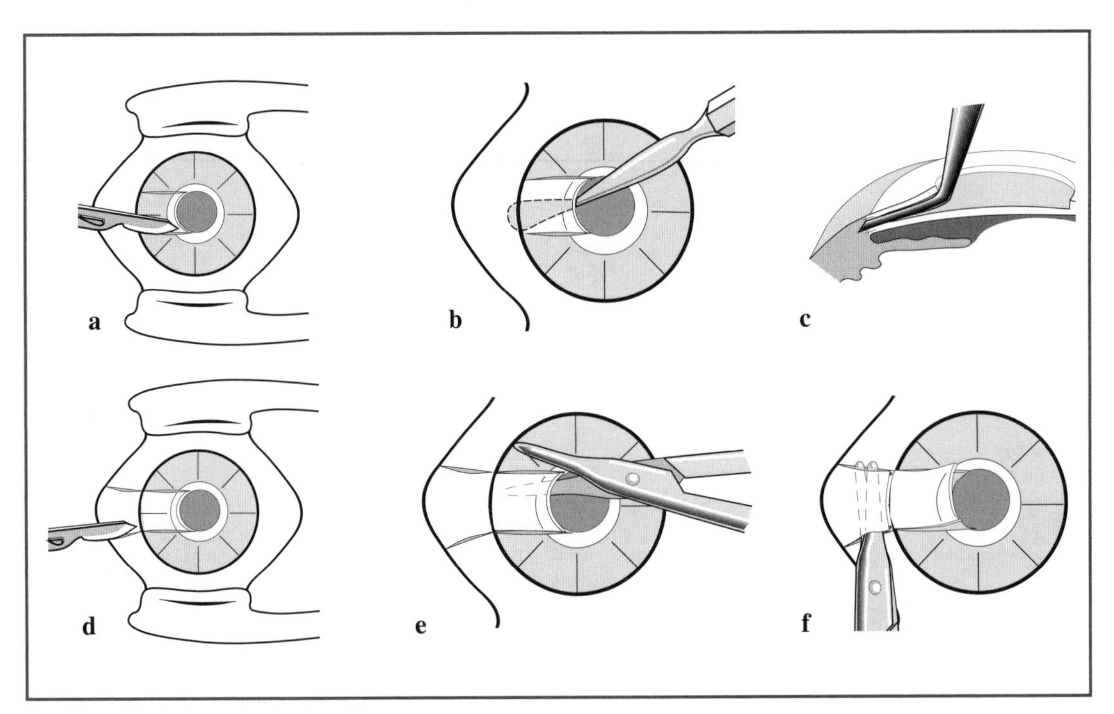

Figure 10-25. Parshall lamellar corneoscleral transposition for deep ulcers. (Part 1)
a. Appearance of deep ulcer is shown in the central cornea. Bard Parker blade marks area of healthy cornea for transposition.
b. Undermining healthy cornea with Martinez corneal dissector
c. Cross-section shows that the dissection is at the depth of the ulcer
d. Scoring the conjunctiva
e. Cutting the undermined cornea free toward the limbus
f. Undermining the conjunctiva between the scored lines

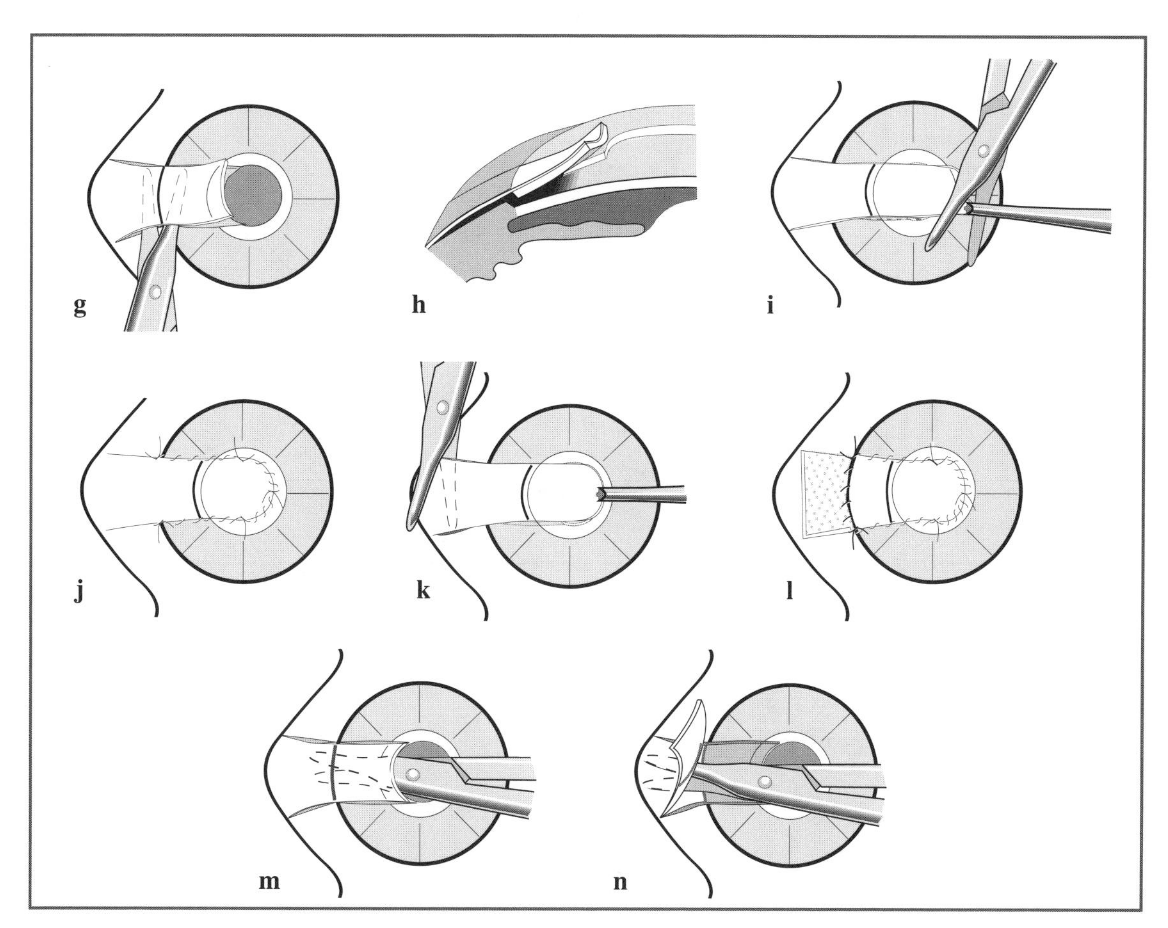

Figure 10-25. Parshall lamellar corneoscleral transposition for deep ulcers. (Part 2)

g. Cutting the limbus free
h. Cross-section shows the conjunctival and corneal flap ready for transposition
i. The transposed tissue is drawn into the defect and the edges of the cornea are trimmed to fit the ulcer
j. Transposed tissue sutured in place - interrupted sutures, or continuous suture pattern with double armed suture tied at 3 o'clock and interrupted cardinal sutures at 6 and 12 o'clock
k. If the cornea cannot be seated properly in the ulcer, the conjunctival flap may be cut at its base
l. Cornea sutured into ulcer and conjunctival graft sutured to cornea and limbus
m & n. Blunt dissection alternative for separation of transposition flap at limbus and undermining conjunctiva.
m. Forcing blunt scissors through limbal cornea into episclera
n. Completing separation of conjunctival flap

DESCEMETOCELE

Descemetocele is protrusion of Descemet's membrane through the floor of an ulcer, forming a transparent vesicle. These occur most frequently in central ulcers of dogs with protruding eyes. Descemet's membrane will bulge into a weakened cornea in dogs but will hold its shape better in horses and cats.

Small, less than 4 mm in small animals; 5 mm in horses

1. Inversion of the descemetocele and suturing the ulcer (Fig 10-26). The vesicle is inverted with an iris spatula and a supportive horizontal mattress suture or sutures are put in the cornea. If the descemetocele is accidentally ruptured, the wound is sutured as quickly as possible.

   After suturing the descemetocele, the third eyelid is sutured over for support if the cornea is edematous. Treat medically the same as you would an ulcer. If the descemetocele ruptures (it usually does), systemic antibiotic is given for three to four days. The third eyelid sutures should be removed in 10 to 14 days.

2. Third eyelid flap only (I cannot recommend this treatment) - Some surgeons position only a third eyelid flap and then treat the eye topically. I would be concerned that the ulcer may still rupture and result in a prolapsed iris that could end up causing loss of sight. It only takes a few more minutes to suture the cornea and I sleep a lot better afterwards.
3. Conjunctival flaps (preferably rotational for central descemetoceles) - A good technique but requires more time than direct suturing of the ulcer

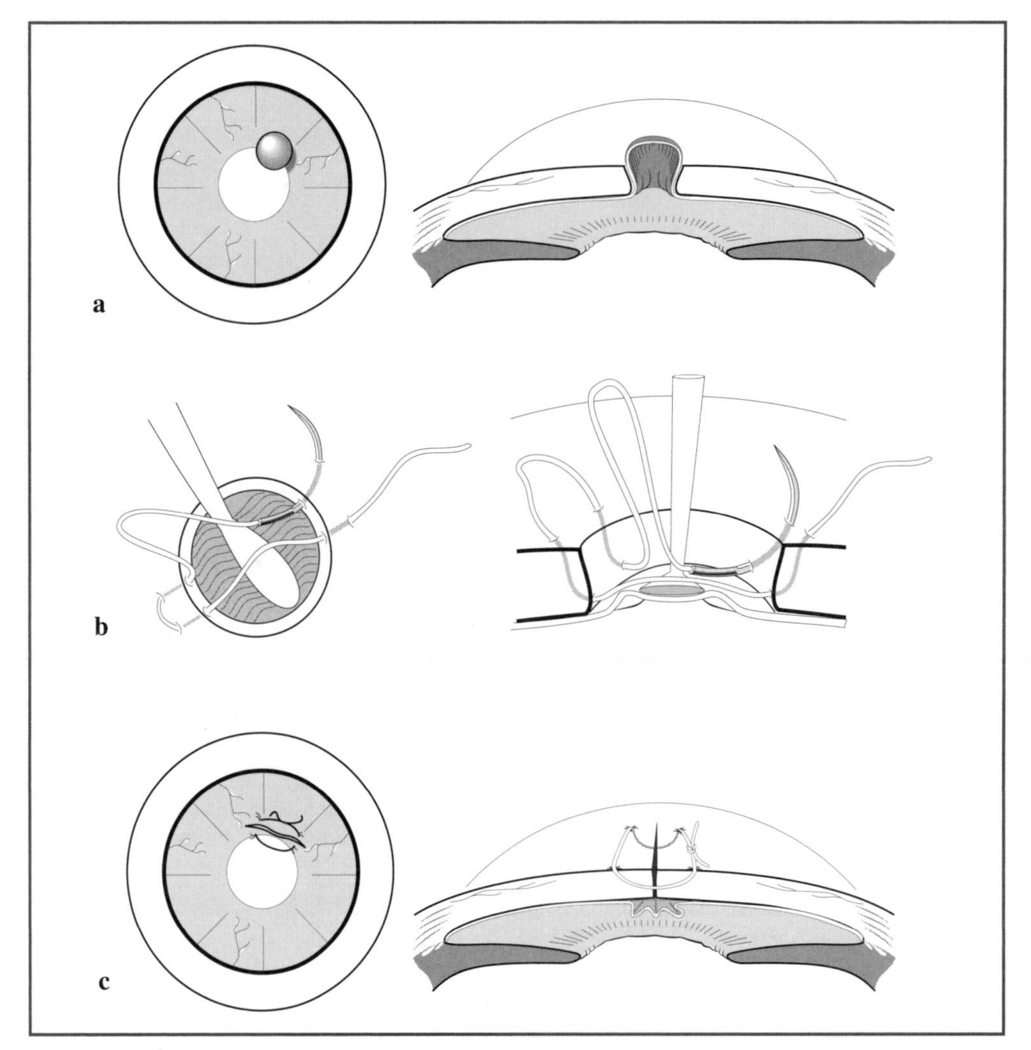

Figure 10-26. Suturing small descemetocele.
- a. Frontal and cross-section view of descemetocele
- b. Descemetocele repositioned with iris or cyclodialysis spatula as mattress suture is placed
- c. Appearance after mattress suture. If ulcer edge is not tightly closed, simple interrupted sutures may be placed as needed.

Large descemetocele

1. Conjunctival flap (in this case a thick flap will result in a stronger cornea than a thin one)
2. Lamellar corneal transplant
3. Corneoscleral transposition if there is adequate healthy cornea

PERFORATING ULCERS

Small perforating ulcer with prolapse of iris (less than 4 mm in small animals, 5 mm in horses)

1. The prolapsed iris can be amputated and the corneal wound sutured. If the cornea is edematous, support with a third eyelid flap is recommended.
   a. Technique (Fig 10-27) - Amputate the prolapsed iris. The iris is freed from the edge of the wound with an iris spatula by rotating it in the wound 360°. If any adhesion of the iris to the corneal wound is present, it is removed. If hemorrhage is severe, the anterior chamber is irrigated through the corneal wound with 1:10,000 epinephrine in PSS until the hemorrhage stops. This will also dilate the pupil. The wound is sutured using mattress or simple interrupted sutures. Two sutures are preplaced and then drawn tight. This should close the wound. Usually the cornea is uneven at this point but it will soon smooth out. Using an air injection cannula, air is introduced through the wound to establish a small air bubble between the iris and the corneal wound (Fig 4-5; Chapter 4, page 144). Do not try to inflate the eye. If the anterior chamber did not form adequately, saline is injected or BSS until the globe is formed. Aqueous production will establish pressure. If there are severe synechia, a 25 to 27 gauge needle is introduced at the limbus and using the needle as an iris spatula, the pupil is carefully shaped and the adhesions broken down. If there is blood or fibrin, intracameral injection of 25 to 50 µg tPA is recommended.
   b. Aftercare
      1) Topical - maintain mydriasis. Treat with antibiotics.
      2) Systemic antibiotics for five days

2. Conjunctival flap - will provide support and immediate blood supply. Scarring and anterior synechia may limit central vision.

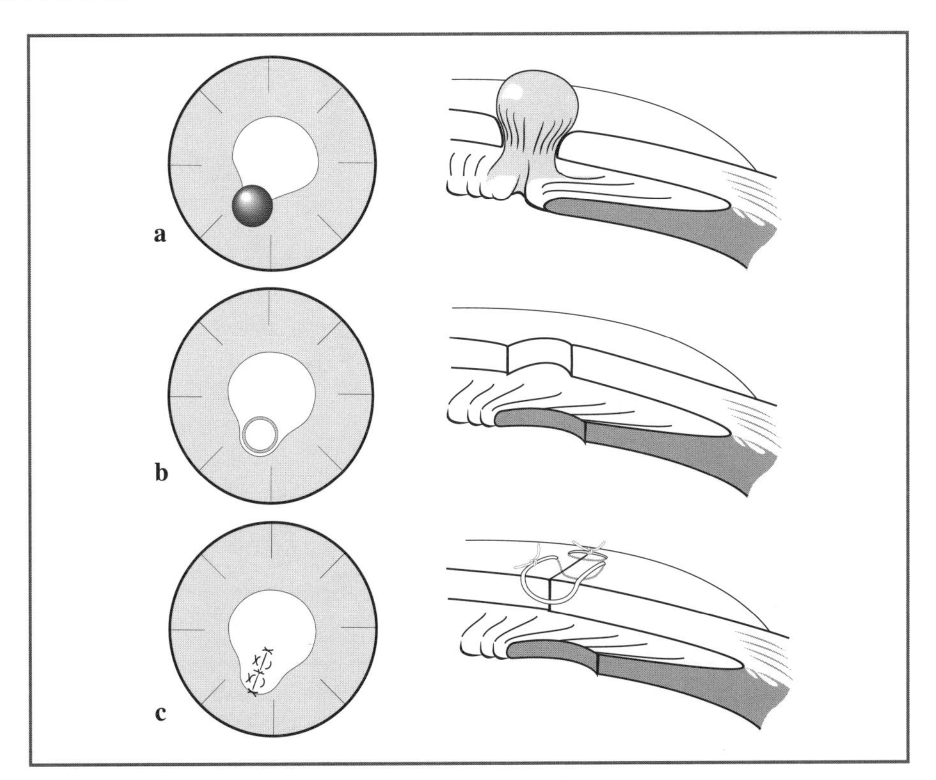

Figure 10-27. Small perforating ulcer with iris prolapse.
- a. Frontal and cross-section view of small perforation with iris prolapse
- b. Prolapse amputated and iris freed from cornea by rotating an iris spatula 360° between iris and cornea
- c. Wound closed with horizontal mattress sutures. Simple interrupted sutures may be added to appose epithelial edges.

Large perforating ulcer with prolapsed iris

These are the most serious. If the eye does not have panophthalmitis, any one of the following may be tried:

- Penetrating corneal transplant
- Parshall corneoscleral transposition
- Conjunctival flap - most frequent treatment
- Suturing eyelids - if owner cannot afford corrective surgery. Some eyes will heal remarkably well.
- No treatment - this is never in the best interest of the patient

If there is panophthalmitis, eye removal may be the best treatment because: 1) stops the pain immediately; 2) no long recovery period; 3) is much less expensive than the procedures to save the eye.

1. Penetrating corneal transplant (Fig 10-28) - The prolapsed iris is amputated and all iris is removed from beneath the area of perforation. A full thickness penetrating corneal transplant is placed in the wound. The transplant is sutured in place. The anterior chamber is re-established. If this is a large transplant, covering with an eggshell membrane held in place with figure-eight sutures may be beneficial or suturing a third eyelid flap. Immediate postsurgical care is the same as described for small perforations. The scars caused by the sutures are very slight.

   The transplant will become opaque in dogs and horses but will give support to the healing eye. In time, the opaque area will become quite small (one-half the size of the original transplant). The patient can usually see around the scar. In cats, the transplant will remain clear and be accepted with a minimal amount of recipient reaction.

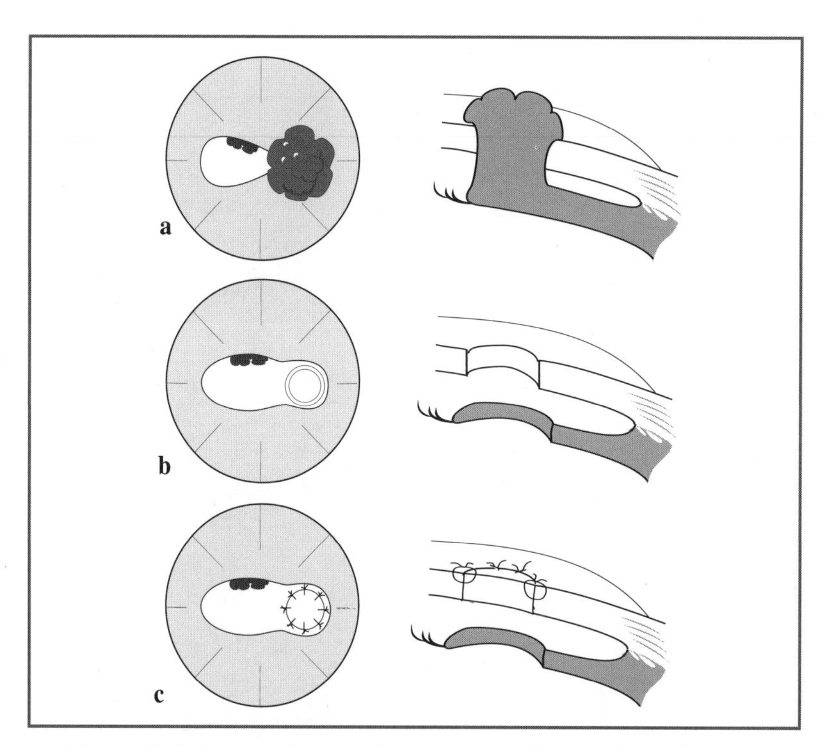

Figure 10-28. Large perforating ulcers treated with corneal transplant.
a. Frontal and cross-section view of perforating corneal ulcer
b. Prolapsed iris has been removed and iris freed from cornea. Edges of the ulcer have been straightened with a corneal trephine.
c. Corneal transplant is positioned and sutured into place with interrupted 7-0 or 8-0 suture (see Figure 10-25c & d).

2. Parshall corneoscleral transposition (Fig 10-25) will work quite well if there is enough healthy cornea to cover the primary lesion. The donor cornea is removed at about two-thirds thickness and it is slid over the perforating ulcer. The technique is the same as described for deep ulcers, except creating a square recipient bed and advancement edge to the transposed cornea that will give the transplant greater stability (Fig 10-29). It will still work even though corneal stroma is exposed directly to the anterior chamber. This works exceptionally well in horses. Be sure the pupil is well dilated and the anterior chamber is formed at the end of surgery. Use the third eyelid or eyelids for additional support.

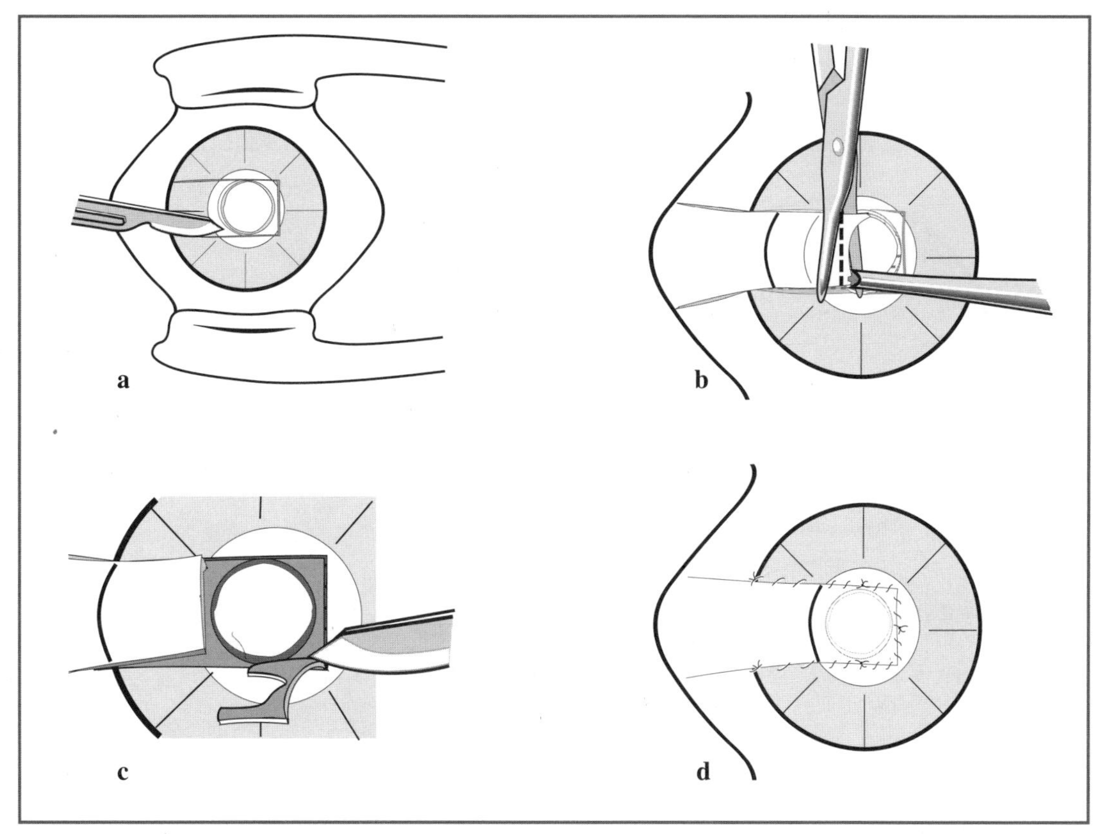

Figure 10-29. Modification of Parshall corneoscleral transposition for perforating ulcers. See Figure 10-26, page 340 for technique to free the corneal-conjunctival flap.

a. Cornea scored slightly wider and beyond the ulcer at a 2/3 to 3/4 depth of cornea
b. Trimming end of mobilized cornea to prepare a square end
c. The recipient ledge is prepared by removing cornea from within the scored area
d. Corneoscleral transposition flap sutured in place. Simple interrupted sutures at the corners and where the ledge is narrow, followed by a continuous pattern using a double-armed suture works very well.

3. Conjunctival flaps - Can be used and are the best treatment if corneal transplanting is not possible. If iris prolapse is minimal, do not amputate it. If amputation is necessary, it is difficult to get a good seal of the conjunctiva to the cornea and the anterior chamber may stay collapsed. Medical aftercare is the same as for transplants. A tarsorrhaphy may be used for additional support.
4. Tarsorrhaphy only - This is sometimes done in large animals to protect the eye when intraocular surgery may be too great a risk to the patient (mares in late foal) or if the expense of the other procedures is prohibitive. It is not the treatment of choice but will have a fairly high percentage of aesthetic looking eyes and about 10 to 15% will even see. The same postoperative medications are used as for transplants. Suture is left in for four weeks.
5. No treatment - Not recommended in small animals because will end up with nearly 100% blind eyes that usually develop phthisis bulbi. Cattle have remarkable healing capability and many will end up with fairly good looking eyes, even though they may be blind.

Large ulcer with small central perforation (Fig 10-30)

1. Large ulcers with small central perforation can be handled with a lamellar corneal transplant technique described for large nonperforating ulcers. The prolapsed iris is removed and the edges of the ulcer cleaned. The anterior chamber is irrigated with dilute epinephrine.

   The perforation is closed with mattress sutures using 8-0 or 9-0 absorbable suture. This suture penetrates the endothelium. The transplant is placed in the ulcer and supported with third eyelid or eyelids. Aftercare is the same as any penetrating transplant. The final scar should not be much larger than the area of perforation.
2. Conjunctival flap or conjunctival graft - If not prepared to do a corneal transplant, a conjunctival flap can be used after the perforation is sutured.

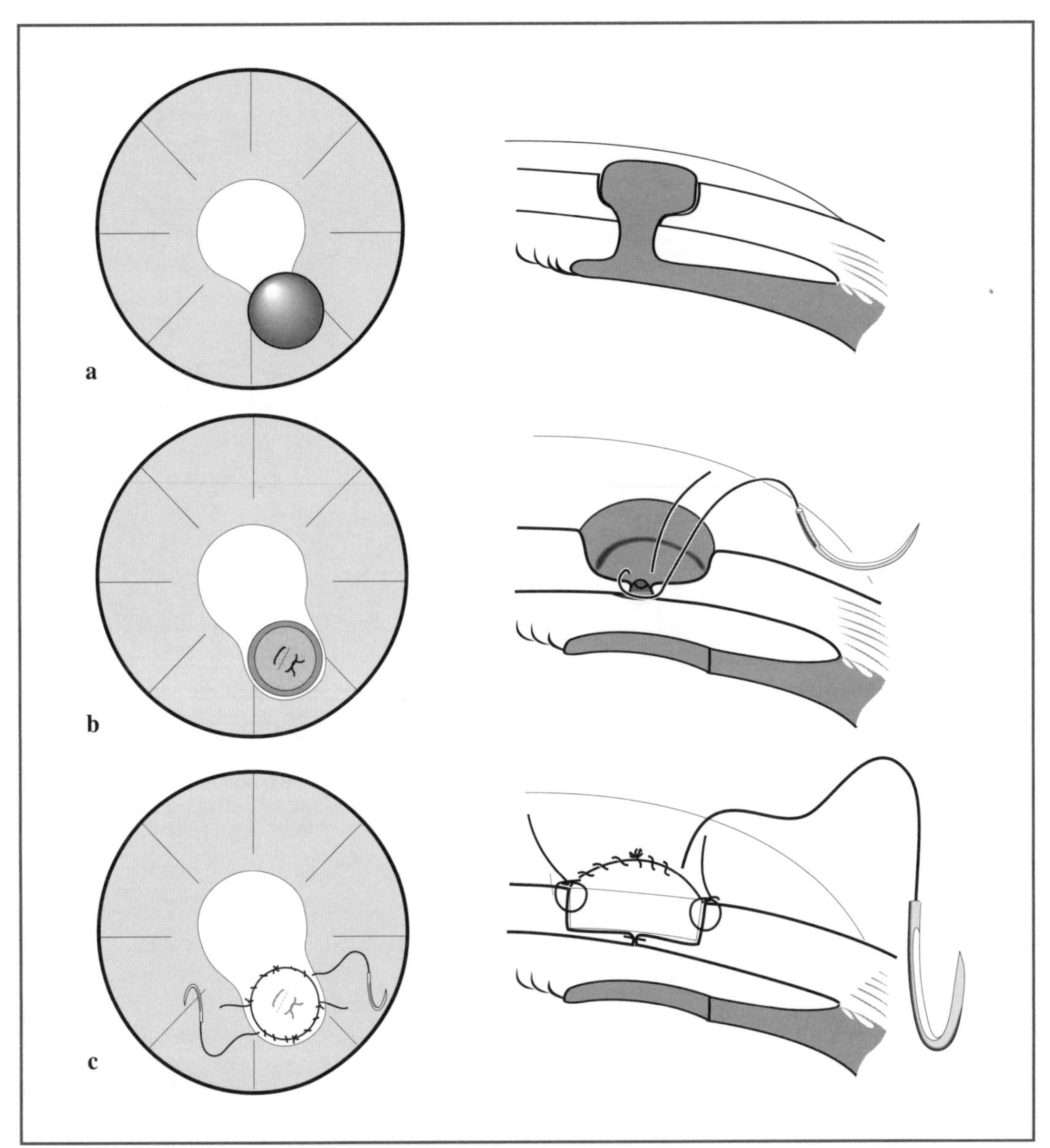

Figure 10-30. Large ulcer with small central perforation treated with corneal transplant.

a. Frontal and cross-section appearance
b. The prolapsed iris has been removed and the corneal wound cleaned up. The wound is closed with a horizontal mattress suture.
c. Corneal transplant sutured in place using interrupted sutures at 3 and 9 o'clock and continuous sutures started at 12 and 6 o'clock.

CORNEAL LACERATIONS - Corneal lacerations are quite common and fortunately the majority do not perforate

Causes

1. Small animals
   a. Cat scratches are the most common cause. This is especially true in young pups with their first encounter with a cat. Also common in cats from fighting.
2. Large animals - Common in horses but rare in cattle
   a. Owner-inflicted injuries are common (striking the eye with whip, stick or other object)
   b. Hitting the head when loading or unloading
   c. Catching the eye on a sharp object in a barn or corral
   d. Fighting with other horses

Types of wounds

1. Superficial - These wounds usually heal in 24 to 48 hours with or without treatment. Will not cause any problem unless the source of the laceration inoculates pathogenic bacteria or fungi into the stroma.
2. Deep but not perforating
   a. Deep penetration with minimal corneal damage, such as a deep cat scratch, is expected to heal with only topical medication. If the wound extends to Descemet's membrane, corneal suturing would be advisable but I have seen wounds heal satisfactorily that were only supported with third eyelid or eyelid suturing.
   b. Deep penetration with severe corneal damage - These should be treated medically like an ulcer and supported with third eyelid or eyelid suturing. If more than 2/3 depth, a conjunctival flap would be the safest treatment. Any fragments of severely damaged cornea should be debrided.
   c. Corneal flaps - Some injuries produce corneal flaps. If these are presented before the cornea becomes edematous, they can be sutured into place with excellent results. If allowed to become edematous, sutures will generally pull out in a few days. If this happens, the edematous flap is debrided and treated as a deep ulcer.
3. Perforating lesions
   a. Small puncture wounds without prolapse of the iris. Loss of aqueous at the time of injury is followed by formation of fibrin-rich aqueous that helps seal the wound.
      1) Signs - This eye is characterized by a pinpoint pupil, plasmoid aqueous, hypotony and severe pain. The wound may be hard to see unless stained with fluorescein. If the wound is still leaking, aqueous rivulets will be seen in the fluorescein.
      2) Treatment - If the anterior chamber is reformed and the iris is not incarcerated in the wound, the corneal wound will not require suturing. Aftercare is the same as for intraocular surgery.
         The eye should be checked every few days to make sure healing progresses as expected. If the wound starts to ulcerate or show stromal abscess or necrosis, corneal suturing or supporting with the third eyelid or eyelids may be needed.
   b. Lacerations with prolapsed iris (Fig 10-31) - The examination is stopped immediately and the patient is prepared for surgery. Further manipulation may cause additional damage to the eye. A raindrop-shaped pupil will result when the iris seals a wound. The iris usually seals the wound soon after injury and the anterior chamber reforms. Mild manipulation will cause the wound to leak aqueous and can cause further prolapse of the iris.
      1) Treatment - If recent (less than one hour) and the iris is in the wound but not severely prolapsed, the iris is replaced into the anterior chamber and the cornea is sutured. If more than one hour or if the prolapse cannot be reduced, the prolapsed iris is amputated.
         The iris is freed from the cornea with an iris spatula by rotating it 360°. The anterior chamber is irrigated with 1:10,000 epinephrine to dilate the pupil and control any hemorrhage. If the pupil does not dilate as much as desired, carefully irrigate the posterior chamber. This is more effective because the epinephrine is applied nearer the dilator muscle.

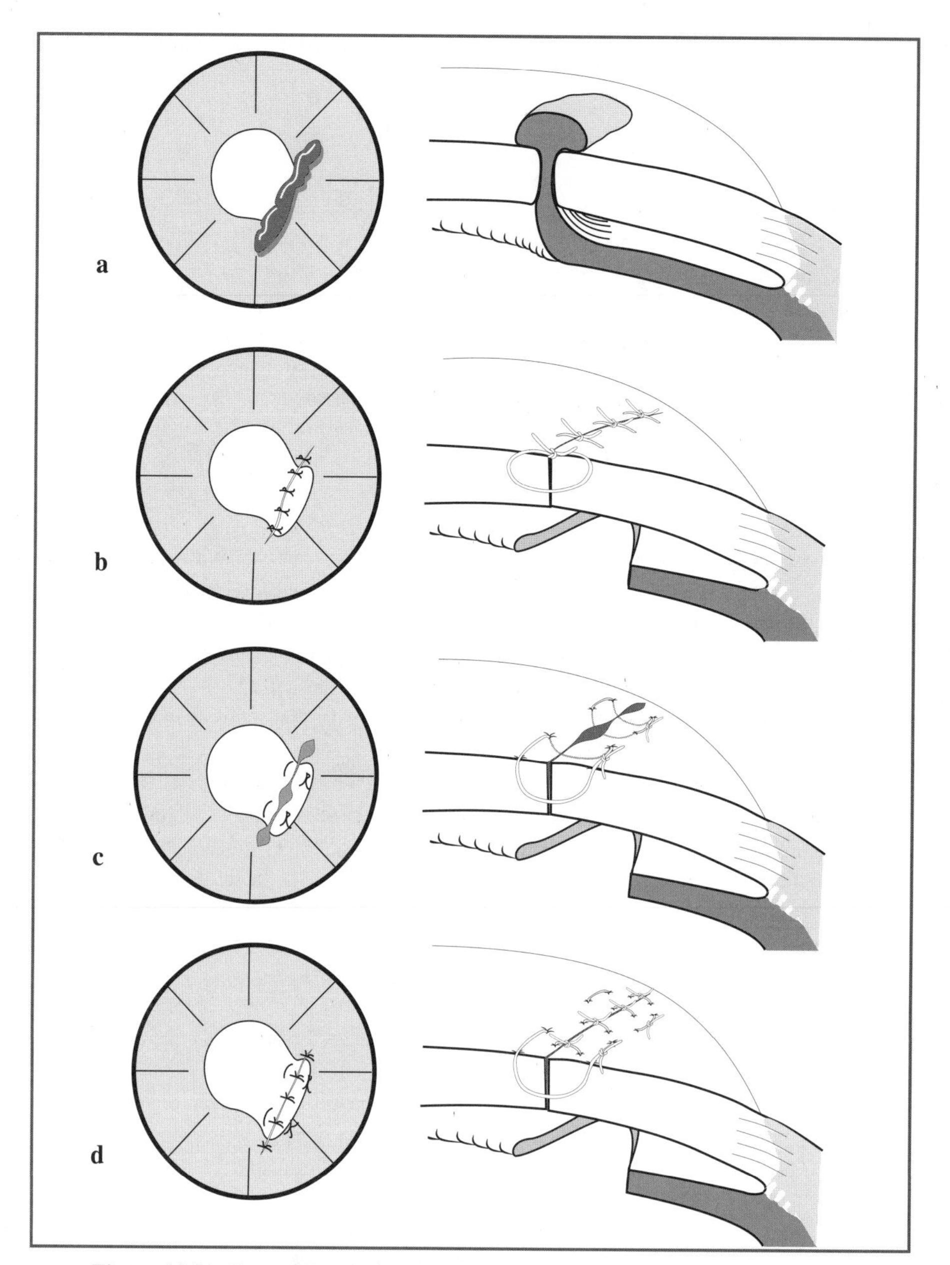

Figure 10-31. Corneal laceration with prolapsed iris.

a. Frontal and cross-section view of perforating corneal laceration
b. The prolapsed iris has been amputated, corneal iris adhesions reduced with an iris spatula and the wound sutured with simple interrupted sutures
c. Eyes with severe corneal edema should be sutured with horizontal sutures. This will seal the endothelial surface.
d. Simple interrupted sutures are placed between the horizontal mattress sutures to close the epithelial edge.

In dogs, simple interrupted sutures going two-thirds of the depth of the cornea are usually adequate. In horses, alternate horizontal mattress and simple interrupted sutures are best. The mattress sutures are placed first. Air placed in the anterior chamber will make suturing easier. The pupil is kept dilated during surgery. Fibrin or blood clots are removed before the final suture is placed, or one can treat with tPA. If hemorrhage occurs every time the iris is manipulated, the blood clots are left alone and suturing the cornea is finished. tPA is injected when surgery is complete.

2) Prognosis - The prognosis of a corneal laceration is dependent on the seriousness of internal injury, not the time elapsed prior to examination or surgery. I have had excellent results suturing lacerations six days after injury.

    Deep injuries may result in lens rupture. When this occurs, the lens must be removed at the same time. The prognosis is guarded in this case.

    Severe contusion, gunshot wounds or deep penetrating objects often cause irreversible uveal and retinal damage. These eyes may develop phthisis bulbi two to three weeks after repair. If deep structures cannot be seen, ultrasound imaging is needed for an accurate prognosis.

    The amount of hemorrhage is of prognostic value. If the hemorrhage is minor, a good prognosis is indicated. In these animals, clots form but clear aqueous can be seen forming in the anterior chamber. The wound seals with fibrin and after a few hours the tear is free of blood. In severe hemorrhage, the anterior chamber remains filled with blood, aqueous cannot be identified and the wound continues to seep blood. This eye has an unfavorable prognosis.

3) Aftercare
    a) Third eyelid flapping or suturing eyelids is indicated if the sutured cornea was damaged and because of this the wound is believed to be weak
    b) Postsurgical medical treatment is the same as for other intraocular procedures

CORNEAL FOREIGN BODIES - Occur in all species. The dog is most frequently affected.

Nonperforating - This is foreign material that adheres to the cornea rather than being flushed away by the tears. Small seeds or plant fragments that have a curvature similar to the cornea are usually the cause.

1. Signs
   a. History - They are usually quite well tolerated and may have a history of chronic eye disease for weeks. The owner will observe chronic epiphora with mild blepharospasm or increased frequency of blinking.
   b. Examination findings
      1) Increased blinking, possible blepharospasm and protrusion of the third eyelid. Mild epiphora.
      2) If recent, no corneal change except possible epithelial erosion beneath the foreign body
      3) If longstanding, there may be several scars indicting the foreign body has shifted its location. Some superficial vascularization may be present.
      4) Topical anesthesia may be needed to overcome blepharospasm
      5) Magnification may be necessary to see small plant seeds
2. Treatment - Topical anesthesia is needed before manipulation
   a. Using a lacrimal needle and saline, one should attempt to wash the foreign material off the cornea. Often a stream of water directed at the edge of the foreign body will lift it up and wash it to the conjunctiva where it can be picked up with forceps.
   b. If it is anchored in the cornea by epithelium growing over it, a probe will be needed to lift it up. A 25 gauge needle is an excellent foreign body probe. Chemical restraint or general anesthesia may be needed.
   c. After removing the foreign body, healing is rapid. Topical treatment is optional.

Perforating - Perforating foreign bodies are usually caused by splinters, thorns or plant fibers. The owner may be aware how it happened.

1. Signs - usually sudden onset and painful
   a. Epiphora, severe blepharospasm and reluctant to have eye examined. May require anesthesia or chemical restraint for examination.
   b. See the foreign body in the cornea
   c. If it perforated the cornea and deeper structures, hyphema and aqueous fibrin clots may be present. A secondary uveitis will also be present.
   d. The cornea will start to show edema quite soon after the perforation
2. Treatment
   a. Premedicate as recommended for intraocular surgery
   b. Small animals - general anesthesia
      Large animals - try topical anesthesia and chemical restraint; give general anesthetic if you suspect corneal sutures will be needed
   c. Remove the foreign body and suture the cornea if there is aqueous loss. If the foreign body is broken or flush with the corneal surface, make a corneal incision parallel to the foreign body and remove using a 25 or 27 gauge needle as a probe. Do not try to grasp with forceps because this may force the foreign body into the anterior chamber. If this happens, incise the cornea, remove the foreign body. From that point on, the eye is handled the same as any perforating corneal laceration.
   d. A foreign body in the anterior chamber should be removed if within the past few days.
      If it has been present for some time and hypopyon has not developed, intensive systemic treatment may control inflammation and infection, and allow the body responses to "wall off" the foreign body, thus eliminating the need for removal.

MYCOTIC KERATITIS

A serious disease with incidence varying with geographic distribution. Uncommon in the Rocky Mountain area, common in warm humid climates. Occurs in horses more than other species. Previous use of topical corticosteroid is a common historical event in most cases of fungal keratitis.

Etiology - Any plant fiber injury is a potential source for pathogenic fungi

1. *Candida* - moderately pathogenic. May be present in conjunctival fluids of normal eyes. Common in some geographic areas but has not been isolated from diseased eyes in our clinic.
2. *Aspergillus* - most frequent causative agent in our clinic. Can cause very severe lesion.
3. *Fusarium* - uncommon. Causes severe lesions, unfavorable prognosis.
4. *Alternaria* - moderate pathogenicity
5. *Mucor* - low pathogenicity, possibly a contaminant
6. Others - nearly a hundred fungal species have been reported in man

Signs

Mycotic keratitis should be suspected in horses with refractory ulcers or keratitis. Many cases have a history of chronicity and have been treated with numerous antibiotics and/or corticosteroids; on presentation they are showing exacerbation with severe corneal damage. The signs are variable but mycotic etiology should be suspected with:

1. Indolent recrudescent course
2. A white or yellowish ulceration with a dry, crumbly, raised surface
3. A crenated edge to the lesion
4. Finger-like extensions into the stroma around the lesion
5. Development of satellite lesions in the cornea
6. Recurrent hypopyon
7. Severe corneal necrosis with a rapidly growing ulcer

Diagnosis

1. Corneal and conjunctival scrapings. Stain and examine for fungal elements. Several scrapings are made and all are examined. If the epithelium has grown over the lesion, debride the epithelium and make impression smears from the exposed stroma.
2. Culture - enriched Sabouraud's agar or blood agar cultures at room temperature and 37°C. Save for two or three weeks. Growth will appear in many cases in five or six days. Some diagnostic laboratories do sensitivity testing of antifungal agents.

Treatment

Aggressive treatment is necessary. There are two schools of thought: 1) very intensive medical treatment (continuous or hourly); 2) immediate debridement, ± superficial keratectomy and a conjunctival flap or keratoplasty.

1. Medical treatment
   a. Topical antifungal agents (see Chapter 2, page 87)
      1) Initial treatment. Readily available OTC 1% myconazole vaginal preparations would be a good presumptive treatment until other antifungals can be located. Other presumptive choices are miconazole 1% ophthalmic solution or 2% ophthalmic ointment (Wedgewood Pharmacy); Fluconazole 0.2% ophthalmic solution (Wedgewood Pharmacy); and Natamycin 5% (Alcon). Atropine, acetylcysteine and antibiotics, if deemed necessary, could be added using concentrated forms. ***If possible, solutions should be administered with an ocular delivery system 0.1 ml every 1 to 2 hours, or continuously 6 to 8 drops (0.25 to 0.33 ml) hourly.***

        2) Maintenance treatment. Identification of preferred drugs may be determined with cytology and culture.
            a) Continuous treatment as previously described.
            b) Intermittent treatment as patient improves.
            c) Maintain treatment with atropine, anticollagenase, and +/- antibiotic.
    b. Systemic medication
        1) Anti-inflammatory drugs (Banamine or Ketofen)
        2) Ketoconazole 4.5 mg/lb may be beneficial in severe cases.
    c. When the corneal fungus dies, there is a severe corneal reaction. Because of this, intensive initial antifungal treatment may result in excessive corneal reaction when compared to gradually increasing the antimycotic drug.
2. Surgery
    a. Surgical debridement of necrotic cornea
    b. Corneal support
        1) Direct corneal support - conjunctival flap or corneal transplant.
        2) Indirect corneal support - third eyelid flap or tarsorrhaphy is a less expensive alternate to direct support.
3. Prognosis - very guarded
    a. If intraocular mycosis can be identified with anterior chamber centesis, enucleation is recommended
    b. Topical treatment should be continued for up to one month after recovery
    c. The owner should be advised that severe scarring and visual impairment are likely.

CORNEAL ABSCESS - Corneal abscesses are common in horses

Etiology

Usually post-traumatic. The owner is often aware of an injury 5 to 15 days prior to the current signs. The patient seemed to improve but now is very painful.

Signs

1. Painful eye - lacrimation, blepharospasm, photophobia
2. Usually chemosis and swollen eyelids
3. Cornea becomes cloudy and yellow to opaque at the abscess site
4. Epithelial erosion may develop
5. Secondary anterior uveitis with aqueous flare and possibly hypopyon

Diagnostic tests

1. Epithelial erosion - cytology and culture from site
2. Deep abscess - incise for cytology and culture for antibacterial sensitivity

Treatment

1. Curet the wound carefully and swab with 1:20 Betadine
2. Treat as stromal ulcer
    a. Topical - antibiotic, anticollagenase, atropine
        1) Extended wear contact lens presoaked with ulcer solution and topical administration q4-6h
        2) Drug delivery system (transpalpebral or nasal) for ulcer solution delivery. Initially q1-2h; reduce to QID as patient improves.
    b. Subconjunctival antibiotic to increase intraocular concentration
3. Systemic anti-inflammatory (flunixin) or prednisolone

Course

1. Will usually heal in two to four weeks but may take longer
2. Owner should be advised of potential for permanent scarring

CHAPTER 11 - ANTERIOR CHAMBER

The anterior chamber is an aqueous-filled space formed anteriorly by the cornea and posteriorly by the iris and lens. Its peripheral limit is the filtration angle. Aqueous flows from the posterior chamber through the pupil, circulates in the anterior chamber and exits at the filtration angle (Fig 11-1).

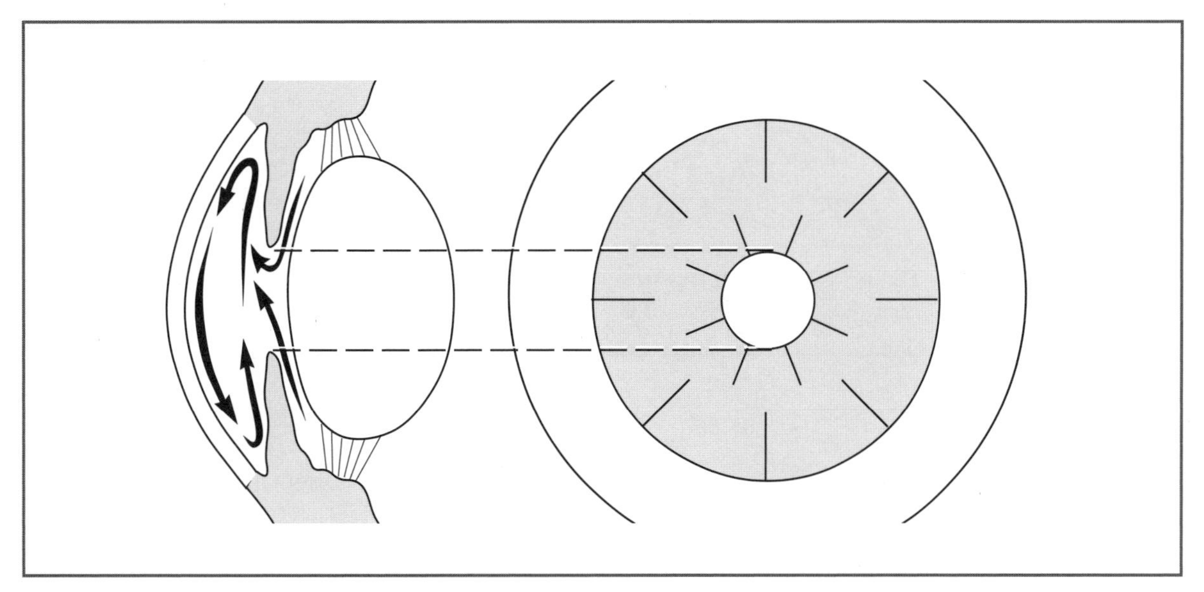

Figure 11-1. Anterior chamber aqueous circulation. Warm aqueous enters from the pupil, mixes with the aqueous next to the iris and rises. Near the cornea the aqueous cools and settles, resulting in a convection current.

The anterior chamber must be examined because changes in it may be observed that are of value in diagnosing diseases in the structures that form it. It should be examined for depth and contents. A goniolens is needed to examine the filtration angle in small animals.

DEPTH

The depth of the anterior chamber is determined by the relationship of the position of the iris and lens in respect to the cornea. The location of the iris is determined by the position of the anterior surface of the lens. Therefore, anterior chamber depth is affected by the:

1. Lens size (Fig 11-2) and position (Fig 13-17 and 13-18; Chapter 13, pages 402 and 403)
2. Primary iris disease - synechia, growths, or inflammatory swelling
3. Enlarged eye (buphthalmos)

Shallow anterior chamber

1. Anterior displacement of the lens forcing the iris forward
2. Enlargement (intumescence) of the lens occurs with some cataracts
3. Iris bombé (forward bulging of the iris) results when a complete annular (ring or circular) synechia seals the edge of the iris to the lens so that aqueous cannot pass through the pupil into the anterior chamber. This accumulation of fluid causes the iris to bulge forward, resulting in iris bombé. In turn, this can cause the base of the iris to obstruct the filtration angle and produce obstructive glaucoma.
4. Neoplasms of the anterior uvea
5. Corneal perforation with loss of aqueous

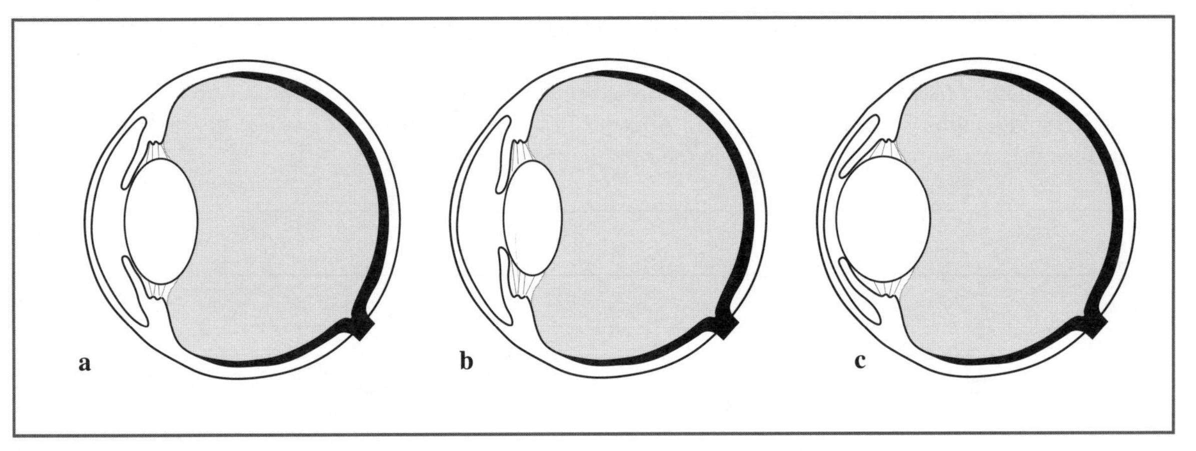

Figure 11-2. Effect of lens size on depth of anterior chamber.
a. Normal lens with normal anterior chamber
b. Deep anterior chamber due to small lens
c. Shallow anterior chamber due to intumescent cataract

Deep anterior chamber

1. Posterior displacement of the lens
2. Small lens - congenital microphakia or absorption cataracts
3. Chronic glaucoma with buphthalmos

Irregular anterior chamber

1. Lens displacement along the equatorial plane results in a shallow chamber in the direction of the displacement and deepening at the point where the lens has pulled away from the zonules
2. Anterior uveal tumors frequently cause an irregular surface to the iris, thereby resulting in irregular anterior chamber depth. This is more frequently seen than a uniformly shallow anterior chamber.
3. Iritis with focal inflammatory swelling or intrastromal hemorrhage
4. Anterior iris synechia - minor synechia may not affect the depth but major anterior synechia will result in a shallow chamber in the area of the synechia

ABNORMAL CONTENTS

Aqueous flare (Fig 1-6, Chapter 1, page 11)

Normal aqueous is optically clear when examined with a transilluminator. If examined with a table slit lamp using a bright narrow slit beam, a faint relucence *may* be seen along the path of light. This is normal and results from light reflected by small particles suspended in the aqueous. Normal aqueous has 20 to 30 mg/dl protein (range 10-50 mg/dl) and occasional cellular debris. When the anterior uvea becomes inflamed, there is an increase in aqueous protein (up to 2-4 gm/dl). This protein will reflect light (Tyndall effect) and is referred to as aqueous flare. Some examiners grade flare from + to ++++, depending on severity. Flare disappears as the uveal inflammation subsides. Examination for aqueous flare should be performed in all animals suspected of anterior uveitis.

Keratic precipitates (Fig 11-3)

These are cellular and fibrinous deposits on the posterior surface of the cornea, occurring after injury or anterior uveitis. They may appear as drops of dew, resemble fat droplets, or have a dark color (black from iris pigment, red from RBC). The aqueous convection currents are responsible for their distribution. The lower half of the cornea is involved first. In severe involvement they occur on the upper cornea as well.

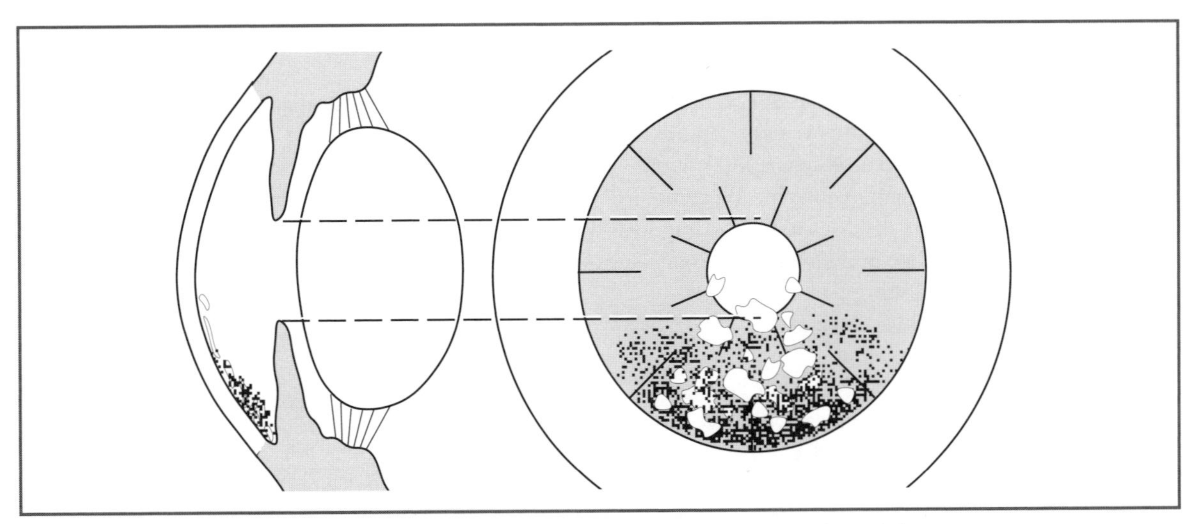

Figure 11-3. Keratic precipitates are shown on the endothelial surface of the cornea. Most of them are on the lower one-half of the cornea.

Hypopyon - pus in the anterior chamber

1. Causes - may be bacterial infection or sterile leukotactic response
   a. Anterior uveitis - most likely cause in cats and food animals
   b. Keratitis (interstitial or ulcerative) - ulcerative keratitis may result in a severe sterile hypopyon - most likely cause in dogs and horses
2. Signs - pus will settle to the lower limits of the anterior chamber. If associated with an ulcer, it will often build up below the level of the ulcer, with a peak resembling sand in an hourglass. When seen with uveitis, it will be level.
3. Treatment
   a. Medical treatment - preferred. Correct the primary cause and hypopyon responds spontaneously.
   b. Surgical - rarely recommended. Surgical removal of hypopyon can result in enough additional irritation to an already acutely inflamed eye to outweigh the benefits of removing it. Do not consider surgery unless the lower portion of the anterior chamber is filled to the level of the pupil and the pus is contacting the lens.
      1) Aspiration at the limbus with a 20 gauge needle. A suture may be needed to close the wound.
      2) Stab puncture at the limbus with a cataract knife or broken razor blade, then hook the material with an iris hook. A mini-tip culturette swab (Becton-Dickinson) can be inserted through the wound into the hypopyon, then twisted and withdrawn. The fibrin in the pus will adhere to the wood and help remove the exudate.
      3) Reform the anterior chamber with intraocular antibiotics
      4) Culture the aspirate to ensure the most appropriate antibiotic is chosen

Hyphema

Hyphema is blood in the anterior chamber and is usually unilateral. It may be acute, chronic or recurring, depending on the type of anterior uveal disease. When the patient is quiet, blood settles in the anterior chamber. With activity it will resuspend in the aqueous. Fresh blood is bright red and will darken if it remains in the anterior chamber. Clotting is reduced by dilution of the blood by aqueous and the release of plasminogen activator by the surface of the iris. Unclotted blood exits via the filtration angle.

1. Causes
   a. Trauma
      1) Perforating wounds
      2) Severe blows to the eye or head (small animals - auto injuries; large animals - owner-inflicted)

3) Choking dogs with a leash or rope (handling vicious animals)

b. Nontraumatic

1) Congenital vascular abnormalities - collie eye, Sheltie eye, Australian shepherd. Severe microphthalmic eyes are predisposed.

2) Anterior uveitis (vasculitis) - acute or chronic. Cats: FLV is probably the most common nontraumatic cause for hyphema; FIP and toxoplasmosis less frequent.

3) Systemic diseases with bleeding disorders

a) Platelet deficiency (immune-mediated, ehrlichiosis)

b) Clotting factor disorders

c) Polycythemia

d) Leukemia

e) Poisons (Warfarin)

4) Systemic hypertension - cats and dogs

5) Neoplasia - anterior uvea

6) Chronic glaucoma - an unfavorable sign. Usually becomes recurrent and eventually persistent.

7) Postcataract extraction - occurs several months after apparently successful surgery

8) Unknown (idiopathic) - adult dogs. Intraocular neoplasia should always be considered. Some adult dogs experience a single episode of hyphema without recurrence. If there is recurrence, warn the owner that the eye may develop a pattern of increased frequency of episodes until constant hyphema persists.

2. Significance - varies with cause. Simple hyphema usually resolves spontaneously without complications in 7 to 10 days.

a. Unfavorable prognosis

1) Severe trauma with "8-ball" hemorrhage - 8-ball hemorrhage refers to an anterior chamber totally filled with darkened blood.

2) Glaucoma

3) Postcataract

4) Intraocular neoplasia

5) The hemorrhage seen with FLV will usually respond dramatically to systemic steroid treatment but the disease warrants an unfavorable prognosis

b. Guarded prognosis

1) Trauma with moderate eye injury - hemorrhage has stopped by the time of examination and areas of clear aqueous are visible

2) Recurring spontaneous

c. Favorable prognosis

1) Choking - is usually normal 24 to 48 hours, with or without treatment

2) Spontaneous - first occurrence

3) Trauma with minor injury to eye

4) Treatable systemic diseases (e.g. immune-mediated thrombocytopenia)

3. Treatment

a. Identify and treat the specific cause

b. Keep the patient quiet (tranquilizers - confinement)

c. Autonomic nervous system drugs (controversial and of NO proven value)

1) Mydriatics vs miotics

a) Atropine 1% - cycloplegic action will reduce filtration angle outflow, therefore increasing danger of glaucoma, but is important in the treatment of anterior uveitis

b) Epinephrine 1% or 2% - vasoconstrictors may reduce hemorrhage and dilate pupil, reducing complications of posterior synechia

c) Pilocarpine 1% - maintains filtration angle outflow. Miotic action increases the iris surface, enhancing fibrinolysin activity. If posterior synechia occurs there is greater chance for interference of aqueous flow through the pupil.

    2) *Comment* - The author prefers topical epinephrine (a weak mydriatic) followed by atropine 24 hours after hemorrhage stops.

  d. Intraocular tissue plasminogen activator (tPA) 25 μg. Will dissolve clots and fibrin, but if the cause is not removed, rebleeding is likely.
  e. Anti-inflammatory - topical corticosteroids that penetrate the anterior chamber (prednisolone acetate, dexamethasone, and prednisolone phosphate).
  f. *Comment*
    1) Mild hemorrhage will clear significantly in 24 hours
    2) Large clots disappear very slowly without tPA
    3) If cause cannot be corrected, relapses are common and eventually will lead to blindness

Fibrin (Plasmoid aqueous)

Fibrin will escape into the aqueous in any condition that decreases the blood-aqueous barrier.

1. Causes
  a. Inflammation of the anterior uvea
  b. Sudden reduction in intraocular pressure
    1) Intraocular surgery
    2) Perforating ocular wound
    3) Anterior chamber centesis
2. Signs
  a. If minor - increased aqueous flare
  b. If more severe - fibrin clots form which may:
    1) Adhere to corneal endothelium and cause leukoma
    2) Adhere to lens and cause capsular cataract
    3) Cause iris to adhere to the lens, resulting in posterior synechia and iris bombé
    4) Obstruct filtration angle and cause glaucoma
3. Significance
  a. Fibrin usually pulls free from fixed structures and absorbs. This may take a few days to a few weeks.
  b. Fibrin that is attached only to one tissue is not harmful (e.g. cornea or iris only)
  c. If severe and not treated, permanent synechia and/or obstructive glaucoma can result
4. Treatment
  a. Identify and treat the cause of the uveitis with anti-inflammatory drugs as previously recommended
  b. Additional treatment
    1) Aqueous flare - not needed
    2) Fibrin clots - intraocular tPA (see page 124)

Lipid aqueous

Free fat (chylomicra) and lipoproteins in the anterior chamber result in aqueous with a milky appearance. This can fill the lower part or all of the anterior chamber. Lipid aqueous is more homogeneous-appearing than fibrin or lens material. Slit lamp examination will reveal that the cornea is normal. Most eyes show signs of mild to acute anterior uveitis.

1. Pathophysiology - The normal blood-aqueous barrier restricts serum lipid and lipoprotein from the aqueous
  a. Particle size limitation of the healthy blood-aqueous barrier is 40 Å
    1) Ciliary body
      a) Capillaries will allow passage of particles up to 250 Å
      b) Nonpigmented ciliary epithelium will restrict molecules larger than 40 Å
    2) Iris - blood vessels will restrict molecules larger than 40 Å

b. Particle size of serum lipid
    1) Lipoproteins - 55 to 90 Å
    2) Chylomicra - up to 5000 Å
c. Anterior uveitis with concurrent hyperlipemia will result in the accumulation of lipid and lipoprotein in the aqueous. Aqueous clearing will result when the uveitis subsides.

2. Clinical signs
    a. Sudden onset of a white-appearing eye. Some animals have a history that this has occurred before and gradually cleared.
    b. If bilateral, dog may appear blind, depending on severity
    c. Signs of anterior uveitis (slight or severe)
        1) Conjunctival hyperemia
        2) Episcleral infection
        3) Photophobia
        4) Low intraocular pressure
3. Treatment
    a. Symptomatic - treat the uveitis
    b. Specific - determine and treat the cause for hyperlipemia

Lens

The lens may luxate into the anterior chamber or rupture and fill the anterior chamber. See lens discussion, Chapter 13, page 401. Ruptured lens cortex must be differentiated from plasmoid or lipid aqueous.

Abnormal growths - Several forms of abnormal tissues may be found in the anterior chamber: anterior uveal tumors, granuloma, anterior chamber pigment epithelium cysts.

1. Anterior uveal tumors - can occur in all species - They may be small masses that are slowly growing or rapidly growing masses that completely fill the anterior chamber in several weeks. They usually begin near the base of the iris.

    Melanoma (benign or malignant) is the most common tumor and can be identified by gross appearance.

    Lymphosarcoma, undifferentiated carcinomas and amelanotic malignant melanomas may appear similar. These must be differentiated from granulomas. Tumors are more likely than granulomas. Aspiration cytology of the mass or aqueous is valuable for specific diagnosis. The cornea usually remains clear even where contacted by the tumor, thus allowing the vascular pattern of the tumor to be clearly visible as the tumor enlarges. Most patients develop a secondary anterior uveitis with circumcorneal injection.

    See Chapter 12, page 378, Anterior Uvea, for treatment of iris tumors.
2. Granulomas - Iris granulomas protruding into the anterior chamber are less frequent than tumors. They will have an associated aqueous flare and possible free fibrin clots.

    Positive diagnosis would be made using aqueous examination (cytology and/or culture). Symptomatic treatment consists of systemic antibiotics and anti-inflammatory drugs. Specific treatment can be started when diagnostic results are available. If medical treatment is not successful after two or three weeks, eye removal should be considered.
3. Pigment epithelium cysts - Cysts are seen in all species; most common in the dog. Pigment epithelium cysts may develop from the iris or ciliary body. They may be attached to the edge of the pupil or pass through the pupil and continue to grow in the anterior chamber. Cysts are dark brown or black and when transilluminated appear hollow. They vary in size and number (singular to many, appearing as fine sand). They are not irritating to surrounding tissue and will not be clinically significant unless large enough to fill the pupillary area. Free floating cysts may persist for months before they rupture. Examinations of the iridocorneal angle may reveal cysts that have adhered, subsequently ruptured and now appear as a black film. An example of this was a Boston terrier with multiple small cysts filling the lower half of the anterior chamber. The dog developed uveitis. When the uveitis was resolved, all of the cysts had disappeared except two that adhered to the corneal endothelium. See also page 366, 376.

Parasites

Aberrant parasite migration may result in migrating parasites (larvae or adults) entering the anterior chamber. The parasites may be quite active and startling to observe. If allowed to remain, they can produce severe uveitis and corneal endothelial damage. This is intensified if the parasite dies.

1. Heartworms - in cats and dogs
2. *Setaria equi* larvae - have been seen in horses, mules and donkeys. This is uncommon in the United States but common in some parts of the world.
3. Ophthalmomyiasis - migration of fly larvae may occur anywhere in the eye
4. Treatment - Surgical removal before they cause irritation can save vision. A limbal incision is recommended. The parasite may flow into the wound for easy removal. If this does not occur, forceps or a blunt iris hook can be used to remove the parasite. Suturing the wound is recommended.

Foreign bodies - Foreign bodies that affect only the anterior chamber are uncommon. Most involve the cornea, iris and/or lens.

1. Etiology - Thorns, slivers or small firearm pellets (BB, airgun, shotgun) that perforate the cornea may lose their momentum so they do not penetrate the lens or iris
2. Treatment
   a. Thorns and slivers presented soon after penetration should be removed. The perforating wound is enlarged or a new wound is made at the limbus, and then a forceps used for removal. Postsurgically they are treated as recommended for other intraocular procedures.

      Organic foreign bodies that have been present for several days warrant a very guarded prognosis. If the foreign body is easily identified and the reaction is minimal, removal would still be indicated. If there is severe inflammatory response, but minimal hypopyon or panophthalmitis, a medical approach with systemic and topical medications can result in the foreign body becoming walled off and the eye remaining visual.
   b. Firearm pellets - if recent, remove through corneal wound and then suture cornea. If longstanding and the pellet is anchored by organized fibrin or secondary scar tissue, do not attempt removal.

CHAPTER 12 - ANTERIOR UVEA

The uvea is the vascular tunic of the eye and consists of the iris, ciliary body and choroid.

TERMS

Anterior uvea - iris and ciliary body
Anterior uveitis - iridocyclitis (the iris and ciliary body are so closely related that inflammation of one is usually associated with inflammation of the other)
Choroiditis - inflammation of the choroid (choroiditis will usually result in a related inflammation of the retina)
Cyclitis - inflammation of the ciliary body
Iridocyclitis - inflammation of the iris and ciliary body
Iritis - inflammation of the iris
Posterior uvea - choroid
Posterior uveitis - the preferred term for inflammation of the choroid (choroiditis or chorioretinitis)
Uveitis - inflammation of the entire vascular tunic

ANATOMY AND PHYSIOLOGY

IRIS - Canine (Fig 12-1), Equine (Fig 12-2)

The iris consists of a delicate network of blood vessels, connective tissue, muscle fibers and nerves. The color varies and is determined by the cellular arrangement of the anterior border layer and the concentration of stromal pigments.

The anterior surface is divided by the collarette into a central pupillary zone and a peripheral ciliary zone.

1. The pupillary zone - is thinner and characterized by small defects that result in a rough (moth-eaten) appearance. The pupillary margin is lined with an extension of pigment epithelium (pupillary ruff) giving it a velvet-like appearance. In herbivorous animals, these are exaggerated to form the granula iridica.
2. Collarette is a slightly elevated area representing where the pupillary membrane was attached to the iris prenatally.
3. Peripheral ciliary zone is smoother and slightly thicker than the pupillary zone. Near the limbus the major arterial circle can be seen within the iris stroma. In animals with a thin iris (blue), these vessels can easily be seen on the surface of the iris stroma.

Wyman divides the iris into four layers:

1. Anterior border area
2. Stroma and iris sphincter (some authors include dilator muscle in this layer)
3. Dilator muscle
4. Posterior epithelium

1. *Anterior border layer* - is composed of an outer layer of fibrocytes (endothelium) and one or more layers of melanocytes. The outer layer is composed of tightly or loosely arranged cells. A tight arrangement provides a smoother, darker surface than the loose arrangement seen in the light-colored iris. The fibrocyte layer is continuous with the endothelium covering the pectinate ligaments and the cornea. The color of the iris varies with the number of melanocytes.
2. *The stroma* - accounts for most of the mass of the iris and contains the sphincter muscle, blood vessels, pigment cells, collagen fibrils, nerves and a matrix of mucopolysaccharides. The shape of the pupil varies with the arrangement of the sphincter muscles. The fibers are circular in the dog, whereas in the cat they are interwoven vertically in the dorsal and ventral regions, resulting in a slit appearance when constricted. The sphincter is smooth muscle originating from the pigment epithelium and innervated by parasympathetic nerves (except in birds, where it is striated muscle).

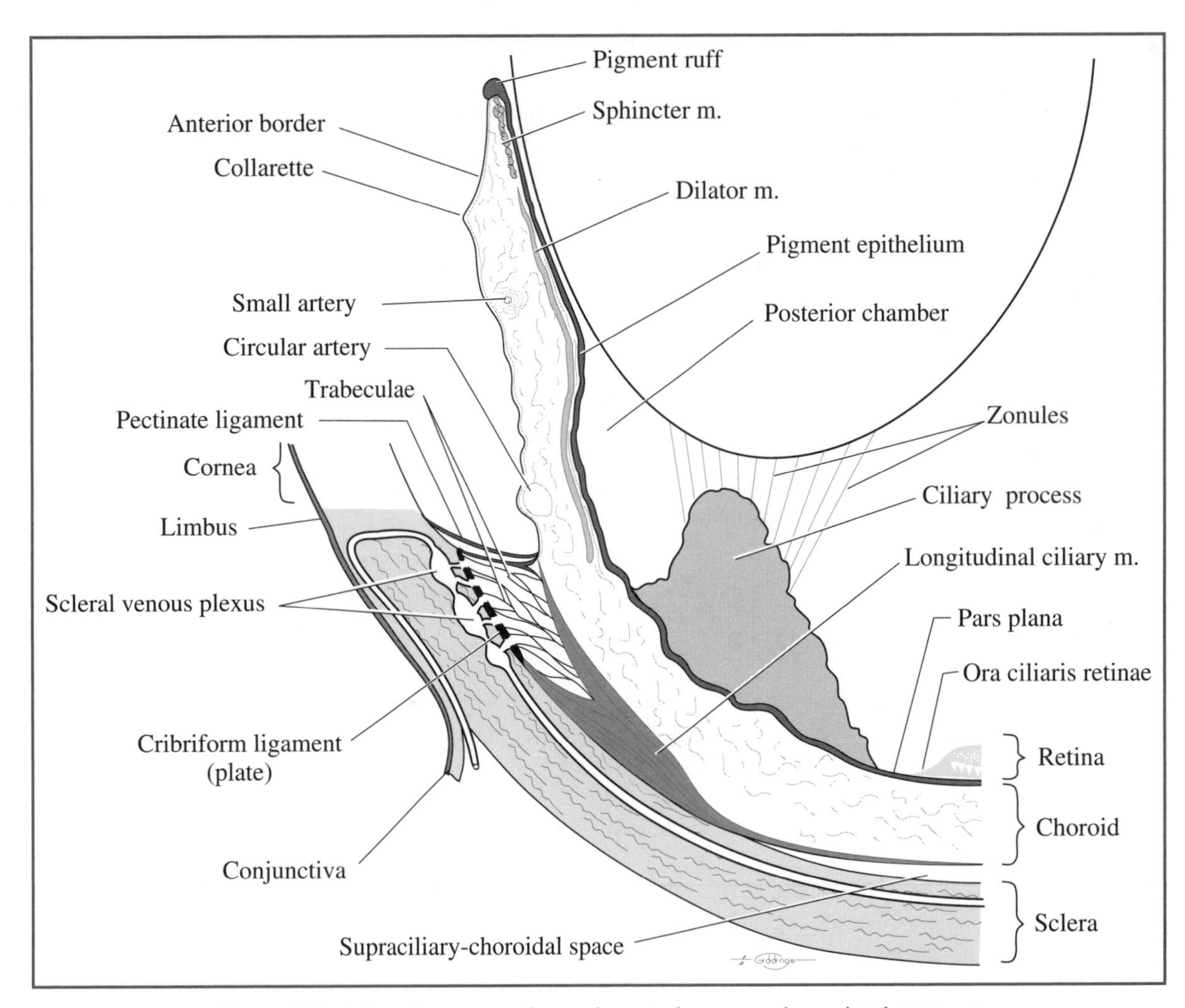

Figure 12-1. Schematic cross-section canine anterior uvea and associated structures.

The major blood supply is by means of the major arterial circle, which is a continuation of the long posterior ciliary arteries. The arteries enter the iris at three and nine o'clock, branch, and continue near the base of the iris to 12 and 6 o'clock. Here they may end or anastomose, making a complete circle. They do not anastomose in the dog, horse and pig.

3. *Dilator muscle* - extends from the base of the iris to the sphincter, separating the stroma from the posterior pigment epithelium layer. The dilator m. is derived from the anterior pigment epithelial layer and contains melanin granules.
4. *Pigment epithelium* - Pigment epithelium originates from the neuroectoderm layers of the embryonal optic cup (Fig 13-2; Chapter 13, page 379), which gives rise to specific ocular structures. Beginning at the anterior portion of the optic cup, the outer anterior epithelial layer is the origin for the dilator and sphincter muscles of the iris and continues posteriorly as the pigmented epithelium of the ciliary body and retina. The inner (posterior) epithelial layer of the optic cup is represented by the pigment epithelial layer of the iris, the nonpigmented epithelial layer of the ciliary body and posteriorly as the neural retina.

   The pigmented epithelium is thick near the pupil and may be seen extending around the edge of the pupil as a black velvet-like border, the pupillary ruff. As previously mentioned, in herbivores it manifests as granula iridica (umbraculum, corpora nigra) along the border of the iris. These consist of pigment epithelium, fine stromal network and small blood vessels. They serve to occlude the central pupil when the pupil is constricted.
5. *Comment* - The iris lies in direct contact with the lens. This contact gives the iris the same curvature as the anterior surface of the lens. Changes in position or size of the lens will result in a change in convexity of the surface of the iris (Chapter 11, Fig 11-2, page 352; Chapter 13, Fig 13-17 and 13-18, pages 402-403).

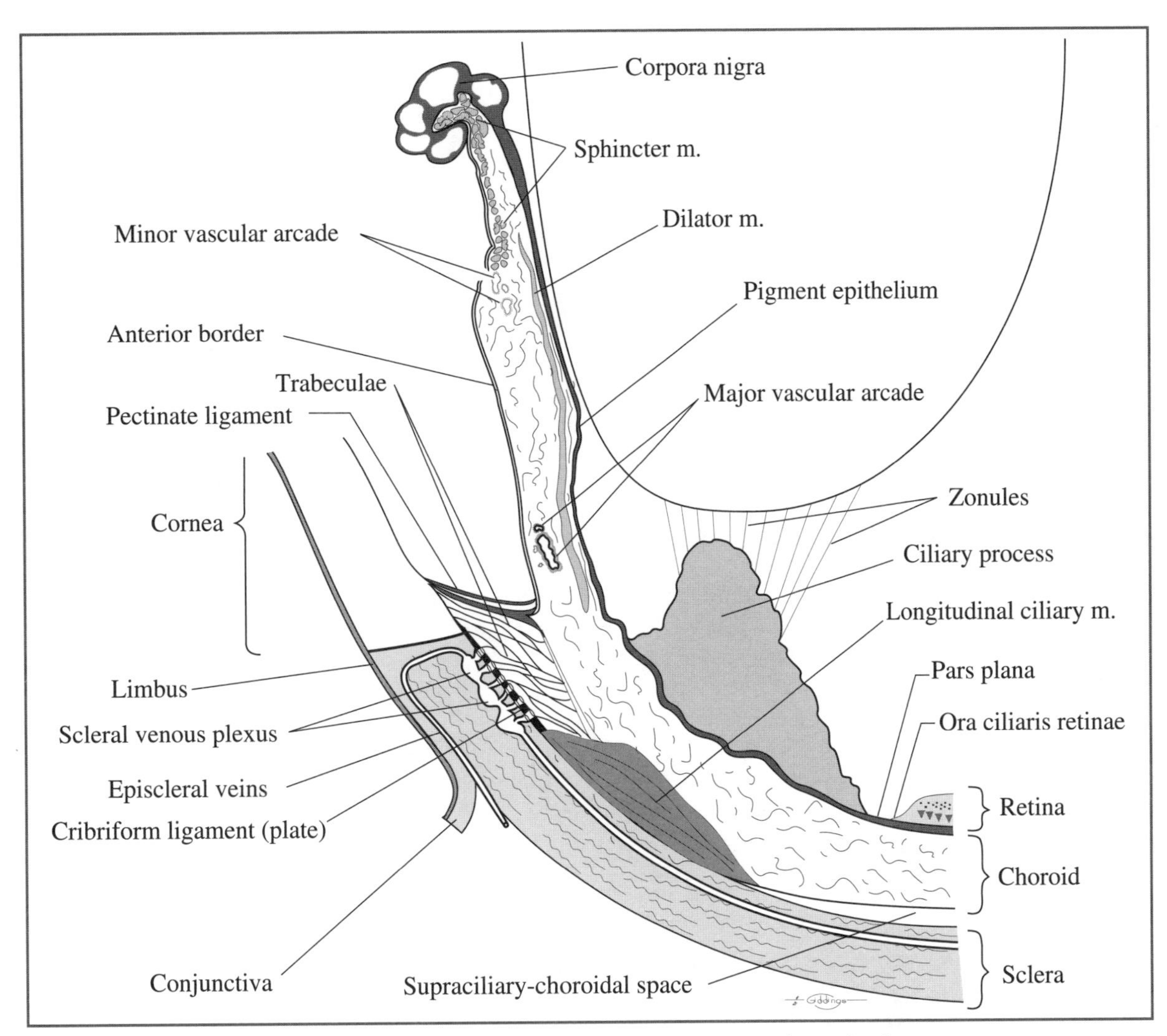

Figure 12-2. Schematic cross-section of equine anterior uvea and associated structures.

Pupillary appearance and shape varies with species (Fig 12-3)

1. Dogs - The iris characteristically has a moderate two-toned effect (this is a normal heterochromia). There is a slightly different shading to the iris central to the collarette than toward the periphery. In some cases, a third, darker zone is seen near the base of the iris. In animals with chronic uveitis the iris typically darkens and the color zones may disappear.

   The pupil is usually central but slight superior nasal deviation is common. The pupil responds quickly to bright light, reducing to 1 to 3 mm in diameter. If the animal is frightened it may be slow to respond. Mydriasis from an unknown cause has been observed in some animals that have normal vision, occasionally in diabetes mellitus before treatment, and in some animals that receive chloramphenicol systemically. The possibility of atropine therapy should be eliminated in animals with dilated pupils.
2. Cats - The iris usually has a single color or mixing of color, without the color zone effect seen in dogs.

   The pupil closes to a vertical slit when miotic and is round when totally dilated. The innervation of sphincter muscle bands in each side are separate. Therefore, injury or intraocular lesions can occur that affect only one side of the pupil. Cats will occasionally have a transient dilated pupil (usually unilateral) without any other signs. The pupil usually returns to normal in two to three weeks, but may take two months. This must be differentiated from mydriasis seen with FLV. Chloramphenicol will occasionally cause transient mydriasis.

   After the pupil has been stimulated by a bright light it is slower to return to normal than in a dog.

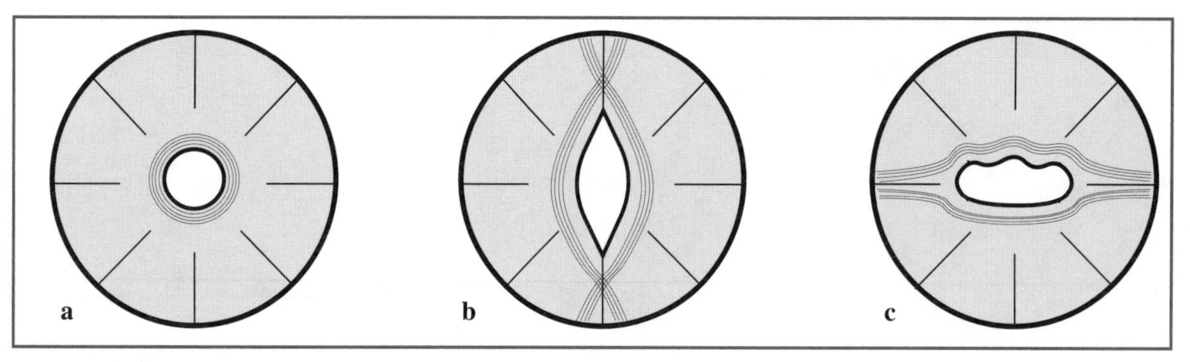

Figure 12-3. Pupil shapes of domestic animals are determined by the type of sphincter muscles.
a. Circular sphincter results in a round pupil (dogs, birds, pig, goat, primates)
b. Vertical slit pupil with interlacing muscles creating a scissors-like pupillary closure (typical of cats)
c. Horizontal pupil characteristic of ungulates (horses, cattle, sheep and llamas)
Modified from Prince JH: Comparative anatomy of the eye. Springfield, CC Thomas, 1956.

3. Horses - The iris is usually evenly colored. Recurrent uveitis will cause darkening of the iris in the affected eye.

   The pupil is round in colts and becomes oval as the animal matures. The granula iridica are most prominent along the upper margin of the pupil. When examined in bright sunshine, the granula may obliterate the central pupil, leaving an opening only at the ends of the pupillary slit. In a darkened room or stall, the pupillary reflexes of horses are the slowest of all domestic animals and will not close as completely as when examined outside.
4. Cattle sheep and goats - Iris similar to equine, with better pupillary reflexes. The granula iridica may be the same size on both sides of the pupil.
5. Llamas - The pupil is similar to cattle except for an extremely prominent pupillary ruff, resulting in an irregular pupil margin, with the upper and lower margins interdigitating.

CILIARY BODY

The ciliary body serves three very important functions: it supports the lens; it is the major site for the production of aqueous; and it is an integral part of the cilioscleral sinus, which is responsible for aqueous outflow.

The anterior portion, *pars plicata (corona ciliaris)*, consists of the ciliary muscles and the ciliary processes; the posterior portion, *pars plana (orbiculus ciliaris)*, extends posteriorly to the choroid. The junction with the choroid and retina is distinct and is called the *ora ciliaris retinae*.

Ciliary processes - are fin-like processes (70 to 100 in number) covered by two layers of epithelium and give the ciliary body a triangular appearance. The processes are highly vascular, with the capillaries separated from the pigment epithelium by a basement membrane and collagen fibrils. The vascular system and the epithelium are responsible for the production of aqueous.

Ciliary muscles - In domestic animals the circular and oblique muscles are poorly developed, thus contributing to poor accommodation. The prominent muscle is the longitudinal ciliary muscle. This muscle arises from the *pars plana* and splits into two layers:

1. The outer layer (cribriform ligament or plate) hugs the sclera and extends anteriorly to Descemet's membrane.
2. The inner layer extends forward to the root of the iris.

This splitting forms the ciliary cleft (cilioscleral sinus). Within the cleft is the ciliary trabecular meshwork, which represents interstitial fibers of the longitudinal muscle.

CONGENITAL DEFECTS

Congenital defects are seen rather frequently. Except for persistent pupillary membranes, the defects usually seen have little or no adverse effect on sight.

HETEROCHROMIA (Fig 12-4)

Heterochromia is difference of color between the irides, part of one iris having a different color, or mixing of colors in an iris. This may be hypopigmentation or variable pigmentation.

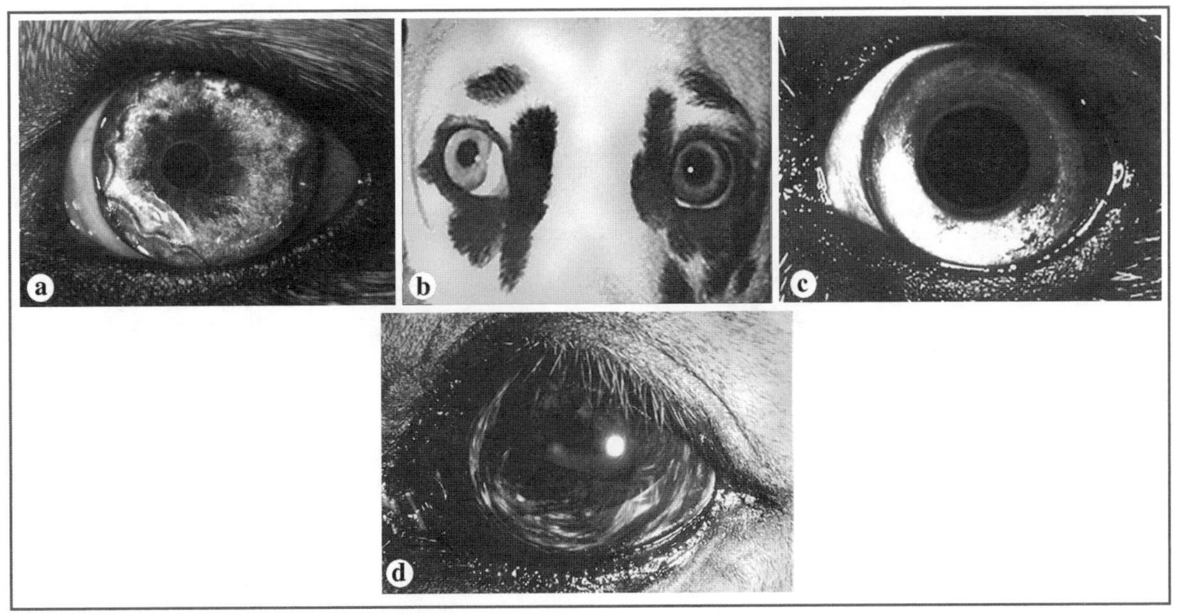

Figure 12-4. Heterochromia.
a. Dog - normal heterochromia color bands from pupil outward: dark, light, dark
b. Dalmatian with blue iris and brown iris
c. Dog - blue and brown iris
d. Horse - variegated brown and orange iris

Hypopigmentation

Hypopigmentation has concurrent iris hypoplasia and is related to haircoat color genetics affecting iris pigment development. It may be seen in subalbinotic or true albino animals.

1. Dogs
   a. Merling genetics (merling genetics are dominant and can be associated with deafness) - collies and related breeds, harlequin great Danes, dappling in Dalmatians
   b. Subalbinism - Siberian huskies and malamutes
2. Cats
   a. Siamese and related breeds
   b. White cats with blue eyes may have unilateral or bilateral deafness. White cats with an eye other than blue will be expected to be deaf on the side of the blue eye.
3. Horses - Pinto, Appaloosa, white and some grays

Terminology for uniocular lesions

1. Walleye - a particolored blue and white iris
2. China eye - a particolored blue iris

3. Watch eye - a particolored blue and yellow or brown iris
4. Piebald iris - any particolored iris

Hyperpigmentation spots

Some animals will have a hyperpigmented area on the iris from birth. When this occurs it is referred to as an iris nevus and should be observed for change that may suggest development of melanoma.

PERSISTENT PUPILLARY MEMBRANE (PPM) (Fig 12-5)

Pathogenesis

In the fetus, the pupil is covered with a thin pupillary membrane that absorbs before birth in precocious animals, such as foals and calves. In dogs, absorption is not complete when the eyes open, and web-like strands are still present. These strands normally disappear by four to five weeks of age. Some small strands may persist longer, disappearing before maturity, but large ones may persist for life. Central anterior capsule pigment deposits can also occur.

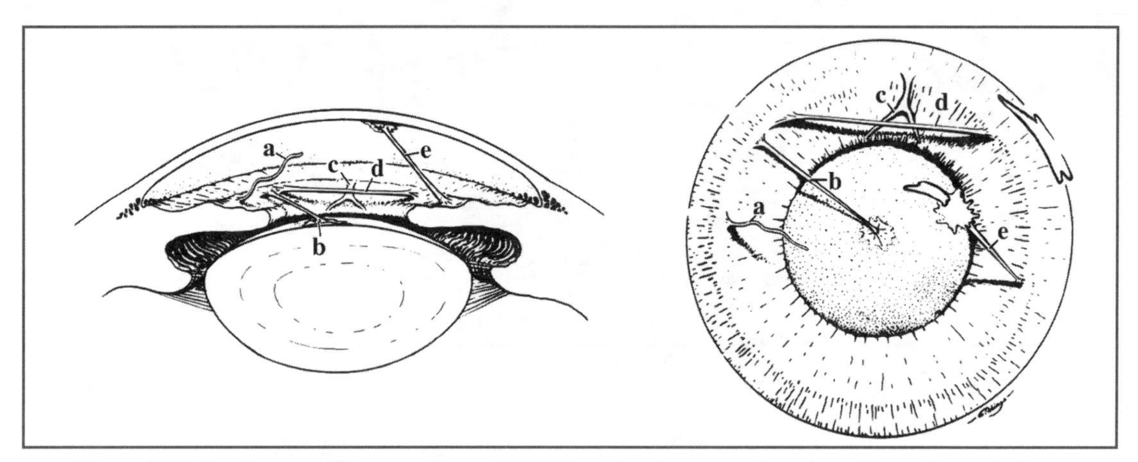

Figure 12-5. Persistent pupillary membrane (PPM) frontal and cross-section views illustrating variations.
a. One end of PPM floating in anterior chamber - no clinical significance
b. Iris to lens - results in capsular cataract
c. "Y" shaped iris to iris band - no clinical significance
d. Single iris to iris band - no clinical significance
e. Iris to cornea - results in adherent leukoma of the cornea

Signs

Signs will vary depending on a) where the strands attach, b) the number involved, and c) how long they persist.

1. Anterior polar capsular pigment deposits - these are common and represent nests of pigment due to incomplete PPM regression.
2. Iris-to-iris - no pathologic change occurs. These are common in young dogs and less frequent in adults. Most are observed as small strands going from one area of the collarette to another. Strands assuming a "crow's-foot" appearance are frequently seen.
3. Iris-to-cornea - pathologic change occurs. This causes corneal endothelial damage, resulting in edema. Severity of the edema is proportional to the number of adherent strands and is most severe in puppies, decreasing with age as the strands regress. Severely affected puppies may be blind and become visual by maturity. Secondary bullous keratitis can occur. Close examination (slit lamp) of the cornea will reveal permanent foci of fibroplasia where the strands attached to the cornea before regression.
4. Iris-to-lens - pathologic change occurs. This causes anterior capsular and/or capsular cortical cataracts at the point of lens attachment. These cataracts are usually stationary; therefore visual impairment is not anticipated. Normal pupillary movement is expected.

Inheritance

1. Basenji - mechanism of inheritance has not been determined. Breeding of Basenji's with any degree of PPM is not recommended.
2. Other breeds that may be inherited or familial predisposition - chow chow, mastiff, dachshund, Cardigan corgi.

Comment

Any dog with PPM causing pathologic changes of the cornea or lens should not be used as breeding stock.

IRIS HYPOPLASIA (Fig 12-6)

Seen concurrently with hypopigmentation in color-dilute animals. These hypoplastic irides may undergo additional primary atrophy early in life, resulting in loss of most of the functional iris tissue. These animals are usually photophobic. When examined with an ophthalmoscope they will have varying degrees of chorioretinal hypoplasia.

Penlight examination will allow light reflected from the tapetum to retroilluminate the iris, making the defect readily visible. These puppies characteristically have an off-centered (ectopic) pupil that is miotic and hard to dilate. Seen commonly in Siamese cats and horses with subalbinotic changes.

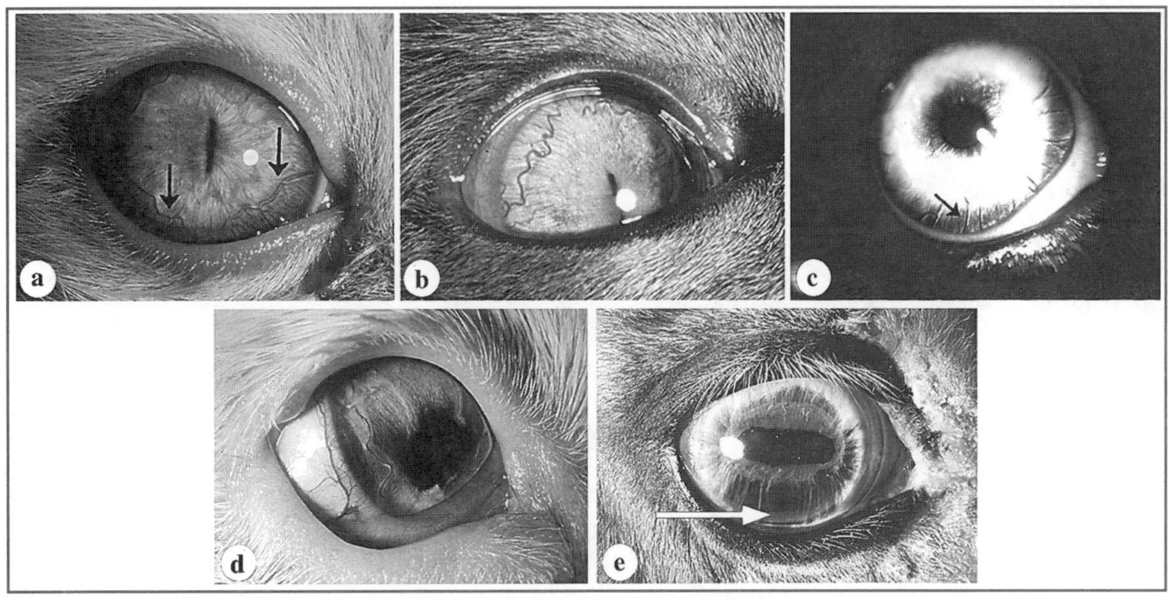

Figure 12-6. Iris hypoplasia.

a. Siamese kitten - iris arteries (arrows) faintly visible
b. Siamese cat with blue iris and clearly visible iris arteries
c. Siberian husky - lens equator (arrow) can be seen through peripheral hypoplastic iris on retroillumination
d. Merle collie puppy - iris hypoplasia and off-centered pupil
e. Twenty year old horse - hypoplasia and secondary iris atrophy resulting in multiple iris perforations. The equator of the lens (arrow) can be visualized through the iris defect.

RARE DEFECTS

Solid iris - no pupil (acorea) results in congenital glaucoma unless small perforations exist

Complete lack of the iris (aniridia)

Ectopic pupil (corectopia) - off-centered pupil

1. Slight corectopia is seen in many dogs without clinical significance
2. Moderate to severe corectopia is usually observed in color dilute dogs (merle collies and Shetland sheepdog, Dalmatian, Great Dane) with or without multiocular changes. See page 435 for multiocular defects.

Polycoria

Polycoria is more than one pupil. This is uncommon. The additional pupil will have sphincter and dilator muscles, giving it reflexes similar to the primary pupil. This pupillary reflex differentiates polycoria from iris atrophy or severe iris hypoplasia. In these conditions, the opening becomes larger when the pupil constricts. This lesion does not have any clinical significance.

Iris coloboma (fissure in the iris) - differs from polycoria in that pupillary membrane constrictor fibers are missing in coloboma. Therefore, the defect becomes larger when the pupil constricts.

Ciliary body pigment epithelium cysts (see also pigment epithelium cysts, page 356, and acquired anterior uveal pigment epithelium cysts, page 376). Although uveal pigment epithelium cysts are usually considered an acquired condition, the author has observed pigment epithelium cysts in golden retriever puppies. They may be single or multiple. The nasal quadrant is frequently affected. In one instance, three-month-old siblings had bilateral posterior chamber cysts that could be seen following mydriasis. In addition, one dog had an equatorial cyst present between the posterior lens capsule and the vitreous.

ACQUIRED DISEASES

ANTERIOR UVEITIS

Mechanisms of ocular inflammation are complex

They may be:

1. The direct response to cell injury from trauma or infection with the release of arachidonic acid and the cascade of events this initiates (Fig 2-14; Chapter 2, Page 91).
2. The response to enzymes and metabolites from inflammatory cells (neutrophils)
3. Immune responses - The eye supports four types of immune responses with types II, III and IV predominating in uveitis. One type of immune response may dominate but several are usually simultaneously involved.
   a. Type I - anaphylactic, mediated by IgE and mast cells
   b. Type II - cytotoxic, mediated by antibodies
   c. Type III - immune complexes, mediated by immune complex deposition and complement activation
   d. Type IV - cell-mediated, mediated by T-lymphocytes
4. The uvea may act as a lymph node - after inflammation, lymphocytes remain in the uvea and when the same antigen recurs at another site in the body, renewed antibody production occurs in the eye, causing an inflammatory response.

Etiology

Anterior uveitis has many causes and, because of this, establishing the exact cause can be one of the most difficult problems in ophthalmology. The causes can be classified as:

1. Exogenous - This is due to direct trauma to the eye or the introduction of infection by perforating wounds. Any form of intraocular surgery will produce some degree of anterior uveitis.
2. Secondary - This results from the spread of inflammation from the sclera or cornea. Deep keratitis and ulcerative keratitis have concurrent anterior uveitis.
3. Specific diseases - Some of the diseases that have been identified are:
   a. Canine - brucellosis, leptospirosis, *Streptococcus* sp, ICH, systemic fungi, heartworms, rickettsia, ehrlichiosis, Rocky Mountain spotted fever, prototheca, toxoplasmosis, *Leishmania donovani*, mycobacteria, rabies, herpesvirus, pyometra, and bacterial septicemia.
   b. Cats - infectious feline peritonitis, feline leukemia virus, feline immunodeficiency virus, toxoplasmosis, systemic fungi, and pyometra.
   c. Equine - see equine recurrent uveitis
   d. Bovine - MCF, prenatal BVD, IBR, toxoplasmosis, complication to IBK, and bacterial septicemia (metritis, severe mastitis)
   e. Sheep and goats - chlamydial infections, *Mycoplasma*, *Elaeophora schneideri*
   f. Llamas - equine herpesvirus-1, septicemia (pneumonia), immunodeficiency syndrome
4. Hypersensitivity (immune-mediated) reactions - This is the most common cause for uveitis seen in dogs and horses. Unfortunately, the exact etiology goes undetermined in most cases.
   a. Local infection elsewhere in the body (tonsils, teeth, anal sacs, uterus or other organs) may result in deposition of immune complexes in the uvea. Later, reinfection may occur and endotoxins or antigenic factors are released from the primary site, reach the uvea, and precipitate an acute allergic response.
   b. ICH ocular reaction in dogs (Arthus type III reaction)
   c. Chronic persistent ocular infection (toxoplasmosis in cats)
   d. Autoimmunity to ocular tissues
      1) Lens protein loss
      2) Uveal or retinal (retinal S antigen) tissues - undergo changes after disease and become antigenic
5. Pigmentary uveitis, in golden retrievers - Characterized by pigment proliferation leading to pigment deposits on the lens with posterior synechia and anterior peripheral synechia predisposing to obstructive glaucoma. Pigment epithelial cysts may also be present.
6. Idiopathic - In many cases a cause cannot be determined.

Species variation

1. Dogs - Hypersensitivity is the most common cause, with exogenous and endogenous causes being next in importance. In the Rocky Mountain area systemic disease is least common.
2. Cats - specific infections are the most common cause; in order of frequency of cause they are: 1) toxoplasmosis, 2) FIP, 3) FeLV (usually a predisposing cause rather than primary). Hypersensitivity seen more in older animals.
3. Equine - Hypersensitivity is the most common cause. The antigen may vary geographically.
4. Bovine - the most common causes are specific infections: MCF, IBR, secondary to infectious bovine keratoconjunctivitis, gangrenous mastitis.
5. Llamas - cause is often obscure

Signs

May be acute or chronic, unilateral or bilateral. If from active systemic disease, usually bilateral; if from hypersensitivity, usually unilateral. One eye may develop signs several days after the other.

1. Animal will exhibit - photophobia, blepharospasm, increased lacrimation and disturbed vision if bilateral.

2. Examination will reveal:
   a. Enophthalmia - due to intraocular pain. There will be an associated prolapse of the third eyelid which will not be improved by topical anesthesia.
   b. Circumcorneal blood vessel injection (ciliary flush) with hyperemia of the conjunctiva
   c. Some cases will even have severe chemosis
   d. Cornea
      1) Varying degrees of corneal edema - This may be severe enough to interfere with visualization of deeper structures.
      2) Cellular infiltrates may give a yellow cast
      3) Neovascularization - amount determined by duration and severity
      4) Keratic precipitates
   e. Abnormal contents anterior chamber - aqueous flare, fibrin clots, hypopyon, hyphema, desquamated pigment epithelial cells.
   f. Iris changes
      1) Iris is rough and swollen in appearance - The iris virtually becomes a waterlogged sponge so full of fluid that its freedom of movement is impaired and the normal pupillary reactions become sluggish or abolished.
      2) Miotic pupil - Pupil constriction results from swelling of the iris and stimulation of the sphincter muscle. The more acute the lesion, the more severe the miosis. Animals with leukemia will have the least pupillary change.
      3) Dull in color and darkened - Ordinarily the iris has considerable luster; this is gone and the iris of the affected eye will be darker than the normal eye.
      4) Vascular congestion - Superficial blood vessels in the stroma become congested and may give a red appearance to the iris if light colored (blue-eyed animals). Superficial hemorrhages may be seen. If the disease becomes chronic, new blood vessels may develop on the surface of the iris (rubeosis iridis).
      5) Synechiae may develop - Exudate may result in adhesion of the iris to other structures. Posterior synechiae are common if treatment is inadequate, started too late, or if the disease is recurrent. Focal adhesions will result in an irregularly shaped pupil and an opacity of the lens capsule at the site of adherence. If the entire pupillary margin of the iris adheres to the lens, an annular posterior synechia occurs (Fig 12-7). This is referred to as seclusion of the pupil. If it prevents aqueous from flowing into the anterior chamber, the iris bulges (iris bombé), the filtration angle is obliterated and secondary glaucoma develops. In some cases the pupillary space may become filled with exudate, which becomes organized into an inflammatory membrane and is referred to as an occlusion of the pupil.

         Anterior synechiae may occur at the base of the iris from permanent organization of inflammatory membranes.
   g. Intraocular pressure. In uncomplicated anterior uveitis, the eye is hypotonic. Inflamed pigment epithelium and vascular congestion result in decreased aqueous production and the aqueous outflow pathway is maximal, resulting in a soft eye. Schiötz tonometer, less than 4 mm Hg (human chart) in acute cases. If the filtration angle becomes obstructed by the iris, fibrin or an inflammatory membrane, obstructive glaucoma will result. Dogs with extreme iris swelling, severe fibrin release, or breeds predisposed to glaucoma should be closely monitored for the development of obstructive glaucoma. An acute anterior uveitis eye with normal pressure suggests impending glaucoma.

Differential diagnosis

Acute anterior uveitis must be differentiated from ulcerative keratitis, acute glaucoma, acute conjunctivitis and episcleritis. The signs these diseases have in common with anterior uveitis are:

1. All have a red eye (circumcorneal injection and/or congested conjunctival blood vessels)
2. Except for episcleritis, all are painful, as evidenced by photophobia and blepharospasm
3. Except for conjunctivitis, all have corneal opacity

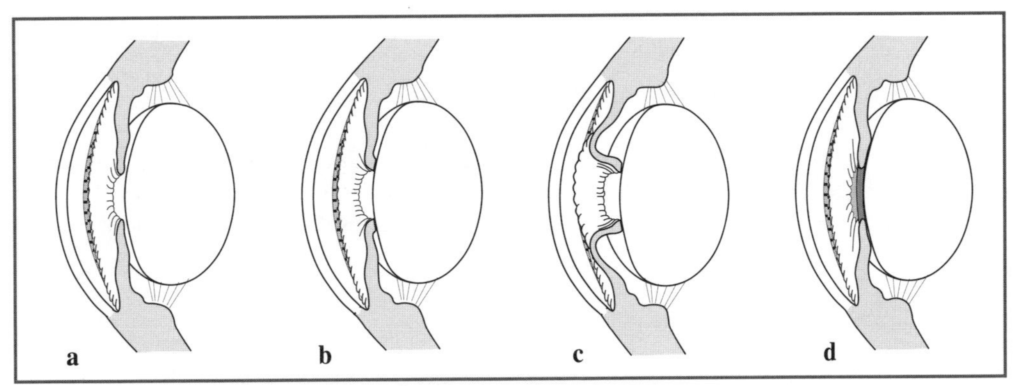

Figure 12-7. Types of posterior synechia.
- a. Normal iris
- b. Secluded pupil - posterior synechia fixing iris to lens prevents iris movement, but does not interfere with aqueous flow
- c. Iris bombé - annular synechia obstructing aqueous flow through the pupil resulting in iris collapse over the filtration angle and secondary glaucoma
- d. Occlusion of the pupil - a secluded pupil with pigment epithelium proliferation filling the pupillary space but does not interfere with aqueous flow

Ulcerative keratitis may result in severe enophthalmia and protrusion of the nictitating membrane, thus hiding the ulcer. Topical anesthesia will relieve the pain so that the eye can be examined.

Acute glaucoma differs in that the pupil will be dilated rather than constricted and the eye is hypertensive rather than hypotensive.

Episcleritis differs in that there is no pain and the iris appears normal.

Acute conjunctivitis will have a mucoid or mucopurulent discharge, the cornea will be clear and the iris will appear normal.

Diagnosis of etiology

1. Clinical signs and history are most helpful
   a. Bilateral suggests systemic disease
   b. Many animals with systemic disease will be presented with additional clinical signs. This is especially true of systemic fungi.
   c. Cats - if granulomatous, is a poor prognostic sign; many will die from the primary disease
   d. Immune-mediated uveitis patients are usually healthy
2. Serology - look for high or changing titers
3. Ocular centesis
   a. Cytology - neoplasia and microorganism
   b. Culture - may be sterile, even with hypopyon
   c. Immunoglobulin levels - In cats when toxoplasmosis is suspected, comparison of serum and aqueous levels of IgM and IgG can be useful in differentiating systemic from ocular produced antibodies. This is also useful in horses with uveitis secondary to leptospirosis.
4. Biopsy - aspiration or excisional
5. Immune profile - to rule out systemic immune diseases

Treatment

Most acute cases are nongranulomatous and respond well to proper treatment.

Granulomatous uveitis does not respond well to treatment and the diseases causing it are usually serious. When it occurs, every effort should be made to determine the exact cause and treat it if possible. Cases that become chronic should be re-evaluated for persistent chronic infectious disease. Treatment with anti-inflammatory drugs may be required the rest of the animal's life.

1. Specific - directed at controlling the primary cause
2. Symptomatic
   a. Anti-inflammatory - corticosteroids and nonsteroidal anti-inflammatory drugs can be administered. They are the most important part of uveitis therapy and in chronic uveitis sometimes the only medication given. They act by inhibiting the inflammatory cascade and immune-mediated uveal response, returning the uveal capillary bed to normal impermeability to protein molecules and red cells, and reducing uveal congestion.
      1) Corticosteroids - are more specific and therefore preferred for acute cases
         a) Systemic prednisolone or prednisone
         b) Topical prednisolone 1% or dexamethasone 0.1% - used concurrently with systemic administration. Initially q2-3h, then QID.
         c) Subconjunctival - may use rapid absorbing for acute or repository combinations for chronic diseases. Indicated when:
            - Systemic is not possible
            - To treat chronic cases where long term systemic medication is contraindicated or cannot be accomplished
            - The patient can only be treated sporadically
      2) Antiprostaglandins are indicated in acute uveitis when corticosteroids are contraindicated. They are often effective to control chronic and/or recurrent uveitis without the side effects observed with extended systemic steroid administration.
         a) Topical antiprostaglandin - Diclofenac 0.1% or Ketorolac 0.5% administered QID
         b) Flunixin meglumine (Banamine) - used in acute ocular inflammation and very effective for controlling ocular pain. It should not be administered for more than five days.
         c) Aspirin - indicated for chronic uveitis in both cats and dogs. It can be given indefinitely. When used for chronic administration, the dosage can frequently be reduced to 1/2 or 1/4.
   b. Immunosuppressants - azathioprine (Imuran) - Systemic azathioprine is indicated in refractory cases when long term therapy is indicated in combination with systemic prednisolone. This reduces the untoward reactions to both drugs while controlling the disease.
   c. Mydriasis
      1) Atropine is the drug of choice - 1% applied every two to three hours until the pupil starts to dilate, then TID. If the pupil does not dilate as well as expected, use concurrent adrenergics. Atropine is beneficial in that it is:
         a) Mydriatic
         b) Cycloplegic - relieves intraocular pain by paralyzing the ciliary muscles
         c) Decongests the iris

         Atropine is contraindicated in glaucoma, therefore it should not be used unless the eye is hypotonic. If the pressure is normal, outflow must be reduced. If mydriasis is deemed necessary, use tropicamide because of its short term effect.
      2) Adrenergic drugs would be indicated in patients where the danger of secondary glaucoma exists.
         a) Epinephrine 1 to 2% - a weak mydriatic
         b) Phenylephrine 2.5 to 10% - a better mydriatic than epinephrine
      3) Combinations - 1% atropine and 10% phenylephrine alternated every one to two hours or mixed together and used every one to two hours. Murocoll 2 (scopolamine and phenylephrine) can also be used. These combinations are useful in severe miosis or to free the iris when

synechiae are present. They will be effective on synechiae that are several days old but will not be effective if longstanding.

d. Fibrin or blood clot lysis
   1) If minimal - no treatment
   2) If severe and threatening complications, intracameral tPA (see page 124).
e. Antibiotics. Less important than atropine and corticosteroid therapy. Many cases are hypersensitization reactions and therefore antibiotics will not alter the course. The acute cases should be treated with antibiotics, even if only as a prophylactic measure. Chronic cases should be examined thoroughly and treated according to individual needs. The acutely inflamed uveal capillary bed will be penetrated by all antibiotics when plasmoid aqueous is being formed. As the case improves, the blood-aqueous barrier to antibiotics returns. By this time the antibiotic has usually served its purpose and can be discontinued.
f. Supportive treatment
   a. Keep in dark room
   b. Warm compresses

Complications

1. May become recurrent or relapsing. Be sure to advise the owner accordingly.
2. Corneal changes
   a. Anterior synechia may cause adherent leukoma
   b. Corneal scarring with a predisposition to corneal vascularization
   c. Corneal endothelial degeneration leading to leukoma and/or bullous keratitis
3. Anterior uveal changes
   a. Synechiae
   b. Secondary atrophy of anterior uvea, leading to phthisis bulbi
4. Lens - Cataract development
5. Secondary glaucoma
   a. Acute obstruction from exudates or the base of the iris
   b. Chronic or recurrent uveitis can lead to progressive filtration angle obstruction and chronic glaucoma

UVEODERMATOLOGIC SYNDROME (VOGT-KOYANAGI-HARADA-LIKE SYNDROME, VKH-LIKE SYNDROME)

VKH-like syndrome is usually an acute onset uveitis with concurrent depigmentation of the skin and hair of the eyelids, nose and lips.

Breed predisposition

1. Most frequently - Akitas, Samoyeds and Siberian husky. Related Akitas have been reported with the disease.
2. Also occurs in Saint Bernard, Shetland sheepdog, Irish setter, golden retriever, Old English sheepdog, Australian shepherd and chow chow.

Age at onset - usually young adults (mean three years)

Signs

1. Ocular
   a. Anterior segment - blepharospasm, conjunctival and episcleral injection, keratitis with vascularization, anterior uveitis, peripheral iris depigmentation and usually poor pupillary reflexes
   b. Posterior segment - chorioretinitis leading to retinal hemorrhage, detachment and/or pigment mottling, optic neuritis, and vitreal exudate and/or hemorrhage
2. Dermatologic
   a. Depigmentation of the skin and hair of the eyelids and lips, and occasionally scrotum and foot pads
   b. Depigmentation and ulceration of the planum nasale and oral mucous membranes

Complications - Hyphema, hypopyon, synechia, cataract, retinal detachment and glaucoma

Diagnosis - is based on history, physical examination and histopathology

1. Skin biopsy reveals a lichenoid dermatitis (intense accumulation of lymphocytes, plasma cells and histocytes along the basement membrane) and marked reduction or absence of melanocytes and melanin
2. Ocular histopathology presents a granulomatous panuveitis, retinitis and focal optic neuritis. Scleral and uveal tissues have diffuse infiltration with a mixed population of mononuclear cells and melanocyte reduction.

Treatment

1. Primary treatment is to control the acute panuveitis (see uveitis for details of treatment)
    a. Corticosteroids - topical and systemic. Pulsed therapy is recommended for peracute cases.
    b. Immunosuppressives - Imuran (azathioprine)
    c. Mydriatic/cycloplegic - atropine: stop immediately if glaucoma develops
    d. Maintenance - as the dog improves, reduce to a maintenance level of corticosteroid and Imuran. Some dogs can be switched to aspirin and/or Imuran.
2. Complications
    a. Acute glaucoma - initiate medical treatment with mannitol, carbonic anhydrase inhibitor and pilocarpine-epinephrine drops
    b. Chronic glaucoma - if visual, medical treatment. If nonvisual, control VKH before pursuing glaucoma treatments
    c. Retinal detachment - if recent, carbonic anhydrase diuretics in addition to uveitis treatment. If chronic, no treatment.

Prognosis - Guarded to unfavorable. Many dogs become blind even with aggressive treatment.

LENS PROTEIN INDUCED UVEITIS

Lens protein induced uveitis results from the formation of excess lens protein antibodies induced by an increased release of lens proteins after injury to the lens capsule, cataract surgery, or the loss of lens protein from cataracts.

Phacoanaphylaxis (phacoclastic uveitis) - is the term for the severe uveitis associated with massive release of lens protein as seen with capsule injury or after cataract surgery when the lens was incompletely removed. Occasionally this occurs with diabetic cataracts.

This results in cellular infiltration of the lens, iris adhesions and a high incidence of obstructive glaucoma (see ruptured lens; Chapter 13, page 403).

Phacolytic (phacotoxic) uveitis - is the milder form of uveitis seen with rapidly developing or hypermature cataracts. This is seen frequently with diabetic cataracts.
This is usually mild uveitis characterized by darkening of the iris, and a mild episcleral injection. Pain will be minimal or absent, and intraocular pressure is decreased.

This type of uveitis can often be controlled with topical corticosteroids and/or oral aspirin.

EQUINE RECURRENT UVEITIS

Equine recurrent uveitis (ERU) is an immune-mediated disease affecting the anterior ocular segment (iris, ciliary body, cornea, lens), the posterior ocular segment (choroid, retina, optic nerve and vitreous) or both. It is the most common cause for blindness in horses and mules. Mules are more resistant than horses.

Synonyms

Recurrent iridocyclitis, periodic ophthalmia, moon blindness. The term moon blindness was given to this disease because the recurring nature suggested it was related to the phases of the moon.

Etiology

Uveitis is the most common intraocular lesion in horses and has many causes: trauma, intraocular surgery, corneal ulcers, interstitial keratitis, local or systemic infection, extension of CNS diseases, immune disorders and severe toxemia. This initial uveitis may heal uneventfully or develop a persistent immune-mediated response resulting in ERU. Often the initiating uveitis may pass unnoticed before the owner is aware ERU exists. Therefore any disease capable of producing a chronic or recurrent sensitization of the vascular tunic of the eye must be considered. Many systemic diseases have been proposed.

1. Deficiency theory - vitamins A, B_2 and C have been suggested but NOT PROVEN.
2. Bacterial
    a. *Leptospira pomona* - has been associated most frequently. Others considered are *autumnalis* and *bratislava*
    b. *Streptococcus equi*
    c. *Brucella abortus* - no longer a significant cause
    d. Others reported *Escherichia coli, Rhodococcus equi, Borrelia burgdorferi* and salmonellosis
3. Viral
    a. Influenza virus
    b. Equine herpesvirus
    c. Equine viral arteritis
4. Parasites
    a. Hypersensitivity to strongyles
    b. *Onchocerca cervicalis* has been proposed as a cause, but the high distribution of this parasite and its incidence in many animals with normal eyes make a causal relationship difficult to establish. It has been demonstrated that when the parasite dies inflammation can occur. Keratoconjunctivitis or keratouveitis have been observed when large numbers of microfilaria migrate into the conjunctiva, superficial stroma of the cornea and intraocular tissues.
    c. Migrating *Setaria* and *Dirofilaria immitis* may gain access to the anterior chamber where they are quite active and startling to see

Signs of anterior segment uveitis

The most frequent observations that cause an owner to have his horse examined include ocular discharge, blepharospasm, change in appearance of the eye (this may be a cloudy cornea and/or a red eye) and less frequently signs of disturbed vision.

1. Acute stage
    a. Early
        1) The horse will be head shy and show photophobia, blepharospasm, enophthalmos, and protrusion of the third eyelid
        2) Catarrhal conjunctivitis with chemosis and epiphora that may become seropurulent after 24 hours
        3) Cornea - may be slightly cloudy
        4) Anterior chamber - slit beam examination will reveal aqueous flare
        5) Iris - swollen, dull in color and a miotic pupil
        6) Tonometry if available will reveal a soft eye
    b. Next one to three days - the eye will change rapidly
        1) Progressive eyelid edema and chemosis

2) Ocular discharge becomes purulent
3) Cornea - edema becomes severe enough to interfere with examination of deeper structures, perilimbal flush as a result of congestion of limbal blood vessels, and keratic precipitates appear
4) Anterior chamber - severe breakdown of the blood aqueous barrier resulting in clotted fibrin and/or blood
5) Iris - extremely edematous and posterior synechia may be forming
6) Intraocular pressure continues to be low

c. After three to six days
1) Cornea - vascularization which proceeds centrally at a rate of 1 mm per day. Severe corneal endothelial damage may result in edema so severe that it will show a ripple effect when the patient blinks. This may progress to bullae formation that ruptures, resulting in corneal ulceration.
2) Anterior chamber - fibrin and blood clots become more organized
3) Iris - posterior synechia develop. Posterior synechia with miosis combined with fibrin obstructing the pupil may cause blindness.

d. If systemic disease is suspected as a cause for ERU, a CBC, urinalysis and blood chemistry are indicated. If infectious diseases such as leptospirosis, brucellosis, toxoplasmosis, systemic fungi or viral are suspected, appropriate serologic tests should be considered.

e. If anterior segment disease were to resolve with treatment at this time, the eye could heal without further deterioration. Unfortunately, in many cases the mechanism for a persisting immune-mediated disease is established and ERU results. Clinical signs may subside and go through quiescent periods, followed by mild recurrent episodes, to acute exacerbations.

2. Quiescent stage - This is the period when the eye is asymptomatic. The length is variable, ranging from weeks to months or even years.

3. Complications
a. Cornea - scarring, residual blood vessels, chronic endothelial degeneration with or without bullous keratitis, anterior synechia with adherent leukoma
b. Iris - One of the most consistent signs of chronicity is darkening of the iris in the diseased eye. It is not unusual to have a horse presented with a history of no previous eye disease and on examination a unilateral dark iris is found that indicates this is ERU and not an initial uveitis episode. Posterior synechia limiting movement of the pupil.
c. Lens and vitreous - complicated cataracts, lens luxation and vitreous opacities
d. Phthisis bulbi - from extensive ciliary body degeneration
e. Obstructive glaucoma from filtration angle obstruction - This is the most common cause for glaucoma in horses.

Treatment of acute anterior segment uveitis

Symptomatic treatment of anterior ERU with anti-inflammatory therapy and mydriatics should be started immediately. Specific treatment is indicated when an etiology has been determined. Anti-inflammatory drugs are the most important part of therapy and often are necessary for several months or longer. Premature discontinuation of anti-inflammatory treatment is a common reason for relapse.

1. Anti-inflammatory drugs
a. Topical prednisolone 1% or dexamethasone 0.1% every four to six hours; or antibiotic combinations
b. Subconjunctival corticosteroids - 20 mg triamcinolone or methylprednisolone, 6-12 mg betamethasone. Subconjunctival repository corticosteroids may be necessary every 30 days for 6 to 12 months.
c. Systemic
1) Flunixin meglumine 1 mg/kg daily for five to seven days. Relief to pain will often be seen in 30 minutes after the IV injection.
2) Ketoprofen can also be used, 1 mg/lb IV daily up to five days
3) Prednisone/prednisolone is used by the author if antiprostaglandins are not effective. Initial dosage - 0.5 mg/lb/day up to two weeks and 0.25 mg/lb/day for three weeks
4) As the patient improves
a) Phenylbutazone 1 to 2 grams BID may be used up to one month and reduced to 1/2 the

dosage for another month

b) The author's choice for convalescence is aspirin, 25 mg/kg (1.1 gm per 100 lbs) BID for one to two months and if there is a history of relapses, reduce to daily indefinitely

2. Mydriatic/cycloplegics
   a. Subconjunctival atropine 1-2 mg and if there is severe miosis add 5 mg phenylephrine
   b. Topical atropine 1% - daily to TID as needed to maintain mydriasis. As the patient improves, atropine is reduced and can eventually be given as infrequently as every four to five days before being discontinued. Atropine will remain longer in the iris of horses than in other species.
3. Systemic antibacterials - if active systemic infection is suspected
4. Symptomatic treatment
   a. Dark stall or cover eye with a hood
   b. Warm compresses are beneficial in the presence of periocular swelling
   c. Topical 5% sodium chloride ophthalmic ointment QID if there is severe corneal edema. Edema is usually transient and will be self-limiting when the corneal endothelium returns to normal. Persistent corneal edema suggests either a continuing endothelial immunologic response or permanent corneal endothelial degeneration. Topical and/or subconjunctival corticosteroids will be beneficial if an active immunologic response exists. If corneal endothelial degeneration has occurred, corticosteroids will not help and an unfavorable prognosis must be given.

Complications to anterior uveitis

1. Relapsing - each attack leads to further damage to the eye and eventually blindness If the eye is blind and constant pain persists, the owner should be advised to consider:
   a. Enucleation - results in immediate relief of pain (see page 497)
   b. Intraocular prosthesis (see page 475)
   c. Intravitreal gentocin injection, 25-50 mg (see pages 77, 475)
2. Cornea - scarring and/or endothelial damage
3. Iris
   a. Darkening color
   b. Synechia
      1) Anterior peripheral leading to glaucoma
      2) Posterior - fixed or irregularly shaped pupil; iris bombé may lead to glaucoma
4. Lens - cataract and/or luxation
5. Vitreous - floaters
6. Phthisis bulbi - from permanent damage to the ciliary body
7. Posterior uveitis

Equine posterior uveitis

Posterior uveitis may occur as a separate entity or concurrent with anterior uveitis. It may be bilateral or unilateral and is rarely presented during the active stage unless blindness results. A blind eye may go undetected by the owner unless the animal involved is a performance horse. Healed lesions are often found as an incidental finding during an eye examination.

1. History - variable
   a. Sudden blindness, but examination reveals one eye has been blind for a long time and now the other eye has recently become blind
   b. Animals with a visual deficiency may be presented with a history of personality change, shying, poor performance or becoming awkward. The blind side may be difficult to examine if blindness is recent and associated with rapid onset.
2. Examination findings - active inflammation
   a. *Optic neuritis* is referred to as papillitis. The optic nerve appears red as a result of congested blood vessels. Small hemorrhages may be seen. The physiologic cup disappears as papillitis progresses. Circumpapillary edema will make the blood vessels near the optic disk appear suspended above the

choroid. Exudate and small blood clots may be seen in the adjacent vitreous.

b. *Active circumpapillary chorioretinitis* will have congested blood vessels, the retina may appear hazy. White infiltrates and small hemorrhages are usually seen. If large areas are involved, subretinal fluid may build up leading to detachment.

3. Examination finding - inactive stage
   a. *Optic nerve atrophy* - will be seen more frequently than optic neuritis. The optic disk appears chalky white and flattened. Blood vessels will be attenuated in early atrophy and absent in advanced atrophy. In rare instances, one-half of the nerve will be atrophied and the remainder normal.
   b. *Retinal degeneration* - As inflammation regresses and the lesion becomes quiescent, this is when retinal degeneration and chorioretinal depigmentation will develop. Later some irregular areas of repigmentation occur and the lesion may take on a butterfly appearance. Tapetal lesions tend to be multiple, more linear in appearance and have areas of hyperreflectivity and pigment reorganization. Rarely is the retinal degeneration extensive enough to cause blindness.
   c. *Retinal detachment* - is usually complete but sectional detachments may occur.
4. Treatment
   a. Acute optic neuritis and chorioretinitis should be treated with systemic prednisolone or dexamethasone and prophylactic antibiotics until laboratory tests are available.
   b. If subretinal edema is present, the patient should receive 0.5 mg/kg of furosemide IV daily to assist removal of the fluid and promote reattachment of the retina.
   c. Treatment is not recommended for patients with optic nerve atrophy, retinal scars or chronic retinal detachment.

ACQUIRED ANTERIOR UVEAL PIGMENT EPITHELIUM CYSTS (see also pages 356, 366)

These are benign cysts that develop from proliferation of ciliary body and iris pigment epithelium.

Occurrence - Most frequent in dogs; less common in cats and horses. Seen in older animals.

Signs

1. Attached to the pupillary border originating from the pupillary ruff
2. Free floating in anterior chamber from pupillary border detachment or passage through the pupil from the posterior chamber. Multiple small cysts are usually formed in the posterior chamber. Sudden motion of the eye will cause cysts to rise up in the aqueous and then settle when the eye is still.
3. Occasionally large cysts will anchor to the corneal endothelium and produce focal corneal edema.
4. They are dark in color and when transilluminated will appear hollow. This differs from solid masses such as tumors or granulomas.

Treatment - Not recommended unless causing pupillary obstruction. Cysts are quite fragile and can be ruptured with a hypodermic needle or 1 mm cataract knife passed into the anterior chamber at the limbus.

IRIS STROMAL CYSTS

Cysts in the iris stroma occur in the equine more than other species. Light-colored irides are usually involved and there is often concurrent stromal atrophy. They may be single or multiple and are located near the base of the iris. Transillumination will result in a hollow appearance. This differentiates the cyst from an iris tumor. Cysts occur more frequently in middle-aged or older horses. Treatment is not recommended.

IRIS ATROPHY

Iris atrophy can occur in aging animals from several causes.

Secondary to iris hypoplasia - Color dilute animals with a thin iris will undergo a generalized iris atrophy

with aging that can result in iris developing a cheesecloth appearance when examined with retroillumination.
Primary iris atrophy - Seen in adult animals that were apparently normal when young. Chihuahua and miniature schnauzer most frequently affected. Multiple holes develop in the iris. These resemble polycoria but become larger when the pupil constricts, thus differentiating them from polycoria.

Pupillary margin atrophy - Seen as an aging change in all species. The pupillary margin becomes irregular. Next, strands of sphincter muscle and stroma become involved, resulting in a larger pupil. In time the sphincter may be totally destroyed, leading to a fixed dilated pupil. There is no treatment. Senile iris atrophy should not be confused with the dilated pupil seen with glaucoma.

ATROPHY OF THE CILIARY BODY PIGMENT EPITHELIUM

Secondary to severe anterior uveitis - This is uncommon. It will lead to decreased aqueous production and eventually phthisis. Seen in all species.

Chronic glaucoma cases occasionally develop epithelial atrophy. The eye becomes hypotonic but remains enlarged unless aqueous production totally shuts down.

TRAUMATIC CYCLODIALYSIS (Ciliary scleral separation)

Severe contusions to the eye cause separation of the anterior uvea from the sclera along the filtration angle. A blow severe enough to do this will be expected to also cause retinal detachment.

One such case in a cat caused permanent separation, traumatic cataract and moderate phthisis bulbi. After traumatic hyphema absorbed, the eye remained aesthetically acceptable and, although blind, was not removed.

ANTERIOR UVEAL NEOPLASIA

The anterior uvea is the most common location for intraocular neoplasia.

The most common primary tumor is melanoma and with exception of the cat, melanoma has a low incidence of metastasis. Terminology for melanomas in animals is inconsistent and for the purpose of simplicity, the following terms will be used for iris pigment proliferation:

Iris freckle (nevus) - a benign focal area of hyperpigmentation that does not change the surface of the iris
Melanosis - progressive hyperpigmentation of the iris that may be diffuse or result from coalescing of freckles, without changing the surface contour of the iris (seen most frequently in cats)
Iris melanoma - a thickened hyperpigmented area with a smooth surface that obscures iris surface, iris detail and has an elevated border

Incidence

1. Dogs
   a. Primary tumors
      1) Melanoma - less than 6% metastatic rate; malignant amelanotic can occur
      2) Ciliary epithelium adenoma/adenosarcoma - more likely to metastasize than melanoma
      3) Rare - hemangiosarcoma, medulloepithelioma (should be considered in nonpigmented masses in the iris of young dogs) and leiomyosarcoma
   b. Secondary tumors - uncommon. Lymphosarcoma, adenosarcomas, transmissible venereal tumor, mammary gland adenocarcinoma, transitional cell carcinoma, fibrosarcoma
2. Cats
   a. Primary tumors
      1) Melanoma - seen in older cats. Iris melanosis may remain benign or develop into iris

melanoma with thickening of the iris. Slit lamp examination often reveals clumps of pigmented cells in the aqueous. The metastatic rate in one group of cats that had their eyes enucleated was 62%. The common ocular complication is glaucoma.
    2) Rare - ciliary epithelial adenocarcinoma, post-traumatic sarcomas (a latent change, blind or phthisical eyes)
  b. Secondary tumors - lymphosarcoma, uterine and mammary adenocarcinomas, squamous cell carcinoma, metastatic hemangiosarcoma
3. Equine
  a. Primary
    1) Melanoma
    2) Rare - medulloepithelioma
  b. Secondary - lymphosarcoma

Signs

1. Visualization of a mass in the iris or through the pupil
2. Secondary changes
  a. Hemorrhage (hyphema or vitreal)
  b. Anterior uveitis
  c. Collapse of the anterior chamber
  d. Erosion through the sclera to produce a staphyloma
  e. Secondary glaucoma

Diagnosis

1. Gross appearance - pigmented, vascular
2. Diagnostic tests
  a. Anterior chamber centesis and cytology
  b. Biopsy
  c. Ultrasound if hyphema

Treatment - With the possible exception of feline melanoma, one should not be in a hurry to operate unless complications are present (glaucoma, hyphema). If available, laser photocoagulation (Argon or Diode) is a modality that may effectively deal with small to midsized benign pigmented tumors.

1. Depends on whether a primary disease or seen with a generalized secondary disease
2. If small, unknown growth rate, or undecided as to cause, document size and re-examine periodically
3. Small iris tumors - sectional iridectomy, laser photocoagulation. This is very effective for canine and equine melanomas. Not recommended for feline melanoma; may increase chance for metastasis.
4. Enucleation
  a. Recommended for a blind painful eye or if tumor is growing rapidly
  b. If still visual, owner may want to wait if metastasis or blindness is not imminent

IRIS GRANULOMA

1. Dogs and cats may be presented with nonpigmented iris granulomas. This clinical condition could be confused with tumors.
2. Anterior chamber centesis and/or granuloma aspiration is recommended.
  a. If the centesis is normal, systemic steroids may cause regression of the granuloma.
  b. If the centesis demonstrates an inflammatory response, systemic steroids and antibiotic should be tried.

CHAPTER 13 - LENS

DEVELOPMENT, ANATOMY AND PHYSIOLOGY

EMBRYOLOGY

The eye is the first organ of the body to develop. It begins with the appearance of the optic sulcus or pit in the anterior neural fold (Fig 13-1). The optic pit develops into the primary optic vesicle, which invaginates to form the optic cup.

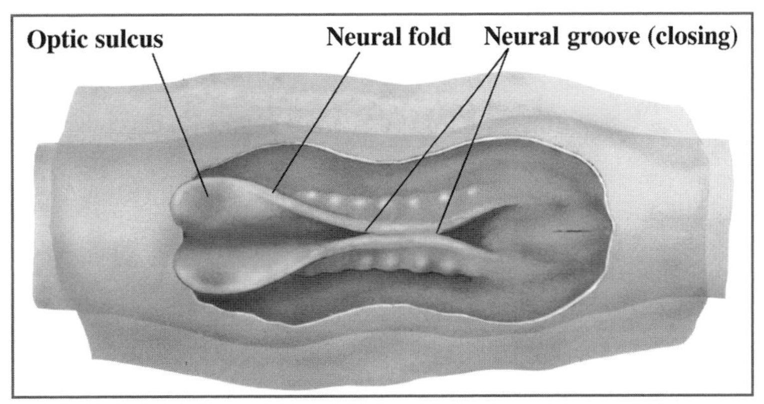

Figure 13-1. Cutaway drawing of 7 somite pig embryo. The optic sulcus (pit) is shown developing on the anterior limit of the neural fold.

The ectoderm over the optic vesicle thickens (lens plate), forming the lens placode in the dog (gestation day 15), which invaginates into the optic vesicle, becoming the lens pit. The lens pit deepens and invagination continues until the lens vesicle is formed (day 19). The lens vesicle separates from the surface ectoderm (day 25) and thereafter develops independently (Fig 13-2).

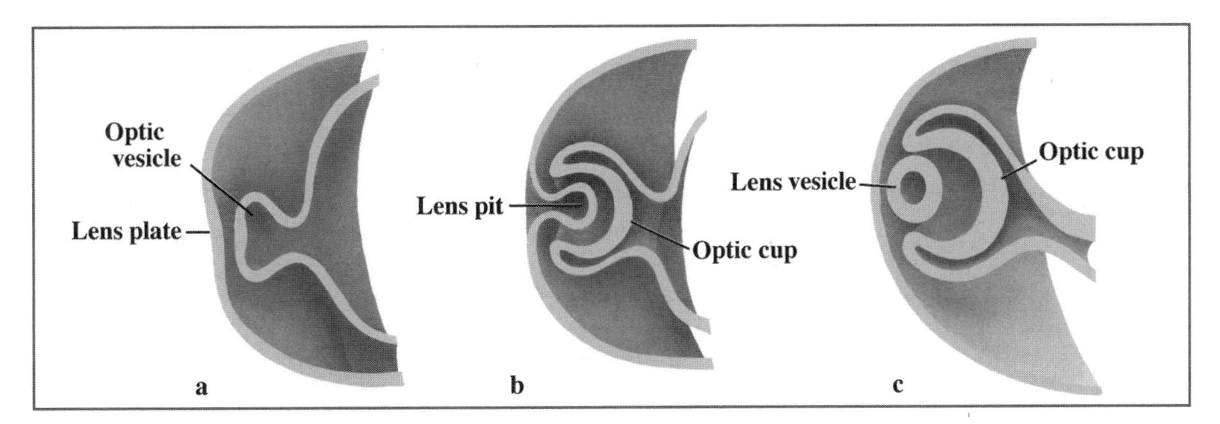

Figure 13-2. Early development stages of the eye.

a. Optic vesicle starting to undergo secondary invagination and formation of the lens plate in the surface ectoderm
b. Invagination of the surface ectoderm to form the lens pit in the developing optic cup
c. Lens vesicle detached from surface ectoderm

The cells of the anterior wall of the lens vesicle persist as the anterior epithelium of the fully developed lens. Cells from the posterior and equatorial wall of the lens vesicle elongate and differentiate to become lens fibers. They elongate anteroposteriorly until the vesicle is filled (day 30) (Fig 13-3). These cells are the primary lens fibers and represent the embryonic nucleus of the fully developed lens.

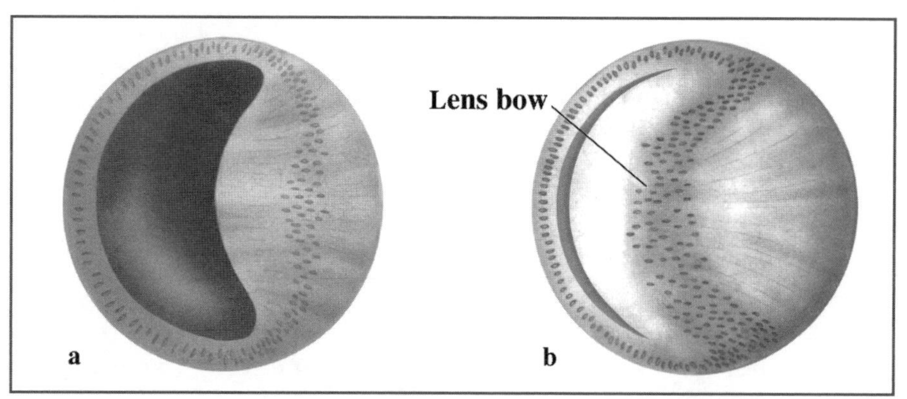

Figure 13-3. Lens formation from the lens vesicle.
a. Posterior epithelial cells elongating to form lens fibers
b. Lens cells elongated to fill the vesicle. Nuclei have formed a lens bow.

Secondary lens fibers form from the cells at the equator and are continually crowded toward the embryonic nucleus by later-forming cells. The new fibers extend anteriorly beneath the anterior epithelium toward the anterior pole and posteriorly toward the posterior pole. As the lens grows, the fibers are not long enough to reach from pole to pole and therefore must join with other fibers in a linear fashion, forming suture lines. With further growth the suture lines develop a Y appearance, with the sutures in the anterior lens appearing upright and those in the posterior lens appearing inverted. The lens has now developed to its postnatal appearance.

The rapid growth of the embryonal lens requires a rich blood supply. This is provided by the hyaloid system (primary vitreous). This system nourishes the rapidly growing lens and, when it has served its purpose, atrophies (Fig 14-1; Chapter 14, page 407).

ANATOMY

The lens is a transparent biconvex body with greater curvature to the posterior surface than the anterior surface. The center of the anterior surface is referred to as the anterior pole and the corresponding posterior surface as the posterior pole. The rounded circumference is the equator. The equator is not a smoothly curved line but has numerous irregularities that represent the areas of attachment of the zonular fibers (Fig 13-4).

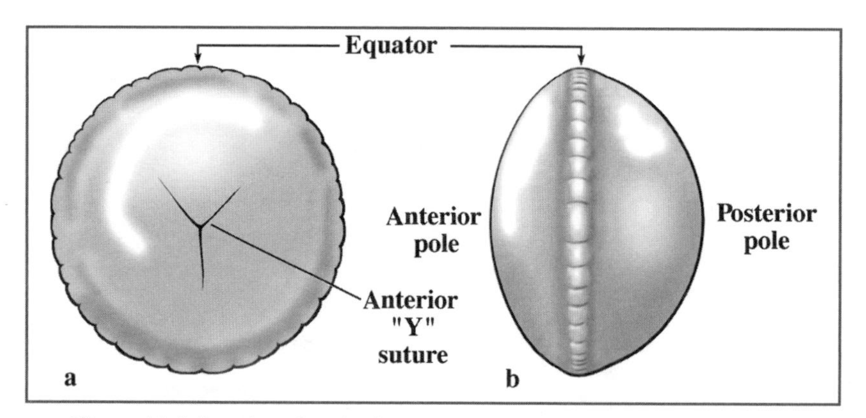

Figure 13-4. Drawing of canine lens.
a. Anterior view showing anterior Y suture and equator
b. Lateral view showing anterior pole, posterior pole and equator

The lens is supported at the equator by the zonules of Zinn (suspensory ligaments), which attach to the ciliary body (Fig 13-5). This mechanism is responsible for accommodation. Contraction of the ciliary muscle allows the lens to become more convex, therefore shortening the focal length of the eye. The ciliary muscle is poorly developed in the dog and other domestic animals, therefore limiting the ability to accommodate (1 to 2 diopters) for near vision.

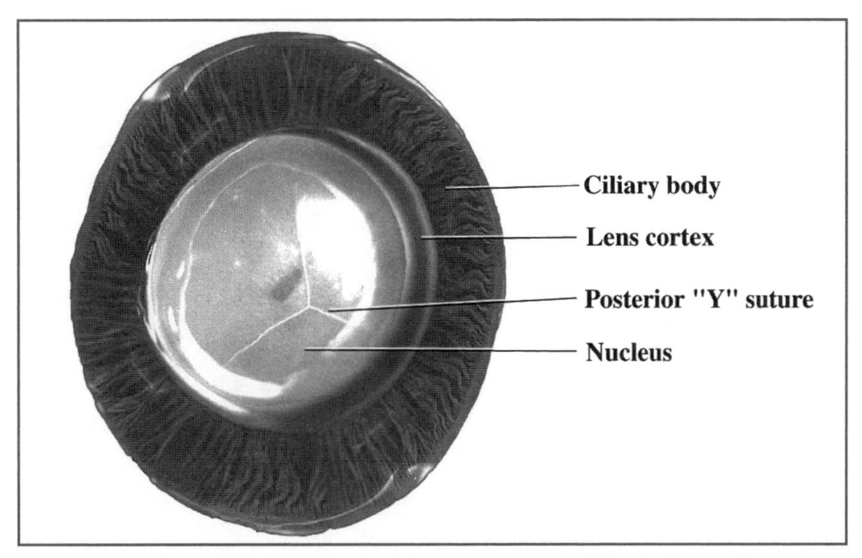

Figure 13-5. Posterior view of adult canine lens and ciliary body attachment.

Accommodation is also limited by the physical size of the domestic animal lens. In all domestic animals the lens is proportionately larger than it is in man. The shape varies between the species, with man having the least spherical lens (Fig 13-6).

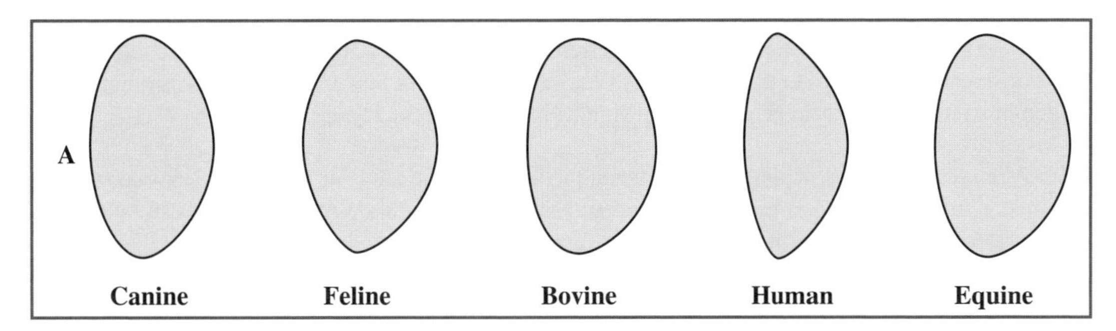

Figure 13-6. Relative cross-sectional appearance of lenses of animals and man. Relative sizes are not in scale. "A" represents the anterior lens surface.

The lens consists of a capsule, the anterior epithelium and lens fibers (Fig 13-7).

Capsule

The capsule is a transparent amorphous elastic envelope that can be divided into anterior and posterior sections. In dogs, the anterior capsule is approximately 50 microns thick and 5 microns at the posterior pole. The equine anterior capsule is 91 microns thick, 20 at the equator and 14 at the posterior capsule. If the capsule is ruptured, it retracts. The capsule provides insertion for the zonular fibers, regulates the transport of nutrients and waste products between the lens and aqueous, and influences the shape of the lens.

Lens (germinal) epithelium

The anterior epithelium is a layer of cuboidal cells beneath the anterior capsule. The lens epithelium is the only lens tissue capable of regeneration. There is no posterior epithelium. The cells near the equator become columnar, elongate and convert to lens fibers. New lens fibers form beneath the capsule at the equator, migrate anteriorly or posteriorly and force the older cells centrally.

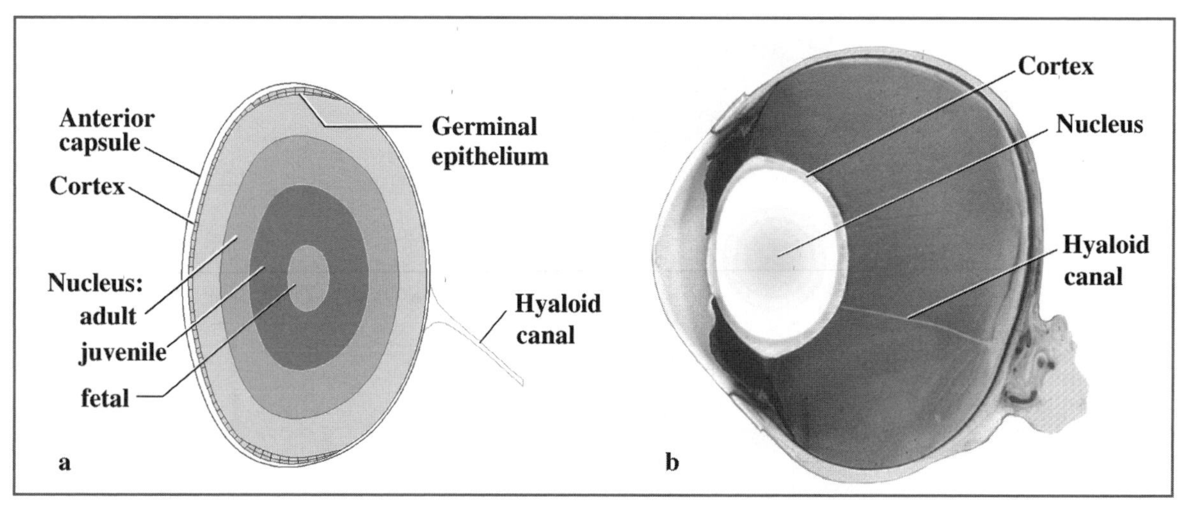

Figure 13-7. Cross-section of lens.
a. Cross-section drawing of adult lens
b. Sagittal cross-section of bovine eye showing layers of lens and hyaloid canal

Lens fibers

The lens fibers make up the substance of the lens and are arranged in layers that can be differentiated into zones indicating when they were formed. The outer younger cells are nucleated and form the cortex. The deeper older cells have lost their nuclei and are referred to as the nucleus. The older cells become sclerotic and less translucent than the younger cells, therefore resulting in layers that are not optically homogeneous and can be demonstrated with a focal or slit beam of light (Fig 1-7; Chapter 1, page 12).

The layers are seen quite well in adult animals when the lens is sectioned (Fig 13-8). The lens continues to grow with age but compacting of cells in the nucleus limits this growth. With age, the relative size of the cortex decreases and the nucleus increases.

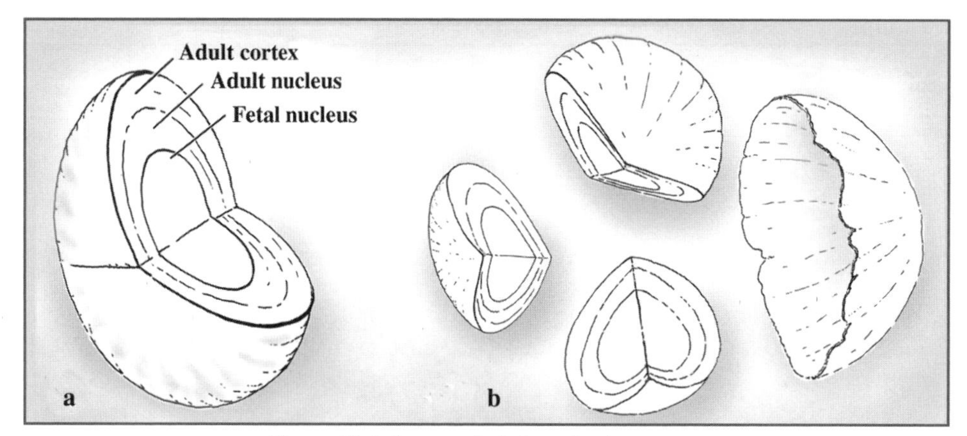

Figure 13-8. Layers of adult canine lens.
a. Appearance of sectioned adult lens
b. Appearance of fractured lens

The lens fibers are hexagonal in cross-section and held together with ball-and-socket interdigitations and cement substance. This is found primarily beneath the posterior capsule, beneath the anterior epithelium and along the central strand. The central strand occupies the axis of the lens, running between the anterior and posterior poles. Coming out from the strand are planes dividing the lens into sections, which are recognized as sutures or lens stars. The suture is an upright Y in the anterior portion of the lens, is inverted posteriorly and can be seen subcutaneously in normal lenses (Fig 13-9). In adult large animals, these sutures show additional segmentation in the subcapsular cortex, which is especially prominent in the equine and bovine lens.

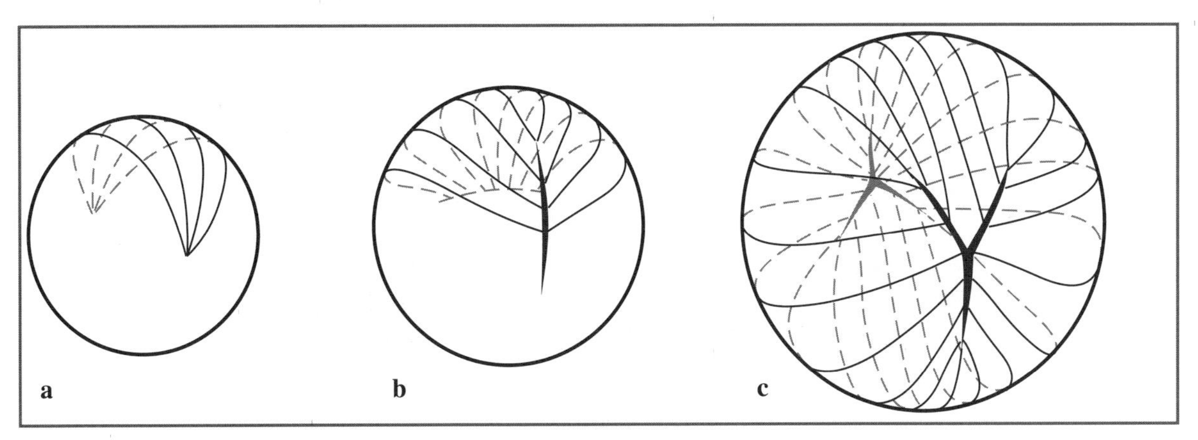

Figure 13-9. The formation of lens sutures.
a. Embryonal lens with all fibers attached along the lens axis
b. Linear suture pattern. Permanent arrangement in lower vertebrates and transitional in the embryonic nucleus of mammals
c. Y suture pattern. Typical lens fiber arrangement in animals.

Comment

The lens is supported by the ciliary zonules and the vitreous. In man, the anterior face of the vitreous develops an anterior limiting layer (membrane) that is attached to the posterior capsule of the lens in the form of a ring, referred to as the hyaloidocapsular ligament of Wieger. The ligament, when viewed with the slit lamp, is identified as Egger's line (Fig 13-10). The vitreous in the dog is securely attached to the entire posterior capsule of the lens, except for a small area at the posterior pole where the hyaloid canal contacts the lens. This junction can be seen as a faint circle with transillumination or slit lamp examination. This difference in the attachment of the vitreous to the lens between man and the dog determines the surgical techniques used to deliver their lenses. In man, the zonules can be lysed with proteolytic agents and the lens readily separated from the vitreous at Egger's line and thereby delivered intracapsularly. In the dog, the lens is still adherent to the vitreous even if the zonules are lysed. An attempt to deliver the lens intracapsularly will result in prolapse of the vitreous (Fig 13-11).

The posterior lens capsule can be separated from the vitreous with greater ease in older cats than in dogs or horses.

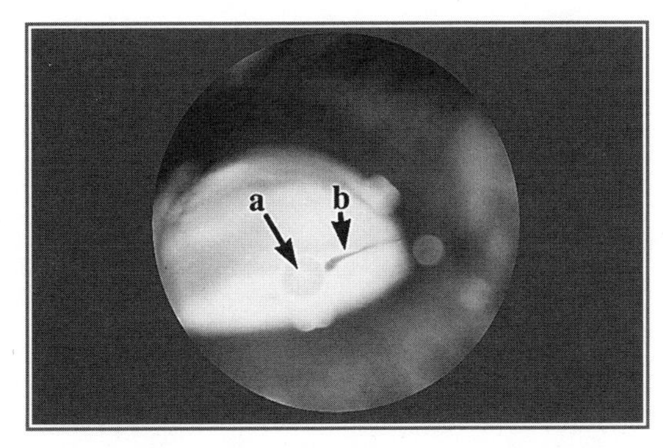

Figure 13-10. Egger's line as viewed with an ophthalmoscope.
a. Egger's line is represented by a faint circle.
b. A small hyaloid remnant can be visualized extending from the posterior capsule a few mm into the vitreous.

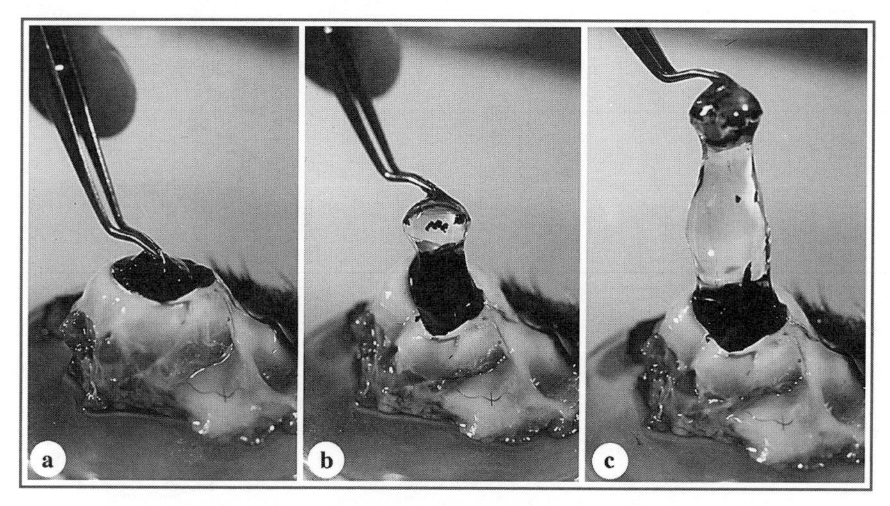

Figure 13-11. Vitreous adherence to the posterior capsule in the canine. The cornea has been removed to better visualize the lens.
a. Anterior capsule grasped with capsule forceps
b. Lens dislodged from ciliary attachment. Some ciliary processes were torn from the ciliary body and remained attached at lens equator.
c. Vitreous body buckles the sclera as the lens is elevated

PHYSIOLOGY

The lens capsule is semipermeable and all metabolites pass through it. The capsule is more permeable in young animals.

The metabolic rate of the lens is low and metabolism is limited to glucose utilization. Glucose in the lens may follow several pathways. Aerobic metabolism is limited to the mitochondria containing lens epithelial cells. Lens fibers metabolize glucose primarily by anaerobic glycolysis (Fig 13-12) which provides more than 70% of the lens energy. Anaerobic glycolysis is regulated by hexokinase. A small amount is metabolized by the hexose monophosphate shunt, which is also controlled by hexokinase. The sorbitol pathway normally accounts for about 5% of the lens metabolism. Ninety percent of the energy used in the lens is for the active metabolic transport. Sodium is low and potassium is high as the result of the Na-K ATPase pump system.

The lens contains a higher concentration of glutathione than any other tissue.

Lens proteins

The lens is high in protein, about 35% protein and 65% water. Most other metabolites are present in levels similar to that of the aqueous and only a trace of minerals are found.

The primary lens proteins are divided into soluble proteins (alpha-crystallin, beta-crystallin and gamma-crystallin) and insoluble albuminoid.

Alpha- and beta-crystallin are further identified into subclasses. Insoluble albuminoid is formed from alpha-crystallin, they have the same primary structure and are similar immunoelectrophoretically. In cataractous conditions and aging, the insoluble albuminoid fraction increases and the alpha-crystallin decreases. In a normal lens, alpha-crystallin decreases going from the cortex to the nucleus, while the proportion of insoluble albuminoid increases.

Antigenicity of lens proteins

Lens proteins are immunologically organ-specific. This indicates that the protein in lenses of different species

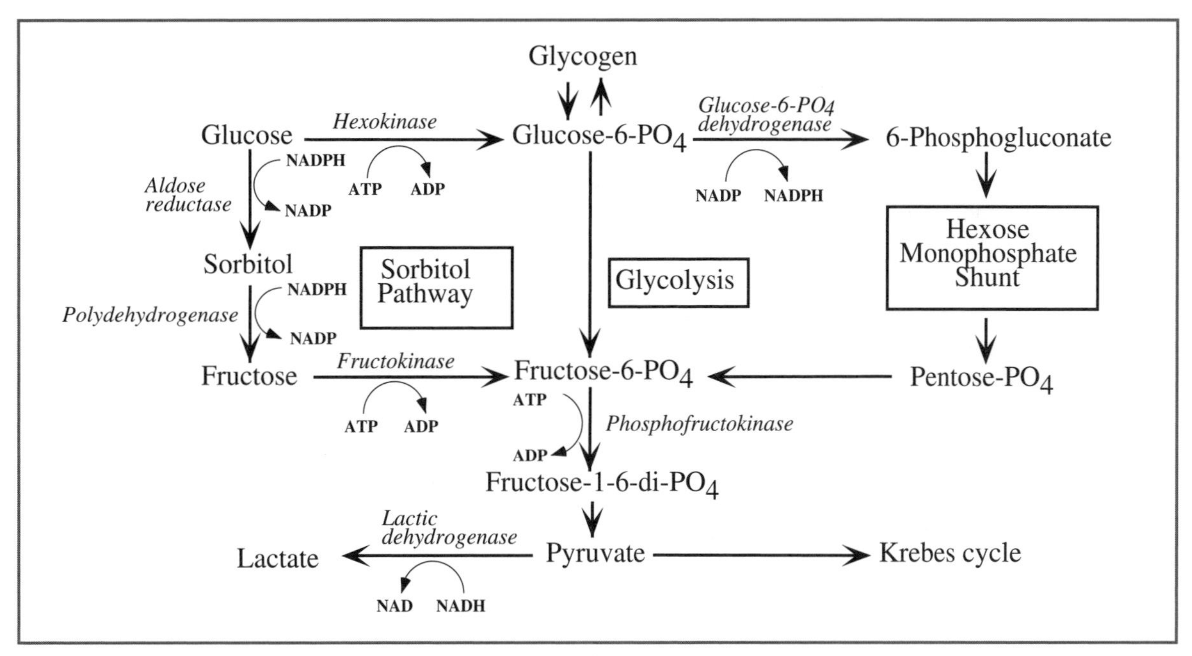

Figure 13-12. Simplified scheme of glucose metabolism in the lens Modified from: Hart W, Jr. Adler's Physiology of the Eye, Mosby Yearbook, 1992.

must be nearly alike. Antigenicity of lens protein is clinically significant. There is a constant low level loss of lens protein from normal lens. This stimulates antilens antibody production, but T suppressor cells prevent this from causing an inflammatory response. Cataracts that are leaking excessive lens protein result in increased lens antibody production that T suppressors cannot override and mild uveitis (lens-induced uveitis) results. With chronicity the lens zonules can break down resulting in lens displacement. If massive amounts of lens protein are released from a ruptured lens, a severe reaction (phacoanaphylaxis) develops in one to three weeks, resulting in synechia, fibroplasia and possibly glaucoma.

Aging of the lens (Fig 1-7; Chapter 1, page 12)

Lenticular sclerosis is the gradual hardening of the central zone of the lens with aging. The most striking changes occur in the nucleus and because of this, nuclear sclerosis is a term frequently used to describe this aging change.

In the dog, at six to eight years of age the nucleus starts to develop a gray haze. With further aging, this haze (sclerosis) becomes more evident. Owners of dogs with lenticular sclerosis will often notice the change, believe it is a cataract and bring the patient in for examination. See page 12, Figure 1-7 for clinical differentiation of cataract and nuclear sclerosis.

Sclerosis is related to the increase in the ratio of insoluble crystallin to soluble crystallins. Gamma-crystallin is the principal lens protein to be affected in sclerosis. Since gamma-crystallin is restricted to the nucleus, sclerosis is limited primarily to the nucleus. This begins in cats at about 13 and horses after 18 years of age.

It is interesting to note that chicken lens does not contain gamma-crystallin and does not develop a nucleus, even in old age.

Transparency of the lens

Normal lens transparency is achieved by dense packing of the individual cells in such a manner that discontinuity is minimal. Vacuolation and precipitation of lens protein will result in loss of transparency and is referred to as cataract.

DISEASES OF THE LENS

The diseases of the lens, listed in order of frequency of clinical observation, are:

1. Cataract
2. Lens displacement
3. Developmental abnormalities - aphakia, microphakia, coloboma, lenticonus
4. Rupture

CATARACT

Cataract is any opacity of the lens or its capsule. It is associated with vacuolation (both cellular and extracellular) and local precipitation of protein.

Pathogenesis

The pathogenesis of cataract development is not fully understood. There are some observed changes in spontaneous and experimental cataracts that are of value in developing some understanding of cataract development.

1. Transparency - Lens fiber transparency is affected by swelling and coagulation
    a. Swelling - If fibers swell from the imbibition of water, the size of the protein micelle will change and opacity will develop. This opacity is reversible.
    b. Coagulation - Opacity occurs when chemical changes occur in the proteins, so that they become insoluble. This opacity is irreversible. Once the process of coagulation begins, it is generally progressive and leads to clinical cataract formation.
2. Biochemical changes - The most outstanding are:

METABOLITE CHANGES OBSERVED WITH CATARACTS

Increased	Decreased
Water	Oxygen consumption
Percent of ash	Glutathione
Sodium	Ascorbic acid
Calcium	Potassium
Insoluble protein	Soluble protein
(albuminoid)	Riboflavin (vitamin B_2)

Classification

Cataracts are classified in various ways and this multiplicity of classification leads to confusion. The following schemes are not mutually exclusive. Cataracts can be classified according to:

How they occur
When they occur
Where they occur
Rate of development
Consistency of the lens
Stage of development of the cataract

1. How they occur
   a. Hereditary - a very important factor. In dogs can be congenital or develop up to five years of age. It is a vital concern to the breeder to determine if genetic factors are involved. A thorough history is needed to better determine inheritance. When questioning the breeder, be sure to determine:
      1) If previous litters by these parents were normal
      2) If cataracts have been previously diagnosed in either bloodline
      3) How many of the litter are affected
      4) What was the survival rate of the litter
      5) If the parents are normal
      6) If the bitch was ill, given medications or had access to chemicals during pregnancy
   b. Acquired - In acquired cataracts the lens has normal development and cataract results from a specific cause.
      1) Senile - the most common cause for acquired cataract in the dog
      2) Radiation - x-ray, gamma ray, microwaves, heat absorption
      3) Inflammatory - result from complications from other ocular diseases. In the United States, anterior uveitis is the most common cause for equine cataracts.
      4) Traumatic - lens capsule lacerations (foreign body, cat scratch laceration) and blunt trauma to the eye. Concussion waves going through the lens after blunt trauma to the eye have been associated with cataracts in horses.
      5) Diabetes mellitus - altered glucose metabolism
      6) Nutritional - milk replacements in orphan puppies, wolves and kittens
      7) Hypocalcemia
      8) Chemicals and drugs - seldom identified. Some include:
         a) High (shock level) doses of corticosteroids can result in transient cataracts in cats
         b) Naphthalene - puppies or kittens getting into mothballs
         c) Dinitrophenol - can cause transient cataracts
      9) Electric - pets chewing on electric cord
2. When they occur
   a. Congenital - lesion present at birth or in neonatal period. These may be inherited or due to *in utero* causes
   b. Juvenile - appear in young to middle-aged patients up to five or six years
   c. Senile - appear as an aging disease, usually after 6 to 8 years in the dog, 12 years in the cat, and 20 years in the equine
3. Where they occur (Fig 13-13)
   a. Structure affected
      1) Capsule - often secondary to abnormalities in adjacent tissue (anterior - iris; posterior - vitreous)
      2) Lenticular - cortex, nucleus. Cortex more frequently involved than nucleus.
   b. Location in the lens
      1) Anterior
      2) Posterior
      3) Equatorial
      4) Polar
      5) Zonular - used to denote that one zone or layer is affected. These are most frequently stationary developmental cataracts (subcapsular, cortical, nuclear)
4. Rate of development
   a. Stationary
   b. Progressive
5. Consistency of the lens
   a. Fluid - juvenile cataracts in horses and toxic cataracts in any animal tend to be fluid
   b. Soft - rapidly developing cataracts tend to be soft - diabetic
   c. Hard - senile and slowly developing inherited cataracts are usually quite hard

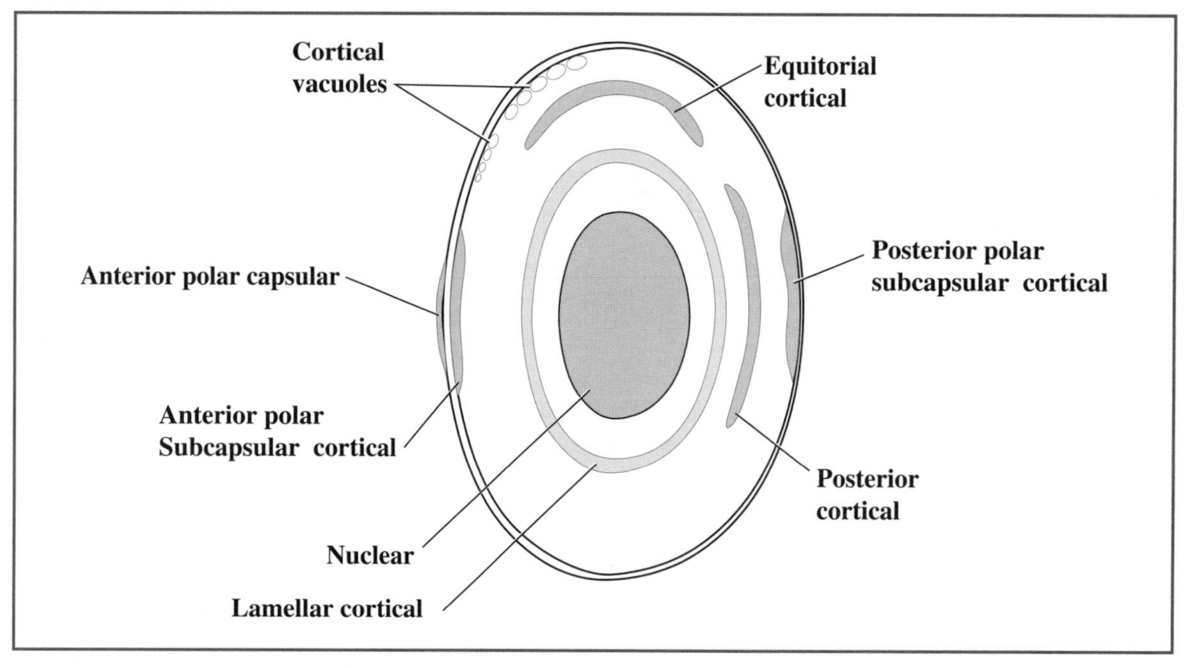

Figure 13-13. Nomenclature of cataracts according to location.

6. Stage of development
   a. Incipient stage - this is the stage of beginning opacity. Frequent areas of development are equatorial cortex, posterior subcapsular polar cortex, and Y sutures. Sight is still normal. The development of incipient nuclear cataract is difficult to differentiate from nuclear sclerosis in old animals. See Chapter 1, Figure 1-7, page 12.
   b. Immature (intumescent) stage - Opacity is more marked and sight may be impaired depending on the location of the cataract. As it progresses the fundus may be indistinctly visualized with an ophthalmoscope. The fundus reflex (tapetal color) with retroillumination is still visualized. This is the stage of marked fluid imbibition and lens swelling referred to as lens intumescence. The swelling of the lens forces the iris forward, resulting in a shallow anterior chamber. Secondary glaucoma has been observed at this stage.
   c. Mature stage - The lens is opaque, firm and excess fluid is disappearing. The fundus reflex is gone, and the fundus cannot be visualized with an ophthalmoscope. The patient is blind.
   d. Hypermature stage - After reaching maturity, some cataracts undergo additional changes as a result of loss of lens proteins. This usually affects the cortex first and last the nucleus.
      1) Shrunken cataract - small, hard, dry-appearing lens with a rough surface. The anterior chamber is deep and there are signs of chronic uveitis (dark iris, low intraocular pressure, and variable miosis and episcleral injection). This lens may spontaneously pull away from the zonules.
      2) Morgagnian cataract - the cortex liquifies, leading to milky texture, and the nucleus gravitates downward. If the head is abruptly moved, the nucleus will float up into the pupillary area and settle down when the eye is motionless.
      3) Resorption cataract - lens material may escape into the aqueous, allowing the lens to decrease in size until only the capsule and small lenticular fragments remain. This may occur even when the lens capsule appears intact. Resorption may lead to a return of vision that is comparable to successful lens removal. Unfortunately, the escaping lens material may cause a lens protein-induced uveitis, resulting in loss of the eye. Resorption occurs most frequently with juvenile cataracts (Afghan hound, cocker spaniel, Siberian husky).

CONGENITAL CATARACTS

Congenital cataracts begin during fetal life and may regress, be stationary or progressive. In calves and foals they may not be noticed before two weeks of age and in small animals until 6 to 12 weeks of age. They may be inherited as a single problem, secondary to other ocular developmental abnormality, or the result of maternal influences. Their etiology will affect their clinical course. When cortical cataracts are the only problem, they usually regress with age as new lens fibers force the cataract toward center (nucleus). Anterior and posterior capsular cataracts are usually stationary.

Dogs

Cataracts presented as the only problem.

1. Beagles - axial anterior subcapsular. A dominant gene with incomplete penetration has been proposed.
2. German shepherd - axial anterior capsular stationary. Dominant inheritance.
3. Miniature schnauzer - nuclear and cortical, progressive. Autosomal recessive inheritance.
4. West Highland white terrier - posterior Y suture, slowly progressive. Autosomal recessive proposed.

Cataracts occurring with other congenital ocular diseases.

1. Persistent pupillary membrane - Stationary anterior capsular cataracts develop if a strand of membrane adheres to the lens. The strand may or may not absorb before maturity; in either case, it will leave a permanent capsular opacity that seldom interferes with vision. If the lens lesion is large enough to disturb vision, topical 1% atropine applied every two to three days will dilate the pupil and help vision. Inheritance should be considered in the Basenji, corgi, and chow chow.
2. Persistent hyaloid system
    a. Small avascular posterior capsule remnants may be seen extending into the vitreous without lens abnormalities and are insignificant.
    b. Persistent hyperplastic primary vitreous/persistent tunica vasculosa lentis.
        1) A single blood vessel attached to the posterior pole of the lens
        2) An artery with a capsular vascular tunic and posterior pole cataract
        3) A vascularized area in the posterior axial cortex - Cortical vascularization will appear as a dark area.

        Congenital cataracts caused by persistent hyaloid are generally stationary. If the lesion is large enough to disturb vision, 1% ophthalmic atropine applied every two to three days will often help vision. Surgical removal of the lens will result in intraocular hemorrhage from the hyaloid artery and therefore cannot be recommended. This is an inherited problem in the Doberman pinscher and Staffordshire bull terrier.
3. Microphthalmia - congenital nuclear and cortical cataracts may be observed in microphthalmic eyes. Microphthalmic eyes are not good surgical candidates. This is inherited in the Akita, Cavalier King Charles spaniel, schnauzer, Australian shepherd, and Old English sheepdog.
4. Anterior polar capsular pigment deposits - common. These are stationary and appear as multiple dots that do not affect sight.
5. Retinal dysplasia
    a. English springer spaniel - usually a slowly growing subcapsular cortical cataract
    b. Old English sheepdog - congenital nuclear/cortical cataracts. The author has observed one litter where nearly the entire lens was involved at five weeks of age. By four months the cataract had regressed and only nuclear involvement remained. The retinal dysplasia was quite severe but the pups were visual. Inheritance was not determined.
    c. Labrador retriever with oculoskeletal dysplasia may have stationary or slowly progressive cortical cataracts, retinal dysplasia, retinal detachment.
6. Maternal influences resulting in congenital cataract are usually stationary or resorbing cataracts. The lens that develops postnatally will be clear and compress the cataract into the nucleus. Causes are:
    a. Maternal infection during pregnancy, parvovirus
    b. Drugs and chemicals should be considered

Cats - Congenital cataracts are rare

1. Eyelid agenesis - may have concurrent iris lesions and cataract. The cataracts are stationary.
2. Persian cats - congenital inherited cataracts have been described

Horses - The lenses of newborn foals may be cloudy for several days. This should not be confused with cataracts. Congenital cataract is the most common ocular anomaly in horses.

1. May occur with microphthalmos
2. Y suture cataracts anterior or posterior are usually stationary. Inheritance is unknown.
3. Posterior subcapsular "starburst" cataracts may be seen that are stationary. Inheritance unknown.
4. Proposed inherited cataracts
   a. Morgan horse - nuclear opacities, stationary, no visual loss (familial)
   b. Belgian - cataracts and aniridia (dominant)
   c. Quarter horse - nuclear, stationary
   d. Thoroughbred - nuclear, stationary (test breeding proved dominant). The horses in this study had severe cataracts at birth and by four to six weeks could see.

Cattle

1. Prenatal BVD - during first trimester; stationary cortical cataract, chorioretinal dysplasia, severe strabismus, optic nerve hypoplasia, and cerebellar hypoplasia.
2. Inherited
   a. Jersey - congenital cataracts, lens luxation, microphakia, $\pm$ buphthalmos; simple autosomal recessive
   b. Hereford - cataracts mature during first year; multiple ocular defects may occur. Simple autosomal recessive.
   c. Holstein Friesian - similar to Herefords
   d. Shorthorn - cataract with multiple ocular anomalies, hydrocephalus, cerebellar hypoplasia and myopathy

NUTRITIONAL CATARACTS

Dogs - Nutritional cataracts have been observed in either orphan puppies or puppies from litters that received supplemental commercial and owner-formulated canine milk replacements. Fast growing breeds appear to be more susceptible. The cataracts regress when the puppy begins pan feeding with a protein-rich diet. Arginine deficiency is probably the cause. Phenylalanine has also been proposed. Canine orphan puppy formulas have been modified to control the problem.

1. Signs
   a. Experimental puppies
      1) Third week - opacity begins and is characterized by a brown-colored layer in the anterior and posterior perinuclear cortex. Involvement of the posterior Y suture results in a feathered pattern. Mild cases may have decreased relucency to the lens.
      2) Fourth week - the opacities become less dense
      3) Fifth week - the bronze coloration disappears, leaving residual white diffuse posterior subcapsular and anterior cortical opacities. Histopathology - vacuolar changes, mainly equatorial and posterior subcapsular.
      4) Six months - prominent nuclear-cortical junction ring
   b. Clinical puppies - similar to experimental puppies, plus:
      1) Bilateral vacuolation and striations at the lens equator and in the posterior cortex near the posterior Y suture
      2) Prominent fetal nucleus-juvenile nucleus junction ring that persists for life and occasionally may have tan coloration

2. Significance - vision is not affected. Must be differentiated from congenital or neonatal cataracts from other causes.

Timber wolves - American timber wolves raised on a canine milk replacer with protein content less than 50% of normal wolf milk developed cortical lens opacities that developed into mature cataracts if the diet was continued through the first two months of life. Cataracts were reversible if the diet was discontinued early or supplemented with normal canine diet. Arginine added to the replacer prevented cataract formation. Additional lactose also prevented lens opacities. It was assumed that lactose acted as a catalyst, assisting in the absorption of arginine.

Kittens - Nutritional cataracts have also been observed in kittens on commercial kitten milk replacers. The cataracts may be related to low arginine concentration. Early signs are diffuse anterior and posterior lens opacification and vacuolation at the posterior Y suture. As the kitten grows, the cataract resolves to a perinuclear halo and occasional incipient cortical opacities.

JUVENILE CATARACTS (Developmental Cataracts)

Dogs

Juvenile cataract is a term usually used to refer to inherited cataracts that appear before six years of age. Hereditary cataracts can be carried by either recessive or dominant genetic factors. The genetics have been proposed for several breeds, but in many cases additional studies will be required to determine the exact mode of inheritance for a particular clinical cataract.

Patients with bilateral juvenile cataracts should not be bred if the eye is normal in all other respects. If there is conclusive evidence that the cataract is secondary to some noninherited cause, then breeding restriction would not be recommended. It will take long cooperative efforts by breeders and veterinarians to solve some of these problems.

The common sites for initial development are the equator, anterior and posterior subcapsular area and along Y sutures, thus affecting the cortex first and nucleus later. As the cataract develops, both areas will be involved.

The typical course of juvenile cataracts is progressive to eventual maturation of the cataract. This may occur in months or take as long as several years. Many juvenile cataracts mature in less than one year. Some animals will develop lens capsule leakage and the cataract will resorb. Others remain as a stable mature cataract without change. If resorption is going to occur, it generally becomes evident within a year. Signs of resorption are deepening of the anterior chamber, decrease in lens diameter and thickness, and corrugation of the anterior capsule. As the lens becomes small, vision can be aided with mydriatics (1% atropine every two to three days). Complete resorption will result in vision comparable to successful lens surgery. Lens protein-induced uveitis may occur and should be treated similarly to any other uveitis. Lens removal is not generally recommended in the presence of uveitis or resorption.

Current beliefs for some of the breeds affected with juvenile and inherited cataracts are presented in Table 13-1.

1. The Afghan hound has a cortical cataract, beginning with vacuolation at the equator and progressing subcapsularly toward the poles. The age of initial signs varies from 4 to 14 months of age. After onset, the cataracts usually progress rapidly. Most clinical cases will have observable signs by two years. Simple autosomal recessive inheritance is proposed.
2. The golden retriever has a cataract that can be observed as soon as the eye can be examined or by one year. This appears as a posterior polar capsular and subcapsular cortical triangular cataract that is stationary or progresses slowly. A juvenile variation appears from six months to three years of age, first in the posterior cortex near the Y sutures and posterior pole, and is progressive. A dominant gene with variable penetrance has been proposed.
3. The Labrador retriever has cataracts similar to the golden retriever.

Table 13-1. Cataract - predisposed breeds

Breed	Mode of inheritance	Age of onset	Position	Rate of progression
Afghan hound	R (?)	6 mo-3 yr	Equatorial cortex	Progressive
Beagle	ID (?)	Congenital	Nuclear and cortical	Progressive
Boston terrier	R (?)	2 mo-5 yr	Posterior cortical	Progressive
Cavalier King Charles	R (?)	Congenital	Nuclear, + posterior lenticonus	Progressive
Chesapeake Bay retriever	ID (?)	6 mo-6 yr	Postaxial and equatorial cortical; nuclear	Variable
Cocker spaniel				
American	R (?)	Any age	Posterior cortical	Variable
English	(?)	Any age	Posterior cortical	Variable
English springer spaniel	(?)	1-2.5 yrs	Posterior cortical	Nonprogressive Slowly progressive
German shepherd	D	Aged	Nuclear and cortical	Slowly progressive
Golden retriever	I (?)	6 mo-3 yrs	Posterior cortical	Stable or slowly progressive
Irish setter	(?)	Congenital-6 yrs	Posterior cortical and nuclear	Slowly progressive
Labrador retriever	(?)	1-7 yrs	Posterior cortical	Stable or slowly progressive
Miniature schnauzer	R	Congenital	Posterior cortical and nuclear	Progressive
Old English sheepdog	R (?)	Congenital	Cortical and nuclear	Progressive
Poodle, miniature	R (?)	Congenital	Nuclear	Nonprogressive
Poodle, miniature and toy	(?)	3-7 yrs	Cortical-striate and clefts	Progressive
Poodle, standard	R	Congenital	Cortical-equatorial	Slowly progressive
Sealyham terrier	R (?)	?	Nuclear and cortical	
Siberian husky	R (?)	1-2 yrs	Posterior cortical discoid	
Staffordshire bull terrier	R	1 yr	Sutural flecks	
Welsh corgi	(?)	6 mo-3 yrs	Equatorial cortical	Slowly progressive
Welsh springer spaniel	R (?)	Congenital	Cortical	Progressive
West Highland white terrier	R (?)	< 1 yr	Posterior suture or complete	Variable
Wire-haired terrier	R (?)	1-6 yrs	Cortical	Progressive

Reproduced by permission from: Wyman M. Manual of small animal ophthalmology, Churchill Livingstone, New York, 1986.

R = recessive; ID = incomplete dominant; D = dominant; (?) = proposed inherited

4. The American cocker spaniel usually has rapidly progressive cataracts that appear first in the posterior cortex and outer nucleus. These can progress to mature cataracts in six to nine months. Occasionally posterior polar cataracts are observed. A recessive mode of inheritance has been proposed.
5. The beagle has axial posterior subcapsular stationary cataracts.
6. The poodle
   a. Miniature and toy breeds are most frequently affected. Most cataracts begin in the cortex. Blindness from cataracts can occur before one year in some dogs but generally it takes one to four years. Occasionally cataracts occur as late as seven years. These cataracts are transmitted recessively. A high incidence of cataract is observed in miniatures and toys with progressive retinal atrophy (PRA).

Metabolites from the degenerating retina may be the cause for some of the cataracts. Poodles with cataracts must be thoroughly evaluated before considering lens removal because of the dual occurrence of these diseases. A history of night blindness or loss of visual acuity prior to the owner observing cataract formation is typical of patients with cataracts that are preceded by PRA. If the cataracts are immature, ophthalmoscopic fundus examinations will be adequate to eliminate advanced PRA. If the fundus cannot be seen, advanced PRA should be suspected if pupillary reflexes are absent or delayed. In early PRA, the pupillary reflex will be within normal limits and an electroretinogram will be needed to determine retinal function.

b. Standard poodle - cataract is uncommon but a progressive equatorial cataract can occur by one year. Autosomal recessive inheritance.
c. German shepherd - slowly progressive posterior Y suture and cortex. May start soon after weaning. Autosomal recessive.

Cats - Juvenile cataracts are rare in cats and when seen are usually secondary to toxic, metabolic lesions or inflammatory process.

Equine - Most cataracts in foals are congenital. Foals will occasionally be presented where the history would suggest a juvenile cataract but in all probability the cataract has been present since birth and is now becoming clinically visible. Inheritance should be considered in foals with congenital or juvenile cataracts but maternal factors can occur. Cataracts in adults are usually postinflammatory or post-traumatic.

Cattle - Most acquired cataracts are postinflammatory.

SENILE CATARACTS

Senile cataracts occur in all species of domestic animals. They are of great clinical importance in the dog, next the horse, then the cat, and lastly the bovine.

Senile cataracts begin in the cortex or nucleus and eventually involve the entire lens. A typical senile cortical cataract will begin at the equator, with opaque streaks or vacuoles extending toward the axis like spokes on a wheel.

Opacification continues until clear areas are present only at the Y suture lines of the cortex. The clear areas are referred to as water clefts and give the lens a segmented appearance. When the lens is uniformly opaque, it has reached the mature state. During the process of cortical opacification, the nucleus is undergoing the same processes. The loss of lens protein into the aqueous frequently results in a lens protein-induced (phacolytic) uveitis. This may be subclinical, resulting only in gradual darkening of the iris. Other animals may develop an acute uveitis.

The mature cataract continues to lose fluid and decrease in size. It is now firm and may remain this way for several years before showing hypermature signs. The most common form of hypermaturity is for the lens to become shrunken and dehydrated. Shrinking can separate the lens from its attachments and cause luxation. Another form of hypermaturity is Morgagnian cataract. The cortex liquifies but the nucleus remains intact and settles to the lowest limits of the lens capsule. Sight returns in this type of cataract similarly to the return of sight in resorption of a juvenile cataract.

Cataracts seldom develop at the same rate, and therefore one cataract generally matures prior to the other. Cataracts may become yellow or green in patients with jaundice or in longstanding cataracts by imbibition of urochrome.

Fibrillar (reticular) nuclear cataracts are occasionally seen. These senile cataracts are stationary and do not interfere with vision. They can be demonstrated by transillumination or slit lamp examination as fine refractile strands in the nucleus with a fibrillar (reticular) pattern.

DIABETIC CATARACTS

Sugar cataracts can be produced experimentally with high sugar diets (galactose, xylose, glucose) or as the result of high glucose levels occurring from diabetes mellitus. The initial changes in the lens are reversible, but when the lens fibers rupture and proteins precipitate, permanent opacity results. The diabetic lens goes through the developmental stages of a rapidly developing senile cataract.

Pathogenesis

1. High blood sugar results in an increase in glucose and to a lesser extent galactose and xylose in the lens. Because of limited hexokinase in the lens, the formation of glucose-6-phosphate for glycolysis cannot increase and glucose metabolism shifts to aldose reductase which converts glucose to sorbitol (galactose to dulcitol, xylose to xylitol). Sorbitol is a polyhydric alcohol (polyol) that cannot escape from the lens fibers. This results in water imbibition, swelling of the lens fibers, cloudiness results, and lens fibers may rupture. If fibers rupture, irreversible cataract results. If blood sugar returns to normal levels during the cloudy stage, the lens will clear.
2. Metabolic changes in the cell membrane also occur resulting in the cell morphologic changes.
3. Polyols interact with lens protein by glycosylation, which is in the attachment of glucose to amino acid residues on the lens crystallines.
4. Oxidation damage to the lens fibers

Signs

1. Early changes are characterized by vacuole formation in the equatorial cortex
2. Rapidly developing bilateral cataracts (3 to 6 weeks)
3. Prominent Y suture "water clefts" (clear areas)
4. Intumescent lens resulting in shallow anterior chamber

Diagnosis

1. Any three year old or older dog with a rapidly developing cataract should be screened for diabetes.
2. History compatible with diabetes - Many people are unaware the dog has systemic disease.
3. The level of glucose in the tears is often high enough to give a positive glucose test using urine glucose test strips (Lilly test tape). A positive test is diagnostic, but a negative test should be followed with blood sugar determination.

Comment

Even if diabetes is diagnosed prior to cataract formation, cataracts will be expected to develop because stabilizing levels of blood sugars are higher than normal.

COMPLICATED AND TRAUMATIC CATARACTS

Cataract may occur after ocular injury, inflammation of adjacent structures, or systemic diseases. The course is variable; the cataract may improve with time, become stationary, or progress, causing blindness.

Anterior uveitis is the most common cause for complicated cataracts in all species. An attack of uveitis usually results in minor posterior synechia and capsular change. If uveitis does not recur, lenticular change is minimal. If uveitis becomes recurrent, total cataracts will result. The feline lens with complicated cataracts will remain functional longer than either the equine or canine.

INCIDENCE OF CATARACT BY SPECIES AT CSU

Dog

1. Juvenile cataracts are most common (this may be biased by the fact that CSU is a referral clinic)
2. Senile (including diabetic cataracts) - Senile cataracts are the next most common cataract seen in the dog. They are usually bilateral with one slightly more advanced than the other.
3. Complicated, traumatic and infectious cataracts comprise the group of least frequency.

Horses

1. Complicated cataracts (secondary to uveitis)
2. Congenital

Cat - uncommon in the cat

1. Complicated cataracts
2. Developmental (toxic and congenital)
3. Senile - very rare

Cattle - uncommon

1. Complicated (secondary to uveitis)
2. Congenital - uncommon

TREATMENT OF CATARACT

Medical

Many medical treatments have been tried but none have proven to be successful. Symptomatic treatment with 1% atropine every two or three days is beneficial in assisting vision in resorption cataracts, stationary axial cataracts, and slowly progressing cataracts.

Surgical

In human ophthalmology, two procedures, phacoemulsification and intraocular lens placement, have revolutionized human cataract surgery. Phacoemulsification permits lens removal with small incisions and minimal surgical manipulation. The development and use of intraocular lenses (IOLs) after cataract removal has become a routine procedure. These advancements have reduced the postsurgical rehabilitation time so that lens removal has become an outpatient surgery with a success rate greater than 95%. After surgery and lens implantation the patient's vision is usually comparable to or better than the patient's precataract vision.

Phacoemulsification and aspiration is adaptable to veterinary ophthalmology, and is having a similar beneficial impact on animal cataract surgery. It reduces surgery time and in turn the secondary inflammatory response. Intraocular lenses have been developed and are being used on an increasing scale.

In addition to phacoemulsification, improved surgical instruments, new suture materials, a better understanding of the mechanism of ocular inflammation and additional anti-inflammatory agents have resulted in modification of previously established techniques and protocols. These advances are increasing surgical success. The lens procedure outlined in this text will describe a surgical technique for the ophthalmic surgeon who does not have a lens fragmentor available.

The author firmly believes that cataract surgery should only be performed by a surgeon who does it routinely and that phacoemulsification should be used whenever possible. The surgical success rate and recovery from surgery is much better with phacoemulsification than with manual extracapsular extraction.

1. Efficacy of cataract surgery on uncomplicated eyes
   a. Dog - manual extracapsular: 80-85%, phaco 95%
   b. Cat - easier than dog, slightly better results
   c. Horses - success closely related to age
      -Foals up to six months: aspiration or phaco 75%
      -Foal 6 to 12 months: aspiration or phaco 60%
      -Adult horses: manual extracapsular 50%, phaco (if available) much better
2. Choosing the patient
   a. The author does not recommend surgery unless there is bilateral involvement or lens-induced uveitis is present or likely
   b. Eliminate the possibility of progressive retinal atrophy (PRA) or retinal disease
      1) If cataract is immature - fundus examination, test for night blindness and visual acuity
      2) If cataracts are mature
         a) Delayed pupillary reflexes are indicative of advanced retinopathy but early PRA may have normal reflexes. Cataracts do not interfere with pupillary reflexes.
         b) Check for dazzle reflex. When a *bright* light is directed at normal retina, the animal will demonstrate photophobia by reflex blinking or blepharospasm. Advanced retinal degeneration will be evidenced by a total loss of dazzle reflex. Early retinal degeneration will still have some response.
         c) Electroretinograms are necessary for accurate retinal evaluation in mature cataracts
         d) Ultrasonic examination will eliminate the possibility of retinal detachment
   c. Choose a healthy patient
      1) Control diabetes mellitus before surgery. All rapidly developing cataracts are potentially diabetic.
      2) Screen for kidney, liver and heart disease
   d. Choose a tractable patient - Do not operate on animals that will be hard for the owner to handle. Over-restraint after surgery may cause retinal detachment or intraocular hemorrhage.

Types of cataract removal

1. Discission - cutting of the anterior capsule and aspiration of the lens contents while continuously flushing the anterior chamber
2. Intracapsular cataract extraction (ICCE) - removal of the lens and its capsule as an intact unit. Difficult in animals because of:
   a. The firm attachment of the zonules to the capsule at the equator. (Proteolytic enzymes have been used successfully in man for zonulolysis, but have no proven value in the dog, cat, and horse.)
   b. The adhesion of the posterior capsule with the hyaloid membrane. Intracapsular removal can be done in dogs with:
      1) Lenticular displacement
      2) Hypermature cataracts that are beginning to separate from the ciliary body
3. Extracapsular cataract extraction (ECCE) - removal of the lens after opening and removing the anterior capsule. The posterior capsule remains. This is the operation that was most frequently performed in animals before phacoemulsification became available. If excess cortex is left adhering to the posterior capsule, a secondary cataract (aftercataract) and/or lens protein-induced uveitis may cause complications. Two techniques are recommended:
   a. Corneal incision
   b. Conjunctival flap with scleral incision
4. Phacoemulsification - this is fragmentation of the lens with an ultrasonic tip and aspiration of the fragments while continuously irrigating the anterior chamber.
5. *Comment.* The immediate results of improved vision and reduced long term complications after phacoemulsification and aspiration are far superior to traditional (manual) ECCE. Because of this, the author feels that ECCE is only indicated in those patients where phacoemulsification is contraindicated.

CATARACT SURGERY IN DOGS

Presurgical treatment beginning five days before surgery

This varies with the surgeon. Phacoemulsification techniques do not require as much premedication.

1. Topical medication
   a. Instill antibiotic corticosteriod combination (e.g. Maxitrol) in the eye QID for three to five days before surgery (an infected eye should not be operated)
   b. Start dilating the pupil with atropine 1% one to three days before surgery
2. Systemic prednisolone or aspirin three to five days presurgery and antibiotic (Cefrazolin, 10 mg/lb) 12 to 24 hours presurgery
3. Premedications day of surgery
   a. Ocufen ophthalmic drops every 30 minutes beginning two hours before surgery
   b. Mannitol IV - 0.5 gm/lb beginning immediately after induction of anesthesia, if ECCE is anticipated, will reduce the danger of vitreous swelling during surgery
   c. Antihistamine administered about the same time as the skin is prepared for surgery will reduce histamine release when the eye is incised
4. Anesthesia
   a. Preanesthetize with atropine and acepromazine
   b. Induce anesthesia with pentothal and maintain on isoflurane. Mask induction is also satisfactory. Isoflurane provides excellent relaxation of the extrinsic ocular muscles.
   c. Clip around the eye and prep with 0.2% Betadine/saline dilution (1:50 saline dilution of 10% Betadine) or similar povidone iodine preparation
   d. Support the head so that the visual axis of the eye is directed as nearly vertical as possible. Dorsal recumbency is usually preferred if both eyes are to be operated.

Surgical procedure - extracapsular cataract extraction using corneal incision (Fig 13-14)

1. A lateral canthotomy is usually needed for good exposure
2. Stabilize the eyelids with sutures or wire speculum
3. Stabilize the globe with 6-0 silk scleral fixation (bridle) sutures near the limbus at the 12 and 6 o'clock positions
4. Neuromuscular blocking agents (atracurium) will facilitate positioning of the eye
5. Make a dorsal incision in clear cornea 1 mm from the limbus (broken razor blades are probably sharpest; #64 Beaver blades are also satisfactory), and extend the wound with corneal scissors. Outlining the course of the incision with the #64 Beaver blade at about 1/3 to 1/2 depth before incising the cornea facilitates extending the wound with corneal scissors.
6. Preplace a suture in the cornea and sclera at the 12 o'clock position with 8-0 vicryl, dexon or PDS suture
7. Extend the wound both ways with corneal scissors until the wound is long enough to deliver the lens. This may be nearly 180° around the limbus if the lens is intumescent.
8. Deliver the lens - grasp the lens with a many-toothed capsule forceps and check to see if the zonule attachments are tight or loose. If loose, deliver intracapsularly with gentle traction on the lens. It will be necessary to cut the vitreous attachments from the lens at the level of the pupil. If tight, incise the capsule with a cystotome and remove as much capsule as possible. Then, using a lens spatula, deliver the cortex and nucleus.
9. Lens fragments can be removed by irrigating with surgical saline solution or intraocular balanced salt solution (BSS). Cellulose spears are useful to remove small lens fragments that remain after irrigation. If the pupil does not dilate properly, irrigation with 1:10,000 epinephrine will enhance mydriasis. If the pupil fails to dilate, perform a sphincterotomy with corneal scissors at the 6 o'clock position, extending from the edge of the pupil to the collarette.
10. The preplaced suture is tied, then the difference is split on both sides with the second and third sutures. An air bubble placed in the eye with a syringe and cannula will generally stay in the eye during suturing.

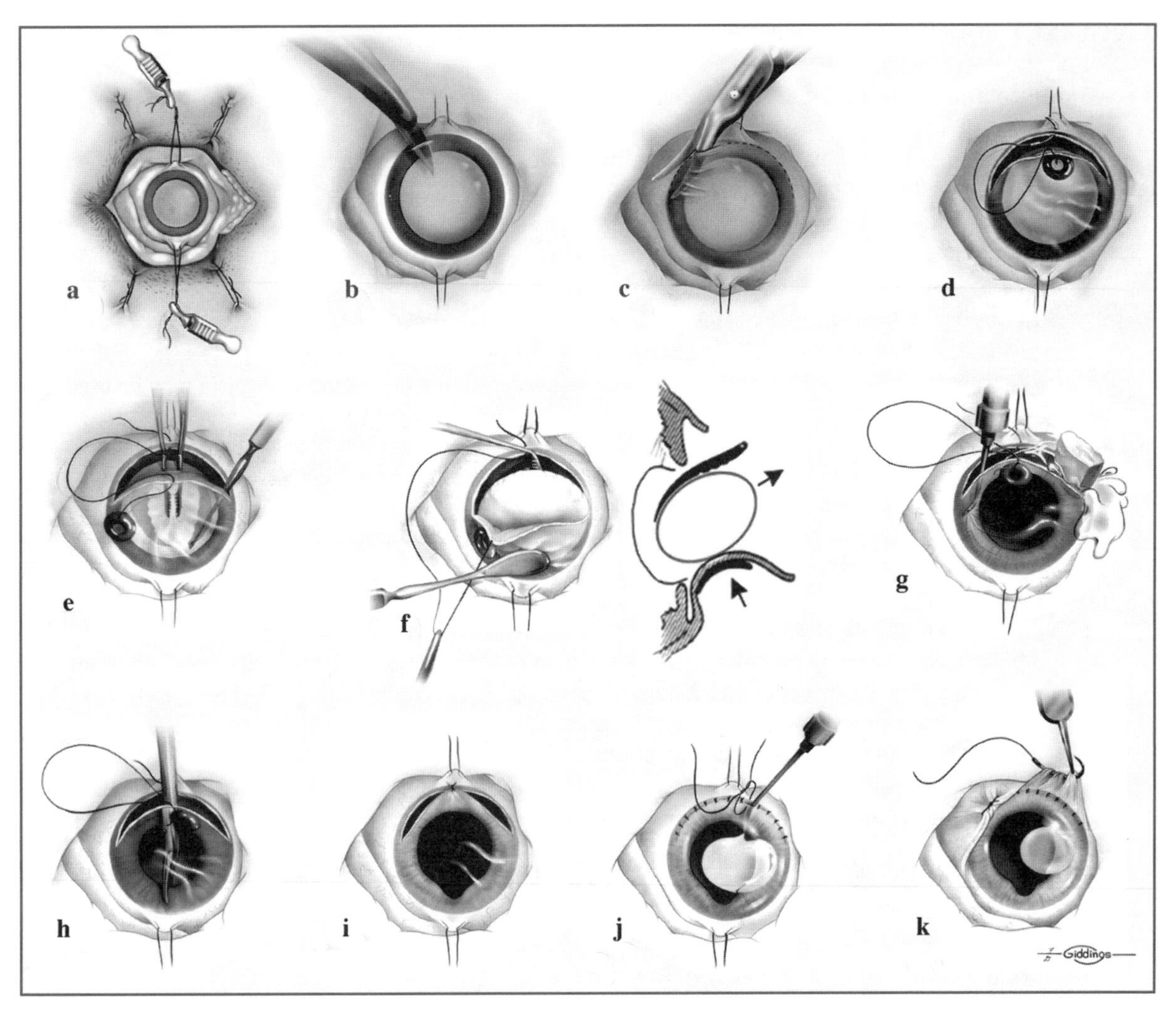

Figure 13-14. Extracapsular cataract removal using a corneal incision.

a. Eyelids stabilized with 4-0 silk sutures and globe with 6-0 silk bridle sutures at 12:00 and 6:00 o'clock. A canthotomy provides good exposure.
b. Incising clear cornea with a broken razor blade
c. Extending the incision with corneal scissors
d. Preplacement of a suture at the 12 o'clock position. A porcelain bead is tied to the end of the suture to prevent it from pulling through. The suture is used to manipulate the cornea and thereby avoid endothelial damage that results from forceps manipulation. 8-0 Vicryl or Dexon are suitable suture material.
e. The corneal incision has been extended halfway around the cornea for good exposure. The anterior capsule is grasped with a many teeth capsule forceps. A cystotome is used to incise the capsule so that it can be removed with a twisting motion.
f. A lens loop is introduced behind the lens and the lens removed leaving the posterior capsule in place. A second spatula can be placed on the cornea to facilitate removal (anterior and sagittal views).
g. Irrigation of lens fragments from capsule bag and anterior chamber.
h. Sphincterotomy at 6 o'clock position is indicated if the pupil closes down
i. Appearance after the preplaced suture has been tied.
j. An air bubble can be placed into the anterior chamber while suturing the corneal wound. This maintains anterior chamber depth.
k. Corneal wound has been sutured with 8-0 suture and the modified conjunctival flap is being positioned with 6-0 or 7-0 silk. Air can be seen in the anterior chamber.

This restores the shape of the globe and facilitates suturing. Before the last suture is placed the air bubble should be re-established so it will hold the iris back. If the anterior chamber appears too deep or the bubble is too large, some air is aspirated and the eye is filled with irrigating fluid until the shape of the globe is restored. The globe should still be hypotonic. A continuous suture is satisfactory after the first three sutures have been placed.

11. Optional - a modified pursestring conjunctival flap folded over the corneal wound with absorbable suture will give added support and eliminate any discomfort the dog may have from blinking over the wound. This flap will retract in about three days, at which time the dog will not show any discomfort.
12. If a canthotomy was performed, it should be closed with 5-0 or 6-0 absorbable suture
13. Aftercare
    a. Continue systemic antibiotics five days
    b. Systemic prednisolone for next two to four weeks, depending on progress. Aspirin may be used instead of prednisolone. Some dogs may require extended anti-inflammatory drugs.
    c. Topical atropine, corticosteroid and antibiotic ophthalmic ointment or drops should be used for the first two weeks, then continued as indicated by the progress of the individual patient.
    d. If animal starts to rub eye, tranquilize or use a protective collar.
14. Complications
    a. Anterior uveitis - the most common and serious complication. This may result from the surgery or from lens fragments remaining in the eye.
        1) Synechia - iris bombé
        2) Cyclitic membrane formation
    b. Secondary glaucoma - many patients develop a mild transient increase in pressure the first 24 hours. Filtration angle obstruction can occur anytime uveitis persists.
    c. Spontaneous hyphema
    d. Wound breakdown

Manual extracapsular cataract extraction using a conjunctival flap with scleral incision (Fig 13-15)

1. A limbus-based conjunctival flap is prepared over the dorsal sclera
2. With a sharp blade or electroscalpel, a groove 0.5 to 0.67 mm of the thickness of the sclera is prepared 0.5 to 1 mm behind the limbus
3. Two horizontal mattress sutures are preplaced to the depth of the grooves. The sutures are looped away from the wound.
4. The incision is completed into the anterior chamber
5. The lens is delivered as previously described
6. The wound is closed and the preplaced sutures tied. The anterior chamber is reformed with air and/or saline solution. The conjunctiva is sutured.
7. Aftercare is the same as before

Comparison of techniques

Both are acceptable and take about the same amount of total time for surgery. The surgeon's preference determines which technique will be used. The author prefers the clear corneal incision.

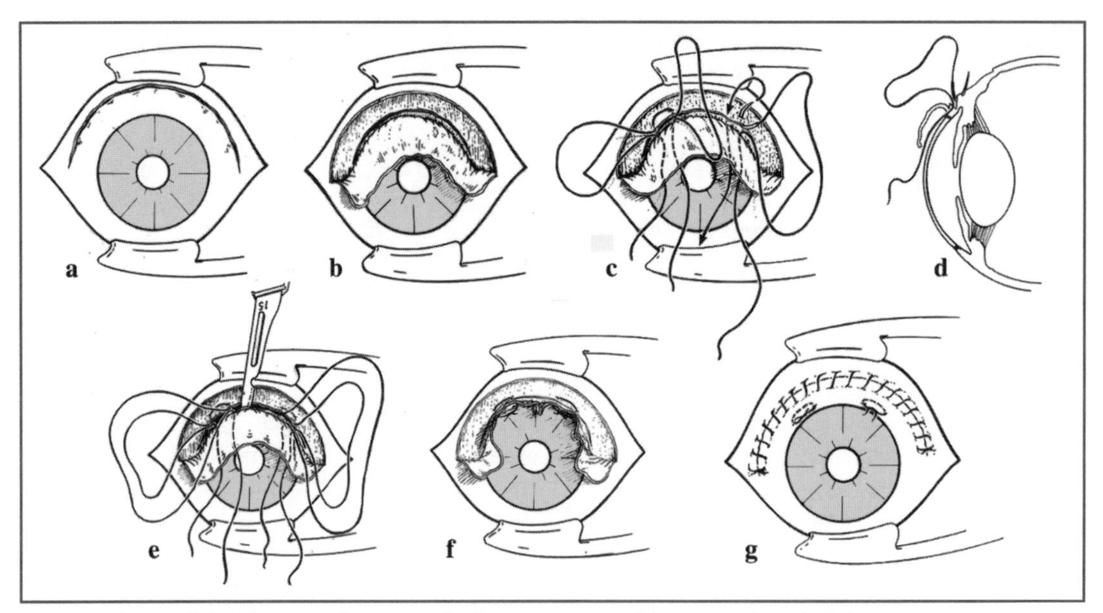

Figure 13-15. Extracapsular removal using a conjunctival flap and scleral incision.

a. Incision for conjunctival flap
b. Conjunctiva reflected to the limbus
c. Incision is made halfway through the sclera. Preplaced sutures are being positioned.
d. Cross-section showing suture placement
e. Sutures are laid to the side and the incision completed. The lens is delivered in the same manner as previously described for the corneal approach.
f. Preplaced sutures are tied closing scleral wound
g. Conjunctiva is sutured with absorbable sutures

CATARACT SURGERY - CATS

Cataracts in cats are usually secondary to chronic anterior uveitis and in these patients complications from uveitis exist, precluding surgical removal of the lens.

In cats with senile cataract or secondary cataract without postinflammatory complications, lens removal can be performed with greater success than in dogs. The technique for removing mature cataracts is the same as in the dog. The large cat eye in relation to the size of the orbit necessitates maximum extrinsic ocular muscle relaxation and good globe positioning.

Cataracts in young cats with toxic or degenerative cataracts will usually be fluid or semifluid. This type of cataract can be treated with discission and aspiration.

CATARACT SURGERY - EQUINE

Congenital cataracts in foals - Phacoemulsification is preferred treatment. Aspiration and irrigation can be performed. The younger the patient the greater the success. Aspiration becomes more difficult by six months of age. After one year the nucleus may not fragment adequately to perform aspiration. When this occurs, the incision needs to be enlarged so that larger fragments can be delivered manually. The anterior chamber collapses when the incision is enlarged, thereby increasing the chance of complications. Aspiration may be accomplished using single or double cannula techniques.

Adult animals with secondary or senile cataracts
Phacoemulsification - several companies offer equipment that accomodates needles of sufficient length to permit adaptation of this surgical technology to horses. The prognosis varies, depending on the cause of the cataract and the age of the horse. Adult horses will have a firm cortex and a hard nucleus. The author has been disappointed in the long-term surgical results in adult horses that had previous anterior uveitis, even if the eye was quiescent at the time of surgery.

LENS DISPLACEMENT

Partial or complete breakdown of the zonular attachments results in displacement of lens.

Etiology

1. Dogs
   a. Congenital - rare. Usually seen with multiple ocular problems.
   b. Traumatic - trauma severe enough to produce luxation will have concurrent ocular damage, resulting in blindness
   c. Spontaneous - breed predisposition. Seen most frequently in terriers (wire-haired fox terrier, Tibetan, Cairn, Sealyham, Welsh and Manchester), less frequently in Boston terrier, poodle, and border collie and associated with poorly developed zonules. Autosomal recessive has been demonstrated for the Tibetan terrier. Usually occurs in young adults (two to five years).
   d. Consecutive luxation (secondary to other ocular disease)
      1) Glaucoma - with buphthalmos probably the most common acquired cause
      2) Chronic uveitis resulting in damage to zonules
      3) Intraocular tumors
      4) Hypermature cataracts
2. Cats - no inherited predisposition. Seen more frequently in older cats and Siamese may be predisposed. May be unilateral or bilateral.
   a. Chronic uveitis - toxoplasmosis is a common cause
   b. Glaucoma - some buphthalmic eyes may return to normal IOP and are blind when presented.
3. Horses
   a. Congenital - rare. But when seen, usually secondary to congenital glaucoma
   b. Spontaneous - rare
   c. Consecutive
      1) The most common cause for lens luxation in the horse is ERU with or without glaucoma
      2) Less frequently - intraocular tumors and hypermature cataracts

Classification and signs

Displacement of the lens is easily determined as long as the cornea is clear.

Examine the iris for abnormal motion and the anterior chamber for depth. The iris moves freely over the anterior surface of the lens and therefore is dependent on the lens for position. Change in size of the pupil is the only normal movement of the iris. If the zonules deteriorate or pull free from the lens, rapid eye movement will cause the lens to oscillate in the patellar fossa. This oscillation will result in iris vibration, referred to as iridodonesis. Iridodonesis is the first sign of impending lens displacement and becomes more evident as the lens continues to loosen from the zonules. Initially the vitreous may swell, forcing the lens forward and resulting in a shallow anterior chamber. Anterior chamber depth is best evaluated by observing the eye from the side rather than eye to eye. If the lens is displaced, iris position will be altered accordingly.

1. Subluxation (Fig 13-16) - The displaced lens remains in the patellar fossa in a plane behind the iris. If the lens subluxates along the equatorial plane, the iris will be convex where it contacts the lens and flat in the area of dislocation. The edge of the lens may be observed in the pupil. The area of the pupil where the lens is missing is referred to as an "aphakic crescent". In mild equatorial subluxation the aphakic crescent may not be observed until the pupil is dilated.

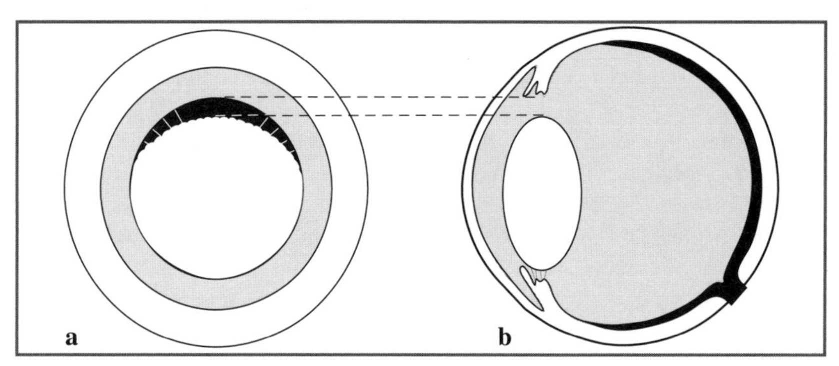

Figure 13-16. Lens subluxation with aphakic crescent.
  a. Frontal view with aphakic crescent. Zonules stretching at periphery of crescent ruptured at the center.
  b. Cross-section demonstrating the zonular detachment in the area of the aphakic crescent

2. Luxation (dislocation) - complete displacement from the patellar fossa
   a. Anterior luxation (Fig 13-17)
      1) Forcing the iris forward - anterior displacement of the lens without passing through the pupil will result in a shallow anterior chamber and increased convexity to the anterior iris surface
      2) Through the pupil - if the pupil dilates, the lens can luxate through the pupil into the anterior chamber. This may be partial or complete. Luxation into the anterior chamber will result in corneal edema where the lens contacts the corneal endothelium, and the iris will be concave where the posterior surface of the lens contacts the iris. There are two methods to determine the limits of the lens when the cornea is cloudy. The focal light source is directed across the eye at the limbus to transilluminate the luxated lens. Light is trapped internally in the lens and produces a reflex arc of light at the equator opposite the light source that can be seen through the cloudy cornea. If this is unsuccessful, the lens can be made to fluoresce using ultraviolet light (Wood's lamp).

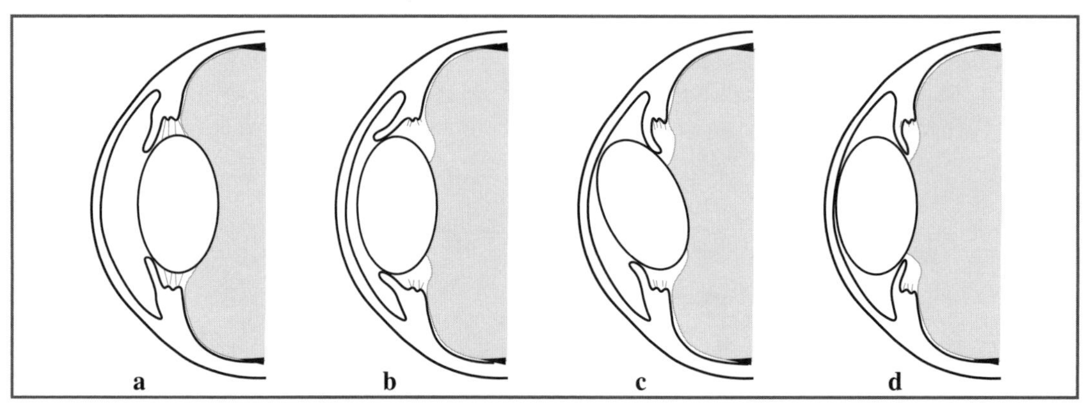

Figure 13-17. Anterior lens luxation.
  a. Normal lens position
  b. Anterior luxation with the lens forcing the iris forward. This results in a shallow anterior chamber.
  c. Lens partially through the pupil, referred to as Marfan's syndrome. If the anterior capsule touches the cornea, edema will ensue.
  d. Complete anterior chamber luxation. The anterior chamber is very deep in this case.

b. Posterior luxation (Fig 13-18) - Increased lens movement causes the anterior vitreous that contacts the lens to separate from the deeper vitreous, allowing more movement of the lens. Eventually the damaged vitreous will liquify and be replaced by aqueous. This process of liquefaction of the vitreous is referred to as a syneresis. Posterior displacement will result in a deep anterior chamber, with the iris appearing flat or concave. Syneresis may continue until most of the vitreous disappears. When this occurs, the lens may settle toward the retina and disappear from the area of the pupil.

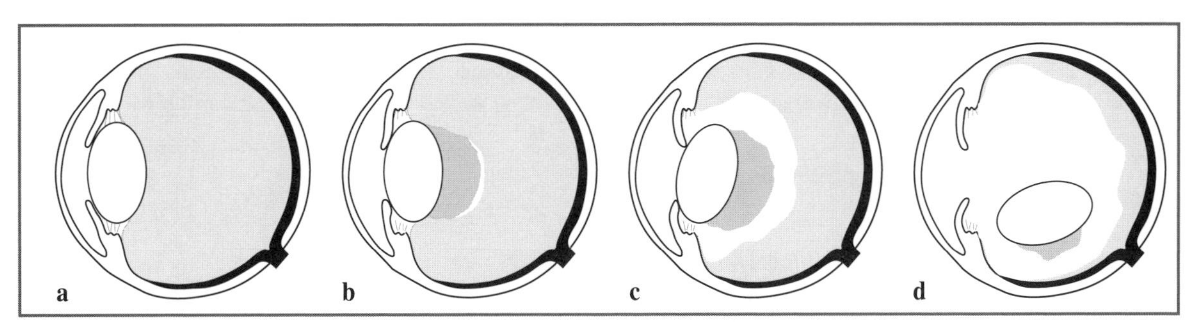

Figure 13-18. Stages of posterior lens luxation and secondary vitreous absorption.
a. Normal lens position
b. Zonules are detached and lens held in place by vitreous attachment. Lens has excess movement but still held in normal position. Sudden eye movement will result in iridodonesis.
c. Vitreous beginning to degenerate, allowing more lens movement.
d. Nearly all vitreous has liquified, allowing lens to settle to lower limit of globe.

3. *Comment* - Lens luxation can cause glaucoma and likewise chronic glaucoma can cause lens luxation. Therefore, it is often difficult to determine which disease is primary. Every effort should be made to establish the primary disease so that proper treatment can be prescribed. Glaucoma is indicated as the primary cause if both eyes have increased pressure and only one lens is displaced. Spontaneous displacement is suggested if both lenses are luxated or permit iridodonesis and only one eye has glaucoma. When glaucoma and displacement are bilateral, the breed of the patient becomes important in establishing the primary cause.

    Anterior lens displacement is the most hazardous form of displacement. It has a high probability of causing glaucoma, and if the lens touches the cornea it will cause endothelial damage, leading to corneal edema.

    Posterior luxation is usually better tolerated by the eye but can also produce glaucoma. It has the constant potential of becoming an anterior luxation.

Differential diagnosis - Anterior luxation with corneal opacity must be differentiated from:

1. Glaucoma
2. Anterior uveitis with corneal edema
3. Corneal endothelial degeneration
4. Interstitial keratitis

Treatment

1. Lens removal of a noncomplicated eye is easier and has a better prognosis than routine lens removal
2. The corneal incision approach for extracapsular cataract removal is recommended
3. Chronic glaucoma will persist even after lens removal

LENS RUPTURE - Lens rupture is uncommon and usually traumatic

Etiology

1. Dogs and cats - gunshot or penetration from pointed object (claws)
2. Horses - severe blow to head is more likely to cause a ruptured lens in horses than in other species

Signs

1. Gunshot - usually has severe hyphema and retinal damage as well. Poor prognosis.
2. Rupture from a blow in horses is easily confused with fibrin in the anterior chamber. Has a granular appearance and will fluoresce in ultraviolet light. May take 7 to 10 days after injury before the ruptured lens fills the anterior chamber.
3. Penetrating sharp object without severe hemorrhage - changes in the lens will be noticed as the eye is examined. Small lens capsule penetrations may seal over and result in a capsular cataract without any further complication. Capsule lacerations that do not seal immediately and continue to leak lens protein will result in a lens protein-induced uveitis in about 14 days. When uveitis occurs, the prognosis for a visual eye is unfavorable.

Treatment

1. Enlarge the wound or make a limbal incision to remove lens material
2. Same aftercare as routine lens removal
3. Fair prognosis if no concurrent intraocular hemorrhage

OTHER CONGENITAL DISEASES

Congenital aphakia (absence of lens) - uncommon. Can occur in all species. Occurs with multiple ocular defects.

Congenital microphakia (small lens) - It may occur as a single lesion or concurrently with other eye lesions. A microphakic lens may have a cataract at birth. Care should be taken to not confuse a resorptive lens with a microphakic lens. If clear, it usually remains clear.

A microphakic lens can be identified by seeing lens equator when the pupil is dilated.

Horses with mild microphakia will have a prominent round nucleus that is easily visualized with transillumination.

Lenticonus (Fig 13-19) - A condition where the surface of the lens protrudes at the anterior or posterior pole in conical form. (Lentiglobus refers to a spherical protrusion.) Anterior and posterior forms have been described in the dog. Posterior lenticonus is most common. The lesion may remain stationary or be predisposed to rupture. Posterior lenticonus can be associated with persistent hyperplastic primary vitreous. Lenticonus internum is a term used to describe a nucleus that is located posteriorly in the lens and possibly touching the posterior lens capsule. It is usually associated with concurrent posterior lenticonus.

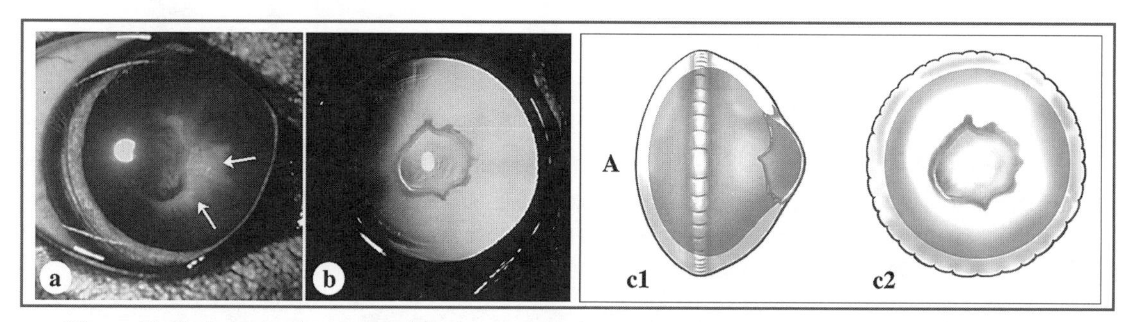

Figure 13-19. Posterior lenticonus with concurrent lenticonus internum.
- a. Lens viewed with transillumination. Posterior cortical cataract areas white. Arrows indicate lenticonus margin.
- b. Cataract appears dark on retroillumination
- c. Drawings made from slit lamp observation depicting shape of lens and the cataract at the junction of normal and abnormal curvatures of the posterior lens surface. "A" = anterior lens surface.
  1) Lateral view
  2) Frontal view

1. Occurrence
   a. Seen most frequently in Siberian huskies with posterior polar cataracts
   b. Can occur at random in any breed
   c. Can occur in animals with other ocular lesions, especially persistent hyperplastic vitreous
2. Significance
   a. Most do not cause any problem except for a concurrent stationary posterior polar capsular and subcapsular cortical cataract. If concurrent lenticonus internum exists, nuclear cataract will also be seen.
   b. The capsule is weak at the polar location of the lenticonus. This weakened area may rupture, resulting in lens material herniating into the vitreous. If this occurs, a severe lens protein uveitis will result, causing a refractory endophthalmitis. When this happens, eye removal or chemical uveoretinal ablation with gentamicin is indicated.
   c. The author has followed Siberian huskies with lenticonus internum and posterior subcapsular cataracts that have developed posterior lenticonus at a later date.

Lens coloboma - Lens coloboma is a congenital defect of the equator of the lens. It is uncommon and does not have clinical significance.

1. Signs - A flattened equatorial section of the lens is seen as an incidental finding when examining an eye with a dilated pupil.

2. Differential diagnosis - Coloboma must be differentiated from an aphakic crescent, which has a circular border compared to the flat border of lens coloboma.

CHAPTER 14 - VITREOUS

Disease of the vitreous is uncommon and of little clinical significance as a primary disease problem.

EMBRYOLOGY, ANATOMY AND PHYSIOLOGY

EMBRYOLOGY

The vitreous goes through three stages of development: the primary vitreous (vascular hyaloidal system), the secondary vitreous (definitive vitreous of postnatal eyes), and the tertiary vitreous (zonules of Zinn or suspensory ligaments of the lens). After birth, these are represented by the hyaloid canal, definitive vitreous body, and zonules of Zinn (Fig 14-1).

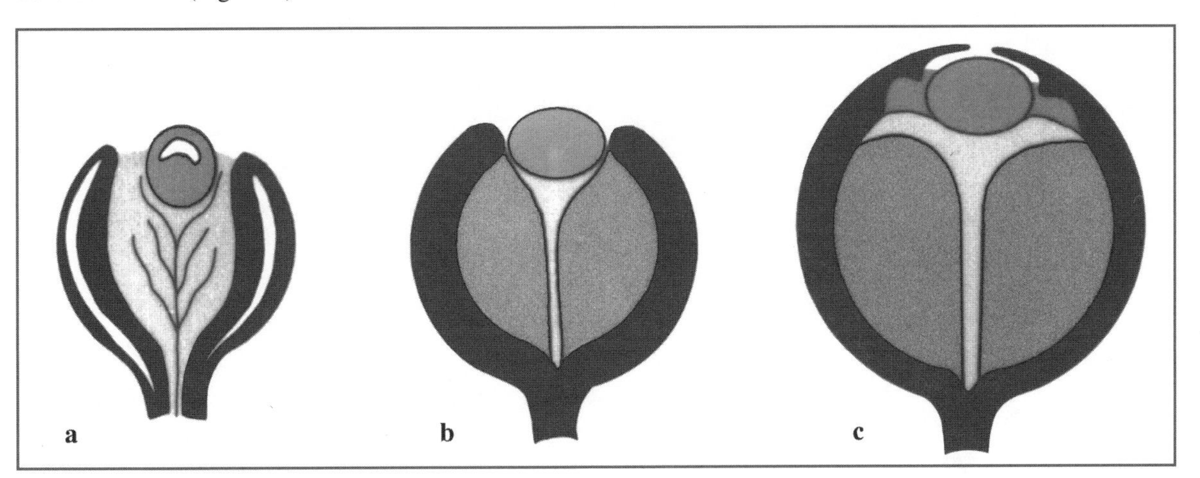

Figure 14-1. Stages of vitreous development.
- a. Primary (hyaloid) vitreous
- b. Secondary (definitive) vitreous fills the posterior globe, forcing the primary vitreous centrally to become hyaloid canal
- c. Tertiary vitreous (suspensory ligaments of the lens) develops at the periphery of the lens. Definitive vitreous and hyaloid canal are shown.

The rapid growth of the embryonal lens requires a rich blood supply. This is provided by the hyaloid system (primary vitreous). The space between the lens vesicle and the optic cup is infiltrated with blood vessels that develop an elaborate vascular tunic around the lens (tunica vasculosa lentis) (Fig 14-2). This system nourishes the rapidly growing lens and, when it has served its purpose, atrophies. The tunica vasculosa lentis is supplied posteriorly by the hyaloid artery and connects anteriorly with the developing anterior uveal circulation. Definitive (secondary) vitreous is secreted by the inner limiting membrane (Müller cells) of the retina, forcing the hyaloid vitreous centrally. As the hyaloid system atrophies, a central canal (Cloquet's canal) remains in the definitive vitreous. The tertiary vitreous is secreted by the neural ectoderm of the ciliary region and differentiates into the zonules of the lens.

ANATOMY AND PHYSIOLOGY

The vitreous is the largest structure of the eye, up to 75% of the ocular volume in domestic animals (80% in man). It is a gel containing 99% water and lacks regenerative ability. The gel-liquid state of the vitreous is referred to as *rheology*. There is a rapid turnover of water (1/2 of the vitreous volume is being replaced every 10 to 15 minutes). Hyaluronic acid provides viscosity and regulates vitreous volume. Its high negative potential is normally neutralized by cations and proteins. If this neutralization is removed, the negative charge of the hyaluronic acid molecules cause them to repel each other, expanding the vitreous. A net positive charge causes the vitreous to collapse.

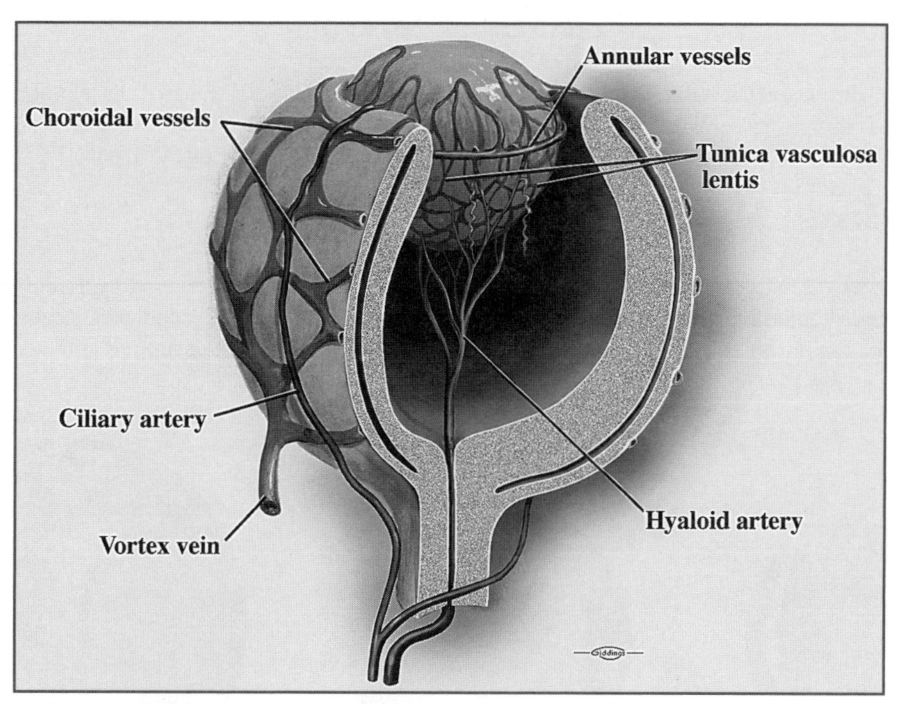

Figure 14-2. Diagrammatic representation of the blood vessels of the embryonic eye.

There is a fine collagen fiber network and a mucopolysaccharide matrix. In areas of contact it is condensed, giving the appearance of a membrane. It is firmly attached at the optic disk, pars plana, and to the posterior surface of the lens (hyaloidocapsular ligament). It is loosely attached to the retina. The hyaloid canal (Cloquet's canal) passes through the middle of the vitreous from the lens to the optic disk. The attachment of Cloquet's at the lens can be visualized as Egger's line (Fig 14-3).

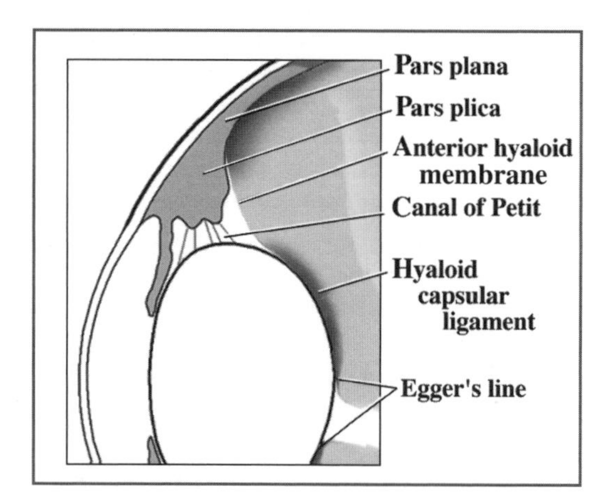

Figure 14-3. Schematic section of canine eye representing vitreous, lens and ciliary body area

Vitreous zones - The vitreous can be subdivided into three zones: **(Fig 14-4)**

1. Cortex - contacts the retina
2. Central channel - containing the hyaloid canal
3. Intermediate zone - (the area between) contains vitreal tracts and membranelles that form funnels packed into one another that diverse from the region of the papilla and extend anteriorly. In man the tracts are preretinal, median and hyaloid surrounding the hyaloid canal.

Consistency of the vitreous

1. Dogs and cats - dense intermediate and liquid cortex
2. Cow, pig and sheep - homogeneous high density
3. Horse - low optical density without separation into cortical and intermediate zones
4. Rabbit - very low density
5. Primates - dense cortex liquid center

When examined with the transilluminator, or slit lamp, cloudy areas will be observed that cannot be seen with an ophthalmoscope. These represent cleavage planes or plicae that are normal and should not be confused with pathologic debris, which can be seen with transillumination and ophthalmoscopy.

When subject to the movement of a dislocating lens, it will become semiliquified in the area of contact. Should the entire vitreous become liquified, it will be replaced by aqueous, and retinal detachment can occur.

The binocular indirect ophthalmoscope is excellent for examining for vitreous opacities.

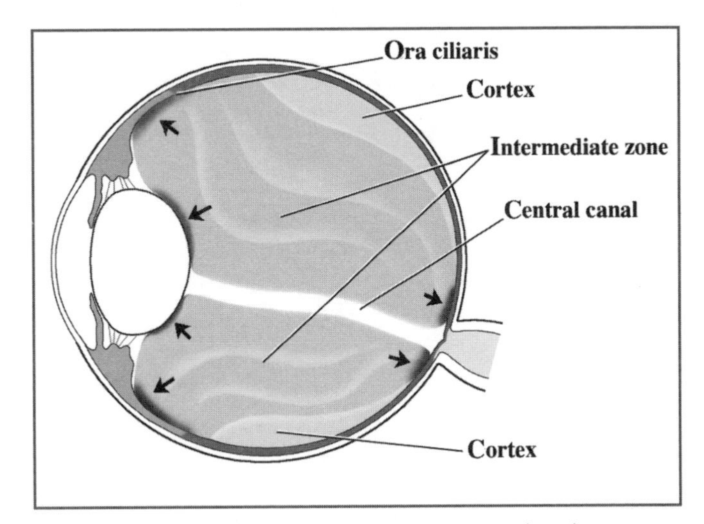

Figure 14-4. Schematic canine eye representing vitreous zones and areas of vitreous attachments (arrows)

PERSISTENT HYALOID ARTERY AND REMNANTS

Varying degrees of persistent hyaloid system may occur. This does not interfere with sight unless areas of the lens are vascularized or cataracts are produced.

Normal remnants

1. Mittendorf's dot (Fig 14-5) - This is a small posterior polar capsular opacity where the artery attached to the lens. Seen most easily in young animals. Located ventral to the junction of the posterior Y sutures.
2. Dense hyaloid canal - This appears as a gray thread or tube extending from the lens to the optic nerve, or as short remnants attached to the lens (Fig 14-6) and/or the optic disk. The remnant attached to the lens may hang down into the vitreous with a "corkscrew" appearance.

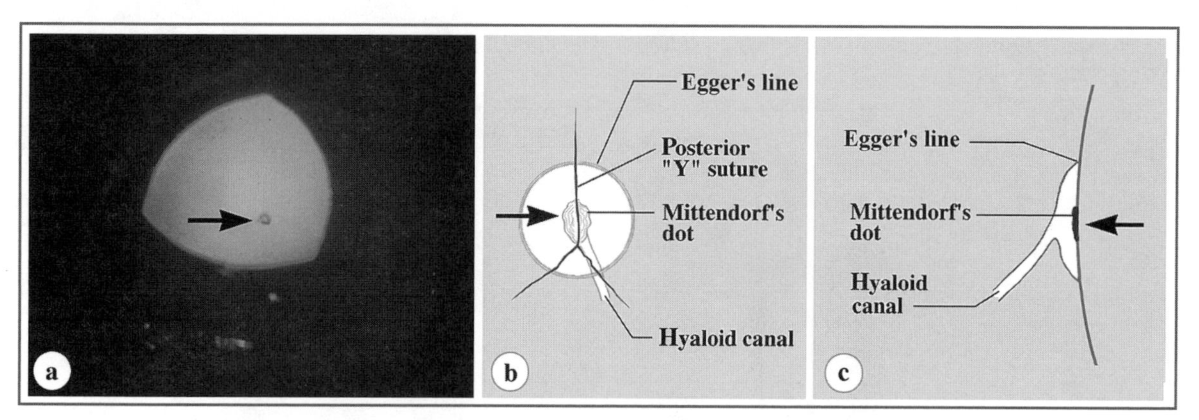

Figure 14-5. Mittendorf's dot.
- a. Retroillumination of canine eye demonstrating Mittendorf's dot as a small posterior capsular opacity (arrow).
- b. Schematic frontal view representing area of Mittendorf's dot.
- c. Schematic sagittal view representing area of Mittendorf's dot.

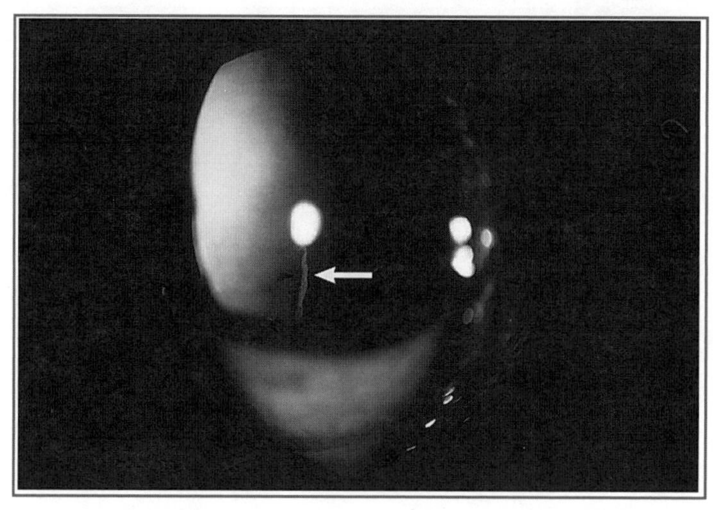

Figure 14-6. Normal adult dog with hyaloid canal remnant attached to posterior lens capsule (arrow).

3. A prominent posterior remnant associated with the optic nerve is referred to as Bergmeister's papilla.
4. Species variations
   a. Dogs - Primary vitreous regression begins after 45 days gestation. Remnants of the tunica are expected to disappear by three to four weeks of age. In beagles, closure of the hyaloid artery occurs 5 to 17 days after birth. Small transparent artery tags on the posterior capsule may be seen with a transilluminator or slit lamp for life. These tags are not seen with the ophthalmoscope and are considered normal.
   b. Cats - Remnants absorb by eight weeks. Adults are less frequently affected with remnants than other species.
   c. Horses - A regressing artery may be seen in newborn foals and will disappear in a few days. All previously described permanent remnants can occur.
   d. Cattle and sheep - Regression is complete by eight weeks of age. Remnants are common. Eighty percent of adult cattle have remnants and 30% of one to two year old sheep. The regressing hyaloid artery contains blood in most of the newborn. The blood disappears quickly, leaving an opaque hyaloid canal and clear ghost vessels that can be seen on the posterior lens capsule for two to four weeks (Fig 14-7).

      An opaque canal remnant usually remains for life. This may be complete, or the central portion may clear, leaving tags at either end. This should not be considered a pathologic finding.

      Short vascularized remnants extending several millimeters into the vitreous from the optic nerve are common; these are not of clinical significance.

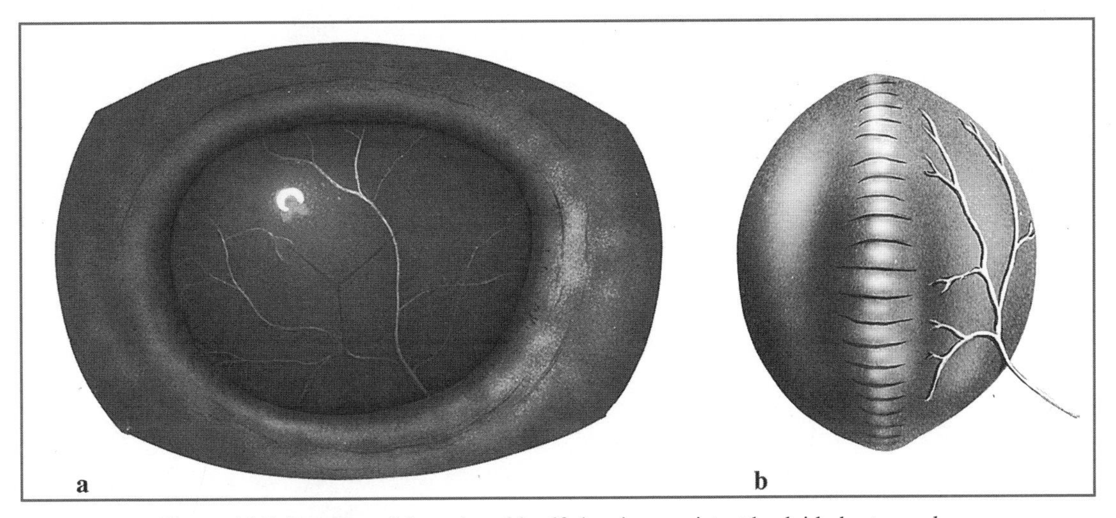

Figure 14-7. Drawing of three day old calf showing persistent hyaloid ghost vessels.
a. Appearance of pupil when examined with transillumination. Ghost vessels can be seen on the posterior capsule.
b. Lateral view showing location of ghost vessels

PERSISTENT HYPERPLASTIC PRIMARY VITREOUS (PHPV) - is persistence of the hyaloid artery leading to vascularization of the lens with or without lens fibroplasia. It occurs in the cat, dog, horse, rabbit and rat.

Dog - the domestic species most frequently affected

1. Clinical signs - unilateral or bilateral. Severity depends on the extent of PHPV and the presence of pleomorphic changes. Patients will be visual, unless the changes are severe.
   a. PHPV changes
      1) Vascular network on posterior lens capsule and visible hyaloid artery
      2) Posterior lens capsule fibroplasia with or without blood vessels. Axial retrolental fibroplasia results in leukokoria (white pupil).
      3) Retrolental pigment deposits

        4) Lenticular hemorrhage
        5) Lens pigment deposits
    b. Pleomorphic changes
        1) Microphthalmia
        2) Retinal dysplasia
        3) Vitreous hemorrhage
        4) Persistent pupillary membranes and/or corneal opacity
        5) Persistent hyperplastic tunica vasculosa lentis (PHTVL)
2. Etiology
    a. Can be spontaneous in any breed
    b. Inherited - autosomal dominant with incomplete penetrance has been proposed for:
        1) Doberman pinscher (Netherlands) - concurrent changes seen included PHTVL, microphthalmia, persistent pupillary membrane, retrolental hemorrhage and pigment, microphakia and lens coloboma
        2) Staffordshire bull terrier (England) - pleomorphic changes similar to the Doberman pinscher were observed
    c. Breed predisposition
        1) Akita - with microphthalmia
        2) Beagle
        3) Standard and miniature schnauzer - sporadic occurrence

Horse and cat - Animals observed by the author were unilateral, had PHPV changes only and were visual.

ACQUIRED DISEASES

OPACITIES

Vitreous floaters or strands - white opacities or strands are suspended in the vitreous

1. Congenital opacities - small opacities are common. They are not considered significant.
2. Precipitates that remain in the vitreous after chorioretinal inflammation - These may appear as suspended masses or strands. Vitreous floaters can be seen in horses with equine recurrent uveitis and in other animals that have recovered from chorioretinitis. Vitreous liquefaction in the area of the opacity may occur, allowing it limited movement of the opacity.
3. Complication - may predispose to retinal detachment if postinflammatory traction bands are present.

Exudates - hyalitis

1. Acute pars planitis and/or posterior segment inflammation may result in exudate that extends into the vitreous. Varies from a faint haze to thick exudate. In some patients it absorbs, while in others permanent opacities remain as floaters (Fig 14-8).
2. Cats - Toxoplasmosis causing a pars planitis is the most common cause for vitreous exudate.

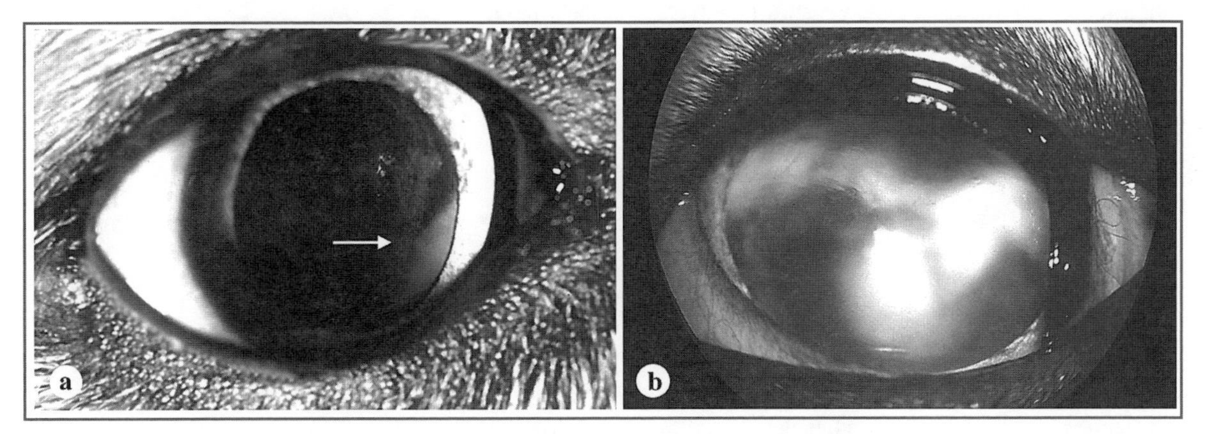

Figure 14-8. Vitreous exudate secondary to pars planitis in a cat with toxoplasmosis
a. Transillumination demonstrates nasal vitreous exudates behind the lens (arrow).
b. Ophthalmoscopic examination reveals extent of vitreous exudates.

Asteroid hyalosis (Fig 14-9) - This is a degenerate disease of the vitreous seen in older animals, especially dogs, and occasionally cats and horses. Characterized by numerous small spherical bodies in the vitreous. They are lipid-mineral complexes rich in calcium. On examination with a penlight or transilluminator, the crystals appear like "stars in the sky" which return to their original position after movement of the eye. When observed *from a distance* with ophthalmoscope retroillumination, they will appear black. When examined with an ophthalmoscope *from less than 5 inches*, they will appear white. If many are present, they reflect enough light when examining the fundus to simulate looking through falling snow. It has no visible effect on sight.

It may occur spontaneously in older dogs or after posterior segment inflammation.

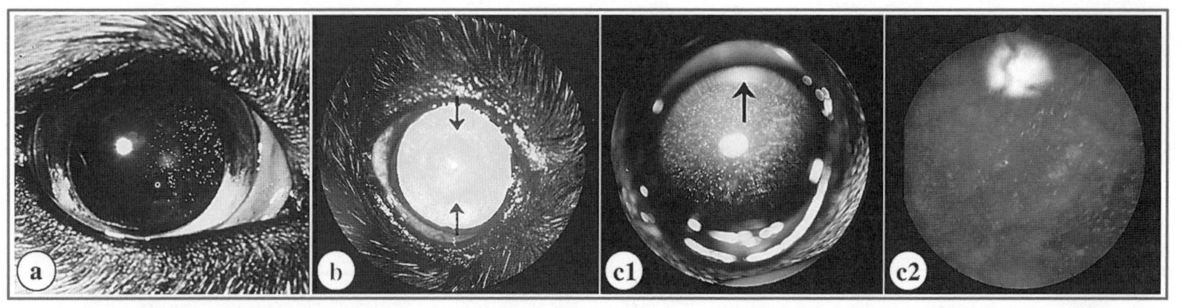

Figure 14-9. Asteroid hyalosis.
a. Asteroid hyalosis in a mixed breed terrier. The asteroid bodies are readily seen in the nasal vitreous.
b. Asteroid hyalosis bodies appear black with ophthalmoscopic retroillumination from 12 inches or more. Note nuclear sclerosis is present (arrow).
c. Ophthalmoscopic examination of asteroid hyalosis from a two-inch distance.
   1) Ophthalmoscope setting at 5 to 8 diopters. Asteroid bodies are clearly seen as white precipitates in the vitreous. Fundus is out of focus. Indistinct optic nerve at 12:00 o'clock (arrow).
   2) Ophthalmoscope setting at 0 diopters. Asteroid bodies are indistinct and make fundus examination appear as if examined through falling snow.

LIQUEFACTION

Terminology - Syneresis: the process of liquefaction of the vitreous

Causes of syneresis

1. Lens motion - most common cause
2. Chorioretinal disease, especially when retinal detachment occurs
3. After vitreous hemorrhage
4. Vitreous degeneration

Signs

When the vitreous liquifies, it will be replaced by aqueous. Because neither aqueous nor vitreous is visible, syneresis will be evident by degenerative vitreous debris (cholesterol complexes) moving freely in the aqueous. The debris remains trapped behind the lens and if the eye is moved, this material will rise and then slowly settle. This falling snow effect is called *synchysis scintillans*.

VITREOUS HEMORRHAGE

Causes

1. Spontaneous - collie eye syndrome
2. Acute retinitis and chorioretinitis - all species
3. Traumatic
4. Hypertension
5. Bleeding disorders

Signs

The anterior chamber usually remains clear. Blood can be seen behind the lens with an ophthalmoscope. The hemorrhage may organize and result in a vitreous floater or a fibrinous band that may contract and cause retinal detachment. Hemorrhage may remain in the vitreous for months.

Prognosis

Hemorrhage is usually associated with serious ocular changes.

CHAPTER 15 - RETINA AND OPTIC NERVE

ANATOMY AND PHYSIOLOGY OF THE RETINA

The retina is innermost of the three tunics of the eye. The neurosensory portion is continuous with the nonpigmented epithelium of the ciliary body, and the retinal pigment epithelium is continuous with the pigmented epithelium of the ciliary body.

The retina has one of the highest metabolic rates of any tissue in the body. In animals with retinal blood vessels, the outer one-half receive nutrition from the choriocapillaris and the inner one-half from retinal capillaries. If either of these are interrupted, complete loss of function will occur. Animals without retinal blood vessels depend on the choriocapillaris and the pecten, a vascular structure near the optic nerve resembling a ciliary process. The pecten nourishes the inner retina via the vitreous.

The retina is a very specialized sensory organ consisting of a three neuron sensory unit which processes stimuli and sends them to the brain for the visual response. It is mature at birth in precocious animals (horses, cattle, sheep, etc) but does not mature until 6 to 9 weeks in dogs and cats.

The retina can be divided into 10 layers from outside inward (Fig 15-1).

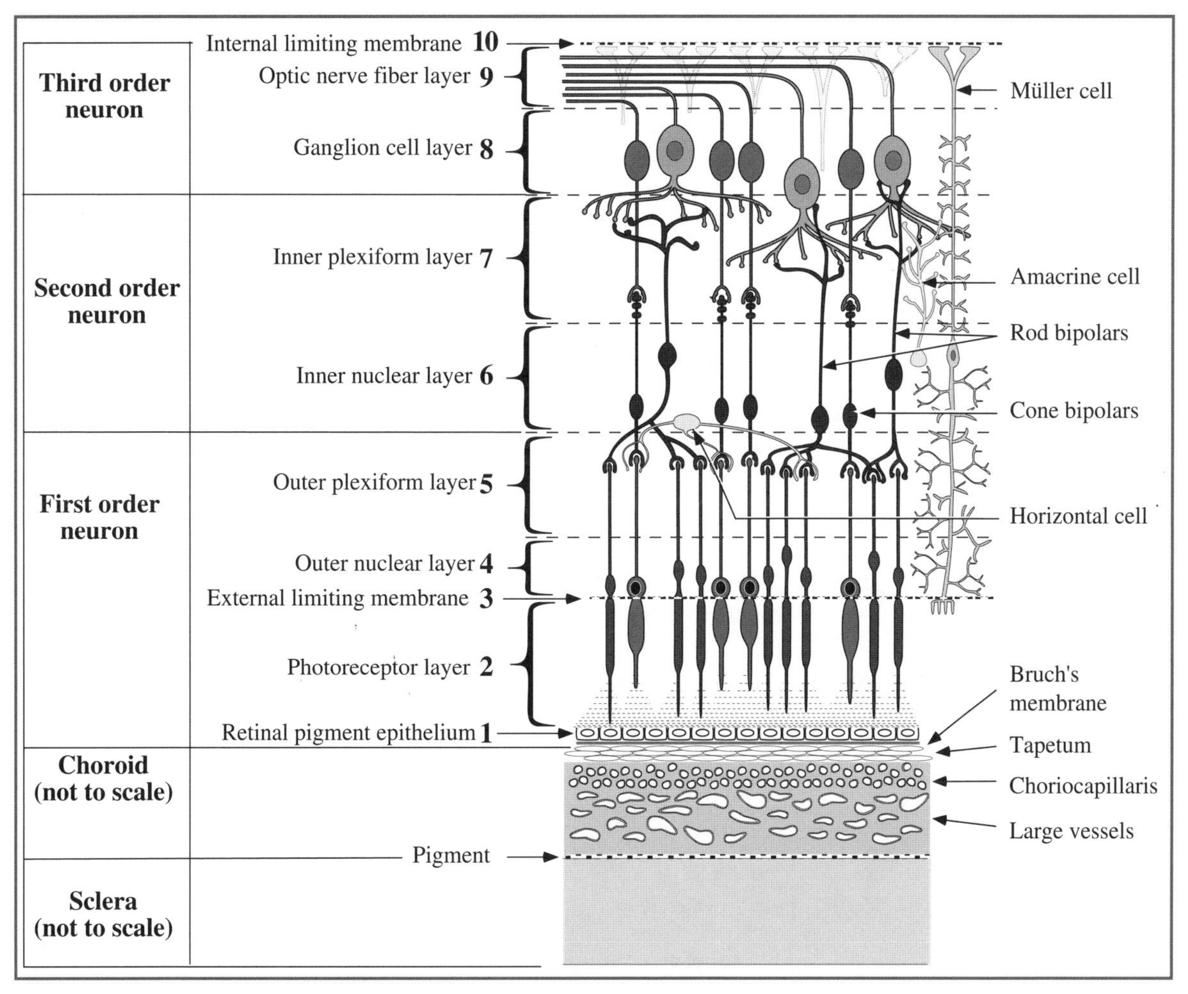

Figure 15-1. Layers of the retina and adjacent choroid.

RETINAL LAYERS

Retinal pigment epithelium

1. Adherent to choroid
2. Pigmented in the nontapetal fundus. Nonpigmented over the tapetum and in albinotic eyes.
3. Acts as a blood aqueous barrier for outer half of retina
4. Important for nutrient transport for the outer layers of the retina and phagocytizes the outer segments that are continuously shed by the photoreceptors.

Photoreceptor layer - This layer consists of the inner and outer segments of the rods and cones.

1. Rods are more sensitive to light and function best in low light. Therefore, they are associated with night vision (scotopic vision). They are more sensitive to short wavelength light (blue). Several rods are connected to a single bipolar cell in the inner nuclear layers and in turn several of these bipolar cells may be connected to one ganglion cell. This is referred to as summation (convergence) and intensifies visual sensitivity in poor light but loses discrimination.
2. Cones are less sensitive to light and function best in bright light (photopic vision). Cones don't have summation, therefore one cone stimulates one ganglion cell. This results in more discrimination.

External limiting membrane - is a thin membrane that separates the inner segment of the rods and cones from their nuclei

Outer nuclear layer - is the cell body for rods and cones

Outer plexiform layer - is the area of synapse between photoreceptors and the inner nuclear area

Inner nuclear layer - contains nuclei for amacrine cells, horizontal cells, bipolar cells and Müller cells

1. Bipolar cells are the connecting cells between photoreceptors and ganglion cells
2. Müller cells are glial cells that are supportive cells of the retina. Their processes extend from the internal limiting membrane to and beyond the external limiting membrane. They are important for internal structural support and nutrition of the retina.

Inner plexiform layer - is the synaptic region between inner nuclear and ganglion cell layers.

Ganglion cell layer - contains ganglion cells, neuroglial cells and retinal blood vessels.

Nerve fiber layer - is made up of nonmyelinated axons going to the optic disk.

Inner limiting membrane - is the basement membrane for the fused terminations of the Müller cells. Vitreal fibrils insert into the basement membrane.

RETINAL VASCULATURE - The retinal blood vessels are the blood-retinal barrier for the inner one-half of the retina.

Holangiotic pattern - provides blood supply to the entire retinal surface. This is the most common vascular pattern in mammals (Figs 1-28, 29, 30, 32, 33; Chapter 1, pages 28-33).

Merangiotic pattern - provides blood supply to a localized region of the retina (rabbits) (Fig 1-34; Chapter 1, page 34)

Paurangiotic pattern - provides blood supply to the peripapillary region (horse, guinea pig) (Fig 1-31; Chapter 1, page 31)

Anangiotic pattern - absence of blood vessels in the retina (birds, reptiles and some mammals)

ANATOMY OF THE OPTIC NERVE

The optic nerve extends from the globe to the optic chiasm and consists of an intraocular, orbital, and cranial portion.

INTRAOCULAR PORTION

Optic papilla (disk) - Appearance varies with the species, depending on the degree of myelination. In the dog, optic disk refers to the elevated area where myelinated ganglion cell axons leave the nerve fiber layer and enter the choroid. It has a central depression (physiologic cup). As it enters, the choroid nerve fibers make a 90° turn and are supported by glial and collagenous elements that allow nerve fibers to enter the sclera. This area is referred to as the choroidal or anterior lamina cribrosa. The sclera consists of laminar sheets with perforations aligned to allow the nerve fibers to pass through and is referred to as the posterior or scleral lamina cribrosa.

There is movement of cellular material continuously within the axon, which is referred to as axonal flow. If intraocular pressure increases, the laminar perforations lose their proper alignment and axonal flow is interrupted throughout the entire optic nerve including the optic disk.

ORBITAL PORTION - covered by the three meningeal sheaths of the central nervous system

THE CRANIAL PORTION - begins at the optic foramen and continues to the optic chiasm

ANATOMY OF THE CHOROID

The choroid is closely associated with the retina and provides it nourishment and support.

Blood vessels are the main substance of the choroid.

Choriocapillaris is a network of small blood vessels that lie beneath the pigment epithelium and is responsible for the nourishment of the outer one-half of the retina.

Tapetum - a light reflecting structure seen in most domestic animals (exception pigs, llamas, and birds). It is located in the upper portion of choroid just behind the choriocapillaris. Its purpose is to reflect light back into the photoreceptors to improve vision in dim light. The color varies with the color coat of the patient.

1. Cellular tapetum seen in carnivores
    a. Dog - high in zinc cysteine
    b. Cat - high in riboflavin
    c. Fish - Guanine crystals
2. Fibrous tapetum - seen in ungulates

DISEASES OF THE OPTIC NERVE

CONGENITAL DISEASES - There are few true congenital lesions of the optic nerve only. Optic nerve lesions are usually secondary to retinal or scleral disease.

Optic nerve hypoplasia/aplasia (Fig 15-2) - The cause is unknown. Probably related to hypoplasia or prenatal atrophy of the ganglion cell layer of the retina. Can occur in all species.

1. Signs - noticed at birth in foals, at three to six weeks in dogs
    a. May be bilateral or unilateral
    b. Vision - may be visual or blind, depending on severity, with corresponding changes in the pupillary light reflex
    c. Ophthalmoscopic changes - the disk may be small or absent at necropsy, with corresponding changes in the optic nerve and chiasm

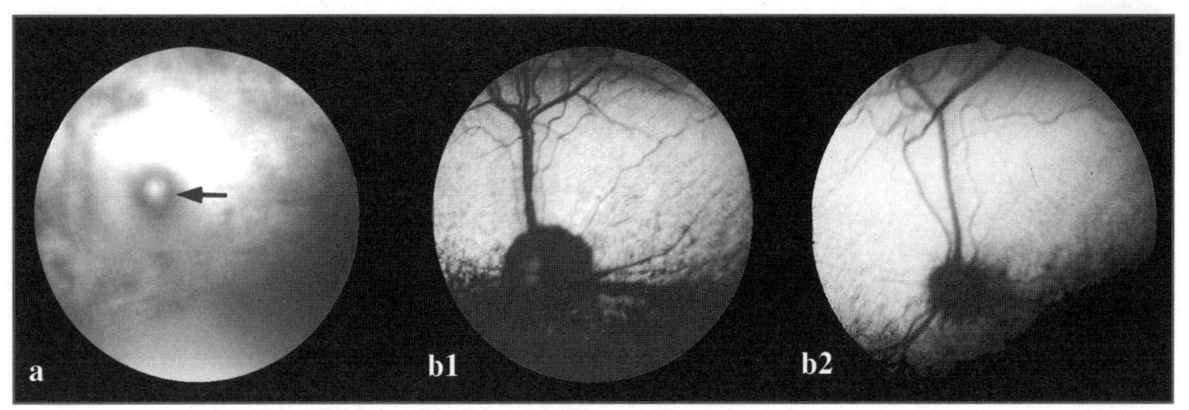

Figure 15-2. Optic nerve aplasia/hypoplasia.
a. Aplasia of optic nerve (arrow) and retina in a dog
b. Hypoplasia of optic nerve in a poodle
1) Right eye normal
2) Left eye hypoplastic optic nerve. Note reduced size of retinal vessels.

1) Hypoplasia - the optic disk will be small, with a normal-appearing fundus
2) Aplasia - the optic nerve will be absent and the retina avascular, dull, and sometimes retinal detachment

2. Differential diagnosis in dogs - Must be differentiated from normal dogs, with limited myelination of the optic disk (micropapilla) resulting in a small depressed disk that is often dark in color due to uveoscleral pigment. At necropsy the retrobulbar optic nerve is normal in micropapilla.
3. Incidence
   a. Dogs - hypoplasia/aplasia can be observed sporadically as a single entity but it is more frequently observed with microphthalmia
      1) Inheritance - has been proposed for the miniature poodle
      2) Breed predisposition - observed in beagle, cocker spaniel, miniature dachshund, Saint Bernard
   b. Cats - rare
   c. Equine - optic nerve hypoplasia and concurrent retinal dysplasia in Quarter Horses and Thoroughbreds (see page 438)
4. Treatment - none
5. Breeding recommendations - affected animals should not be bred

Coloboma - is a congenital fissure, pit or excavation. *Typical* optic nerve coloboma results from incomplete closure of the optic fissure and is restricted to the ventral portion of the optic disk. *Atypical* coloboma refers to a peripapillary or scleral coloboma.

1. Incidence
   a. Dogs
      1) Common - in collie eye anomaly; less frequently seen in Shetland sheepdog and border collie
      2) Basenjis - has been observed with persistent pupillary membrane; inherited
      3) Color-dilute dogs - occurs with multiple ocular defects
   b. Cats - infrequently seen
   c. Cattle
      a. Dominant inheritance in Charolais and albino Hereford
      b. May occur in animals with multiple ocular lesions
   d. Horses - uncommon; can occur with retinal dysplasia/optic nerve hypoplasia in Quarter Horses
2. Signs (Fig 15-3)
   a. Vision - not affected unless lesion is larger than the normal optic nerve. Large lesions will have a visual field deficit related to the size of the coloboma.
   b. Ophthalmoscopic appearance is variable, depending on the location and size of the lesion
      1) Optic disk colobomas - may involve only a small portion of the papilla to the entire papilla.

Small lesions are difficult to differentiate from normal variations in the physiologic cup and vascular pattern. When examining with direct ophthalmoscopy, the lesion is out of focus in relation to the rest of the fundus. Retinal blood vessels may be followed into the defect by examining with negative diopter lenses (approximately 3-D change for 1 mm change in depth). Indirect ophthalmoscopy will allow examination with the entire lesion in focus.

2) Peripapillary lesions may involve an area much larger than a normal optic disk and subsequently cause a significant defect in the visual field.

Close examination will often reveal the optic nerve at the bottom of the coloboma.

In young animals, the choroid will contact the rim of the coloboma. As the animal ages, choroidal blood vessels will retract from the rim, exposing a white avascular scleral border.

Retinal detachment may be observed at the rim of the coloboma and extend down into the coloboma. It is not unusual for the retina to reattach at the rim as the dog ages.

3) Scleral colobomas near the equator are seen in Australian shepherds and homozygote merles

3. Treatment - none
4. *Comment* - breeding is not recommended when seen in dogs and horses

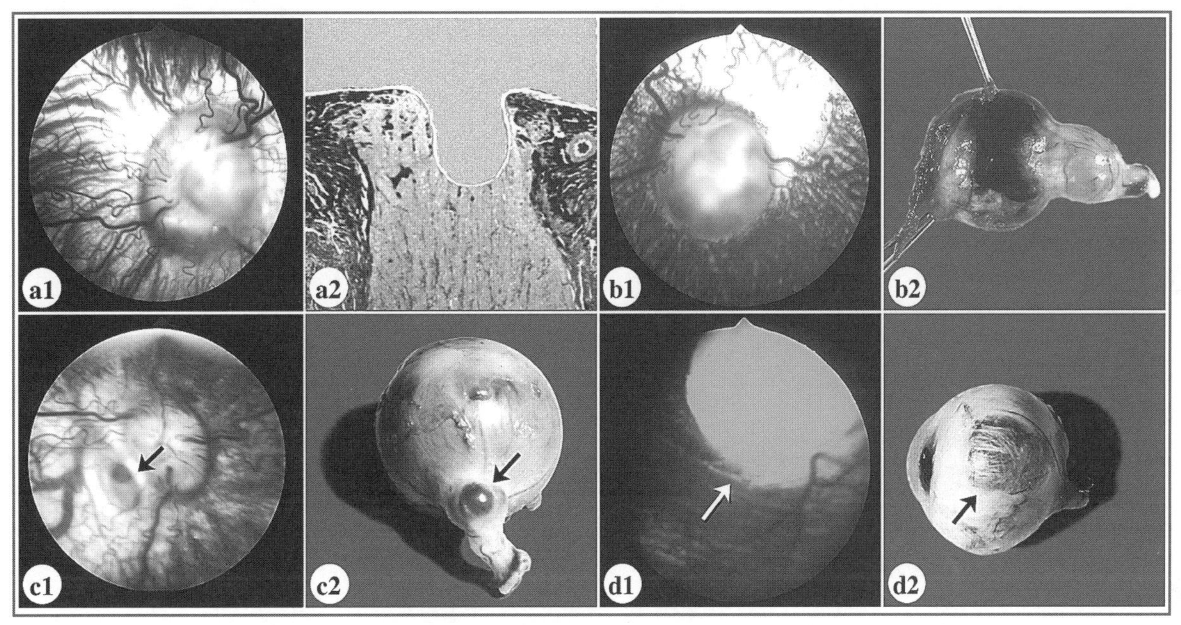

Figure 15-3. Variations in appearance of colobomas
- a. Optic nerve with small coloboma
  - 1) Ophthalmoscopic view
  - 2) Cross-section
- b. Large coloboma involving optic nerve and surrounding sclera
  - 1) Ophthalmoscopic view
  - 2) Lateral view
- c. Scleral coloboma adjacent to optic disc
  - 1) Ophthalmoscopic view
  - 2) Lateral view
- d. Scleral equatorial coloboma - Shetland sheep dog
  - 1) Ophthalmoscopic view
  - 2) Lateral view

ACQUIRED DISEASES

Optic neuritis (papillitis) - Occurs in all species and can be unilateral or bilateral, may be seen in association with retinitis, and causes blindness in the affected eye

1. Etiology - may occur as a primary ocular disease or in association with CNS and systemic diseases. Any disease that can cause retinitis may cause optic neuritis.
   a. Infections
      1) Systemic disease (also see retinitis, page 440) - Borna disease in horses, canine distemper in dogs.
      2) Localized infections - posterior episcleritis, postorbital abscesses or cellulitis, guttural pouch infection
   b. Toxic - ethyl and methyl alcohol, lead, arsenic, thallium and quinine, male fern ingestion in cattle
   c. Neoplasia - orbital neoplasia
   d. Granulomatous meningoencephalitis (GME)
   e. Traumatic - foreign body wounds, trauma to the orbital area (especially in horses) orbital hemorrhage
   f. Horses with severe acute blood loss, with or without blood transfusion, will sometimes develop acute bilateral exudative optic neuritis within 24 hours. Close examination of the fundus will invariably reveal inactive chorioretinitis lesions. The author believes this previous inflammation in some way presensitizes the eye to respond with a fulminating optic neuritis. Acute hemorrhage in 28 experimental horses with normal eyes did not cause any lesions.
   g. Unknown - this may be a hypersensitization reaction. Many animals fall into this unknown category.
2. Signs
   a. If bilateral involvement, dilated pupils, disturbed vision
   b. If unilateral involvement, loss of direct PLR, may not show any subjective signs
   c. If from orbital trauma or disease, the eye may appear normal except for optic neuritis
   d. May be incidental finding during routine ophthalmoscopic examination
   e. Ophthalmoscopic signs - (Fig 15-4) if only retrobulbar optic nerve is involved, the optic disk will appear normal
      1) Papillitis - The optic nerve will appear red and swollen. Many small congested blood vessels will be visible and small hemorrhages may be seen. The physiologic cup disappears when the optic nerve swells.
      2) Circumpapillary retinal edema - The blood vessels leaving the disk appear as if they are floating in space above the fundus.
      3) Circumpapillary retinal hemorrhage - Small blood clots may also be seen in the vitreous. This is most likely in horses.
      4) Exudates on and around optic disk that may extend into the adjacent vitreous

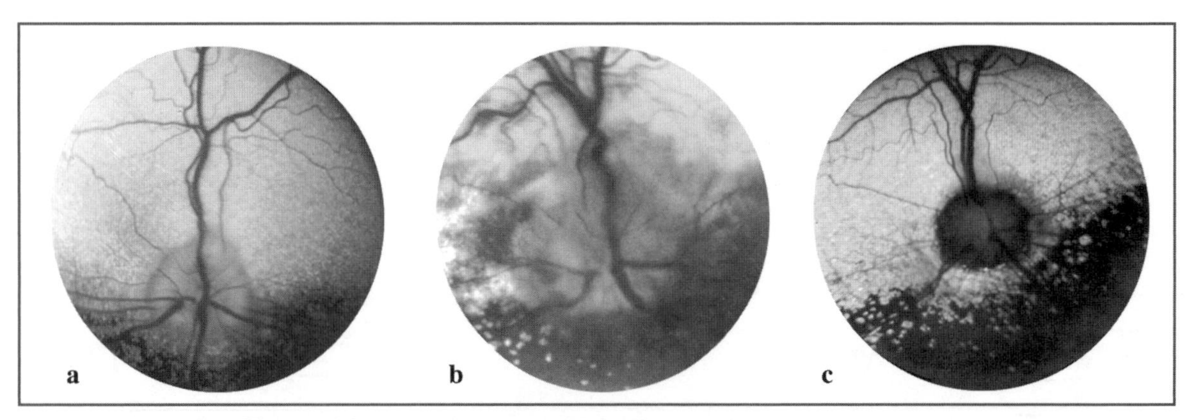

Figure 15-4. Unilateral optic neuritis leading to optic nerve atrophy
a. Normal right eye
b. Acute optic neuritis, left eye
c. Recheck four months later. Marked optic nerve atrophy with minimal attenuation of retinal blood vessels

3. Differential diagnosis
   a. Papilledema - does not cause blindness. The ophthalmic examination is normal except for swollen optic nerve.
   b. SARD - normal optic disk, retinal changes not compatible with the degree of blindness exhibited by the patient. If still in doubt, ERG (absent if SARD; normal if optic neuritis).
   c. Severe retinal disease - if severe enough $\pm$ cause blindness; marked ophthalmoscopic changes
   d. Cortical blindness - intact PLR, normal fundus
4. Treatment - specific treatment if cause is known. Symptomatic treatment immediately to restore vision (this can be risky with some infections).
   a. Small animals
      1) Acute cases will benefit from pulsed corticosteroid administration (Chapter 2, page 94). Less severe cases can be treated with systemic administration at anti-inflammatory levels with a gradually reducing dosage. If long term treatment is needed, aspirin or immunosuppressant drugs may be needed.
      2) Systemic antibiotics are indicated if bacterial or fungal infection is suspected
      3) GME patients respond best to high level dexamethasone. When the lesion has been controlled, radiation therapy is recommended to prevent recurrence.
   b. Equine
      1) Immediate - systemic Banamine, ketoprofen, Butazolidin or prednisolone with gradually reducing dosage
      2) Long term - aspirin
5. Course and prognosis
   a. If sight does not return to normal in two weeks, very unfavorable. The author has never seen an animal that was blind for one month regain its sight. The acute exudative optic neuritis seen in horses after acute hemorrhage is nonresponsive to treatment and should always be given an *unfavorable* prognosis.
   b. May become recurrent, requiring continuous anti-inflammatory or immunosuppressive therapy
6. Sequelae
   a. Optic nerve atrophy (Fig 15-4c)
   b. Circumpapillary scarring
   c. Exudative optic neuritis *might* be an initiating cause for some cases of proliferative optic neuropathy of horses

Papilledema - Papilledema (choked disk) is noninflammatory (passive) swelling of the optic disk that does not affect vision

1. Etiology
   a. Increased cerebrospinal fluid pressure
      1) Brain tumors - most common cause
      2) Hydrocephalus
   b. Space-occupying lesions of the orbit
   c. Hypertension and hyperviscosity syndromes
   d. Early vitamin A deficiency in cattle
2. Signs - bilateral indirect ophthalmoscopy is recommended
   a. Swelling of the optic disk
   b. Disappearance of the physiologic cup
   c. Peripapillary subretinal edema
   d. Blood vessels are congested and appear elevated over the disk and the area of peripapillary edema
   e. Occasionally small disk and peripapillary hemorrhages
3. Differential diagnosis
   a. Heavily myelinated optic disk (pseudopapilledema) - physiologic cup lacks edema or vascular congestion
   b. Optic neuritis - blind, marked inflammatory response
4. Treatment - correct the primary cause

Proliferative optic neuropathy in horses

1. White proliferations are observed on the optic nerve of horses. These are vascularized and have a cauliflower-like appearance. The remainder of the optic nerve appears normal. Vision is unaffected. The lesions are stationary. We observed one horse for 20 years without change.
2. The etiology is not known. Saunders and Rubin proposed that it is a storage disease similar to xanthelasma in man.
3. The lesion does not have clinical significance but the owner should be advised of it for sale or insurance purposes.

4. *Comment* - A cat was examined at CSU with a lesion that appeared the same ophthalmoscopically as the equine lesions just described. The eye was visual but pupillary and menace reflexes were diminished when compared to the normal eye. There was no history of previous ocular or systemic disease. No histopathology was available.

Optic nerve atrophy - Optic nerve atrophy is seen in all species and results in blindness of the affected eye. If unilateral, the animal may not show any definite signs. Horse owners may notice a change in temperament or the animal becoming skittish when approached from the blind side. If bilateral, the owner is aware when they become blind.

1. Causes
   a. After optic neuritis (especially equine recurrent uveitis)
   b. Post-traumatic
      1) Prolapsed eyes in dogs and cats may or may not develop atrophy, depending on how near the eye the optic nerve ruptures
      2) Severe trauma to the head and eye in horses may be followed by optic nerve atrophy. After rearing and severely striking their heads or falling over backward, horses may develop an immediate or delayed blindness. This injury may result in:
         a) Circulatory interference to the orbital portion of the optic nerve and peripapillary retina or,
         b) Direct damage to the orbital optic nerve due to a contrecoup effect.

         Immediately post-trauma the fundus and optic nerve may appear normal, except for small hemorrhages involving the disk. If injuries are reversible, the optic nerve will return to normal and vision remains normal. If the optic nerve is irreversibly damaged, the vascularity decreases in a few days and by 30 days the optic nerve is avascular and atrophied.

         Blindness can also result from brain hemorrhage involving the visual pathway or hemorrhage along the floor of the cranium damaging the cranial portion of the optic nerve. Cranial damage will not result in immediate optic nerve change. Optic nerve atrophy may develop as a latent change (6 months or more).
   c. Chronic exophthalmos from orbital deformity or space-occupying lesion (equine chronic frontal sinusitis causing orbital deformity)
   d. Idiopathic - no observable cause or history that would suggest the etiology. Middle-aged to old horses with subalbinotic eyes seem to be predisposed to atrophy.
2. Signs - The affected eye is blind and has lost its direct pupillary response. The ophthalmoscopic signs are (Fig 15-4c)
   a. Decrease in size of optic disk
   b. Disk becomes chalky white and granular in appearance
   c. In some animals myelination may disappear, revealing a dark lamina cribrosa
   d. Blood vessels
      1) Equine becomes totally avascular
      2) Other animals - retinal blood vessels are slightly decreased in size. If there is a concurrent retinal atrophy, retinal blood vessels may disappear.
3. Treatment - none

Cupping of the optic disk in chronic glaucoma (Fig 15-5)

1. Cupping of the optic disk is seen with prolonged increased intraocular pressure in cats and dogs. The disk appears deeper and flattened posteriorly as a result of optic nerve atrophy.
2. The optic disk in normal cats has a flattened appearance because of lack of myelination that should not be confused with glaucomatous cupping.

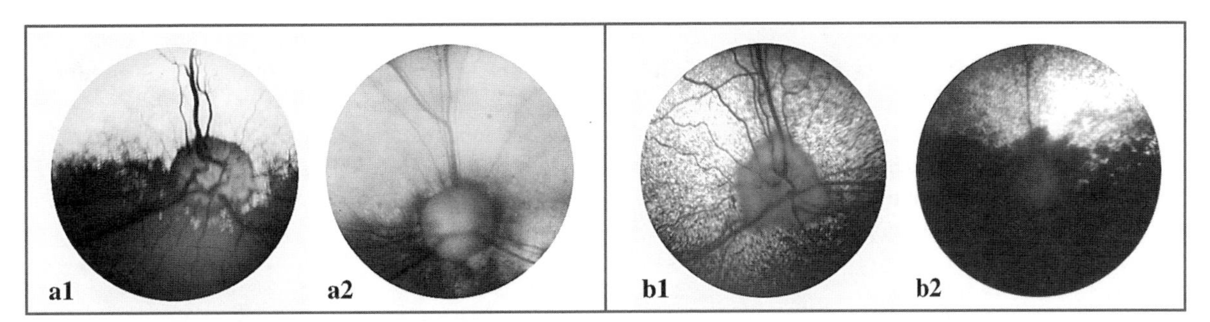

Figure 15-5. Cupping of the optic disc

a. Unilateral chronic glaucoma in a Chesapeake Bay retriever
   1) Normal eye
   2) Cupping optic nerve. Note blood vessels dropping down into the cupped disc. Slight corneal edema interferes with observing fundic detail. No hyperreflectivity.

b. Unilateral glaucoma with advanced changes
   1) Normal eye
   2) Glaucomatous eye, with advanced changes - severe optic nerve atrophy, fundus hyperreflective, and marked vascular attenuation

CONGENITAL AND INHERITED DISEASES OF THE RETINA OF DOGS

Congenital and inherited diseases of the retina are more common in dogs than other species. Some are present at birth (dysplasia, collie eye, retinal detachment), while others (degenerations) develop clinical and ophthalmoscopic signs later, often after maturity.

TERMS

Atrophy is a loss of tissue mass usually resulting from diminution and size of constituent cells. It is usually a reversible process.

Degeneration is a broad category more complex in that the tissue remains viable for a time but metabolism is disturbed. It is usually irreversible. Two categories of degeneration are:

- abiotrophy: premature loss of vitality after normal development
- dystrophy: degeneration before cells reach maturity

Dysplasia is abnormal embryonic development

Retinal dysplasia is abnormal differentiation of the layers of the retina and is characterized by the formation of folds and rosettes in its mild form and if severe, retinal detachment will be seen. It may occur as a single entity or with other ocular abnormalities.

CANINE RETINAL DYSPLASIA - Reported in 33 of the 114 breeds of dogs listed in the Guidelines Used By the ACVO Genetics Committee for Breeding Recommendations. See appendix IV, page 519

Etiology

1. Genetic - is the most common cause
   a. Simple autosomal suspected or proposed in:
      1) Akita - microphthalmia
      2) American cocker spaniel
      3) Australian shepherd - multiple ocular changes
      4) Bedlington terrier - vitreoretinal dysplasia
      5) Beagle
      6) Doberman pinscher - multiple ocular changes
      7) English springer spaniel
      8) Labrador retriever
      9) Rottweiler
      10) Old English sheepdog - microphthalmia
      11) Sealyham terrier - microphthalmia
      12) Yorkshire terrier - in Europe
   b. Oculoskeletal dysplasia - dominant autosomal gene proposed. Heterozygous animals have only ocular changes, which are usually mild. Homozygous have skeletal changes and mild to severe ocular changes. Retinal dysplasia is more commonly seen than oculoskeletal dysplasia.
      1) Labrador retriever
      2) Samoyed
   c. Means of inheritance not determined in many breeds (e.g. Borzoi, Brittany spaniel, English cocker spaniel, golden retriever, Gordon setter, Great Dane, and saluki)
2. Infection - systemic viral diseases, with "mitolytic" capability, occurring prenatally or neonatally while the retina is still developing
   a. Canine herpesvirus
   b. Canine parvovirus
   c. Possibly canine adenovirus
3. Other factors
   a. Irradiation

   b. Drugs - seen most frequently in drug trials, uncommon in clinical practice: antiherpes drugs, actinomycin D, methyloxymethanol, chlorambucil
   c. Intrauterine influences - fetal nutrition, trauma, hypoxia
4. *Comment* - Normal puppies may have transient retinal folds that disappear within a few weeks to several months. These folds probably represent varying growth in the inner and outer layers of the optic cup that is self-correcting. Observed most frequently in beagles, collies and Shetland sheepdogs.

Pathogenesis

1. Retinal dysplasia occurs in the developing retina *in utero* and/or *neonatally*, depending upon the species
   a. The retina is fully developed at birth in cattle and horses, therefore when seen, dysplasia results entirely from intrauterine influences
   b. The dog and the cat retina are immature at birth, therefore lesions can start *in utero* or postnatally until adult characteristics are present. The neonatal retina has adult architecture by 42 days and the tapetum is fully developed by four months
2. Theories as to the mechanism of development
   a. Faulty obliteration of the optic vesicle
   b. Imbalance in growth of scleral, choroidal and retinal layers
   c. Localized overgrowth of the outer nuclear layer of the retina
   d. Excessive growth of mesodermal layers of the eye
   e. Vitreoretinal developmental abnormalities

Signs

Lesions may be mild with multifocal retinal folds and normal vision or can be generalized with large areas of hyper-reflectivity, retinal detachment, and/or cataract, resulting in visual loss proportional to the severity of the lesions.

1. Ophthalmoscopic examination - fundus
   a. Dysplastic areas in tapetal fundus
      1) Small oval hyperreflective foci with or without central pigment
      2) Linear hyperreflective folds (streaks) that may be vermiform, V- or Y-shaped. The area where most lesions will be concentrated varies with breeds.
      3) Small to large hyperreflective lesions with or without infiltration of pigment resembling inactive areas of chorioretinitis
   b. Dysplastic areas in nontapetal fundus appear as gray to white folds
   c. Optic disk appears normal
   d. Blood vessels appear normal in size and number
2. Retinal detachment - may be partial to complete
   a. Perivascular cuffing involving arteries and veins near the optic disk. These are usually stationary lesions.
   b. Bullous detachments - usually stationary
   c. Total detachment resulting in leukokoria. Tears are common.
3. Concurrent lesions
   a. Cataract - several types have been observed
      1) Young puppies can have posterior Y suture cataracts characterized by a small “arrow tip” appearance. These may persist or disappear with age. They are not progressive.
      2) Cortical cataracts occur that are slowly progressive, leading to blindness
      3) Congenital nuclear cataracts - these usually regress with age but never disappear totally
   b. Microphthalmia - usually seen with severe changes
   c. Persistent hyperplastic primary vitreous
      1) When this is observed with dysplasia, severe lesions usually result. This is especially true when vascular remnants of PHPV exist.
      2) Persistent opaque hyaloid remnant is seen in some breeds without complications
   d. Vitreal hemorrhage
   e. Nystagmus may occur in puppies blind since birth

Breed characteristics

1. Bedlington terriers have a vitreoretinal dysplasia with leukokoria (due to retinal detachment), entropion, blindness, altered pupillary light reflexes, intraocular hemorrhage and slight microphthalmia
2. Sealyham and Yorkshire terriers may have similar signs as those reported in Bedlington terriers
3. Beagle - usually has mild lesions. Multifocal retinal folds in tapetal and nontapetal areas. Mildly affected animals will improve with age. No visual deficit.
4. American cocker spaniel - usually has mild lesions with folds in tapetal and nontapetal areas. When only a few lesions are present, they tend to occur in the peripheral tapetum. They may clinically disappear with age (3 to 5 years). No visual deficit in mild lesions.
5. English springer spaniel - majority have mild lesions with normal vision
   a. Mild - multifocal lesions predominantly in central tapetal area. May have mild perivascular cuffing of the blood vessels immediately dorsal to the optic disk. Small arrow-shaped cataracts at the tip of the posterior Y suture can occur in some animals. These cataracts may disappear with aging.
   b. Severe - larger "medallion" lesions, perivascular cuffing leading to bullous retinal separation near optic disk and central tapetum. Detachment is usually nonprogressive after three to four months of age. Therefore, total detachment with blindness is rare. Slowly progressive cortical cataracts may be seen.
   c. Persistent opaque hyaloid remnants are occasionally seen but are not complicated by PHPV.
6. Labrador retriever - signs vary with clinical form of the disease
   a. Early onset dysplasia - seen in puppies six to eight weeks of age. Severe lesions may be present resulting in visual problems that may be passed off by the owner as "clumsiness". Retinal detachment, cataract, intraocular hemorrhage, nystagmus and microphthalmos can occur.
   b. Multifocal retinal dysplasia - described in field trial Labrador retrievers. Characterized by small retinal folds with hyperreflectivity and pigment changes. Vision is not affected.
   c. Oculoskeletal dysplasia - visual problems may be initially passed off by the owner as "clumsiness"; limited lameness can occur before the owner is aware of skeletal abnormality
      1) Ocular changes - Severe retinal lesions are common. These are characterized by large hyperreflective lesions near the optic disk, retinal folds, and bullous or complete retinal detachment with tears. Cataracts, vitreous strands and persistent hyaloid remnants are common. Visual deficits will be determined by the extent of the lesions.
      2) Skeletal changes - The radius and ulna are most severely affected and, to a lesser extent, the tibia. This gives the front legs a shortened appearance. Lameness will be more severe in rapidly growing puppies. The forehead may have a shallow stop, with wide-set eyes and moderate exophthalmos.
7. Samoyed - ocular lesions are variable. Retinal folds, delayed retinal detachment, congenital cataracts and persistent hyaloid artery have been observed with some animals showing skeletal dysplasia.
8. Old English sheepdog - mild to moderate multifocal areas with large hyperreflective areas and nuclear cataracts. At birth, the cataracts affect the entire neonatal lens. As the animal grows, new lens fibers are normal, resulting in clear cortex. The nuclear cataract regresses and progressive visual improvement results.
9. Greyhound, Doberman pinscher and Airedale terrier - have PHPV with retinal dysplasia. These breeds have multiocular defects that may include microphthalmia, cataract, abnormal vascularization of the lens and other embryonal remnants of the primary vitreous, retinal detachment, and retinal dysplasia.

Treatment - none

Prognosis - depends on severity of the disease

Significance - do not breed affected dogs.

POSTINFLAMMATORY RETINAL DYSPLASIA DUE TO NEONATAL PARVOVIRUS IN DOGS

Pathogenesis - puppies infected with acute parvovirus while the retina and choroid are still developing. After the retina and choroid are structurally mature, they will not be affected by the virus.

Signs

1. Young dogs
    a. Tapetal areas can develop large hyperreflective lesions with choroidal pigment exposed centrally (medallion lesions), areas of generalized mottling and hyperreflectivity
    b. Some attenuation of retinal vascularization
    c. Nontapetal fundus may have moderate depigmentation, resulting in tigroid changes
    d. Optic nerve may appear pale, be poorly myelinated and resemble early optic nerve atrophy
    e. Retinal detachments - bullous or total
    f. Stationary cataracts - generally affecting posterior capsule and equator
2. As severely affected animals age, slow progressive changes can be observed. Retinal degeneration progresses, leading to night blindness and eventually poor bright light vision. The cataracts progress, making fundus examination difficult.

Treatment - none

RETINAL DEGENERATION

Retinal degeneration (retinopathy) leading to blindness is common in the dog. A problem in differential diagnosis exists when trying to differentiate inherited retinal degeneration from acquired retinal degeneration that may be postinflammatory, metabolic, nutritional, toxic, or a spontaneous aging change.

Generalized progressive retinal atrophy (GPRA)

1. Terminology - This is not atrophy, but degeneration, and therefore would be more correctly called progressive retinal degeneration.
2. General - Originally reported in the Gordon setter (1911). By 1988 PRA had been reported in 86 breeds, including mongrels. It includes a group of diseases with similar signs, therefore resulting in variability in age of onset and rate of progression, leading to three clinical groupings.
   a. Early onset, rapid progression
   b. Early onset, slow progression
   c. Late onset, slow progression
3. Pathophysiology - biochemical, morphologic and electroretinographic defects have been characterized in some breeds
   a. Irish setter and collie - increased cyclic guanosine 3',5' monophosphate (cGMP) is present due to lack of an enzyme activator
   b. Types of cell deficits
      1) Photoreceptor dysplasia
         a) rod-cone dysplasia type 1 (rcd-1) - Irish setter
         b) rod-cone dysplasia type 2 (rcd-2) - collie
         c) rod dysplasia - Norwegian elkhound
         d) early receptor degeneration - Norwegian elkhound
         e) photoreceptor dysplasia - miniature schnauzer
         f) cone degeneration - Alaskan malamute
      2) Later-onset photoreceptor degenerations
         a) progressive rod-cone degeneration - miniature and toy poodles, English and American cocker spaniels, Labrador retriever
         b) progressive retinal atrophy - Akita, Tibetan terrier, miniature longhaired dachshund, Samoyed
      3) Retinal pigment epithelial dystrophies
         a) retinal pigment epithelial dystrophy - Briard
         b) central progressive retinal atrophy - Labrador retriever, collie

4. Inheritance - It has been shown to be autosomal recessive in miniature and toy poodle, collie, cocker spaniel, Akita, Norwegian elkhound, Tibetan terrier and Irish setter. The recessive nature makes this disease extremely difficult to eliminate from affected blood lines, especially in breeds with late onset signs. The Siberian husky has an X chromosome-linked PRA. Therefore it is not recessive.
5. Clinical signs
   a. History
      1) Personality changes - reluctance to go outside at night or down a dark stairway
      2) Night blindness occurs early in the disease due to rod degeneration. Poor vision in reduced light. Dog appears nervous and moves cautiously under these conditions.
      3) As the pupil begins to dilate, the owner may notice increased tapetal reflectivity
      4) Owner may identify loss of peripheral vision
      5) Total blindness - owner may not be aware of this until dog is placed in unfamiliar surroundings
   b. Examination findings - *always a bilateral disease.* Early signs may be subtle and as the disease progresses signs become obvious.
      1) Ophthalmoscopic
         a) *Retinal blood vessels* - attenuated blood vessels, most apparent in arteries. Vessels become lighter in color and eventually lose essential reflexes. Blood vessels do not

extend as far toward periphery as in normal dogs. This change is most noticeable along dorsal limits of tapetum.

b) *Tapetal fundus* - increased tapetal reflectivity. The initial change may be very subtle. An early change may be irregular hyperreflectivity of the peripheral tapetum, characterized by parallel bands of hyperreflectivity that seem to appear and disappear with patient eye movement or slight movement of the viewing lens when performing indirect ophthalmoscopy. This change will be followed by generalized hyperreflectivity with possible change in tapetal color.

c) *Nontapetal fundus* - no changes early in the disease. As the disease progresses, close examination of the nontapetal area will reveal decreased pigmentation.

d) *Optic disk* - attenuated blood vessels. Small arteries become indistinct until only veins will be seen. In time the veins may disappear. The disk becomes white, losing the normal pink color. As the disease progresses, myelin retracts at the edge of the disk, developing a scalloped appearance.

e) *Advanced changes* - blood vessels nearly gone, they may appear as ghost vessels without blood. Highly reflective tapetum, appears more granular. Nontapetal area much lighter, with patches of dark pigment granules.

2) Pupillary light reflexes become delayed. The dog will be nearly or completely blind before they are completely abolished.

3) Vision tests - obstacle course and gradually reducing light. Any time we can see better than a dog in a darkened room, the dog has a problem. One must be sure to allow the dog time to dark adapt. Night blindness may be quite marked in a dog with normal pupillary light reflexes.

4) Bright light photophobia (dazzle reflex) disappears in advanced cases.

5) ERG - the best single means of early clinical diagnosis. Accurate when clinical signs are still questionable. Will be extinguished as the clinical signs become pronounced.

6) *Comment* - A combination of ophthalmoscopic examination, dark room obstacle course and ERG is the most accurate means of early diagnosis.

6. Age of onset of clinical signs varies with breeds and in some cases within a breed. Breeds more frequently involved are:

a. Early onset, rapidly progressive (onset to blindness < 1 year)

1) Collie - ERG reduced as early as 16 days. Earliest date for light microscopy diagnosis 42 days, ideally 49 days. Ophthalmoscopic diagnosis by 14 to 16 weeks. Some puppies are night blind by six weeks.

2) Irish setter - ERG has change by 24 days. Clinical onset between 3 to 12 months and usually blind before maturity. Latent PRA has been reported occurring at six to eight years. This is probably a rod-cone degeneration.

3) Cardigan corgi

b. Early onset, slowly progressive (onset < 1 year of age, blindness after 1 year)

1) Akita - ERG changes 4 to 18 months. Ophthalmoscopic changes 6 to 18 months. Earliest ophthalmoscopic changes are seen in animals with a horizontal bar. Night blind in one to three years, with blindness developing as early as two years in some dogs.

The author has seen one dog with ophthalmoscopic signs at 2.5 years that still had good vision at seven years, and a littermate that was totally blind at 3.5 years.

2) Miniature schnauzer - considerable variation

3) Norwegian elkhound - there are two distinct variations. Early onset, slowly progressive is the most common and was originally reported. More recently, early onset, rapidly progressive has been reported.

4) Tibetan terrier - ERG amplitudes reduced at 10 months, gone at 30 months. Night blind at 8 to 15 months. Delayed pupillary light reflexes by two years.

5) Dachshund

6) Gordon setter

c. Late onset, slowly progressive (onset after two years, usually blind by four years but some as late as six to eight years)

1) Afghan hound

2) Border collie
3) Cocker spaniel, American and English - American cocker spaniels have an earlier onset than English cocker spaniels
4) Chesapeake Bay retriever
5) English springer spaniel
6) Golden retriever
7) Irish terrier
8) Labrador retriever
9) Miniature and toy poodles - most common reported breed. Rod-cone degeneration. Onset for ophthalmoscopic changes three to five years. May not go blind until after six years. ERG changes in some dogs as early as 10 weeks, but others may not have change until one year.
10) Standard poodle
11) Saluki
12) Samoyed
13) Shetland sheepdog
14) Cross breeds - cross breeding cocker spaniels with miniature or toy poodles will result in affected offspring

7. Complications - Cataracts are seen concurrently in many poodles and less frequently in other breeds. If cataract development is minimal, ophthalmoscopic changes are adequate to determine the presence of GPRA. If cataracts are advanced and the pupillary light reflex is still normal, an ERG or determination of photophobia with a bright examining light is needed to determine retinal function.
8. Treatment - none
9. Prevention - selective breeding
   a. Do not breed animals that have not been examined
   b. Do not breed littermates or parents of affected dogs
   c. Avoid breeding dogs with a history of the disease in their backgrounds
   d. Test mating of normal-appearing animals with affected dogs will determine the status of suspected carriers. This is very beneficial in early onset, rapid development breeds, but expensive and time-consuming in late onset breeds.
   e. Irish setters - blood based DNA test. Irish setters suspected to have rod cone dysplasia PRA (rcd-1) can be identified as genetically normal, affected, and carrier dogs. The test is administered by canine DNA Registry which is affiliated with the Canine Eye Registry Foundation (CERF). Information concerning this test, including application forms and other data, can be obtained through the Canine DNA Registry (phone: 317-494-8179; FAX 317-494-9981) or by writing the Canine DNA Registry at 1235 SSC-A, Purdue University, West Lafayette, Indiana 47907-1235.

Central progressive retinal atrophy (CPRA, Retinal pigment epithelium dystrophy)

1. CPRA is a pigment epithelium dystrophy, beginning with hypertrophy and hyperplasia that eventually progresses to involve the visual retina
2. Incidence - not observed as frequently as PRA and occurs in older animals. More common in the United Kingdom than in the United States.
3. Breeds reported to be affected - border collie, rough collie, German shepherd (in Europe), golden retriever, Irish setter, keeshond, Labrador retriever, redbone coonhound, Shetland sheepdog
4. Inheritance - dominant, with variable penetrance has been proposed for Labrador retriever and Shetland sheepdog. Assumed to be same in other breeds.
5. Clinical signs
   a. History
      1) Good peripheral vision and can see moving objects
      2) Trouble with central vision, especially stationary objects in bright light
      3) As the disease progresses, vision decreases, but rarely does the dog go blind
   b. Examination findings - always bilateral
      1) Begins with small pigmented areas in the area centralis; these generally enlarge and increased reflectivity develops between them

2) As the lesion advances the pigment patches move peripherally and the area of central reflectivity enlarges
3) Late in the disease, blood vessels become smaller and optic disk may atrophy
4) Nontapetal area remains normal until disease is advanced, then becomes much lighter in color

c. Diagnostic tests
1) Obstacle course less effective because most still have peripheral vision
2) ERG no value early in the disease, but may change when disease is advanced
3) Fluorescein angiography will demonstrate defects in the retinal pigment epithelium

6. Differential diagnosis
a. Table 15-1 compares PRA and CPRA
b. Central progressive atrophy should not be confused with severe retinal dysplasia. If in doubt, re-examine later. CPRA is *progressive;* retinal dysplasia is *nonprogressive* and, in fact, may show slight improvement year to year

7. Treatment - none
8. Prevention - examine animals annually until five years of age. Do not breed animals that are affected or their progeny.

Table 15-1. Comparison of clinical features of progressive retinal degeneration. Modified from Slatter, Fundamentals of Veterinary Ophthalmology, WB Saunders Co., 1990.

	PRA	**CPRA**
Breeds affected	All breeds possible	Mostly working breeds
Visual defect	Poor night vision early; difficulty seeing moving objects; total blindness eventually	Early loss of central vision with temporary retention of peripheral vision; moving objects seen well; difficulty with stationary objects; good vision in dim light but day vision gradually lost; total blindness unusual
Direct pupillary reflex	Eventually lost	Some activity usually retained
Retinal vessels	Attenuated early	Normal until late in course
Tapetal fundus	Hyperreflectivity	Focal hyperpigmentation with some hyperreflectivity later
Optic disk	Pale as disease progresses	Normal until very late in course
Nontapetal fundus	Focal depigmentation and mottling later	No significant changes
Lens	Cataracts frequent later in disease	Cataracts rare
ERG	Useful in diagnosis	No use in diagnosis
Inheritance (if known)	Recessive	Dominant with incomplete penetrance

HEMERALOPIA - Hemeralopia is day blindness and results from cone degeneration beginning at birth and continuing until all cones disappear.

Breeds affected - Malamute and miniature poodle

Inheritance - Autosomal recessive in the malamute

Signs - Day blindness usually occurs soon after weaning (two months) but may or may not be detected until as late as six months of age. Animals have normal rod function, therefore normal reduced light and night vision.

Examination - ophthalmoscopically normal. Pupillary light reflexes are normal.

Diagnosis

1. Vision testing - vision improves in reduced light when dark adapted
2. ERG - dogs have scotopic (rod) response; no photopic (cone) response. Rod response is enhanced with blue light and the flicker fusion response ends at 20 Hz.

Treatment - none

Prevention - do not breed affected dogs

CONGENITAL STATIONARY NIGHT BLINDNESS IN THE BRIARD

This is a defect in essential fatty acid metabolism or absorption. The onset of night blindness is at about six months of age. The ERG is flat. A rapid vertical pendular nystagmus may be present. Ophthalmoscopic changes are linear depigmentations of the nontapetal fundus and slight tapetal hyperreflectivity. Plasma arachidonic acid levels are doubled. Systemic lipemia is present and histologically lipid inclusions are seen in the pigment epithelium.

COLLIE EYE ANOMALY (CEA, COLLIE ECTASIA SYNDROME, SCLERAL ECTASIA SYNDROME)

An inherited disease of the eye in collies, Shetland sheepdogs and border collies. The disease is characterized by abnormal development of the connective tissue tunic (sclera).

Breeds affected

1. Collies - very common in USA. Seen in > 80% of the collies in the CSU practice area.
2. Shetland sheepdog and border collie - seen in < 10% of the shelties in the CSU practice area

Inheritance - simple recessive

Signs

1. Clinical appearance of the eye
   a. Small eyes (microphthalmia) is common in many collies. Wyman had a collie eye research colony in which all dogs had normal-sized eyes. He feels microphthalmia is related to color-dilute changes and not part of CEA. Unfortunately, the collie standard emphasizes an "almond"-shaped eye, which in turn has resulted in selective breeding of small-eyed dogs. Dogs with microphthalmia will have a prominent third eyelid.
   b. Red fundus reflex - occurs with choroidal hypoplasia and vitreous hemorrhage. Some owners will use a penlight to screen sable and tricolor puppies for a prominent red fundus reflex.
2. Fundus changes - These have been subdivided into grades denoting degree of severity of the lesions. The only value of grades is to describe the lesion. ***The owner should be advised that any abnormal eye represents affected breeding stock.***
   a. *Grade I* - tortuous retinal blood vessels. The optic disk is often covered with an extensive network of blood vessels in addition to severe tortuosity seen in retinal vessels. This is a ***subjective*** diagnosis. If an eye is normal in all other respects, it would be advisable to recommend test breeding to determine if the dog is affected.
   b. *Grade II* - chorioretinal hypoplasia. This is the most common lesion observed. If mild, it appears as a pale pink area temporal and dorsal to the optic disk. The tapetum and retinal pigment are not developed, which allows choroidal blood vessels and sclera to be seen. Small lesions may fill in with age. When this happens, the eye will appear normal. Extensive lesions can affect a large portion of the fundus. Color-dilute animals (merles) may have similar decreased pigmentation and/or lack of tapetal development related to color genetics. This can be differentiated from primary choroidal hypoplasia by the choroid vascular pattern. Normal choroid blood vessels are evenly spaced and similar in size, with a parallel arrangement radiating from the optic disk. In collie eye, this vascular pattern is altered, resulting in fewer but larger blood vessels in a disorganized pattern. Color dilution may vary from mild depigmentation to an eye without visible pigment or tapetum.
   c. *Grade III* - coloboma. This may affect the optic disk or be located in the sclera near the disk. The size may vary from small excavations or pits to large colobomas affecting an area two to four times the size of a normal disk. Some animals with severe colobomas will have a clinical visual deficit because of the blind spot caused by the coloboma.
   d. *Grade IV* - retinal detachment. This is a secondary lesion and may be partial (bullous) or complete; unilateral or bilateral. The lesions are usually stationary. Unless animals have bilateral total detachment, the owner is unaware of a vision deficit. We had a collie as a teaching dog that at six weeks had a circumpapillary detachment in the right eye and total detachment in the left. At one year of age, the circumpapillary detachment reattached and the left eye never changed.
   e. *Grade V* - intraocular hemorrhage. This may occur into the vitreous from the retina or from the anterior uvea into the anterior chamber.
      1) Vitreous hemorrhage may lead to retinal detachment (if not already present)
      2) Hyphema is usually recurrent or constant, and warrants an unfavorable prognosis
   f. *Comment* - The eye is graded relative to the most severe lesion present. Most owners are aware that grades I and II do not affect vision and grades III, IV and V may affect vision.

g. Juvenile streaks (folds) are occasionally seen in collie puppies. They appear similar to the retinal folds of retinal dysplasia but disappear as the eye matures. They are believed to be nonpathologic retinal folds that smooth out as the eye grows. Occasionally they will be seen in other dogs that are examined before the eye matures. When seen, advise the owner the eye should be rechecked at six to eight months. If they disappear, the lesion was juvenile folds. If they persist, retinal dysplasia should be considered.

3. Other eye lesions may also be seen that indicate abnormal development, but are not part of collie eye anomaly.
   a. Corneal opacities (Seymour R. Roberts felt this was stromal fibroplasia)
   b. Persistent pupillary membrane
   c. Iris coloboma
   d. Cataract
   e. Persistent hyaloid remnant
   f. Distichiasis

OCULAR ABNORMALITIES ASSOCIATED WITH COLOR DILUTION - Multiple ocular abnormalities and deafness have been observed in color-dilute dogs

Inheritance and breed predisposition

1. Autosomal recessive
   a. Confirmed - Australian sheepdog, with incomplete penetrance
   b. Proposed - collie, Shetland sheepdog, Dalmatian, Great Dane
2. Means of transmission - associated with subalbinotic genetics
   a. Merle - Australian sheepdog, collie, Shetland sheepdog
   b. Harlequin - Great Dane
   Comment - A predominantly white haircoat as the result of subalbinotic genetics suggests a homozygous merle and increases the risk. In other breeds (poodle, Samoyed, etc) white haircoat does not signify a color-dilute animal and therefore does not predispose to ocular disease.

Signs - are bilateral and may be asymmetrical

1. General examination - changes may vary from moderate microphthalmia with a basically normal, sighted eye to a severely deformed, blind eye
   a. Eyelids - small palpebral fissure and prominent third eyelid
   b. Microphthalmia - varies from mild to gross deformity
   c. Cornea - small, irregular shape and may have opacities
   d. Iris - heterochromia (blue), corectopia, coloboma, aniridia, and/or hypoplasia
   e. Lens - cataracts. Most are slowly progressive.
   f. Leukokoria - due to detached retina
   g. Intraocular hemorrhage
2. Ophthalmoscopic examination - the smaller the eye, the greater the difficulty to examine. Pupils may be hard to dilate due to poor development of dilator muscle.
   a. Lens - cataracts tend to be predominantly cortical
   b. Hyaloid remnants - are frequently seen
   c. Detached retina
   d. Coloboma/staphyloma - equatorial are most common
   e. Retinal dysplasia
   f. Choroid hypoplasia

Diagnosis - based on breed predisposition and examination findings

Treatment - none

Breeding recommendations - affected dogs should not be bred

Prognosis - Animals with mild involvement make good pets. Some Australian shepherd breeders euthanize newborn puppies with more than 50% white haircoat because of the higher incidence of deafness and significant visual deficit.

CONGENITAL AND INHERITED DISEASES OF THE RETINA OF THE CAT

RETINAL DYSPLASIA

Etiology

1. Most common cause - infectious feline enteritis virus
   a. Prenatal exposure - Most queens that develop feline enteritis during pregnancy abort, but if they do not, cerebellar hypoplasia and/or retinal dysplasia may result.
   b. Neonatal exposure - Kittens that are infected before six weeks of age usually die; if they survive, retinal dysplasia will result.
2. All noninfectious causes listed for dogs should also be considered.

Signs

1. General examination
   a. Prenatal infection - during early pregnancy will result in cerebellar hypoplasia and retinal dysplasia. Later infection will result in retinal dysplasia only.
   b. Neonatal infection - Kittens that survive will frequently have malabsorption signs for several months and occasionally for life. This may result in slow growth, but these kittens have a good appetite and are active.
2. Ocular examination
   a. Multiple vermiform and spherical dysplastic lesions in the tapetal and nontapetal fundus. Tapetal lesions are most obvious. Small lesions fill in as the animal matures.
   b. Vision - usually no visual deficit

Treatment - none

Prevention - vaccinate queens before breeding

RETINAL DEGENERATION IN ABYSSINIAN CATS IN SWEDEN (NARFSTROM)

Incidence - reported to be 40% in three year olds during survey in Sweden

Inheritance - simple autosomal has been proposed; therefore, do not breed affected animals

Signs

1. Initial - ophthalmoscopic signs seen at 1.5 to 2 years of age. The tapetum develops grayish appearance, with attenuated blood vessels noticeable in the peripheral tapetum.
2. By three to four years there is tapetal hyperreflectivity, marked attenuation of blood vessels. This progresses to total loss of the blood vessels and depigmentation in the nontapetal fundus.

RETINAL DEGENERATION IN PERSIAN CATS (RUBIN AND LIPTON)

Incidence - reported in two litters of sibling Persian kittens

Inheritance - autosomal recessive proposed

Signs

1. Examination - beginning at 12 to 15 weeks of age
   a. Moderate mydriasis with nearly normal pupillary light reflexes
   b. Cautious movement in unfamiliar environment

   c. Increased tapetal reflectivity
   d. Decreased caliber of retinal blood vessels
   e. Optic disk paler and seems smaller
2. Begins with nyctalopia, proceeding to blindness
3. ERG is reduced early (15 weeks), absent later

Differential diagnosis - must be differentiated from generalized nutritional retinal degeneration. Age and history are important differentiating features.

Treatment - none

Prevention - do not breed affected animals

RETINAL DEGENERATION IN DOMESTIC SHORTHAIR CATS (WEST-HYDE AND BUYUKMIHCI)

Early onset retinal degeneration with blindness was described in a queen and her four kittens. When one of the kittens was bred by an unrelated tomcat, one of three kittens developed similar lesions.

Inheritance - suspected but not classified

Clinical signs in kittens

1. 3 weeks - dilated pupil and sluggish pupillary light reflex
2. 6 weeks - blind behavior and slight attenuation of blood vessels
3. 8 weeks - tapetum developed ground glass appearance and marked attenuation of blood vessels
4. 16 weeks - hyperreflective tapetum and severe attenuation retinal blood vessels

Special examinations

1. Vision impaired by six weeks and blind by four months
2. ERG - diminished at four weeks and extinguished by eight weeks

Pathogenesis - resembles rod-cone dysplasia seen in dogs

Differential diagnosis - must be differentiated from generalized nutritional retinal degeneration. Age and history are important differentiating features.

Treatment - none

Prevention - do not breed affected cats that have early onset (six weeks) retinal degeneration

CONGENITAL AND INHERITED DISEASES OF THE OPTIC NERVE AND RETINA OF HORSES

RETINAL DYSPLASIA/OPTIC NERVE HYPOPLASIA

The author has observed optic nerve hypoplasia and concurrent retinal dysplasia in Quarter Horses and Thoroughbreds.

Etiology - Inheritance is proposed

1. One group of affected Quarter Horses was inbred, with all affected animals related to one affected mare.
2. A normal Thoroughbred mare with an affected colt had another affected colt when rebred with the same stallion, but subsequently had three normal foals from different stallions.

Signs

1. Affected animals vary from diminished vision to total blindness
2. Pupillary light reflexes - delayed or absent
3. Microphthalmos - possible but uncommon
4. Ophthalmoscopic findings
    a. Predominantly blue to yellow tapetum and focal areas of hyperpigmentation
    b. Focal retinal detachments
    c. Optic nerve hypoplasia and/or coloboma

Treatment - none

Prevention - do not breed affected animals

CONGENITAL RETINAL DETACHMENT

Seen occasionally as a unilateral or bilateral, partial or total lesion. Severity will determine the effect on vision. If blind, nystagmus will be anticipated. Leukokoria and/or visual deficit may be noticed by the owner.

CONGENITAL STATIONARY NIGHT BLINDNESS (EQUINE NIGHT BLINDNESS)

Incidence - most common in Appaloosa

Inheritance - recessive proposed for Appaloosa

Signs - congenital and nonprogressive

1. Moderate to total night blindness (nyctalopia)
2. Severely affected animals may have bilateral dorsomedial strabismus and appear apprehensive in bright light conditions
3. Ophthalmoscopic examination - normal

Diagnosis

1. Subjective signs are quite diagnostic
2. Definitive diagnosis - ERG is characteristic with absence of the B wave (only a negative deflection)

Treatment - none

CONGENITAL AND INHERITED DISEASES OF THE OPTIC NERVE AND RETINA IN CATTLE

OPTIC NERVE COLOBOMA AND CHAROLAIS CATTLE

Inheritance - dominant with complete penetrance in bulls and incomplete penetrance in cows

Signs - typically bilateral

1. Usually a small coloboma on inferior optic disk
2. Severe lesions may involve entire optic disk with visual impairment

Treatment - none

Prevention - do not breed affected animals

MULTIPLE OCULAR CONGENITAL DEFECTS

Multiple ocular congenital defects can occur in purebred and mixed bred cattle. In some instances, inheritance has been determined. Some examples are listed below.

Shorthorn cattle - hydrocephalus ocular syndrome - Ocular changes usually cause blindness and consist of retinal dysplasia, optic nerve hypoplasia, microphthalmia and cataracts

Jersey cattle - Recessive proposed. Changes consist of large pupil, rudimentary iris and cataract.

Mixed breed - Brahman/Santa Gertrudis bred to a Hereford - Kaswan et al, 1989 described lesions including microphthalmos, cataracts, retinal detachment and dysplasia. Possible dominant characteristic.

PRENATAL BVD OCULAR CHANGES - Natural and experimental infection of fetuses with BVD virus have resulted in multiple ocular lesions that may cause limited vision or blindness. Signs vary depending on the stage of pregnancy where the fetus is exposed to the virus.

Exposure before 150 days gestation

1. Cerebellar hypoplasia
2. Generalized retinal dysplasia with large areas of hyperreflectivity and abnormal coloration in the tapetal area. The nontapetal fundus is depigmented with a mottled appearance.
3. Optic nerve hypoplasia
4. Retinal blood vessels are small and few in number
5. Cataracts range from small linear cortical opacities to diffuse cortical cataracts
6. Nystagmus and lateral strabismus is common in severely affected animals
7. The lesions are stationary and most animals have some vision

Exposure during the last trimester - Signs are milder and can be associated with complications of anterior uveitis

1. Corneal opacity
2. Synechia
3. Cataracts

Treatment - none

ACQUIRED DISEASES OF THE RETINA AND CHOROID

INFLAMMATORY DISEASES OF THE RETINA AND CHOROID - The retina and choroid are so closely related that inflammation of one will affect the other.

Chorioretinitis - primary choroidal lesion
Choroiditis - inflammation of the choroid
Retinitis - inflammation of the retina
Retinochoroiditis - primary retinal lesion. This is the most common lesion seen.

Etiology - the exact cause often goes undiagnosed. The causes listed for anterior uveitis should be considered.

1. Infections
    a. Viral - viral retinitis occurs in all species. The important recognized ones are:
        1) Dogs - canine distemper, parvovirus, herpesvirus
        2) Cats - feline panleukopenia virus, FIP, FeLV, FIV
        3) Cattle - BVD, rabies, MCF
    b. Bacterial - septicemia and extension from other tissues
        1) Dogs - brucellosis, tuberculosis
        2) Cats - tuberculosis
        3) Horses - leptospirosis, *Streptococcus equi, Actinobacillosis equuli, Actinomyces sp*
        4) Cattle - *Haemophilus somnus*, listeriosis, tuberculosis. They are one of the most susceptible species to septic emboli (scours, mastitis, navel ill)
    c. Rickettsia
        1) Dogs - ehrlichiosis, Rocky Mountain spotted fever
    d. Systemic fungi - any fungus can potentially occur in all species. They may affect the choroid initially and the retina secondarily. The inflammatory response may be granulomatous or nongranulomatous.
        1) Blastomycosis - most common in the dog
        2) Coccidioidomycosis - seen in southwestern USA; dog more frequently involved
        3) Cryptomycosis - most common in cats
        4) Histoplasmosis
    e. Protozoa - toxoplasmosis - seen in all species - most common in the cat
    f. Migrating parasites
        1) Dogs - migrating toxocara larvae, fly larvae (*Dioptera sp*)
        2) Cats - migrating fly larvae
        3) Horses - *Onchocerca cervicalis*
        4) Cattle - bot fly larvae
        5) Sheep, goats and wild ruminants - *Elaeophora schneideri*
    g. Algae - protothecosis in dogs
2. Trauma
    a. Blunt trauma - especially proptosis
    b. Surgery
    c. Foreign bodies
3. Immune-mediated disease
    a. Nonspecific immune-mediated reactions of unknown etiology are the most common cause of retinochoroiditis in dogs and horses
    b. Systemic immune-mediated disease - often affects anterior uvea simultaneously
        1) Immune-mediated thrombocytopenia
        2) Autoimmune hemolytic anemia
        3) Systemic lupus erythematosus
        4) VKH-like syndrome
        5) Gammopathies (hyperviscosity syndrome)
4. Primary vascular disease

a. Hypertension
   1) Renal disease
   2) Hyperthyroid
   3) Hypothyroidism
   4) Hyperparathyroidism
   5) Arteriosclerosis
   6) Adrenal neoplasia - hyperaldosteronism
   7) Primary (essential) hyperthyroidism
b. Chronic anemia in cats
c. Preretinal loops

5. Neoplasia - retinal and choroidal neoplasms usually stimulate a granulomatous inflammatory response
   a. Reticulosis (pseudotumor)
   b. Lymphosarcoma
   c. Metastatic tumors
   d. Choroidal melanoma

Presenting signs

1. Blindness will not usually be present unless both eyes are severely involved
2. The eye should be examined thoroughly when a patient has a systemic disease that may cause chorioretinitis or retinochoroiditis

Ophthalmoscopic findings - are nonspecific in relation to cause. They vary, depending on the stage of the disease when the patient is examined. Inactive lesions with or without clinical signs are more frequently seen than active lesions.

1. Active inflammation
   a. Retinal edema - dull-appearing areas that are easiest to see in tapetal area. Distinct lines of demarcation may be seen. The fluid may develop subretinal bullae, predisposing to retinal detachment.

      In cats, retinal vasculitis may cause edema to develop along small capillaries that will be seen as a reticular pattern in the retina. These lines may be hyperreflective or light-absorbing, depending on how the examining light strikes them. This is seen in acute retinitis from FIP, but can also occur with other infections.
   b. Exudate - inflammatory elements may appear as gray or white areas, seen most easily in the non-tapetal area. Exudate may organize as focal granulomatous elevations in the retina or escape into adjacent vitreous.
   c. Vascular changes
      1) Blood vessels may appear congested, with red-tinged transudate surrounding them
      2) Active perivascular cuffing (sheathing) occurs, resulting in a white appearance and less distinct vessel margins. Sheathing may be followed by sclerosis.
      3) Retinal hemorrhages vary in appearance, depending on location (Fig 15-6)
         a) *Preretinal* - blood trapped between internal limiting membrane and vitreous gravitates and gives a "keel boat" shape (Fig 15-7)
         b) *Intraretinal* - if superficial in nerve fiber layer, has a "flame" (brush) appearance (Fig 15-8); if deep, develops a dot appearance (Fig 15-9)
         c) *Subretinal* - is between the sensory retina and the pigment epithelium elevating the retina (Fig 15-10)
         d) *Intrachoroidal* - appearance will vary between tapetal or nontapetal areas. Retinal features are not changed (Fig 15-11)
      4) Elevation of retinal blood vessels - may result from:
         a) Detachment; subretinal masses in choroid
         b) Subretinal mass in choroid or sclera
         c) Extraocular mass collapsing the globe
      5) Size of blood vessels - enlarged with papilledema, hypertension, hyperviscosity

6) Color
   a) Increased - hypertension, polycythemia, hyperviscosity
   b) Decreased - anemia, atrophy
   c) Pink (lipemia retinalis) - increased serum lipid

d. Serous retinal detachment - occurs if edema becomes excessive

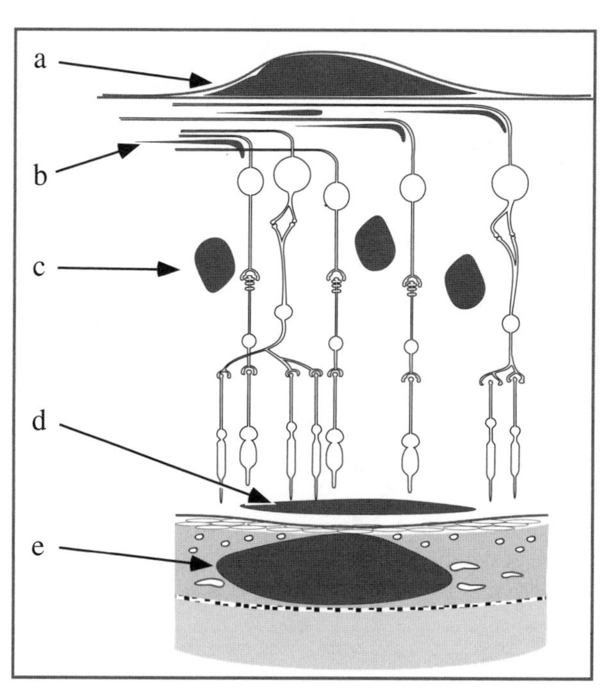

Figure 15-6. Posterior segment hemorrhages vary in appearance according to their location. Small hemorrhages are usually in the retina.
a. Preretinal hemorrhage between outer limiting membrane and vitreous
b. Nerve fiber layer - flame appearance
c. Midretinal - small and round
d. Subretinal between rod-cone layer and pigment epithelium - leads to retinal detachment
e. Choroidal - may be large, retina appears normal

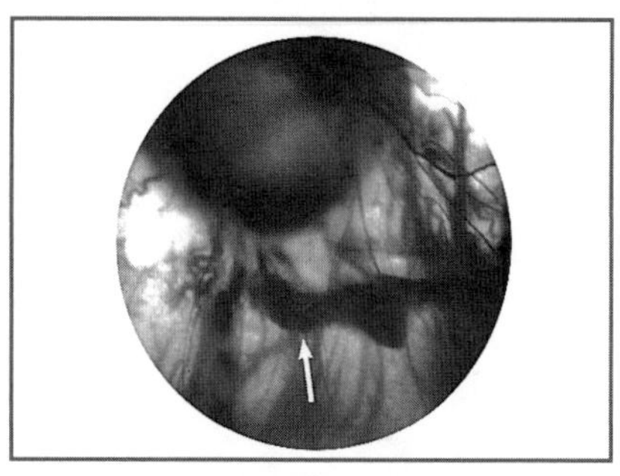

Figure 15-7. Collie with coloboma and preretinal hemorrhage. Note "keel boat" appearance (arrow).

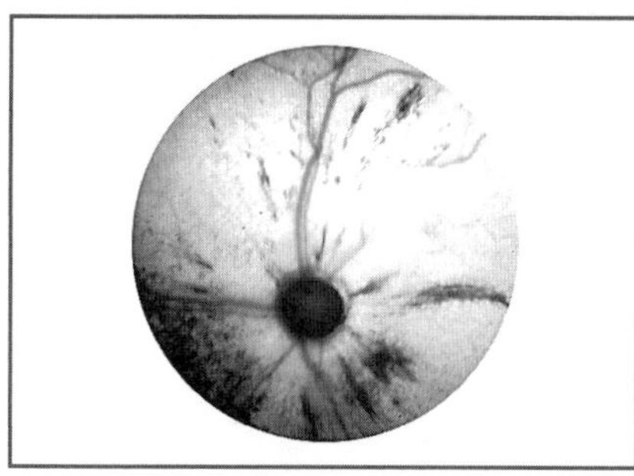

Figure 15-8. Cat with anemia and flame hemorrhage in nerve fiber layer.

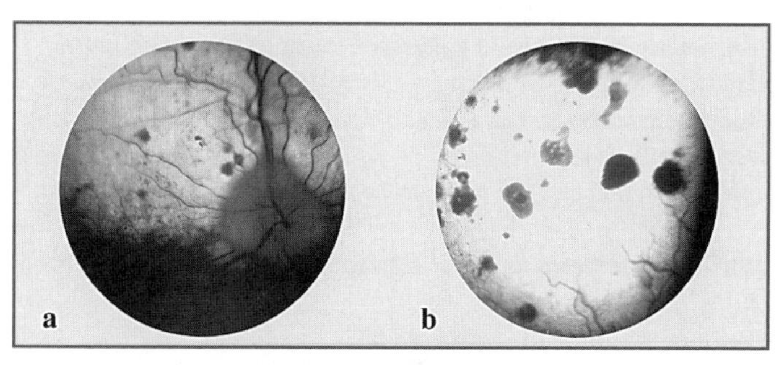

Figure 15-9. Midretinal hemorrhages.
a. Dog with postradiation retinopathy and small hemorrhages
b. Dog with hyperviscosity syndrome due to multiple myeloma

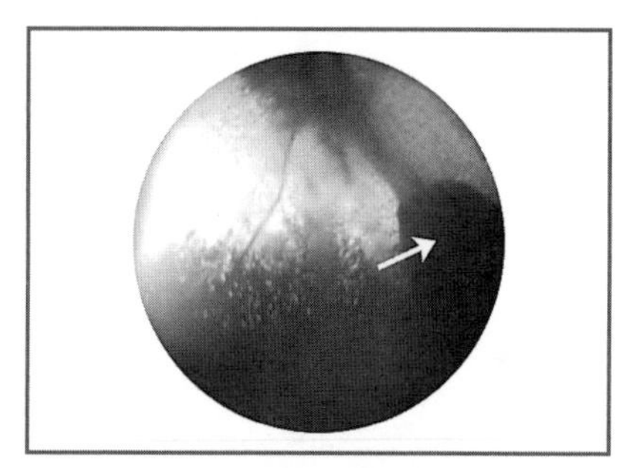

Figure 15-10. Cat with orbital abscess and post-traumatic subretinal hemorrhage. Retinal detachment is visible over the hemorrhage (arrow).

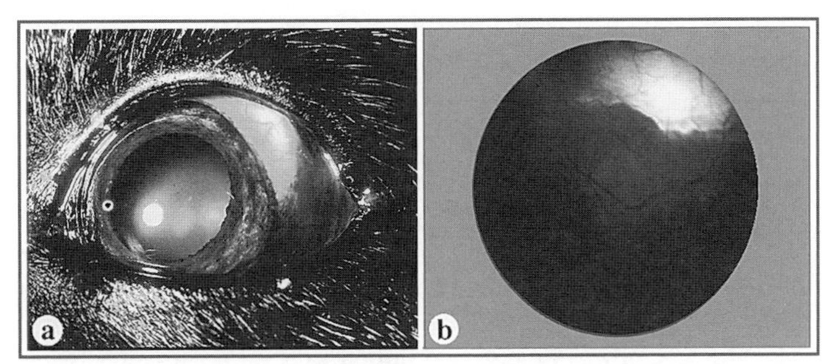

Figure 15-11. Dog with post-traumatic choroidal and episcleral hemorrhage.
a. Appearance of episcleral hemorrhage
b. Choroidal hemorrhage. Retina intact.

Appearance after one to two weeks

1. Edema and exudates - may absorb or persist
   a. If absorbed, the retina will be smooth, but small white or gray areas of debris may still remain. In some cases, linear folds and irregular opacities will be seen. This is most prominent in the non-tapetal fundus.
   b. If the edema has persisted, retinal detachment may be present. This can lead to static detachment, with the formation of folds, or a progressive detachment eventually leading to total detachment.
2. Blood vessels may have returned to normal size. If severe, there may be generalized permanent damage leading to attenuation of the blood vessels.
3. Hemorrhages are usually regressing. If primary vascular disease, new hemorrhages appear as old ones regress.
4. Hyperreflective areas will develop where retinal damage occurred. This is due to thinning of the retina. These lesions become more prominent in time, leading to scars typical of inactive lesions.

Inactive lesions (retinopathy)

1. Tapetal area
   a. Increased reflectivity due to retinal atrophy in the area of the lesion
   b. Migration of pigment epithelium as a healing change may result in an increase of pigment around the periphery of the lesion
   c. Tapetal color of the lesion may change, giving sharply contrasting colors in and around the lesion
   d. As the tapetum degenerates, choroidal pigment will be seen in the center of the lesion
2. Nontapetal area - pale depigmented areas develop, with irregular patches of pigment epithelium hyperplasia, resulting in a mottled appearance
3. Blood vessels - the lesion is less vascular. Blood vessels crossing hyperreflective lesions appear smaller as a result of hyperreflectivity
4. *Comment* - healed scars are a common incidental finding in the ophthalmoscopic examination of apparently normal animals
   a. Dogs - lesions are most noticeable in the tapetal fundus. Prior to the advent of MLV distemper vaccine, most hyperreflective retinal lesions were sequelae to canine distemper and referred to as "medallion" lesions because of their distinct dark border and hyperreflective tapetum
   b. Cats - small postinflammatory lesions are less common than in dogs. Temporal tapetum is affected more frequently than nasal
   c. Horses examined at CSU - circumpapillary scars are present in many horses eight years or older. Small scars are of no significance. Large scars may cause some vision loss. Concurrent optic nerve atrophy will result in visual deficit.
   d. Cattle
      1) Generalized scars may be present from prenatal BVD
      2) Focal scars can occur and tend to locate along the area centralis, similar to the location for scars in cats with central retinal atrophy

Differential diagnosis - It is important to establish the etiology, therefore a good clinical workup is essential, combined with screening tests for systemic diseases common to the geographic area and appropriate for the age of the patient.

1. Vitreous centesis for cytology, culture and/or serology is recommended for severely involved eyes
2. Immune panel

Treatment of acute retinitis/chorioretinitis - Systemic medications are essential

1. Specific treatment - identify the primary cause and initiate specific treatment. If infection is suspected, systemic antibiotics should be given until the cause is determined.
2. Symptomatic treatment
   a. Systemic anti-inflammatory medications
      1) Initial treatment - the author prefers prednisolone at anti-inflammatory levels, 0.5 mg/lb BID, then reducing dosage according to the response to treatment
      2) Long-term treatment (if needed) - change to aspirin to avoid secondary problems from long term corticosteroid therapy
   b. Immunosuppressives are indicated for long term therapy in immune-mediated diseases. Imuran (azathioprine) is very beneficial.
   c. Diuretics - for retinal edema or retinal detachment. The benefit is controversial. The author feels diuretics are beneficial for edema and early detachment but of little or no value after a retina has been detached one week.
3. Eye removal may be the most appropriate treatment for uncontrolled panophthalmitis or neoplasia

Granulomatous retinitis/chorioretinitis - Granulomatous chorioretinitis generally warrants an unfavorable prognosis because of the serious nature of the etiologies. Most are chronic lesions.

1. Mycotic - histoplasmosis, cryptococcosis, blastomycosis
2. Toxoplasmosis
3. Neoplastic diseases

ACQUIRED NONINFLAMMATORY RETINAL DISEASES

This includes a group of retinopathies with varied causes and significance. The lesions may be stationary or progressive, and focal without a visual deficit or generalized, leading to blindness. The most common diseases are taurine deficiency in cats, sudden acquired retinal degeneration in dogs, and vitamin A deficiency in cattle.

ETIOLOGY - The following is a partial list of nutritional, toxic and metabolic storage diseases that have been associated with retinopathy

Nutritional deficiencies

1. Taurine - cats
2. Thiamine - cats
3. Vitamin A - cattle and pigs
4. Vitamin E - dogs

Toxic

1. Drug administration
   a. Ketamine and/or methylnitrosourea (cats, rabbits)
   b. Hexachlorophene (sheep, cattle)
   c. High oxygen concentration (kittens, dogs)
   d. Rafoxanide (sheep, dogs)
   e. Ivermectin (dogs - especially collies and related breeds)
   f. Others - zinc chelating agents, chloroquine, diaminodiphenozyalkanes, ethambutol
2. Plant toxicity
   a. Locoweed poisoning (horses and cattle)
   b. Bracken fern (bright blindness disease in sheep)

Metabolic diseases with secondary retinal changes

1. Dogs
   a. Global cell leukodystrophy (Krabbe's disease) - beagle, cairn terrier, West Highland white terrier, blue tick hound
   b. GM_2 gangliosidosis - German shorthaired pointer
   c. Neuronal ceroid lipofuchsinosis (Kuf's disease) - Chihuahua, English setter, Australian blue heeler, border collie, saluki, and Tibetan terrier
2. Cats
   a. Mucopolysaccharidosis - Siamese
   b. GM_1 and GM_2 gangliosidosis - Siamese, domestic shorthair
   c. Mannosidosis - Persian and domestic shorthair cats

TAURINE DEFICIENCY IN CATS - Taurine deficiency in cats can cause central and generalized retinal degeneration. The generalized form cannot clinically be differentiated from inherited progressive retinal atrophy.

Etiology - Taurine was not identified as a dietary requirement in cats until 1975 and a minimal daily requirement was not recommended until 1981. The taurine available for retinal metabolism is dependent on several factors:

1. The amount available in the diet
   a. Dry dog food has little, if any, taurine
   b. Commercial cat foods now have added taurine, but dry foods historically had marked variation in the amount
   c. Fish and meat are high in taurine
2. Availability for intestinal absorption is reduced by high fiber diets
3. Tissue storage - liver and retina. Kittens have minimal storage compared to adults and therefore are more subject to dietary variations.
4. General health and appetite - sick animals appear to have greater susceptibility to developing ocular lesions
5. Bile acid conjugation - taurine is used exclusively for conjugation in cats. Other animals can switch to glycine conjugation.

Incidence - higher in neutered cats and Siamese

Clinical signs

1. Central retinal degeneration
   a. Vision - no visual deficit with small lesions. If lesions are extensive, night blindness occurs
   b. Ophthalmoscopic - Aguirre proposed five stages from an incipient lesion to generalized retinal degeneration. The lesions are characterized by hyperreflectivity (Fig 15-12).
      Stage I: Initial changes - slight granularity and beginning hyperreflectivity in the area centralis
      Stage II: Focal hyperreflectivity in the area centralis. This can be round or ellipsoidal
      Stage III: Ellipsoidal lesion in area centralis and a second, usually smaller, hyperreflective lesion nasal to the optic disk. If degenerative lesions are not extensive, blood vessels will appear normal in size, except over the hyperreflective lesions
      Stage IV: Single lesions extending across the tapetum and parallel to the tapetal/nontapetal junction. This may be a narrow band, in which case the retinal blood vessels are still normal in size. If the lesion involves a large portion of the tapetum, a generalized attenuation of the tapetal retinal blood vessels will be seen and the pupillary light reflex is delayed.
   c. Pupillary reflexes - normal in Stages I-III; may be delayed in Stage IV

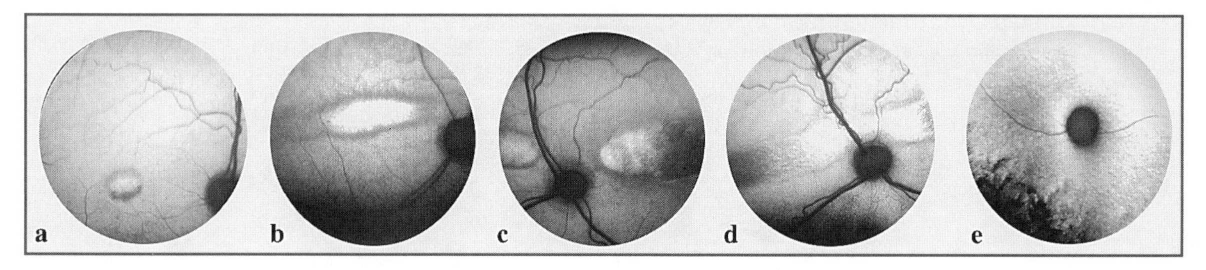

Figure 15-12. Feline taurine deficiency central retinal atrophy.
a. Beginning lesion in area centralis
b. Ellipsoidal lesion in area centralis
c. Ellipsoidal lesions both sides of optic nerve
d. Single lesion extending across the tapetum
e. Generalized retinal degeneration with marked vascular attenuation. Only two small retinal veins are present. Cat was presented blind. Diet was dry dog food.

2. Generalized retinal degeneration (Aguirre Stage V)
    a. Vision - visual deficit begins with nyctalopia and progresses to total blindness
    b. Pupillary light reflex - diminished early, fixed dilation later. Pupils dilated under normal light.
    c. Ophthalmoscopic - generalized tapetal hyperreflectivity. Early in the disease retinal blood vessels are attenuated and in advanced cases are nearly nonexistent.
    d. ERG - absent
3. *Comment* - The author feels central lesions are the result of subacute or recurring deficiency, whereas generalized degeneration (Stage V) occurs as an acute generalized retinopathy associated with acute taurine deficiency.

Diagnosis - clinical signs and diet history

Treatment

1. Correct the diet
2. Supplement taurine if the animal has active deficiency (tablets or 1/8 teaspoon of taurine powder daily)

Prognosis

1. Depends on stage of the disease
2. Favorable for central
3. Guarded to unfavorable for generalized. Some with acute blindness may regain day vision if taurine replacement is started soon enough.

VITAMIN E DEFICIENCY RETINOPATHY - has been produced in pups fed a diet deficient in vitamin E. Lesions begin to develop three months after weaning and by four months the pups were blind. The fundus became mottled and developed hyperreflectivity.

VITAMIN A DEFICIENCY IN CATTLE - Young animals develop signs more rapidly and severely.

Maternal vitamin A deficiency - Calves born from cows with vitamin A deficiency may be congenitally blind as a result of optic nerve atrophy (hypoplasia).

Cattle less than two years - The younger the animal the more rapidly signs develop

1. Incidence - Steers more predisposed than heifers. Heifers apparently can produce vitamin A by *in vitro* biosynthesis of beta carotene and enzymatic conversion to vitamin A by the corpus luteum.
2. Ocular changes
   a. Night blindness develops first, followed by total blindness if the deficiency is not corrected
   b. Pupillary light reflex - delayed or absent if blind
   c. May have corneal edema and/or exophthalmos
   d. Papilledema - the first objective sign. The disk will appear enlarged and elevated. Small hemorrhages will be present on or adjacent to the disk. Longstanding cases may develop atrophy. Papilledema is thought to result from two changes:
      1) Thickening of the dura mater which in turn results in an increase in CSF pressure
      2) Altered development of the sphenoid bone with subsequent narrowing of the optic foramen and compression of the nerve
   e. Retinal changes include preretinal and flame hemorrhages, extensive depigmentation of nontapetal area, and in the tapetal area focal orange hyperreflective areas
3. Systemic changes - Vary with severity of deficiency and may include seizures, ataxia, unthrifty animals, diarrhea and pneumonia

Cattle over two years - Signs are much milder

1. Night blind
2. Papilledema without nerve constriction
3. Fundus changes - tapetal color changes and mottling nontapetal pigment
4. Systemic changes same as seen in young animals

Diagnosis

1. Signs
2. Vitamin A levels - plasma below 20 µg/dl; liver 2 µg/gm

Treatment - if blind, not reversible

1. Vitamin A - 440 IU/kg IM or PO
2. Correct and supplement diet

SUDDEN ACQUIRED RETINAL DEGENERATION (SARD)

This may be one disease or possibly several specific aging retinopathies.

Synonyms - silent retina syndrome, metabolic toxic retinopathy

Incidence

1. Older dogs - 6 to 14 years, average age 10 years
2. Breed predisposition - none
3. Sex - females more frequently seen

Etiology - unknown. Several theories have been proposed but no consistent finding has been identified.

Most animals are in good health but many have the complaint of polyphagia, weight gain, polyuria, and polydipsia. However, this may be nothing more than a stress reaction to sudden blindness.

1. Cushing's disease
2. Immune-mediated
3. Neurotoxic reaction

History

1. Sudden onset - 24 hours to several days. After being questioned, many owners believe the dog may have had trouble several days before they realized it was totally blind.
2. Nyctalopia may precede total blindness

Examination findings

1. Pupils dilated but will respond to bright light
2. Dazzle reflex - absent
3. Fundus examination
   a. Normal at onset; after several days may have subtle hyperreflective changes
   b. After 30 days - signs of generalized degeneration are more obvious, but the changes seen are insufficient to account for the degree of blindness
   c. Advanced cases will appear similar to generalized progressive retinal degeneration
4. ERG - absent

Treatment - none

Comment - Sudden blindness disorients older dogs more than young ones, but given time, most old dogs will usually become well adjusted pets.

RETINAL DETACHMENT

Retinal detachment can occur from several causes. It is common and will cause clinical signs only if bilateral.

Causes - are multiple

1. Congenital
   a. Collie eye anomaly
   b. Prenatal intraocular infections resulting in abnormal eye development
   c. Retinal dysplasia in dogs
   d. Spontaneous - seen occasionally in foals
2. Acquired - any of the inflammatory causes listed earlier for inflammatory retinitis. The most common are:
   a. Trauma - severe blows resulting in tears and/or dissecting hemorrhage
   b. Vascular disorders leading to edema or hemorrhage
   c. Hypertension with or without retinal disease
   d. Infectious chorioretinitis
   e. Immune-mediated retinochoroiditis - this is probably the most frequent cause for sudden onset retinal detachment in dogs. Concurrent anterior uveitis may also be present.
   f. Traction on the retina from:
      1) Loss of vitreous during surgery, especially in horses
      2) Contraction of inflammatory membranes or hemorrhages in the vitreous
   g. Spontaneous - some adult animals develop bilateral detachment without any observed cause

Signs

1. History
   a. If complete
      1) If pupil is dilated, owner may notice the pupil has a white or gray appearance (leukokoria)
      2) Bilateral detachment will cause blindness
   b. If incomplete - generally no signs observed by the owner
2. Examination findings
   a. Pupillary reflexes
      1) Usually normal, unless patient has concurrent optic neuritis
      2) Reflexes disappear only when the detached retina undergoes degeneration. A CSU cat, used for teaching students, that has complete bilateral postinflammatory detachment still has good reflexes after 10 years. Horses develop retinal degeneration faster than other species.
      3) If there is concurrent optic neuritis, the pupils will be dilated and fixed.
   b. Pupils are dilated with Mydriacyl (tropicamide 1%)
   c. Examination with a transilluminator and loupe (Optivisor)
      1) Total detachment with syneresis of the vitreous - The retina is seen as a white membrane floating behind the lens. Blood vessels appear dark. Exudate, hemorrhage and adhesions may be seen. The retina may touch the peripheral portions of the lens and centrally present a "cone" appearance where it is anchored to the optic disk.
      2) Incomplete detachment - If the retina is in its approximate normal position, nothing abnormal will be seen with a transilluminator.
   d. Direct ophthalmoscopic examination
      1) Examination at two inches working distance is difficult because retina near the lens is seen clearly at +10 and +12 diopters while retina in a nearly normal position is seen best at 0 to -3 diopters.

2) A good way to examine this eye is to set the ophthalmoscope at 0 diopters and begin the examination 16 to 18 inches from the patient. Retina near the lens is clearly visible at this distance. One then moves progressively closer to the patient. This moves the focal point of the eye progressively deeper, until the optic nerve is seen when the examiner is two to three inches from the patient. This procedure gives a continuous view from the lens to the optic disk without changing the lenses in the ophthalmoscope.

3) Incomplete detachment with bullae formation - Detached areas will lack detail. Positive diopter lenses will permit clear focus of blood vessels in the detached area. These vessels lose their essential reflex and are much darker. Detached retina loses transparency, giving it a cloudy appearance.

e. Indirect ophthalmoscope examination - This is the best method to evaluate detachment. The entire area from the lens to the fundus is clearly seen.

Treatment - Success of treatment varies as to the cause and duration of the detachment.

1. Congenital detachment - usually stationary when presented. Treatment is not advisable.
2. Traumatic detachment - generally associated with hemorrhage and nonresponsive to treatment
3. Bullous detachment in a noninflamed eye - usually stationary, but if the owner wishes, reattachment with laser technique has been successful
4. Serous detachment with active inflammation - treat as soon as possible. Most of these are nonspecific immune-mediated diseases with or without anterior uveitis
   a. If a specific cause can be identified, systemic treatment is started for the primary disease
   b. Symptomatic treatment
      1) Anti-inflammatory - systemic prednisolone at anti-inflammatory level (0.5 mg/lb BID) for seven days; reduce as case improves
      2) Diuretics - this may or may not help, but cannot do any harm. I feel it helps.
      3) If concurrent anterior uveitis - topical treatment with atropine and 1% prednisolone acetate
   c. *Comment* - We have had about 50% reattachment and return of vision, if treated within five days of onset of blindness. Retinal atrophy may occur later but further detachment is not likely. If reattachment is going to occur, it will begin within the first week. If there is no improvement in two weeks, the prognosis is unfavorable. Patients with concurrent optic neuritis should be given a more guarded prognosis. I have seen the retina reattach, only to have the optic nerve become atrophied.

CHAPTER 16 - GLAUCOMA

Glaucoma is increased intraocular pressure and if not controlled, will lead to blindness. A thorough understanding of the formation and flow of aqueous is necessary to interpret and treat glaucoma.

NORMAL ANATOMY AND PHYSIOLOGY

AQUEOUS HUMOR FORMATION

The exact nature of the formation of aqueous is not fully understood, but the major mechanisms are known. Aqueous production by the ciliary processes is by passive diffusion, ultrafiltration and active secretion. The formation is constant at a rate of about 2% of the anterior chamber volume per minute (dog 2.5 µl/min, cat 15 µl/min).

Control of passive diffusion and ultrafiltration

The control of passive diffusion of water and substances from the anterior uveal capillaries to the aqueous is referred to as the blood-aqueous barrier. This barrier is primarily a function of the tight junctions of the non-pigmented epithelium.

All substances seen in blood are seen in the aqueous. They can be divided into three categories according to how freely they pass into the aqueous.

1. Large molecules (such as plasma proteins) penetrate so slowly as to give the impression there is an absolute barrier. Thus, the concentration of plasma proteins is about 1/200 the amount seen in blood (0.01% to 0.05% in the aqueous). In the presence of increased permeability, plasma proteins can pass into the aqueous, resulting in "plasmoid aqueous". Permeability is increased by:
   a. Inflammation of the anterior uvea
   b. Rapid decompression of the anterior chamber
2. Smaller molecules or ions usually penetrate more rapidly
3. Lipid-soluble molecules and water cross the barrier rapidly

Secretion is the primary source of aqueous production. The pigment epithelium has several transport systems that have been identified. These account for the osmotic pressure of the aqueous being higher than that of the plasma.

1. Carbonic anhydrase - the main enzyme transport system. It results in the secretion of bicarbonate ions into the aqueous.
2. Several pump systems have been identified. Some move constituents into the aqueous and others move them out.
   a. Sodium is secreted into the posterior chamber under the influence of Na-K activated ATPase found along the membranes of the inner nonpigmented epithelium
   b. Ascorbate
   c. Amino acids
3. Beta receptors - a positive resting tone involved in maintaining secretion

AQUEOUS HUMOR FLOW

Aqueous outflow occurs via two basic pathways (Fig 16-1). The mechanisms involved for each pathway are not completely understood.

Conventional outflow - through the filtration angle (ciliary cleft) and across the corneoscleral trabecular meshwork (cribriform plate) into the scleral venous plexus. Aqueous passage across the corneoscleral trabecular meshwork is mediated by beta receptors on the trabecular meshwork cells and involves pinocytosis-like transport process. This is the primary pathway in companion animals.

Unconventional (uveoscleral) outflow - through the filtration angle (ciliary cleft) and ciliary muscle interstitium into the suprachoroidal space and across the sclera. In horses, this may be as or more important to aqueous drainage than the conventional outflow route. It is likely that uveoscleral aqueous outflow increases with uveal inflammation and this may partially explain why glaucoma is uncommon in horses.

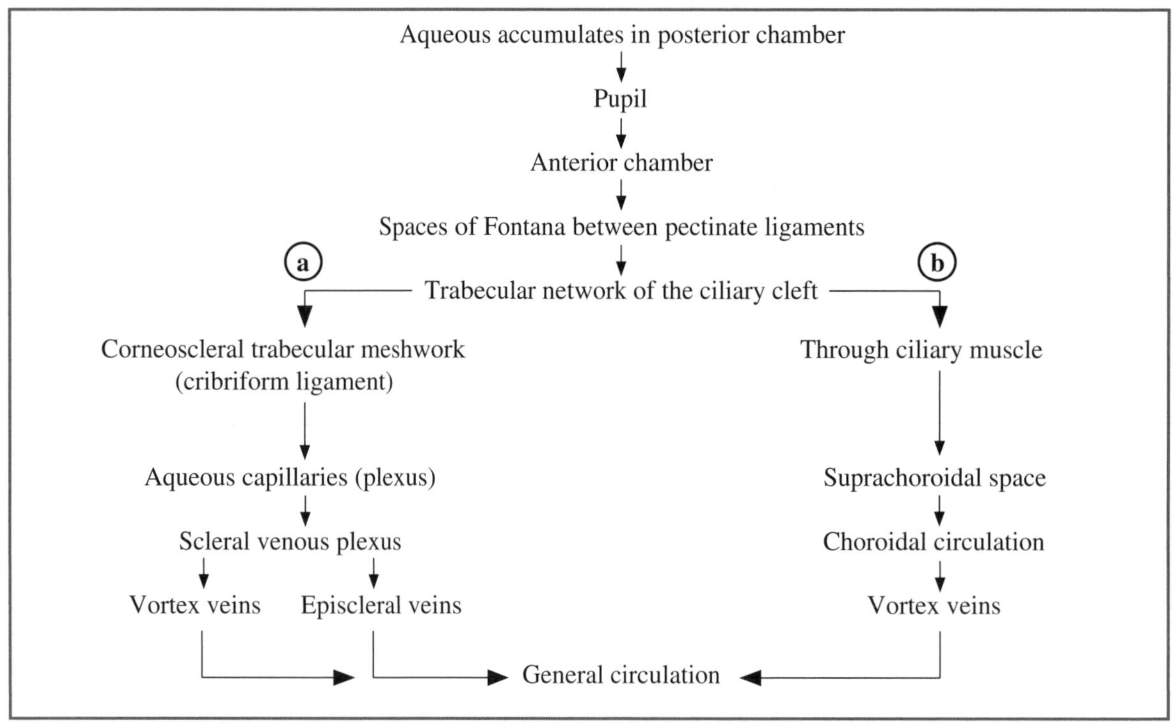

Figure 16-1. Flow of aqueous humor
a. Conventional outflow through corneoscleral trabecular meshwork (cribriform plate)
b. Unconventional outflow through ciliary muscle interstitium into the suprachoroidal space

FUNCTIONS OF AQUEOUS HUMOR

Aqueous maintains intraocular pressure and therefore affects the shape, size and turgidity of the eye. Intraocular pressure is dependent on equilibrium between the rate of formation and the ease of outflow. In a normal eye, formation is quite constant and the resistance to outflow through the trabeculae regulates intraocular pressure.

1. Rate of formation is related to:
   a. The circulation to the uvea - systemic hypotension (dehydration/shock) reduces aqueous production
   b. The activity of the secretory epithelium
   c. Integrity of the blood-aqueous barrier
2. Outflow is related to:
   a. Open communication through the pupil

b. An open filtration angle
c. Unobstructed flow through the ciliary-scleral pathways. Inflammation of the anterior uvea or sclera will increase uveoscleral outflow.

3. Effect of inflammation in IOP. When inflammatory disease of the anterior uvea is present, the total production is altered. Active secretion decreases while passive formation increases slightly, resulting in a net decrease of aqueous formation. This, combined with increased outflow, results in a hypotonic eye.

Aqueous carries metabolites for vitreous lens and cornea (oxygen, glucose, amino acids, etc)

Aqueous removes waste

EFFECT OF DRUGS ON INTRAOCULAR PRESSURE

Sympathomimetic drugs (epinephrine/dipivefrin hydrochloride)(see Chapter 2, page 109) - There is an initial increase in aqueous production followed by decreased production. Outflow is increased by apparent direct action on the innervation of the trabecular meshwork.

Beta-Adrenergic blocking agents - (see Chapter 2, page 110) block the resting positive beta receptor tone of the ciliary process epithelium, decreasing cAMP and lowering aqueous production

Miotics - (see Chapter 2, page 106) produce miosis through contraction of the iris sphincter and contraction of the longitudinal ciliary body musculature, thereby increasing tension on the scleral spur, in turn enlarging the sclerociliary cleft and opening the trabecular network to facilitate aqueous outflow. Uveoscleral outflow is decreased.

Carbonic anhydrase inhibitors (acetazolamide, dichlorphenamide, dorzolamide, methazolamide)(see Chapter 2, page111) - can reduce active aqueous formation from the ciliary body epithelium by 50 to 60%

Systemic osmotic diuretic agents (see Chapter 2, page 112) - reduce intraocular pressure by creating a hyper-osmotic state within the extracellular fluid compartment, thus drawing water from the vitreous chamber and decreasing the passive formation of aqueous humor

Prostaglandins (see Chapter 2, page 112) - reduce intraocular pressure by increasing uveoscleral outflow.

Parasympatholytic drugs (atropine/tropicamide) - (see Chapter 2, page 108) ***do not affect intraocular pressure in normal dogs***. They may increase intraocular pressure in dogs with an abnormal filtration angle. The cycloplegic effect on the longitudinal ciliary muscle and paralysis of the iris sphincter muscle may permit the base of the iris to restrict aqueous flow through the filtration angle. Uveoscleral outflow is increased.

CLASSIFICATION OF GLAUCOMA

The human classification of glaucoma does not work well in veterinary medicine because of anatomical differences seen between species. Several classifications have been proposed for animals and therefore, are controversial.

PRIMARY GLAUCOMA

Beagle - Primary (open angle) glaucoma is increased intraocular pressure without antecedent ocular disease and is bilateral. The filtration angle is open, thus an obstruction to outflow exists at the level of the venous plexus within the scleral side of the filtration angle. This type of glaucoma is characteristic of beagles with autosomal recessive inheritance. It occurs about six to eight months of age and secondary changes occur by two to three years of age. Glycosaminoglycan alterations are suspected.

Cocker spaniels and Samoyeds have been classified as primary glaucoma because as young animals the filtration angle may appear normal or nearly normal and as the animal ages, the angle becomes progressively more dysgenic.

Siamese cats - The author has seen related Siamese cats with apparent primary glaucoma.

Mesodermal dysgenesis/goniodysgenesis occurs in dogs

1. Bilateral and genetic predisposition - dominant proposed for English springer spaniel
2. The significance of mesodermal dysgenesis is not clearly defined at this time but affected breeds are predisposed. Anterior uveitis is often antecedent to glaucoma development in these animals.
3. The age of onset of glaucoma is variable (months to years). Therefore some authors question whether this should be considered in the congenital glaucoma category.
4. Clinical appearance of the filtration angle varies from shortened ligaments that may get broader with age (e.g. Arctic Circle breeds) to areas where a sheet of tissue may cover the pectinate ligaments with only occasional "flow holes" for the aqueous to pass through to the trabeculae (e.g. basset hound).

SECONDARY GLAUCOMA

Secondary glaucoma is increased intraocular pressure with antecedent ocular disease.

Lens - luxation (pupillary block/collapse of filtration angle), intumescence

Vitreous prolapse - secondary to luxation/postsurgical

Complications to anterior uveitis

1. Inflammatory debris
2. Synechia - posterior > iris bombé; anterior peripheral (horses)

Hyphema - anterior uveitis, bleeding disorders, tumors, hypertension

Acute trauma

Intraocular neoplasia - infiltrating filtration angle

Pigment deposition - a proliferation of pigment in the filtration angle. Golden retrievers with pigmentary uveitis.

CONGENITAL GLAUCOMA

Glaucoma at birth - Animals are rarely born with glaucoma. When seen it may be bilateral or unilateral.

INCIDENCE OF GLAUCOMA

Dogs - most common, may be acute or chronic
Cats - less common than dogs and usually presents as a chronic disease
Horses - uncommon, often unilateral, secondary to anterior uveitis and presented as a chronic problem with buphthalmos

CANINE GLAUCOMA

Acute glaucoma is an emergency problem that requires quick assessment and appropriate therapy if function is to be restored to the globe. By definition, glaucoma exists if the intraocular pressure elevation is sufficient to cause loss of vision, either temporary or permanent. Usually intraocular pressures > 30 mm Hg are consistent with a diagnosis of glaucoma. Some cases will have glaucoma signs but have intraocular pressures within the 20 to 30 mm Hg range when examined. Pressure should be measured in both eyes because the difference may be more significant than the absolute values in low pressure glaucoma.

SIGNS - Glaucoma typically presents as an acutely painful, red, blind eye, with a dilated pupil and a cloudy cornea.

Acute glaucoma early signs - noted within two to three hours of onset

1. Pain
   a. Epiphora
   b. Blepharospasm and exaggerated menace or avoidance response when the eye is examined
   c. Protrusion third eyelid
2. Red eye - mild conjunctival hyperemia, chemosis, and episcleral injection, which quickly become severe
3. Cornea - may be clear or slightly cloudy from edema
4. Iris - pupillary light reflex may be intact but sluggish. If seen early the pupil may be miotic. The pupil is usually dilated when presented. Checking for an indirect pupillary light reflex in the opposite eye is of prognostic value (Fig 16-2).
5. Fundus - will appear normal
6. Vision - this will depend on IOP. If moderate elevation (< 40 mm Hg) the eye should be visual. If severe elevation (> 60 mm Hg), anticipate blindness.

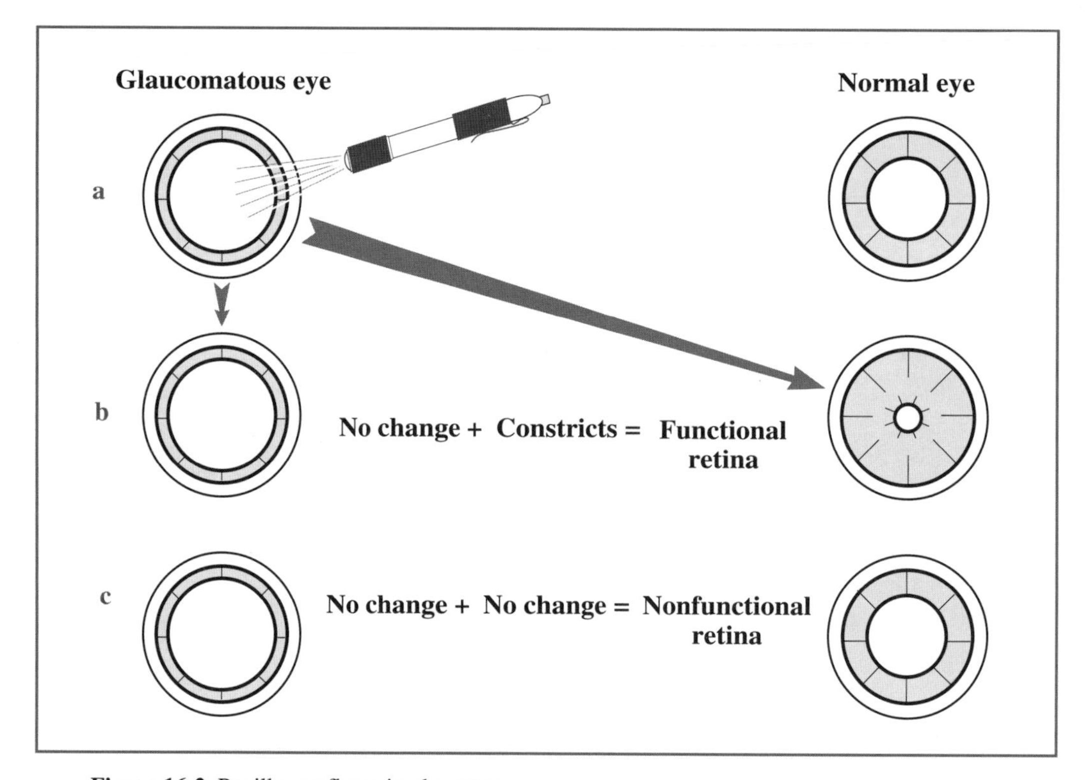

Figure 16-2. Pupillary reflexes in glaucoma
a. Appearance before pupillary light reflexes are tested
b. Indirect reflex is present if glaucomatous eye has functional optic nerve
c. Indirect reflex is absent if optic nerve is nonfunctional in glaucomatous eye

Advanced signs - these may occur in a few hours to days after onset of glaucoma

1. Pain persists
2. Red eye - marked conjunctival and episcleral congestion (i.e. dilated blood vessels), thus imparting a striking red appearance
3. Corneal opacity - edema due to increased hydrostatic pressure at the endothelial surface of the cornea is a consistent finding. Vascularization and pigmentation of the cornea also occur in more chronic cases.
4. Dilated pupil
5. Fundus - increased size of the optic disk physiologic cup and reduced optic nerve diameter. Peripapillary retinal thinning.
6. Blindness - The eye is blind due to pressure-induced compromise of the optic nerve (mechanical pressure pushes the nerve caudally and results in vascular ischemia and blocked axoplasmic flow)
7. Normal ERG

Late or chronic signs (Fig 16-3) - these changes require days, weeks, or even months to occur

1. Minimal pain
2. Buphthalmos - chronic glaucoma causes stretching of the ocular tunics, resulting in an enlarged globe. Even if the intraocular pressure is normal at the time of examination, buphthalmos signifies that glaucoma has been present. Buphthalmos predisposes to exposure keratitis. Puppies develop buphthalmos quickly because of their thin cornea and sclera.
3. Corneal striae (Haab's striae) - buphthalmos causes stretching and often rupture of Descemet's membrane. As this membrane heals, a leukoma tract is left.
4. Optic nerve atrophy - elevated intraocular pressure stops axoplasmic flow along the axons of the ganglion cells, resulting in nerve atrophy. The optic disk will appear sunken (glaucomatous cupping) and gray to white in color (Fig 15-5; Chapter 15, page 423).
5. Retinal atrophy - elevated intraocular pressure destroys the ganglion cell quickly. Initially, this change cannot be appreciated with an ophthalmoscope. With continued elevation of the eye pressure, degeneration of the photoreceptor layer of the retina occurs as well. After a period of three to six weeks, generalized retinal thinning results in tapetal hyperreflectivity. The retinal blood vessels become attenuated in response to the decreased metabolic demand of the degenerating retina.
6. ERG - decreases as retinal atrophy develops; absent at end stages

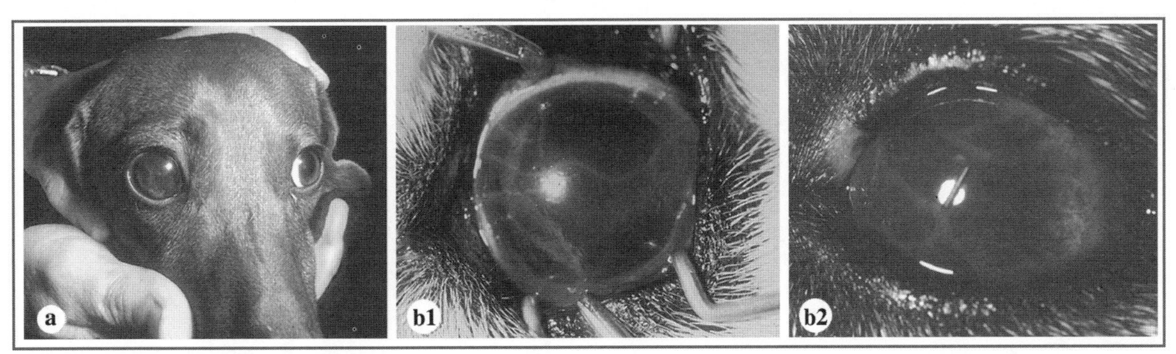

Figure 16-3. Signs of chronic glaucoma
- a. Dog with unilateral buphthalmos of the right eye.
- b. Siberian husky with Haabs striae due to chronic glaucoma
  - 1) Appearance on presentation. Note dilated pupil, cloudy cornea and multiple white striae.
  - 2) Same dog after glaucoma controlled by cyclocryosurgery. Pupil was normal and cornea clear except for striae.

DIAGNOSIS - Glaucoma can be confirmed by measuring the *intraocular pressure* using tonometry

Tonometry

1. Digital - Although some clinicians attempt digital tonometry by palpating the globe, this method is crude and can be misleading. Digital tonometry should not be performed by simply retropulsing the eye. After topical anesthesia, slight pressure can be applied directly to the globe with a moistened finger, cotton swab, or blunt instrument (tip of a curved mosquito hemostat). The resistance to indentation of the fibrous tunics of the eye should be noted and the corneal surface should be watched to get a visual impression of the amount of indentation.
2. Schiötz indentation tonometry (page 44) - The Schiötz tonometer is accurate but the conversion table that comes with it is calibrated for the human eye and yields pressure readings that are lower than the actual pressure in cats and dogs. When using the table that comes with the tonometer, pressures for the normal dog are 15 to 27 mm Hg. Conversion tables are available for dogs and cats (Tables 1-2 and 1-3; Chapter 1 pages 46 and 47). The instrument is accurate if an effort is made to keep the scale reading between 3 and 12 by using one of the several loading weights that accompany the device. Eyes with normal pressure typically have scale readings equal to the plunger mass load ± 2 units. Technique is important to avoid introducing error.
   a. The cornea is anesthetized by applying several drops of proparacaine HCl 0.5%, waiting 30 seconds or so between drops
   b. The animal should be looking at the ceiling so the direction of gaze is parallel with the force of gravity. In some animals this can be done by dorsoflexing the head, while in others it is easier to lay the animal on its side or back.
   c. The tonometer is placed on the cornea, taking care to not touch the third eyelid, eyelids or lashes. ***The instrument must be vertical when placed on the corneal surface***. Only the weight of the instrument should be rested on the globe. This is best accomplished by allowing the sliding finger hold to glide midway along the range of movement.
   d. The tonometer measures the corneal indentation caused by the plunger. Each scale unit is equal to 0.05 mm of indentation of the plunger on the cornea. The scale readings are inversely proportional to the intraocular pressure.
3. Applanation tonometry - A variety of mechanical and electronic devices are available to measure the force necessary to flatten a 1 mm diameter area of the corneal surface. The flattening force is proportional to the intraocular pressure. These instruments are expensive.

Gonioscopy - Examination of the filtration angle with a contact lens is a specialized method of assessing the possible cause of glaucoma and the potential response of the eye to the various methods of treatment. See Fig. 1-55 (Chapter 1, page 53) for normals. Abnormal filtration angles are seen in Fig. 16-4.

1. Direct lenses - Examination of the angle is possible by directly looking into the lens at a 30 to 45° angle. In this way the angle can be visualized. Useful lenses include Franklin, Cordona, Koeppe, and Lovac Barkan.
2. Indirect lenses - In this situation mirrors are built into the lens that reflect light and allow viewing of the angle. Other lenses are available that allow an indirect ophthalmoscope to be used in conjunction with the lens, thus increasing magnification and stereoscopic vision.

Ophthalmoscopy - If optic nerve cupping and/or retinal atrophy are present, glaucoma has been present for some time. In chronic cases, the intraocular pressure may currently be normal.

TREATMENT - After making a diagnosis, either medical or surgical therapy must be instituted. The choice of treatment depends upon the type of glaucoma and the stage of the disease at which diagnosis is made.

1. Eyes with potential for vision - the response to medical therapy can be frustrating because long term control is difficult to maintain. Surgical procedures thus are frequently required (i.e. cyclocryotherapy, cyclophotocoagulation, filtering procedures, and drainage implants)

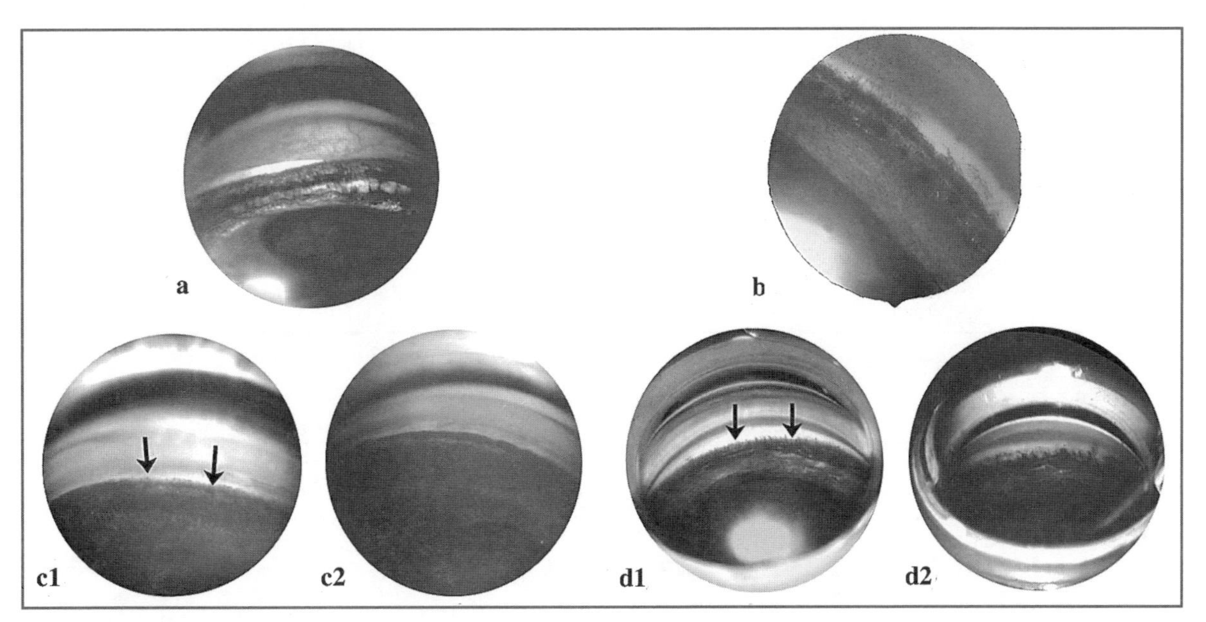

Figure 16-4. Filtration angle abnormalities
- a. Cocker spaniel with narrow angle with variation in width and length of pectinate ligaments
- b. Basset hound with goniodysgenesis. Note flow holes through the sheet of abnormal tissue.
- c. Samoyed with goniodysgenesis and glaucoma.
  1) Area with limited outflow (arrows)
  2) Area with complete obstruction
- d. Springer spaniel with secondary glaucoma after acute anterior uveitis. Peripheral anterior synechia is obstructing the filtration angle.
  1) Normal eye - note the lack of corneal pigment where pectinate ligaments attach to cornea (arrows)
  2) Glaucomatous eye - peripheral synechia obstructing filtration angle

2. Irreversibly blind eyes - treatment should be to relieve chronic pain and/or provide a cosmetic eye

MEDICAL TREATMENT OF ACUTE GLAUCOMA

Acute glaucoma is an emergency - Emergency medical treatment should always be attempted in cases that are acute to subacute. The case should be reevaluated several times during the initial 12 to 48 hours to assess response to medical therapy and also whether surgery is indicated. If a surgical procedure is opted for, it should be performed within the first few days of the hypertensive crisis. The higher the pressure, the sooner irreversible damage will occur. A pressure > 50 mm Hg for two to three days may result in irreversible nerve damage. Medical treatment should be directed at decreasing ocular inflammation as well as reducing the elevated intraocular pressure (Table 16-1). Initial medical treatment can be divided into five broad categories that:

1. Reduce inflammation
2. Absorb fluid from the eye
3. Reduce aqueous production
4. Assist outflow
5. Calcium channel blockers reduce optic nerve damage

Anti-inflammatory agents - Anti-inflammatory agents can be based on steroidal or nonsteroidal agents and are useful if inflammation is a significant factor of the disease. Corticosteroids are effective but have been documented to elevate the intraocular pressure in primates, rabbits, and cats. This problem has not been reported in dogs, but the author has seen transient glaucoma in cocker spaniels after subconjunctival methyl prednisolone. If severe inflammation exists, controlling the inflammation outweighs the danger of corticosteroids causing glaucoma. Nonsteroidal antiprostaglandin agents (such as aspirin and flunixin meglumine) have been used successfully. Topical nonsteroidal agents (diclofenac 0.1%, flurbiprofen sodium 0.03%), are available and may be helpful in case management.

Table 16-1. Drugs used for treatment of glaucoma. Modified from Ophthalmic Drug Facts; Facts and Comparison, 111 Westport Plaza, St. Louis, Missouri.

Drug	Strength/ Dosage	Route	Duration Hours	Frequency of administration	Decrease aqueous production	Increase aqueous outflow	Pupil
Sympathomimetic							
Apraclonidine-Iopidine (Alcon)[1]	0.5-0.1%	Topical	7-12	TID	+++	NR	Dogs
							Cats
Epinephrine-Many sources	1.0-2.0%	Topical	12	Daily/BID	+	++	Dilate
Dipivefrin-Propine (Allergan)	0.1%	Topical	12	BID	+	++	nil
Beta Blockers							
Betaxolol-Betoptic (Alcon)	0.25-0.50%	Topical	12	BID	+++	NR	NR
Carteolol-Ocupress (Otsuka)	1%	Topical	12	BID	+++		NR
Levobunolol-Betagan (Allergan)	0.25-0.5%	Topical	12-24	Daily	+++	NR	NR
Metipranolol-Optipranolol (Bausch & Lomb)	0.3%	Topical	12-24	BID	+++	NR	NR
Timolol-Timoptic (Merck & Co)	0.25-0.5%	Topical	12-24	BID	+++	NR	NR
Miotics, Direct-Acting							
Acetylcholine-Miochol-E (Ciba-Vision)	0.1%	Intra-ocular	10-20 min		NR	+++	Miosis
Carbachol-Isoptocarbachol (Alcon)	0.75-3.0%	Topical	6-8	TID	NR	+++	Miosis
Pilocarpine-Many sources[2]	0.25-10%	Topical	4-8	QID	NR	+++	Miosis
Miotics, Cholinesterase Inhibitors							
Physostigmine-Eserine (IOLAB)	0.25-0.5%	Topical	12-36	Daily	NR	+++	Miosis
Demecarium-Humersol (Merck & Co)	0.125-0.25%	Topical	Days	1-3 days	NR	+++	Miosis
Echothiophate-Phospholine Iodide (Wyeth-Ayerst)	0.03-0.25%	Topical	Days	1-3 days	NR	+++	Miosis
Carbonic Anhydrase Inhibitors							
Acetazolamide-Diamox (Storz Ophthalmics)	10 mg/kg	Oral; IV	8-12	BID or TID	+++	NR	NR
Dichlorphenamide-Daranide (Merck & Co)	2-4 mg/kg	Oral	6-12	BID or TID	+++	NR	NR
Dorzolamide-Trusopt (Merck & Co)	2%	Topical	5 hrs	TID	+++	NR	NR
Methazolamide-Neptazane (Storz Ophthalmics)	5 mg/kg	Oral	10-18	BID or TID	+++	NR	NR
Osmotic Agents[3]							
Mannitol-Various sources	1.5-2 gm/kg	IV	~4	BID			NR
Sodium ascorbate-Various sources	2 gm/kg	IV	~4	BID			
Glycerin-Various sources	1.5 gm/kg	Oral	4-6	BID-QID			
Isosorbide-Ismotic (Alcon)	1.5 gm/kg	Oral	4-6	BID-QID			
Prostagiandins $F_{2\alpha}$ Analogue							
Latanoprost - Xalatan (Upjohn)	0.005%	Topical	12-24	BID	NR	+++	NR
Combination Agents							
Epinephrine-Pilocarpine (Various sources)	E1%-P2% and lower %	Topical	4-8	BID-QID	+++	+++	Miosis
Cosopt - Dorzolamide and timolol (Merck)	2% 0.5%	Topical		BID	+++	+++	NR
Calcium Channel Blockers[4]							
Amlodipine besylate-Norvasc (Pfizer)	1.25-2.5 mg	Oral		Daily			
Diltiazem HCl-Cardizem (Lederle)	0.5-1.5 mg/kg	Oral		TID			
Verapamil-Various sources	3 mg/kg	Oral		TID			

Affect in man: +++ = significant activity; ++ = moderate activity; + = some activity.
NR = no activity reported; ND = no data available
[1]Intraocular administration only for miosis during surgery
[2]Also available as a gel and an insert; the duration of these forms is longer than solution
[3]Reduces ultrafiltration and draws fluid directly from eye
[4]Treatment of ocular hypertension and other symptoms of glaucoma (optic nerve damage)

Osmotic agents - to absorb fluid from the vitreous and aqueous. These drugs become less effective with chronic use. Water should be withheld two to four hours after administration.

1. Mannitol (IV 1-2 gm/kg) for immediate effect. Effect may last six hours or more and can be repeated BID or TID.
2. Sodium ascorbate (IV 1-2 gm/kg) for immediate effect. This osmotic agent is not confined to the vascular compartment and is less effective than mannitol, especially if anterior uveitis is present.
3. Glycerin (oral 1-2 ml/kg) for maintenance. If causes vomiting, dilute with equal amount of skim milk.

Drugs that reduce aqueous production

1. Carbonic anhydrase inhibitors - are necessary in immediate and long term treatment. In the latter, they can sometimes be titered to PM treatment only. The author prefers methazolamide for small breeds and dichlorphenamide in dogs over 40 pounds.
    a. Methazolamide - 5 mg/kg BID
    b. Dichlorphenamide - 2.5 mg/kg BID or TID
    c. Acetazolamide - 10 mg/kg BID. Acetazolamide produces adverse side effects more rapidly than either methazolamide or dichlorphenamide, therefore the author recommends acetazolamide only when the others are not available.
    d. Dorzolamide - 2% ophthalmic solution BID.
    e. Adverse effects - electrolyte imbalance may result in anorexia, vomiting, diarrhea, panting, lameness, weight loss and/or depression
2. Sympathomimetics - have a modest inhibiting effect
    a. Epinephrine - 0.5-1%
    b. Dipivefrin HCl 0.1% (Propine) - an epinephrine prodrug that penetrates the cornea 17 times as readily as epinephrine and is converted to epinephrine in the uvea. Minimal mydriatic effect.
3. Sympatholytic drugs (beta blockers) - timolol maleate 0.25 to 0.5% (Timoptic), betaxolol HCl 0.5% (Betoptic) and levobunolol 0.25 to 0.5% (Betagan). This class of drugs is more effective in primates than the domestic animals we commonly deal with because of few receptor sites in dogs and cats. Use of the more concentrated solutions may be more effective. In man, these drugs are currently the most frequently prescribed topical medications to treat primary glaucoma. In certain select cases, these drugs may be worth using along with other agents.

Drugs that assist outflow at the filtration angle

1. Parasympathomimetics
    a. Pilocarpine 1 to 2% - short duration therefore QID; Pilopine-HS gel 4% every 24 hours
    b. Carbachol 0.75 to 3% - QID
    c. Echothiophate iodide (Phospholine iodide) 1/32 to 1/16%; demecarium HCl (Humorsol) 0.125 to 0.25%. Prolonged duration, therefore daily or BID
2. Sympathomimetics - increase aqueous outflow and uveoscleral output

Drug combinations - The response to a single autonomic nervous system drug is limited and therefore combinations are frequently recommended. A combination of pilocarpine 2%-epinephrine 1% (P_2E_1). QID is more effective in dogs than pilocarpine only, but is becoming difficult to find. If the patient develops sensitivity a reduced strength can be used ($P_1E_{1/2}$). Mixing equal parts of pilocarpine 4% and epinephrine 2% can be used to make P_2E_1. This combination frequently results in a red stain to the tears at the nasal canthus, causing the owner to become alarmed, believing there is blood in the tears. This is a reaction between the tears, drugs and light.

Medical plan for treating acute glaucoma - A combined therapeutic plan is frequently required to control the intraocular pressure successfully. A suggested plan is outlined below.

1. Systemic acute inflammatory therapy - if no uveitis, systemic Banamine; if uveitis - systemic prednisolone should be considered
2. IV mannitol to drop pressure rapidly - follow with oral glycerin for maximum of one week. Discontinue when normal pressures can be maintained for 48 hours.
3. Oral carbonic anhydrase inhibitor - start BID or TID, maintain BID until pressures are stable for one week. In some cases reduce to daily for one to three weeks. ***Consider discontinuing only if patient is doing well and initiating cause has been corrected.***
4. Topical medications - initially P_2E_1 q2-4h and concurrent beta blocker BID. As pressure responds, reduce P_2E_1 to QID. If sensitivity to P_2E_1 occurs, reduce concentrations to $P_1E_{1/2}$ and continue with a beta blocker. If sensitivity persists, discontinue $P_1E_{1/2}$ and start Propine and Pilopine gel 4% or an indirect parasympathomimetic.
5. If the pressure is not dropping or is still greater than 50 to 60 mm Hg after two to four hours, surgical procedures should be considered and if available, a veterinary ophthalmologist should be consulted. Remember high pressures can result in permanent optic nerve and retinal damage in 24 hours.

Prophylactic treatment - of the unaffected eye in breeds predisposed to glaucoma is recommended but probably of limited value, delaying onset of glaucoma.

SURGICAL TREATMENT OF AN EYE WITH VISUAL POTENTIAL

Anterior chamber centesis (Fig 1-40; Chapter 1, page 38) - ***this is a very controversial procedure***. Acute glaucoma with high pressure that is not responsive to aggressive medical treatment due to sphincter paralysis and secondary collapse of the filtration angle may respond to pilocarpine and open the angle when pressure is reduced. Centesis combined with medical treatment can give time until surgery can be performed. Withdrawal of 0.1 ml of aqueous with a 25 or 27 gauge needle and followed by subconjunctival leakage of aqueous will gradually reduce pressure and may allow medication to keep pressure down. The goal is to reduce the IOP to the normal range (approximately 15 mm Hg). Sudden removal of an excess amount of aqueous will result in profound hypotony (less than 4 mm Hg) leading to plasmoid aqueous (excess fibrin content) and/or hyphema. If pressures begin to rise above normal, definitive surgical procedures are indicated.

Secondary glaucoma with a correctable cause - recommend glaucoma surgery within 24 hours

1. Lens luxation - lens displacement may cause glaucoma or be the result of chronic glaucoma. Gonioscopic examination of the other eye and close examination for impending signs of lens luxation (iridodonesis/abnormal chamber depth) may help to determine if the lens luxation is causing glaucoma or the result of it. Early lens removal is essential and the prognosis is dependent on the condition of the filtration angle.
2. Iris bombé - Anterior chamber injection with tPA 25 µg should be tried. If this is not effective a multiple iridotomy will allow aqueous to escape into the anterior chamber. This can be done in several ways (Fig 16-5). Small wounds tend to close down but large ones will often stay open.
   a. Multiple iridotomy with von Graefe cataract knife
   b. Iridotomy with DeWecker iris scissors - these special scissors can be introduced through a small limbal wound. The iris is incised to make a large wound or wounds. If the major vascular arcade near the base of the iris is cut, hemorrhage may fill the anterior chamber. Intracameral tPA is indicated after surgery.
3. Filtration angle obstruction with fibrin or blood - medical treatment for glaucoma and inflammation combined with chamber injection of tPA 25 µg

Glaucoma operations

There are many procedures that have been tried in man and animals. They are often promising for several weeks or months and then may fail. These procedures fall into three categories. Those that:

- Reduce aqueous production (cryosurgery/laser photocoagulation)
- Open existing drainage channels (cyclodialysis)
- Create an alternate drainage pathway (filtering procedures/shunts)

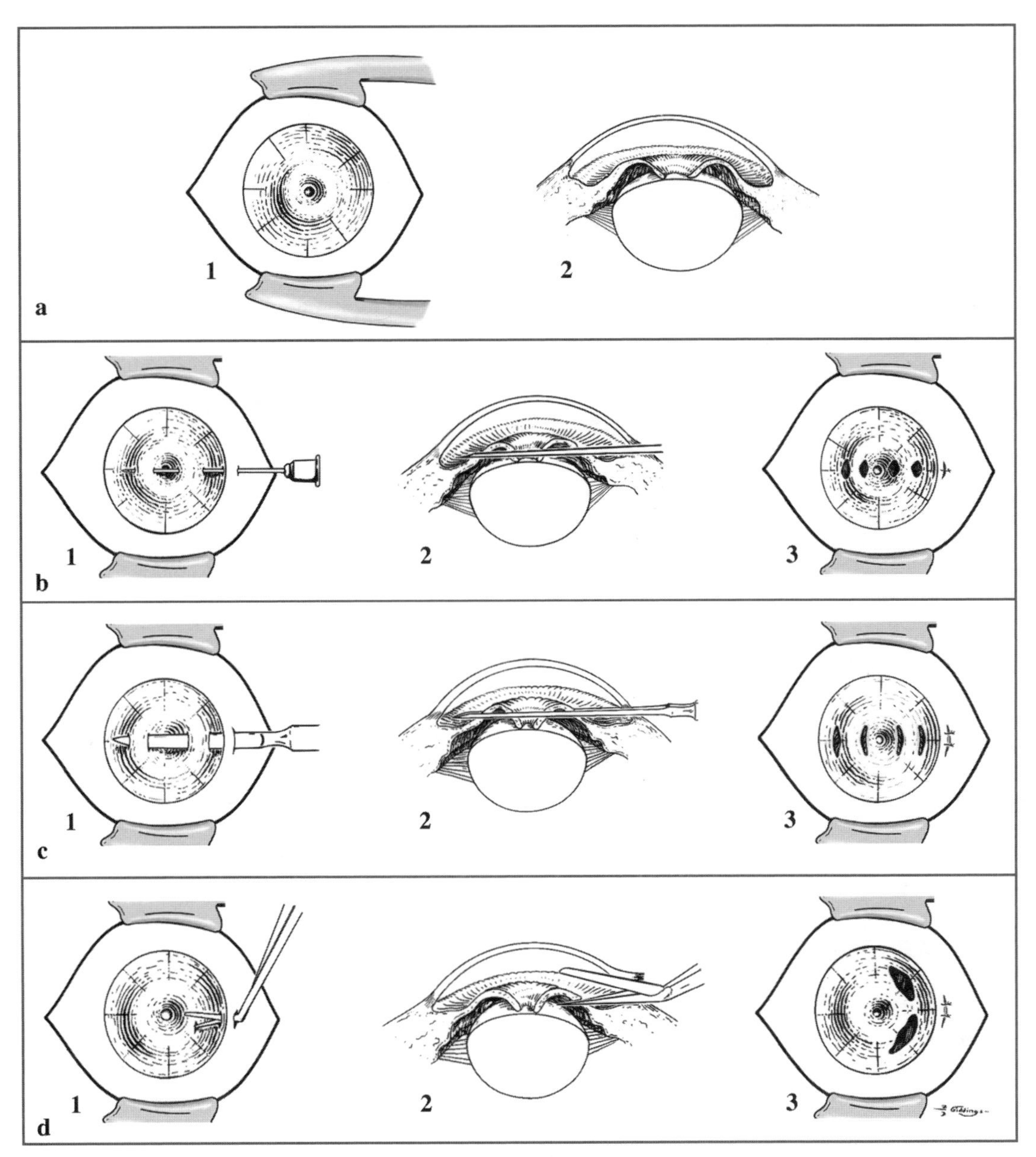

Figure 16-5. Iridotomy techniques for iris bombe´

a. Views of iris bombe´
   1) Frontal
   2) Cross-section

b. Needling the iris
   1) A 20-gauge needle is introduced at the limbus and passed through the iris on both sides of the pupil
   2) Cross-section view
   3) Appearance after the needle is withdrawn

c. VonGraefe knife iridotomy
   1) The knife is introduced at the limbus and directed through the iris on both sides of the pupil
   2) Cross-section view
   3) Appearance after the knife is withdrawn

d. Multiple iridotomies with DeWecker scissors
   1) The sharp point is forced through the iris and the round tip is kept in the anterior chamber
   2) Cross-section view
   3) Appearance after two iridotomies have been made

1. Cyclocryotherapy (Fig 16-6)
   a. Liquid nitrogen has been more successful than nitrous oxide because it will provide freezing to -20°C, which is needed to be cryotoxic to the ciliary body
   b. Technique will vary with the cryogen and probe size. Premedication with corticosteroids or antiprostaglandins is recommended. A freeze-thaw-freeze technique is recommended with nitrous oxide and/or small probes. If liquid nitrogen and a large probe are used, single freezes may be adequate. The probe should be centered over the ciliary body (approximately 5 mm posterior to the limbus) and the freeze continued until the iceball extends 1 mm into the cornea. Depending on the size of the eye, 4 to 6 sites should be frozen. Freezing over the long posterior ciliary arteries at the 9 and 3 o'clock positions should be avoided. This may result in intraocular hemorrhage. The intraocular pressure will rise immediately after freezing and remain elevated up to three days. Therefore, carbonic anhydrase inhibitors should be used until the pressure drops. Subconjunctival short-acting corticosteroids and/or systemic corticosteroids are helpful. Severe chemosis is immediate and will take several days before it disappears. Anterior chamber shunts are helpful to manage postcryosurgery IOP increase.
   c. Complications
      1) Intraocular hemorrhage (hyphema/intravitreal)
      2) Anterior uveitis
      3) Retinal edema > detachment. This usually reattaches.
      4) Increase in pressure for several days may damage an already compromised retina
      5) Inadequate cryotherapy may not control glaucoma
      6) Excess cryotherapy may cause phthisis bulbi

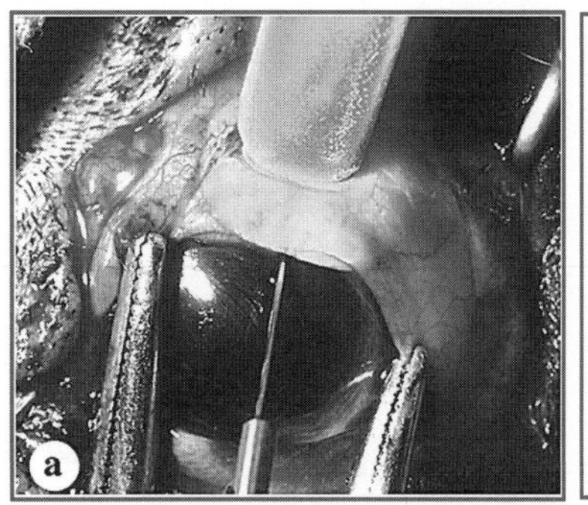

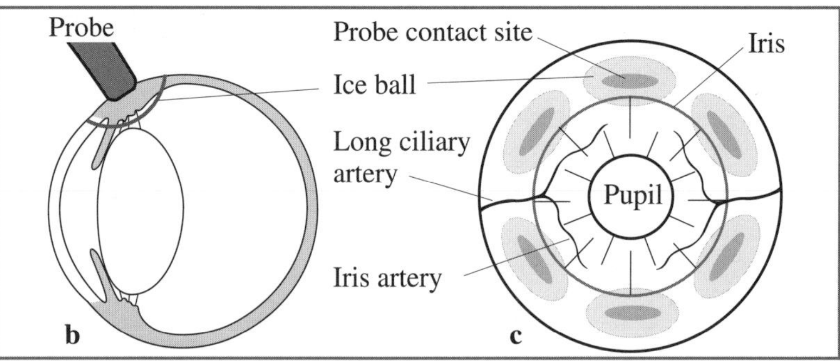

Figure 16-6. Cyclocryosurgery for glaucoma
   a. Probe centered over the ciliary body until ice ball proceeds 1 mm into the cornea
   b. Side view schematically representing size of ice ball
   c. Probe placement for freezing 6 sites. Freezing over the ciliary arteries at 9 and 3 o'clock is avoided

2. Transcleral laser therapy (cyclophotocoagulation) - Laser therapy provides a noninvasive means of reducing aqueous formation when directed over the ciliary body or increasing outflow when directed over the pars plana. This is a very promising technique that avoids the edema and discomfort seen with cryotherapy. If retreatment is needed, it is easier to perform.
   a. Aftercare
      1) Mild uveitis occurs, therefore topical corticosteroids are indicated
      2) There is a transient IOP increase post-laser surgery; if severe, anterior chamber centesis may be indicated.
3. Cyclodialysis - opening existing drainage channel. Cyclodialysis is separating the ciliary body from the sclera with a semisharp spatula. In this procedure the filtration angle is also opened when breaking down the pectinate ligaments so the base of the iris can pull away from the sclera.
4. Iridencleisis - creating an alternate drainage pathway. These are filtering procedures whereby aqueous drainage is channeled subconjunctivally through a limbal scleral wound that the iris has been sutured into, to make a fistulous tract. This procedure rarely remains patent more than a few months.
5. Combination cyclodialysis-sclerotomy and peripheral iridectomy (Fig 16-7) is the most successful filtering procedure.

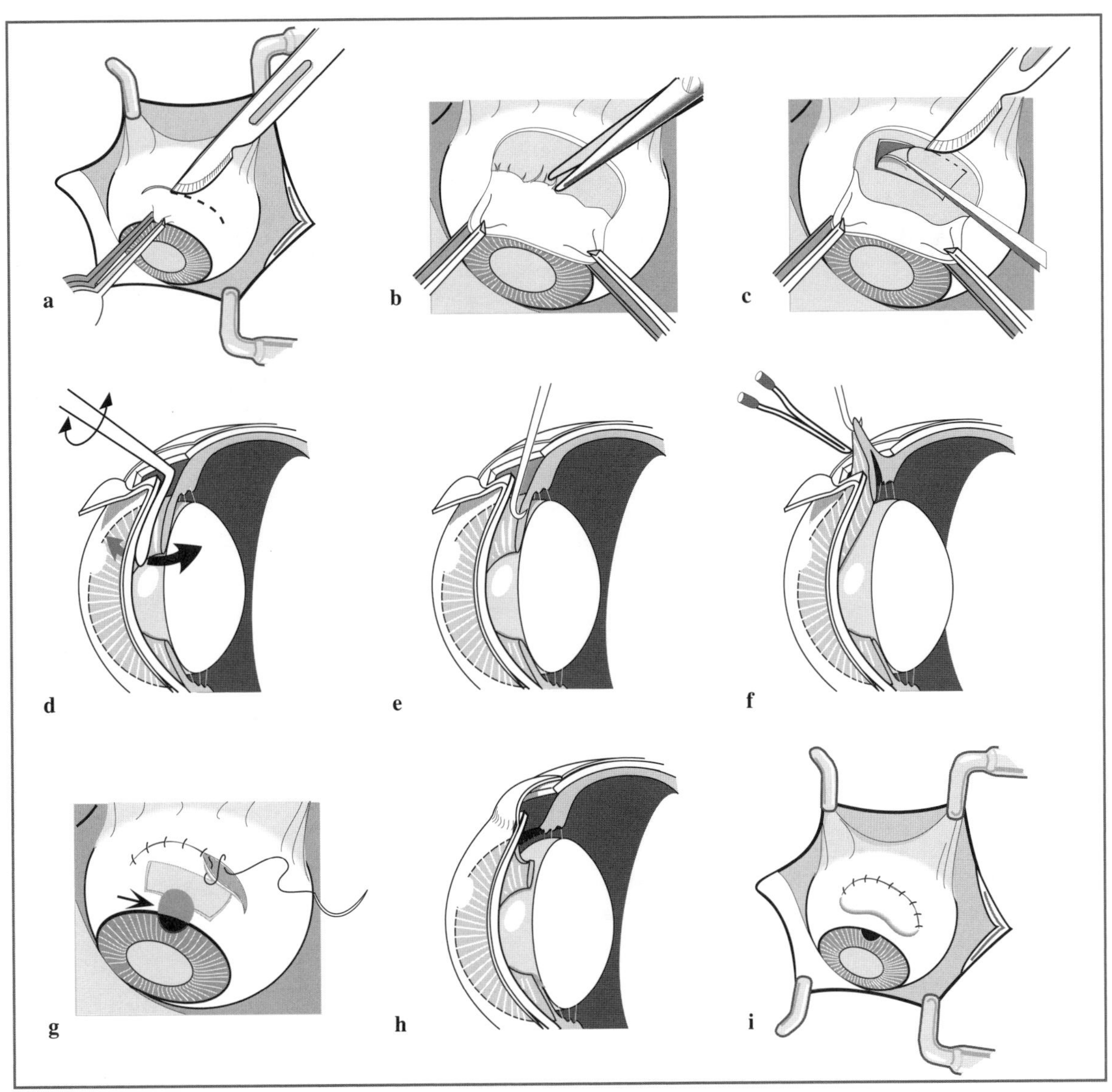

Figure 16-7. Combination of cyclodialysis-sclerotomy and peripheral iridectomy technique of Vainisi

a. Preparing limbal-base conjunctival flap
b. Flap undermined to the limbus exposing sclera
c. Incision through sclera, exposing ciliary body
d. Sclera removed and cyclodialysis spatula passed into anterior chamber from supraciliary space. A sweeping action is used to separate the choroid from the sclera for about a 120° arc
e. The base of the iris caught with an iris hook
f. Peripheral iris and adjacent ciliary body are retracted into the scleral wound and excised with electrocautery
g. The conjunctival wound is closed and the anterior chamber restored with BSS or air. Shaded area (arrow) represents where the iris and ciliary body have been removed. If a canthotomy was needed it will be closed now
h. Cross-section showing completed surgery
i. Anterior view of completed surgery

6. Subconjunctival shunts - This may be a simple subconjunctival drainage tube placed through the limbal sclera into the anterior chamber or an implant that maintains IOP by regulating subconjunctival aqueous flow. The immediate effect is excellent but tube obstruction or fibrosis around the implant frequently causes problems. Early glaucoma cases or cases implanted prophylactically demonstrate less fibrosis around the implant. This is likely due to less aqueous humor cytokines. The use of antimitotic drugs (mitomycin) injected at the implant site will reduce this reaction. Noninflamed eyes will show less reaction than those with any degree of anterior uveitis. The author's experience is limited to the Ahmed valve (New World Medical Inc) (Fig 16-8).

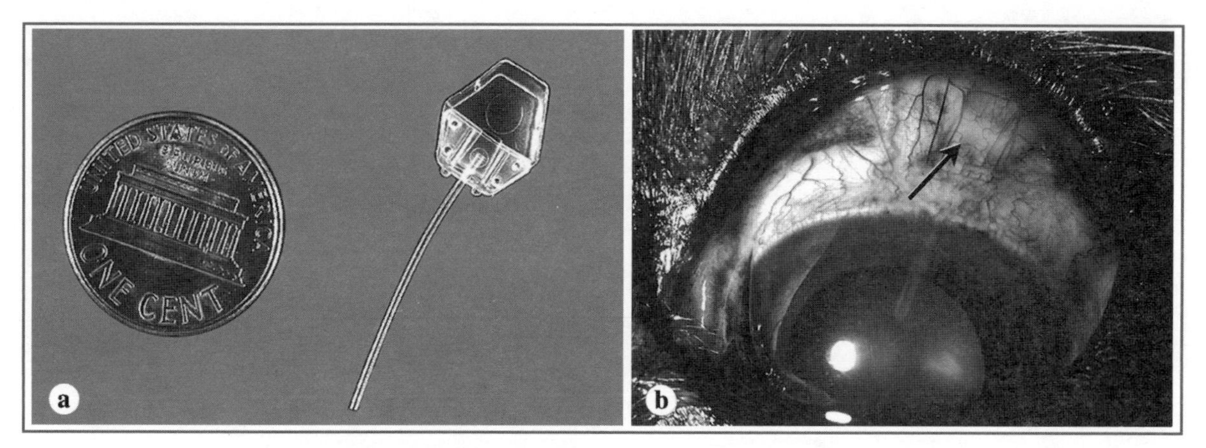

Figure 16-8. Ahmed glaucoma valve
- a. Ahmed valve and penny to illustrate size of valve
- b. Ahmed valve implanted in glaucoma eye; 30-day follow-up. Valve tube visible in the anterior chamber. Edge of aqueous pocket over valve (arrow)

TREATMENT OF CHRONIC GLAUCOMA - The intraocular pressure of dogs with chronic glaucoma can rarely be controlled with medical treatment and when they respond, usually require systemic and topical treatment for the rest of their lives. These animals routinely have good days and bad days.

Visual eyes that have fluctuation of pressure should be treated surgically before irreversible damage occurs

Blind eyes - medical treatment cannot be recommended. The owner should consider surgical treatment, which will stop further pain and discomfort to the patient (e.g. enucleation, intraocular prosthesis, oculotoxic gentamicin injection).

TREATMENT OF IRREVERSIBLY BLIND EYES - Medical treatment for blind dogs with absolute glaucoma should not be recommended except as a temporary measure in painful eyes while the owner is considering choices of surgical treatment.

Enucleation (see Chapter 17, page 495 for enucleation techniques) - a hard decision for many owners to make but an excellent one because all pain and discomfort is gone within hours after surgery. The author has never had a client state disappointment about removing the eye. In fact, the frequent comment is that the dog was more active and playful the day after surgery than it had been for a long time, thus giving the owner a feeling of guilt that the eye had not been removed sooner. An orbital prosthesis is always recommended to maintain a full appearance to the orbit.

Intraocular prosthesis - Evisceration and intraocular implant will provide a pain-free cosmetic eye. Plastic and silicone rubber implants (Jardon) are available. The author uses black silicone rubber implants.

1. Selection of implant size - prosthesis should be the same as or 1 mm greater than the horizontal corneal diameter of the normal eye. A buphthalmic globe begins to adjust to the size of the implant in 4 weeks.
2. Surgical technique (Fig 16-9)
   - a. The area is clipped and sterile surgical preparation is performed.
   - b. An eyelid speculum is positioned. Animals with a small eyelid aperture may need a canthotomy for good exposure.
   - c. The eye can be stabilized with bridle sutures, fixation forceps or hemostats placed near the limbus at 9 and 3 o'clock.
   - d. A conjunctival incision is made 4 mm dorsal and parallel to the limbus extending from 10 to 2 o'clock. The conjunctiva should be undermined a few mm toward the equator of the globe and the free edge tagged at 12 o'clock with forceps or suture.

e. Using a scalpel, incise the sclera 5 mm from the limbus in the same manner. The globe will collapse when the sclera is incised. Because of this surgical scissors may be preferred to extend the wound from 10 to 2 o'clock.

f. Starting at the iridocorneal angle, the anterior uvea is separated from the sclera. An iris spatula, cyclodialysis spatula, or Green lens spatula works well to separate these tissues. This results in considerable hemorrhage, therefore, *aspiration if available is useful*. Next, the choroid is separated from the sclera until the only attachment is the optic nerve. Carefully cut the choroid free with small scissors. If excess tension is applied to the choroid, the optic nerve will buckle the sclera, which in turn can result in cutting the sclera when the optic nerve attachment is severed.

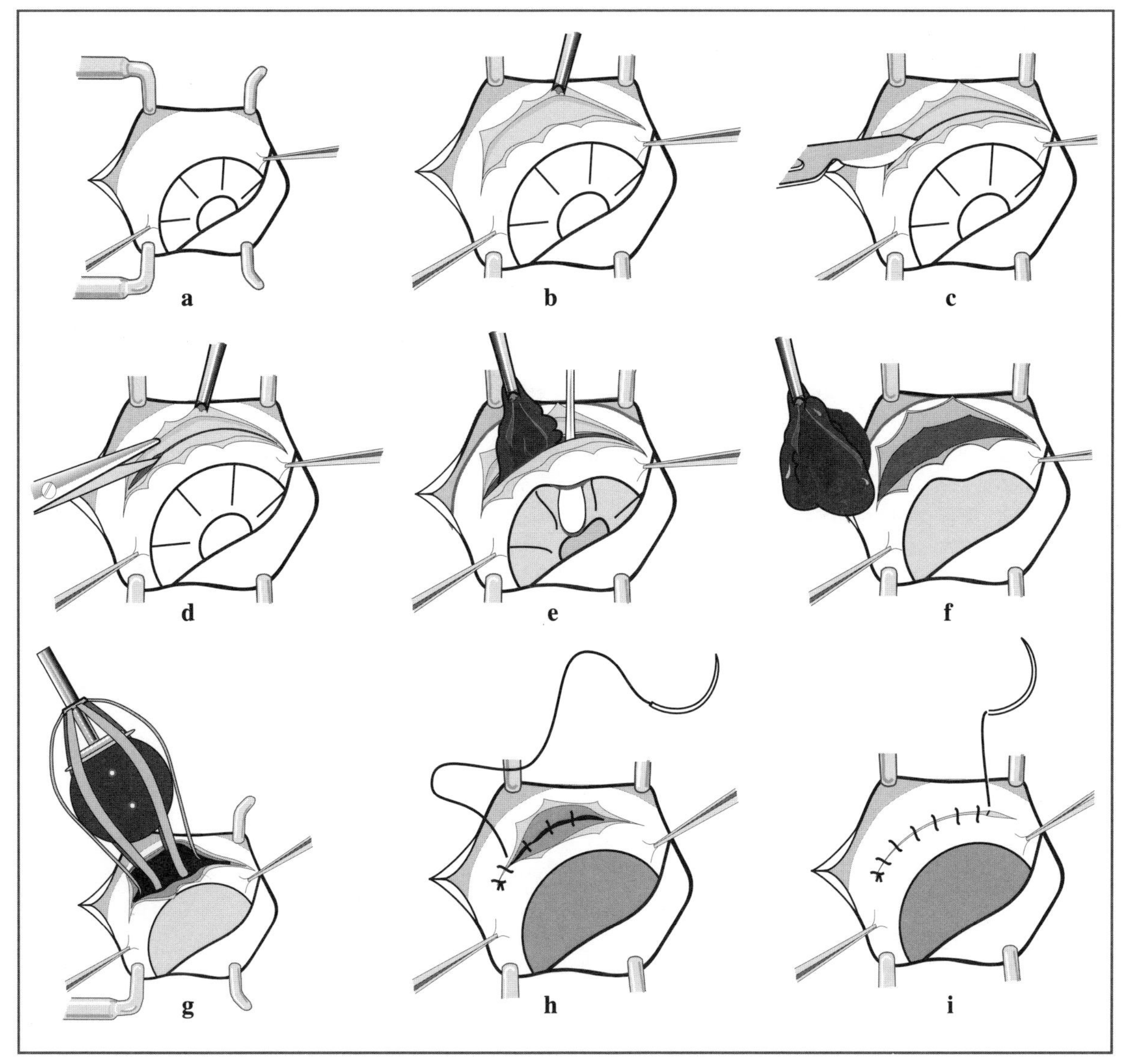

Figure 16-9. Intraocular prosthesis for blind glaucomatous eye

a. Eye prepared for surgery. Lateral canthotomy and eyelid speculum provide exposure. Eye stabilized with fixation or mosquito forceps at 9 and 3 o'clock
b. Conjunctival incision completed and sclera exposed
c. Scleral incision initiated with scalpel results in collapse of eye
d. The incision can be completed from 10 to 2 o'clock position with Mayo scissors
e. Ciliary body separated from sclera with Green spatula
f. Appearance of eye after evisceration. Ocular contents visible to the left of the globe
g. Carter sphere introducer with silicone rubber sphere ready to transfer to globe
h. Sclera sutured with continuous pattern after 3 appositional sutures are placed. Note eye filled with blood
i. Continuous suture pattern in conjunctiva

g. The eye is now ready to have the implant inserted. Grasping the scleral wound edges at 12 o'clock will stabilize the wound making it easier to place the tip of the inserter into the corneoscleral shell. After the inserter tips are in the wound, the plunger is pushed, stretching the wound as the implant is inserted into the corneoscleral shell. The scleral wound should be extended if more than moderate pressure is needed to insert the implant. Excess pressure may tear the sclera resulting in a wound that will be difficult to suture.
h. Several techniques have been described for suturing the wound. I prefer a two layer closure. Using 6-0 absorbable suture, the scleral wound is approximated with 3 equally spaced simple interrupted sutures followed by a continuous suture pattern placed the entire length of the incision. Next, the conjunctiva is closed with 6-0 or 7-0 absorbable suture in a continuous pattern.

3. Aftercare - postsurgical pain is moderate and chemosis is quite severe. This can be reduced by premedication with flunixin meglumine.
    a. A tarsorrhaphy is recommended for buphthalmic eyes for 7 to 10 days
    b. Systemic antibiotics, flunixin meglumine, and analgesics are recommended for several days
4. *Comment*
    a. Blood will remain in the globe for several weeks
    b. Cornea - will develop marked interstitial keratitis with vascularization. If scarring is present, the cornea may remain white. By two months the interstitial keratitis will subside and the globe will have its final appearance.
    c. Prosthesis rejection is uncommon

Cyclocryosurgery (Fig 16-6)

1. If the pressure returns to normal, buphthalmos will persist. With low pressure the eye may return to normal or develop phthisis bulbi.
2. Ciliary body regeneration may occur, resulting in recurrence of glaucoma and necessitating an additional freeze
3. Latent hyphema may occur

Chemical ablation with intravitreal gentamicin - Intravitreal injection of 8 to 20 mg (12-15 average) of gentamicin will be toxic to the ciliary body pigment epithelium and retina, and will reduce IOP in a few days. The pressure stabilizes in one to two weeks. Gentamicin injection is an alternative to enucleation or intraocular prosthesis. The owner must be advised that gentamicin injection is also toxic to the retina and will result in blindness to a visual eye.

1. Advantages - inexpensive, can be done quickly, relatively nonpainful (combining 1 mg of dexamethasone further reduces pain)
2. Disadvantages - dosage varies with individuals
    a. Too little - elevated IOP persists
    b. Too much - extreme hypotension resulting in phthisis bulbi
    c. Secreting epithelium may regenerate and glaucoma return later
    d. May produce cataracts, especially if lens is luxated
3. Technique - aspirate a volume of aqueous from the anterior chamber (Fig 1-40; Chapter 1, page 38) equal to the volume of gentamicin mixture that will be injected into the vitreous (Fig 1-41; Chapter 1, page 38).

GLAUCOMA IN CATS

Cats are less predisposed to glaucoma than dogs because of their relatively large iridocorneal angle and ciliary cleft.

CLASSIFICATION

Primary glaucoma - is rare in cats. The author has worked with a blood line of Siamese cats in which primary glaucoma was diagnosed and responded well to medical treatment with epinephrine 1% and oral Neptazane.

Secondary glaucoma

1. Usually due to inflammatory changes (chronic lymphocytic-plasmacytic uveitis) - rule out toxoplasmosis
2. Neoplasia - especially iris melanoma; lymphosarcoma uncommon
3. Lens luxation - may cause glaucoma but more frequently is a complication of chronic glaucoma

SIGNS - Often chronic, bilateral and has buphthalmos **(Fig 16-10)**

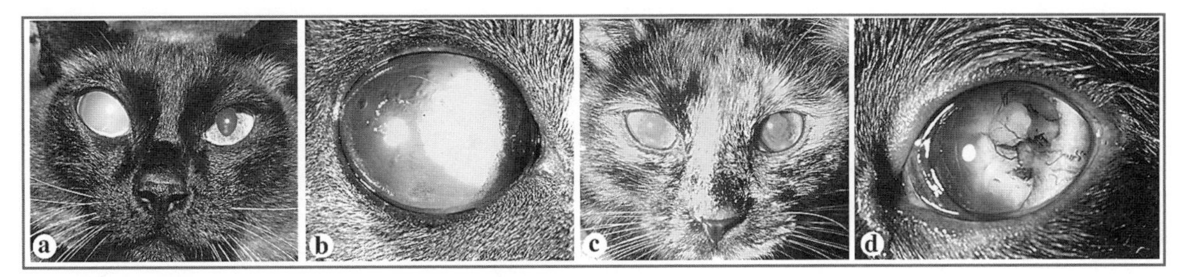

Figure 16-10. Clinical signs occurring with feline glaucoma
- a. Siamese cat with buphthalmos secondary to chronic glaucoma
- b. Chronic glaucoma with buphthalmos, secondary lens luxation and degenerative keratitis (pigmentation, bullous keratitis)
- c. Domestic shorthair cat with bilateral uveitis and secondary glaucoma in the right eye. Cat was FeLV positive.
- d. Intraocular tumor resulting in secondary glaucoma

Insidious - onset with owner unaware disease exists until eye shows buphthalmos, secondary corneal changes and lens displacement

Pain - minimal; usually lack of epiphora and blepharospasm

Cornea - minimal (if any) edema. Chronic scarring and vascularization may occur.

Lens luxation - due to buphthalmos. This may occur with a clear cornea.

Ophthalmoscopic examination

1. Retinal degeneration with vascular attenuation and areas of tapetal hyperreflectivity
2. Optic nerve is cupped. This is difficult to evaluate because of the cat's normally flat optic nerve.

Vision - Cats, even with obvious buphthalmos, will remain visual much longer than dogs. Tonometry - pressure seldom exceeds 40 to 50 mm Hg.

MEDICAL TREATMENT

The cause should be determined and eliminated. If cause can be eliminated, pressures are more apt to return to normal and remain normal without further treatment than secondary glaucoma in dogs.

Anti-inflammatory - If due to inflammatory changes, systemic corticosteroids are very beneficial.

Antiglaucoma drugs

1. Cats respond to mannitol, methazolamide, epinephrine or Propine, and apparently beta blockers.
2. Cholinesterase inhibiting miotics should be avoided because they can be cumulative and toxic to cats.

SURGICAL TREATMENT - usually considered only when the eye is blind

Enucleation (see Chapter 17, page 495, for enucleation techniques)

Evisceration and intraocular implant - Cats with buphthalmos have a higher incidence of implant extrusion; this is probably due to scleral thinning due to buphthalmos. A risk of postsurgical sarcoma may also exist.

Intravitreal injection with gentamicin - This may predispose to intraocular sarcoma formation.

EQUINE GLAUCOMA

Glaucoma is uncommon in horses and appears to be related to their high unconventional aqueous outflow. When seen, glaucoma is usually secondary.

CLASSIFICATION

Congenital - rare **(Fig 16-11)**

1. Present at birth and may be unilateral or bilateral
2. Marked buphthalmos with secondary luxation of a microphakic lens

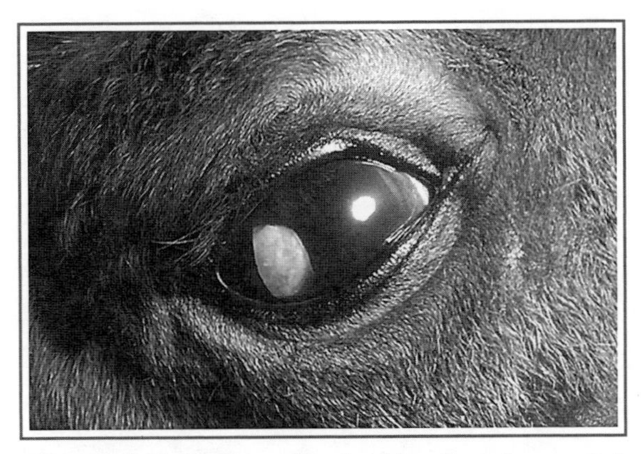

Figure 16-11. Five day old colt with unilateral congenital glaucoma, buphthalmos, lens subluxation and cataract. Note the lens is microphakic indicating intrauterine lens growth stopped when the pressure became elevated.

Primary - rare

The author has seen two cases - one unilateral and the other initially unilateral that became bilateral in eight months.

Secondary - compromise of aqueous outflow

1. After inflammation - recurrent uveitis most common
   a. Peripheral anterior synechia
   b. Iridis rubeosis with a preiridal fibrovascular membrane that is proposed to obstruct the filtration angle
   c. Inflammatory exudate
2. Intraocular neoplasia
3. Post-traumatic

SIGNS - chronic glaucoma is most common

Acute glaucoma

1. Ocular pain (epiphora, blepharospasm)
2. Vascular injection (conjunctival and episcleral)
3. Corneal edema
4. Anterior chamber and iris
   a. Primary - normal depth and mydriasis
   b. Secondary - swollen iris with shallow anterior chamber. Pupil may be small with iris bombé.
5. Vision - usually blind

Chronic glaucoma - most cases are chronic when presented **(Fig 16-12)**

1. Little or no pain
2. Buphthalmos - this is what the owner is often most concerned about
3. Conjunctival-scleral injection - absent to mild
4. Cornea
   a. Corneal edema is proportional to pressure and endothelial damage
   b. Vascularization - minimal, if any
   c. Corneal striae (Haab's striae) - *interconnecting parallel lines that are equally spaced* due to rupture of Descemet's membrane. These are not to be confused with *striae that vary in width* and are occasionally seen in the cornea of normal eyes.
5. Anterior chamber is deep
6. Iris - mydriasis with poor or absent pupillary reflex. Posterior synechia can affect pupil size and shape. Iridodonesis may be present if there is lens displacement.
7. Lens ± cataract or displacement from zonule degeneration
8. Fundus examination - optic nerve atrophy and sometimes area of retinal atrophy. Retinal detachment may be an incidental finding.
9. IOP - affected eye usually elevated but may become hypotonic from ciliary body atrophy

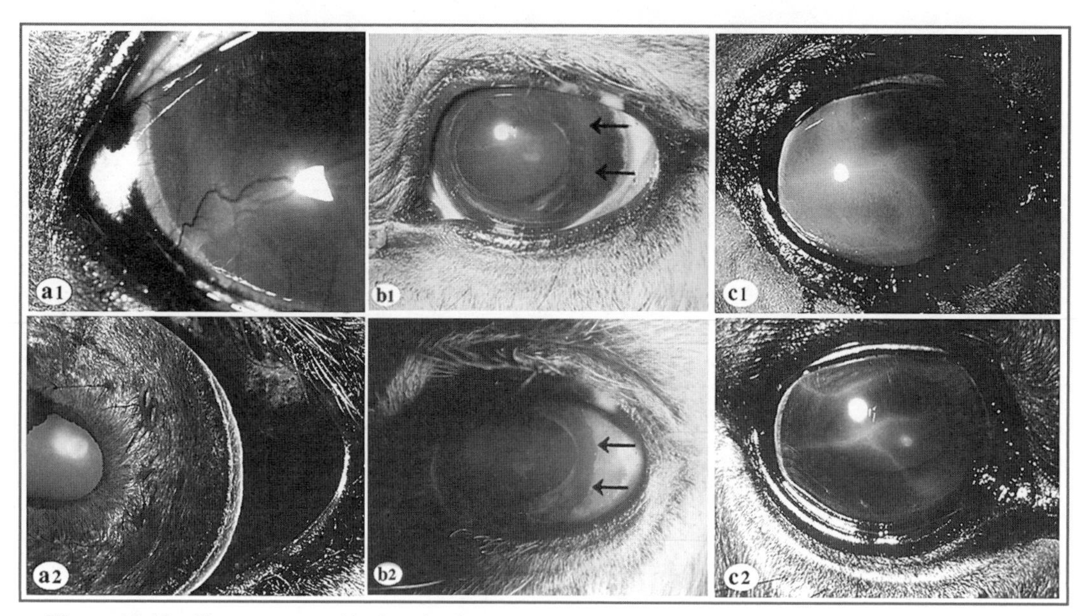

Figure 16-12. Changes seen with chronic glaucoma
a. Chronic glaucoma right eye, left eye normal
   1) Right eye showing filtration angle obstruction
   2) Left eye normal filtration angle
b. Bilateral chronic glaucoma both eyes; left eye shown. History of equine recurrent uveitis.
   1) Direct illumination showing moderate mydriasis, dark iris and faint temporal corneal edema (arrows)
   2) Transillumination reveals extensive anterior peripheral synechia (arrows)
c. Horse presented with acute uveitis and secondary chronic glaucoma right eye
   1) Eye at presentation - epiphora, generalized corneal edema prominent near corneal striae and dark iris
   2) Appearance after treatment with systemic flunixin meglumine and topical demecarium (Humersol) BID. Pressure now normal and clinical signs disappeared except striae.

TREATMENT

Primary glaucoma - has responded to demecarium bromide (Humersol) 0.5% BID. Pilopine-HS gel 4% should be effective but has not been used by the author.

Acute secondary glaucoma - treat the primary *uveitis*. Systemic anti-inflammatory agents. Anterior chamber injection of 25 to 50 μg tPA for fibrin, hemorrhage, or synechia. Miotics can be used if the pupil is unobstructed.

Chronic secondary glaucoma - visual eye - value is questionable

1. Systemic - aspirin daily to reduce recurrence of uveitis
2. Topical - demecarium bromide (Humersol) 0.5%, dipivefrin (Propine) 0.1%, or Pilocarpine gel 4% (Pilopine-HS gel 4%) BID
3. Cyclocryotherapy - author has had success but horses are more prone to post-cryohemorrhage than dogs and cats. Technique is the same except cryoprobe placed 7 mm from limbus dorsal and ventral and 3 mm nasal and temporal (Fig 16-13).
4. Transcleral cyclophotocoagulation (laser).

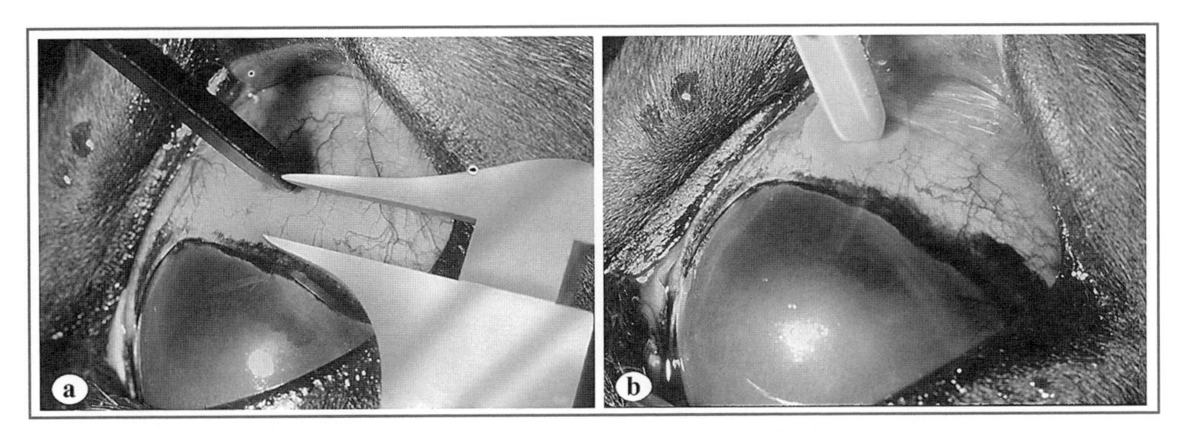

Figure 16-13. Cyclocryosurgery for chronic glaucoma of visual eye
a. Measuring 7 mm from limbus for dorsal placement of cryoprobes
b. Freezing ciliary body. Ice ball has progressed to 1 mm of the limbus.

Chronic secondary glaucoma - blind eye

1. If nonpainful, not subject to recurrent uveitis or ulcers; the owner may choose not to treat
2. Intravitreal Gentocin, 25 to 50 mg - will relieve pain and control pressure; same technique and complications as stated for dogs (Fig 1-40 and 1-41; Chapter 1, page 38)
3. Evisceration and intraocular sphere implant - this procedure offers a cosmetic eye and no pain after several days. The technique is the same as previously described for small animals (Fig 16-8, page 468), except for the scleral incision. In the equine the parallel scleral incision needs to be nearly 180° (9 to 3 o'clock) to allow introduction of the implant. An alternative technique is a "T" incision combined with a 10 to 2 o'clock parallel incision (Fig 16-14). After the parallel incision has been made, a perpendicular scissors incision is made at 12 o'clock and extended to the equator of the globe. After intraocular contents have been removed, the perpendicular incision is closed before the parallel incision. The author prefers 5-0 absorbable suture for the sclera and 6-0 for the conjunctival closure.
4. Enucleation with orbital implants (see Chapter 17, page 495, for enucleation technique).

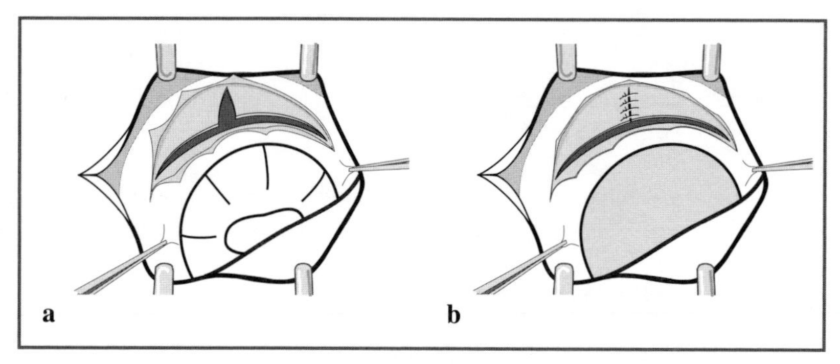

Figure 16-14. "T" scleral incision for equine intraocular implant

a. A scleral incision is started at the 12 o'clock position and extended toward the equator of the globe

b. The incision is closed with interrupted sutures before closing the parallel incision

CHAPTER 17 - DISEASES OF THE ORBIT AND GLOBE

ANATOMY

BONY ORBIT

Horses and ruminants

1. The bony orbit is complete in horses and ruminants
2. The eyes are placed laterally, giving a very wide field of vision, but limited binocular vision

Dogs and cats

1. In dogs and cats, the bony orbit is incomplete in the dorsolateral area, which is filled in with the supraorbital ligament extending from the zygomatic process of the frontal bone to the frontal process of the zygomatic (malar) bone. This and the depth of the orbit predisposes the cat and dog to traumatic proptosis of the eye.
2. The depth of the orbit varies with skull type
   a. Brachycephalic - a shallow orbit with anteriorly placed eyes, providing better binocular field but predisposing to eye proptosis
   b. Mesocephalic - a deeper orbit, more lateral position of the eyes with less binocular, a wider visual field, and reduced chance for proptosis
   c. Dolichocephalic - deepest orbit, extreme laterally positioned eyes, poor binocular visual field and rarely seen with proptosis

ORBITAL TISSUES

Periorbita - The connective tissue sheath of the orbit

1. It lines the bones of the orbit and becomes thicker in areas where bone is absent
2. Continuous with the periosteum of the bones of the orbital rim and septum orbitale

Dura of optic nerve - Divides into two layers as it enters the orbit **(Fig 17-1)**

1. Outer portion - is the periorbita
2. Inner portion - is Tenon's capsule. Tenon's capsule covers the extrinsic ocular muscles and extends to the limbus where it joins the conjunctiva and anchors to the globe. Conjunctiva can be easily separated from Tenon's capsule about 2 mm from the limbus.

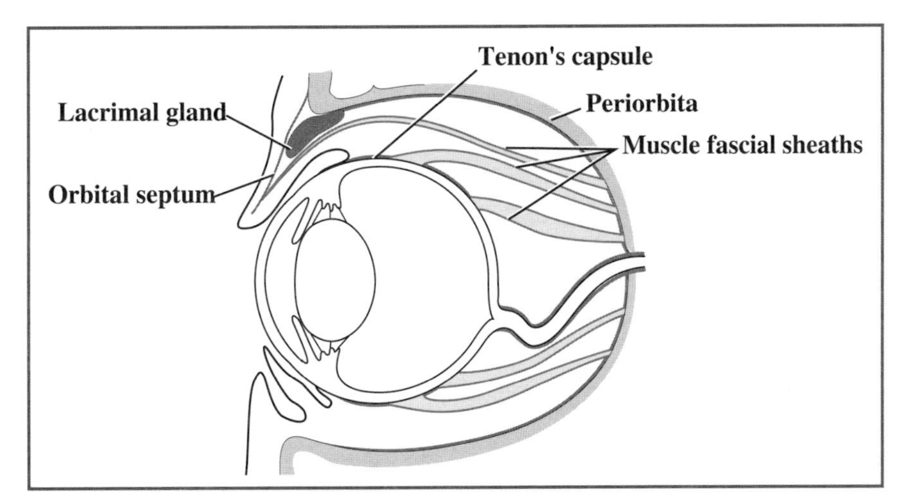

Figure 17-1. Divisions of orbital fascia.

Orbital fat pad - Located between orbital wall and periorbita

Extrinsic muscles of the eye and levator palpebrae superioris - The extrinsic muscles are the dorsal (superior) rectus, medial rectus, ventral (inferior) rectus, lateral rectus, dorsal (superior) oblique, ventral (inferior) oblique, and retractor oculi (bulbi). The dorsal oblique passes through a trochlea in the dorsomedial portion of the orbit. All but the ventral oblique originate at the optic foramen, it originates from the medial wall of the orbit near the lacrimal fossa (Fig 17-2).

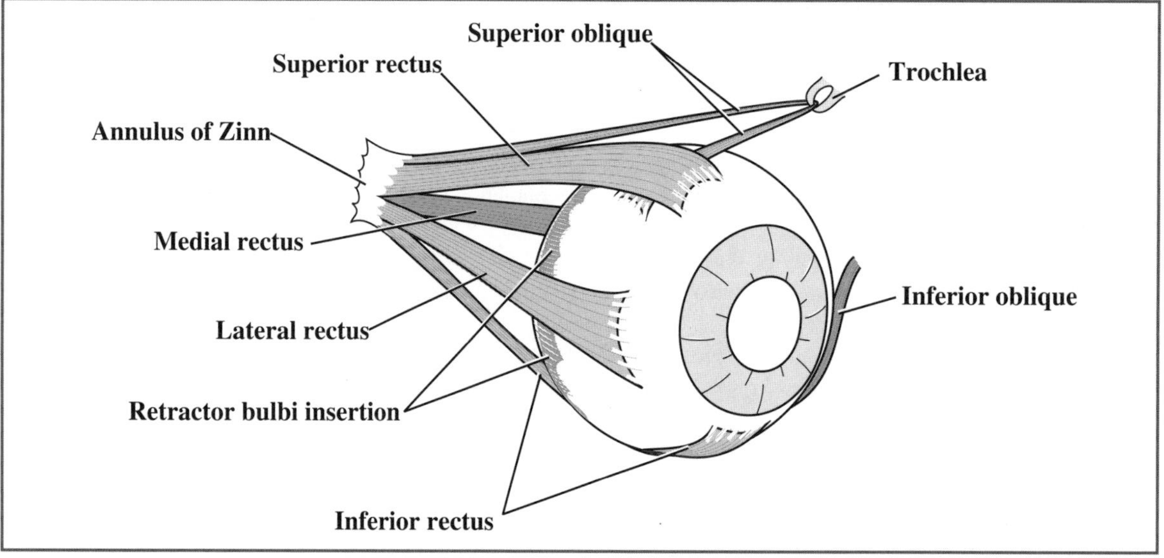

Figure 17-2. Arrangement of orbital muscles Modified from Prince JH et al: Anatomy and histology of the eye of domestic animals. Charles C. Thomas, Springfield, IL, 1960.

Glands

1. Lacrimal gland inside the dorsal lateral rim of the orbit. Very large in horses.
2. Zygomatic salivary gland - outside the periorbita below the level of the zygomatic arch and covered by the temporal and masseter muscles. The duct opens near the last molar.
3. Gland of the third eyelid

THE PROMINENT EYE

CAUSES FOR A PROMINENT EYE

Exophthalmos - a normal sized eye that is pathologically forced forward

1. Space-occupying lesion in the orbit
   a. Abscess/cellulitis (abscessed tooth root, zygomatic sialoadenitis, foreign bodies)
   b. Retrobulbar neoplasia (primary/secondary)
   c. Retrobulbar hemorrhage (trauma, blood dyscrasias, clotting defects)
   d. Cysts (zygomatic/orbital mucocele)
   e. Granuloma/edema (immune-mediated)
   f. Arteriovenous fistula (very rare)
2. Deformity of the orbit
   a. Fracture
   b. Orbital neoplasia (bone, sinuses, nasal and oral cavity)
   c. Chronic frontal sinusitis in horses
   d. Mandibular hypertrophic osteoarthropathy in terriers
3. Muscle disease
   a. Eosinophilic myositis (muscles of mastication, ocular muscles)
   b. Degeneration of extraocular muscles (horses)

Breed predisposition

1. Brachycephalic dogs/cats with shallow orbit
2. Toy breeds with large eyes

Buphthalmos - an enlarged eye from chronic glaucoma

INCIDENCE OF PROMINENT EYES EXAMINED AT CSU-VTH

Dogs

1. Breed predisposition
2. Buphthalmos
3. Retrobulbar abscesses/cellulitis
4. Trauma with edema and hemorrhage
5. Orbital neoplasia

Cats

1. Trauma with hemorrhage/edema
2. Chronic glaucoma
3. Retrobulbar abscess/cellulitis
4. Orbital neoplasia

Equine

1. Buphthalmos
2. Inflammation/edema
3. Retrobulbar neoplasia
4. Trauma (fractures/hemorrhage)
5. Deformity (chronic sinusitis)

Cattle

1. Buphthalmos after infectious bovine keratitis
2. Acute cellulitis/edema
3. Retrobulbar neoplasia (orbital lymphosarcoma, invasive squamous cell carcinoma)

DIFFERENTIAL DIAGNOSIS OF A PROMINENT EYE

Rule out anatomic causes

1. Brachycephalic breeds with shallow orbit
2. Small breeds have a large eye in proportion to the size of the head (Chihuahua, Pomeranian, toy poodle, etc)

Measurement - if in doubt about buphthalmos, measure the corneal diameter and compare it with the normal globe

Displacement (small animals) - look at the cornea from the top of the head and compare the anterior placement of each eye

Retropulsion

1. Exophthalmos - retropulsion may vary from reduced to total absence (exception equine muscle degeneration)
2. Buphthalmos - retropulsion restricted in proportion to size of the eye
3. Breeds with shallow orbit - retropulsion limited, but same in both eyes
4. Small breeds - eye easily repulsed

Nictitans protrusion

1. Exophthalmos - nictitans protrusion is present and may precede globe displacement
2. Buphthalmos - no or minimal nictitans protrusion
3. Breed predisposition - normal position of third eyelid

DIFFERENTIAL DIAGNOSIS OF EXOPHTHALMOS

Trauma (fractures/hemorrhage) - history of injury and appearance of the patient

Infection (abscess/cellulitis)

1. Rapid onset
2. Painful
3. Systemic signs (increase temperature and WBC)

Noninflammatory (neoplasia, cysts)

1. No significant history
2. Nonpainful
3. Gradual development

RETROBULBAR ABSCESS

Occurrence - seen most frequently in small animals

Etiology

1. Abscessed zygomatic salivary gland

2. Migrating foreign bodies
3. Post-traumatic - fighting is the common cause in cats
4. Hematogenous - bacteremia in calves
5. Dental abscesses

Signs

1. Signs of acute infection - fever, increased WBC
2. Protrusion of third eyelid - lids may be normal or have moderate edema
3. Chemosis and conjunctivitis
4. Deviation of gaze
5. Corneal and anterior uveal changes ***may*** be seen
6. Vision is anticipated to be normal
7. Opening mouth very painful in small animals
   a. Oral palpation reveals swelling behind last molar
   b. Visual examination may demonstrate discoloration of oral mucous membrane where abscess is pointing

Treatment - dogs and cats

Establishing drainage, followed by systemic antibiotics is most successful.

1. General anesthesia
2. Drain into the mouth (Fig 17-3) or into the region of the zygomatic arch. The weakest spot in the orbit is immediately behind the last molar and nearly all abscesses will surface at this area.
   a. Tap the abscess with a 16 or 18 gauge needle and aspirate a small amount to determine that the lesion is an abscess; withdraw the needle.

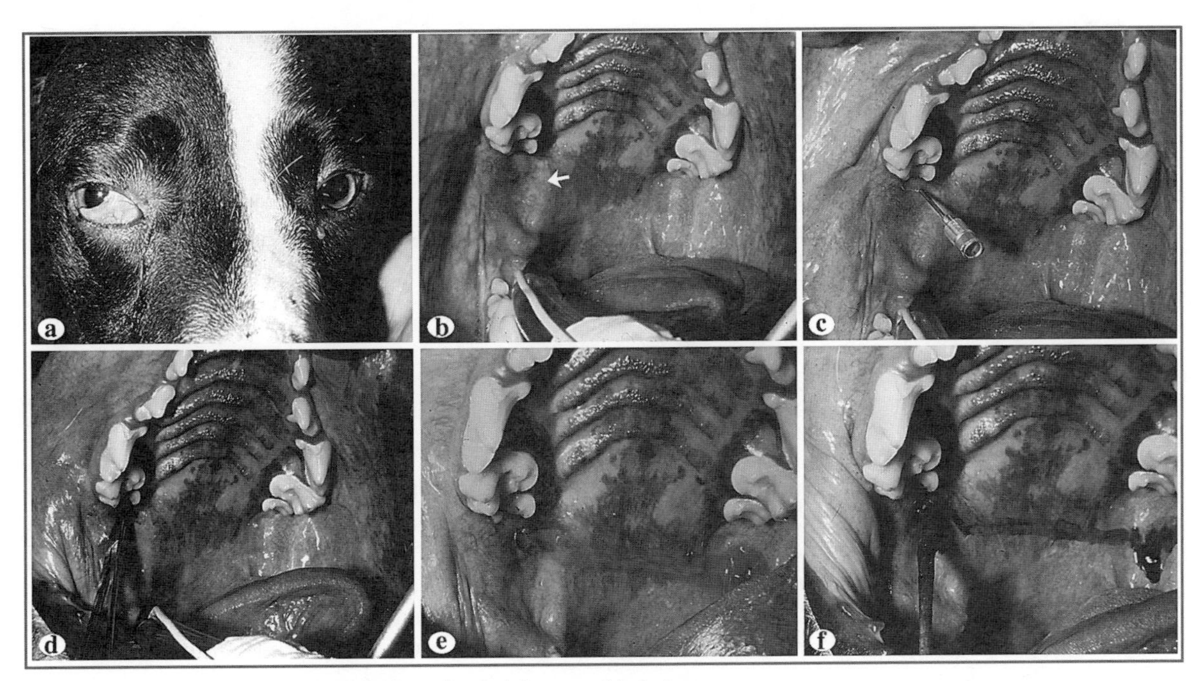

Figure 17-3. Technique for draining an orbital abscess.
a. Appearance at entry - note protrusion of the third eyelid and exophthalmos
b. Swelling in the area of the palatine fossa (arrow)
c. Eighteen gauge needle introduced into abscess
d. Establishing drainage with mosquito forceps
e. Pus draining from the wound
f. Swabbing abscess with Betadine swab

        1) Advance the tip of a curved hemostatic forceps through the needle track, then open the forceps and withdraw it. This will bluntly enlarge the wound and establish liberal drainage.
        2) An alternate method would be to incise into the abscess with a scalpel blade, followed by enlarging the incision with a hemostatic forceps.
    b. Swab out the abscess with a 1:50 dilute Betadine-soaked swab
    c. Start systemic antibiotics
    d. If uveitis is present - systemic prednisolone
    e. Topical antibiotic/steroid if secondary conjunctivitis
    f. Warm compresses will help reduce swelling
    g. Diseased teeth should be extracted if involved

Prognosis

1. Favorable - if drainage is established
2. If drainage cannot be established and only systemic antibiotics are given, recurrence is common
3. Optic neuritis is rare, but can lead to atrophy and blindness

Treatment in horses

Lance and drain temporal or dorsal to the globe. Treat like any other abscess.

ORBITAL CELLULITIS - seen more frequently in cats

Signs - compared to retrobulbar abscess
1. More swelling and discoloration of eyelids
2. Severe chemosis
3. Minimal exophthalmos
4. Minimal or negligible pain on opening the mouth

Treatment

1. Systemic antibiotics
2. Hot compresses
3. If cellulitis localizes, it will drain around the eye. Purulent discharge over the eye does not cause any harm.
4. If diseased teeth, especially dogs, provide appropriate dental care and swelling disappears in a few days.

Prognosis - favorable

RETROBULBAR NEOPLASIA

Etiology

1. Dogs - as dogs live longer, more neoplasia is diagnosed. Orbital neoplasia includes nasal adenocarcinomas, osteosarcoma, malignant melanoma, hemangiosarcoma and mast cell sarcoma. Optic nerve meningeoma is the most common ocular tumor.
2. Cats - orbital lymphosarcoma most common
3. Cattle - orbital lymphosarcoma and invasive squamous cell carcinoma
4. Horses - invasive squamous cell carcinoma, angiosarcoma, adenocarcinoma lacrimal gland, and optic nerve meningioma.

Signs

1. Slowly progressive exophthalmos - direction of deviation of the eye often indicates the location of the tumor
    a. Anterior - indicates a mass behind the eye

   b. Dorsal - a mass ventral to the globe
   c. Lateral - a mass medial to the globe
   d. *Comment* - tumors of the orbital rim lead to enophthalmos
2. No pain when opening mouth
3. Orbital deformity may be present
4. Globe - may develop exposure keratitis and conjunctivitis
5. Vision - blind if optic nerve is involved or exophthalmos is severe
6. Third eyelid is usually very prominent except when tumor is associated with optic nerve

Diagnosis

1. Clinical signs
2. Fine needle aspiration
3. X-rays - will identify bony involvement
4. Ultrasound - useful in large and small animals (CT scan will provide better orbital imaging)
5. CT scan - if available is excellent for small animals

Treatment - Many orbital tumors are invasive and/or malignant, and will require multiple therapy techniques. Referral or consultation with an oncologist is recommended. Aggressive treatment may prolong life but quality of life should be seriously considered before treatment is started.

1. Surgery - varies with the cell type and location of the lesion
   a. Enucleation or exenteration for tumors within the orbital cavity, especially optic nerve meningioma originating at the globe.
   b. Orbitotomy provides the opportunity to examine the orbit for retrobulbar tumors that may be operable and perform exenteration
   c. Orbitectomy - combined with exenteration when the bony orbit is involved. Radiation or chemotherapy will also be indicated.
   d. Chemotherapy - if cell type is known, chemotherapy can arrest some tumors
   e. Radiation - megavoltage radiation for orbital, nasal, and paranasal cavity malignant neoplasms has had limited success but may cause severe ophthalmic changes if the eye and adnexa are in the radiation field

ORBITAL CYSTS AND MUCOCELES (Uncommon)

Etiology

1. Congenital - likely to occur concurrently with microphthalmia and dermoids
2. Acquired
   a. Zygomatic salivary gland
   b. Lacrimal gland (orbital or gland third eyelid). The author has seen two gland of the third eyelid cysts in dogs. Cysts involving the lacrimal canaliculi or sac are rare.
   c. Post-traumatic
   d. Retrobulbar hydatid cysts have been reported in horses

Zygomatic salivary gland mucoceles

1. Incidence - rare. The author has seen three zygomatic salivary cysts.
2. Signs of zygomatic salivary gland cyst
   a. Slowly progressive, nonpainful, exophthalmos, and marked protrusion of the third eyelid
   b. Oral examination
      1) Two dogs has marked swelling of the palatine fossa. The mucous membranes were normal in one dog and in the other appeared thin with an amber shading. Aspiration yielded thick amber fluid.
      2) The third dog did not have swelling in the postmaxillary area. The cyst was aspirated through the skin from below the zygomatic arch

Treatment

1. Mucoceles with swelling of the palatine fossa - After incising the mucosa, the cyst was separated from the mucosa and digitally stripped free from the muscle and adjacent tissue until the gland could be palpated and removed. The mucosal wound was sutured and healed uneventfully.
2. Mucocele without oral swelling - This cyst could be palpated adjacent to and deep to the zygomatic arch. It was drained and a Penrose tube was placed in the cyst cavity and secured to the skin. The cyst recurred in 45 days. At that time a decision was made to do an orbitotomy with zygomatic arch resection. Using this technique, the cyst was visualized and removed with the associated gland. The dog recovered uneventfully.
3. Aspiration and intralesional injection with oxytetracycline has been described, but has not been used by the author.

ACUTE EOSINOPHILIC MYOSITIS

An acute plasmacytic, lymphocytic and eosinophilic infiltration of the muscles of mastication.

Etiology - cause unknown, but thought to be an immune-mediated reaction of the type 2M fibers of the muscles of mastication

Incidence - any breed, but primarily German shepherd, German shepherd crosses, Samoyed, and Doberman pinscher

Signs
1. All of the muscles of mastication are swollen and firm
2. Pain on opening the jaw
3. Ocular
   a. Exophthalmos - due to swollen muscles forcing orbital fat forward
      1) Keratitis
      2) Conjunctivitis
   b. Prolapse third eyelid
   c. Vision - may be blind if optic neuritis occurs
4. Systemic signs - variable
   a. May have myositis of other muscles
   b. Enlarged lymph nodes

Diagnosis
1. Clinical signs
2. Laboratory findings during acute stage - elevated creatine phosphokinase (CPK), eosinophilia, and muscle biopsy showing increased eosinophils

Treatment

Systemic prednisolone, with reducing dosage for several months. Then treated according to response.

Sequelae - Recurrent attacks leading to muscle atrophy, trismus and weight loss

CANINE EXTRAOCULAR POLYMYOSITIS (BILATERAL EXTRAOCULAR POLYMYOSITIS [BEP])

Etiology - Cause unknown, but thought to be an immune-mediated disease restricted to the extraocular muscles (extrinsic muscles of the eyes), which are type 1M fibers.

Incidence - Usually young dogs, large breeds (golden retriever most frequently affected), females predisposed 2:1, and may be preceded by stress.

Signs
1. First sign is chemosis of the bulbar conjunctiva.
2. Exophthalmos - two to eight days after onset of chemosis. Always bilateral, but not necessarily symmetrical.
3. Other signs - variable
   a. Scleral exposure/upper eyelid retraction.
   b. Mild resistance to retropulsion.
   c. Moderate increase in IOP.
   d. Visual impairment (reversible with treatment).
   e. Fundus - tortuous retinal veins, focal retinitis, optic neuropathy.

Treatment
1. Oral prednisolone with reducing dosage up to six weeks.
2. Oral azathioprine - not as effective as prednisolone. It can be used with prednisolone allowing reduced dosage of both medications if long-term treatment is needed.

Course - Relapse is common, up to 60-80%, and may correlate with stress (e.g., estrus, kenneling).

MUSCLE DEGENERATION IN HORSES

The author had a case of unilateral exophthalmos in a horse that was progressive for seven months, leading to exposure keratopathy and recurrent ulcers. When the eye was removed, the orbit was normal but the extrinsic muscles were thin and flabby. Histologic examination revealed muscle degeneration. An etiology was not determined.

ORBIT DEFORMITY FROM CHRONIC SINUSITIS IN HORSES

Signs
1. Exophthalmos - chronic and progressive. If allowed to continue, ***chronic sinusitis can cause blindness due to optic nerve atrophy.***
2. Physical examination
   a. Bulging of the skull over the sinus area
   b. Percussion of the sinus area - dull due to fluid
3. Diagnostic examination
   a. X-ray and ultrasound - reveals fluid distended sinuses with lateral deviation of the nasal orbital wall, which in turn results in exophthalmos.
4. Digital examination of the orbit under anesthesia - outward deviation of the bony orbit over the sinus

Treatment
1. Drain the sinus
2. If the eye is blind and severe corneal ulcers are present, eye removal may be indicated

CONGENITAL HYDROCEPHALUS

Enlargement of the calvarium from congenital hydrocephalus can result in the distortion of the dorsomedial orbit resulting in moderate exophthalmos and lateral-downward strabismus.

ORBITAL GRANULOMAS

We have had two horses in which needle aspirates revealed inflammatory reaction with large numbers of eosinophils. Antibiotic and concurrent steroid therapy brought about regression of signs within 14 and 20 days respectively.

ORBITAL EDEMA

Incidence - all species

Etiology - usually results from orbital circulatory disturbance or acute allergy
1. Unilateral - anticipate local cause (e.g. orbital tumor, trauma)
2. Bilateral - anticipate systemic cause (circulatory interference, allergy)
3. "Downer" and moribund septicemic large animals
4. We had a horse suspended in a sling that would rest its head on the manger, resulting in severe venous congestion of the head, leading to extreme transient orbital and eyelid edema.

Signs - severe edema in and around the orbit
1. Chemosis
2. Swelling of the eyelids
3. Variable exophthalmos

Treatment - identify and treat the primary cause

THE DEEP-SET EYE

CAUSES FOR THE DEEP-SET EYE

Enophthalmos
1. Dehydration
2. Decreased orbital fat (cachexia, traumatic loss of fat)
3. Increased tone to extraocular muscles
4. Fibrosis of the muscles of mastication
5. Breed predisposition - breeds with a deep orbit
6. Posterior episcleritis

Small globe size

THE SMALL EYE

TERMS

Anophthalmos - Absence of a true eyeball. Except for swine, an extremely rare condition. Histologic examination of orbital tissues will usually reveal some vestigial ocular tissues.
Microphthalmos - An abnormally small eyeball. Seen sporadically in all species and most commonly in dogs.
Nanophthalmos - A nonfunctional microphthalmic eye. Term is infrequently used.
Phthisis bulbi - A shrunken, fibrotic globe resulting from injury or intraocular inflammation.

MICROPHTHALMOS

Incidence and cause
1. Dogs - common. Usually genetic predisposition.
    a. Color dilute genetics (merle genetics in collie and related breeds, harlequin in Great Dane). Homozygote merles are more severely affected.
    b. Inherited in many breeds. See Appendix IV, ACVO table of inherited eye diseases.
    c. Drugs - griseofulvin
    d. Sporadic from unknown causes
2. Cats - rare
3. Horses - rare
4. Cattle
    a. Hereford - has been associated with muscular dystrophy and hydrocephalus
    b. Guernsey, white Shorthorn, and Hereford - inheritance has been proposed
5. Sheep, goats, llama - uncommon

Signs - variable from small normal eye to an eye with multiple defects and blindness
1. Small eyelid opening - size of eyelid opening is related to size of the eye
2. Protrusion third eyelid - may interfere with vision in some patients
3. Globe - may be small with normal vision or have multiple dysplastic changes resulting in blindness

Treatment - none

PHTHISIS BULBI

Incidence - occurs in all species

Etiology - occurs after severe damage to the ciliary body, thereby decreasing aqueous production

1. Trauma
2. Panophthalmitis
3. As a sequelae to chronic glaucoma with severe ciliary body atrophy

Signs

1. Onset after severe uveal damage
    a. Animals less than four months old - 2-4 weeks
    b. Adults - 1-2 months
2. Small globe with opaque cornea. As the globe shrinks, the sclera contracts more rapidly than the cornea, resulting in the cornea becoming globus (Fig 17-4). This exaggerates the difference in globe curvature at the limbus.
3. Adnexa and face - as the globe contracts, the eyelids lose their support. This results in increased ocular discharge, contraction of the eyelids and in some cases entropion.
    In large animals, the ocular discharge leads to severe summer fly problems as well as being unsightly.
4. Pain - the eye is not acutely painful but secondary keratoconjunctivitis and blepharitis can be troublesome.

Treatment - none, if no secondary problems

1. If causing problems, the best treatment from the patient's standpoint would be to remove the blind eye and position an orbital implant before closing the wound. See enucleation, page 495.

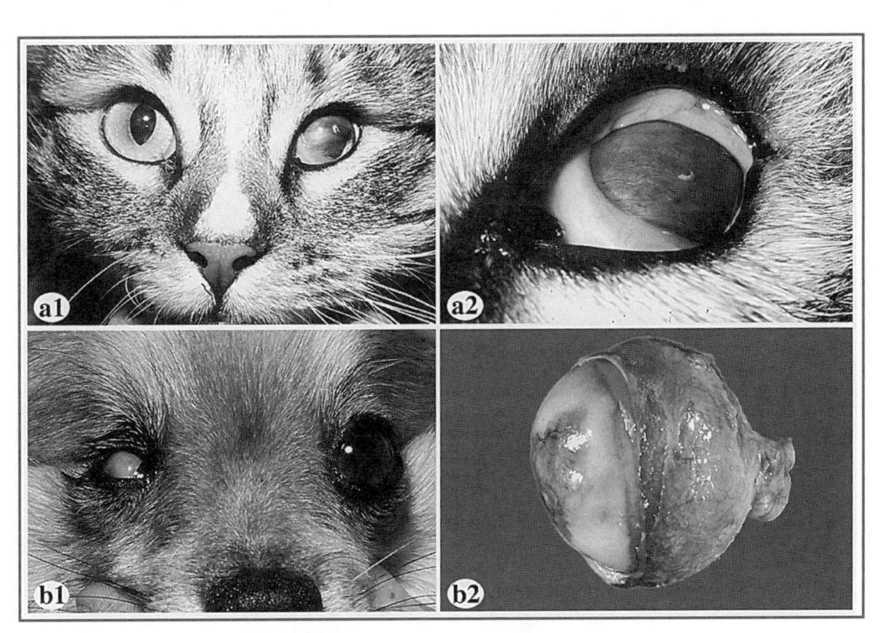

Figure 17-4. Phthisis bulbi.
- a. Cat with phthisis bulbi of left eye after corneal injury
    1) Frontal view
    2) Close up - note clear cornea and visible iris
- b. Pomeranian with phthisis bulbi after replacement of proptosed eye
    1) Frontal view - note corneal edema
    2) Cross section of eye after enucleation - note keratoglobus as a result of sclera contracting faster than the cornea

2. If cosmetic appearance is a factor, the owner may choose a corneoscleral prosthesis (Fig 17-5). This is the treatment of choice for moderate phthisis bulbi.

A successful corneoscleral prosthesis is dependent on normal eyelids and well defined superior and inferior fornices. Fabrication of a successful prosthesis requires close cooperation between the veterinarian and an ocularist. CSU works with Walter Johnson (Denver Optic Co) and William Trawnik (Dallas Eye Prosthetics).

a. Materials needed (these are usually available from the ocularist)
   1) Casting impression trays (Denver Optic) or molded by the veterinarian from Orthoplast (Johnson & Johnson orthopedic)
   2) Casting material (a fast-setting alginate)
   3) Dental stone casting material
   4) Distilled water, 20 cc syringe, mixing bowl and a sealable plastic bag for shipping the cast made of the eye

b. Casting technique (Fig 17-5)
   1) Restraint - A shortacting general anesthetic is desirable for making the cast. After one has done this procedure several times, castings can be made from calm horses using a palpebral nerve block, topical anesthetic and chemical restraint.

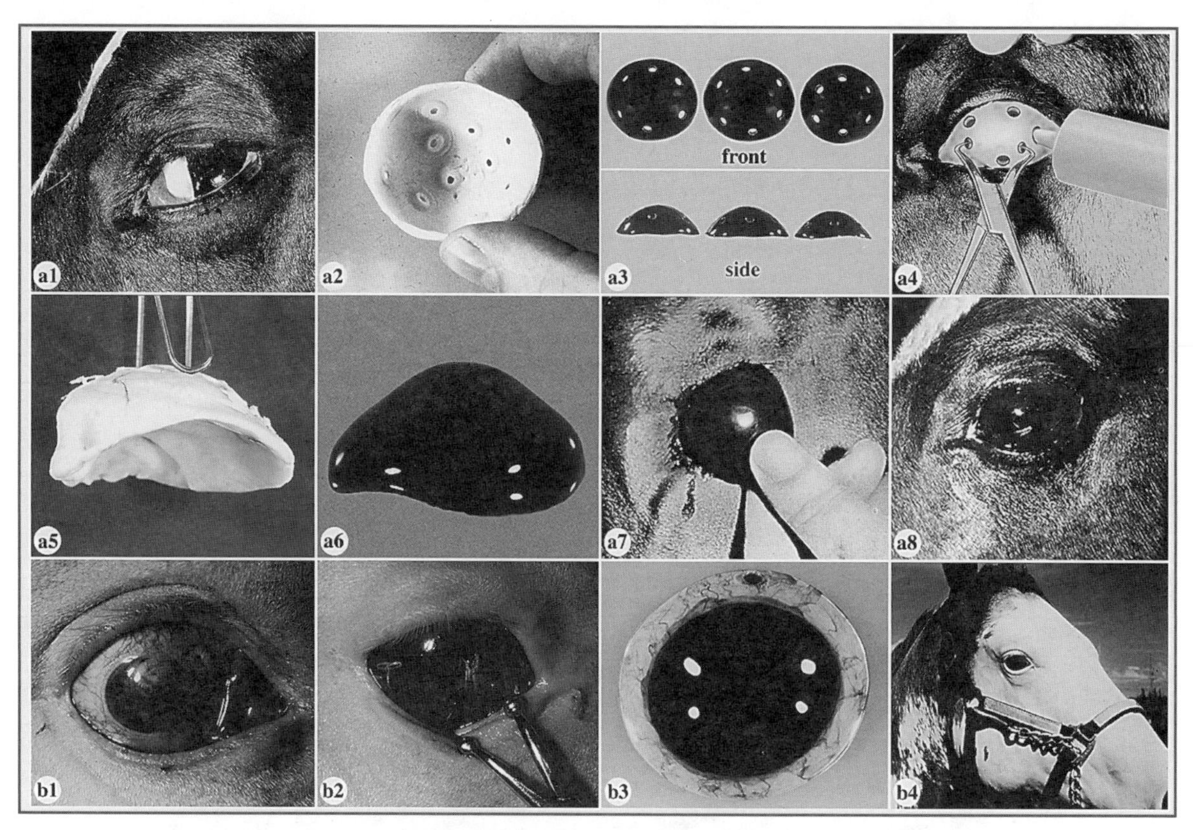

Figure 17-5. Corneoscleral prosthesis.

a. Quarter Horse with phthisis bulbi
   1) Eye at presentation
   2) Impression tray molded from Orthoplast
   3) Impression trays available from Denver Optic
   4) Molding material injected through an opening in an Orthoplast impression tray
   5) Appearance of mold when removed from orbit
   6) Finished prosthesis
   7) Insertion of prosthesis below upper eyelid
   8) Appearance of horse after prosthesis placement

b. Appaloosa with blind eye after perforating ulcer
   1) Eye at presentation
   2) Denver Optic impression tray positioned behind eyelids
   3) Finished prosthesis - note blood vessels represented by fine red thread
   4) Appearance of horse after prosthesis placement

2) Alginate preparation - The ophthalmic alginate is prepared by carefully following the manufacturer's instructions. The warmer the temperature, the faster the alginate sets up.

3) A 20 cc syringe is filled with alginate

4) Molding the eye - The template is positioned behind the eyelids. The template is held with a towel clamp that has had the tips clipped and blunted. The template is elevated away from the phthisic globe until the eyelid and the template appear similar to the position of the normal eye. It is best to have the template position appear slightly enophthalmic or normal. If the template is pulled excessively toward the lids, it will result in a casting that is too thick and will make the prosthesis appear exophthalmic. A thick prosthesis may be too heavy for the lids to hold in proper position. A template is chosen that can be slipped through the eyelid opening without using excess force. Remember, it will be necessary to place and remove the final prosthesis in a conscious patient. The alginate is injected through one of the holes in the template. The injection is continued until the space between the template and the eye has been filled. Care should be taken not to inject excessive casting material that would result in forcing the template excessively against the eyelids. The template and associated casting will be ready for removal when the alginate left in the mixing bowl has "set up" (3-5 min). This will be indicated by a dry, soft texture that when pressed with your finger will indent and then spring back without leaving an imprint. Before removing the casting, the template is marked with the position of the temporal and/or nasal canthus. The casting should be carefully worked out between the eyelids. The template will represent the anterior surface of the prosthesis and the molding material will have an exact imprint of the phthisical eye, third eyelid and conjunctiva.

c. Preparation of the casting for shipment to the ocularist. Two methods are possible, therefore check with the ocularist for his preference.

1) Sending the casting and impression tray. After removal of the casting from the eye, any irregularities are trimmed from the casting with a scalpel blade or scissors. The impression tray and casting are covered with moistened cotton or sponges and placed in a sealable plastic bag with a few cc's of water or PSS before packaging for shipment.

2) Preparing a dental stone mold from the casting. The dental stone casting material is mixed with water and gently agitated or tapped to bring air bubbles to the surface. A two piece dental stone investment (casting) is made by filling a paper cup one-third full with casting material and slightly embedding the posterior impression surface into the casting material as it would normally be positioned within the orbit. Fifteen minutes is allowed for cast setting. A thin layer of liquid soap is then applied on top of the investment surface. The anterior impression surface is carefully covered with casting material, making a second investment. The investments should completely cover the impression at a thickness of 1 to 2 cm. After setting is complete, the investments are separated (the layer of soap prevents adherence of the two portions) and the portion representing the socket surface is carefully examined. To aid the ocularist in the final prosthetic fabrication, the nasal, temporal, and third eyelid locations are labeled on the surface of the investment cast. The entire procedure is repeated if the impression or investment is imperfect. Accurate impression and investment will prevent secondary problems related to poor prosthetic fit. The impression and investment are sent to the ocularist. Two weeks should be allowed for the ocularist to fabricate a temporary prosthesis.

d. Prosthesis fitting - Sedation is recommended for the first fitting. If the horse is tractable, topical anesthesia may be all that is needed. The prosthesis will be white and will have a mark indicating how it is to be positioned in the socket. The adnexa is irrigated until all foreign material has been washed from the eye. A liberal amount of antibiotic corticosteroid ointment is applied to the prosthesis and eye socket. The prosthesis is slipped in by pushing it upward beneath the upper eyelid. The prosthesis is passed through the eyelid opening until the lower edge of the prosthesis falls behind the lower eyelid. Passing through the eyelid opening should be a snug fit. The prosthesis should then sit in a position with the posterior surface matching the contour of the globe and the third eyelid.

If the owner wants a pupil on the prosthesis, the prosthesis is marked at the nasal and temporal canthus with permanent marking pen. A circle is drawn on the prosthesis representing the desired pupil position. The owner can then check for any prosthesis rotation during the trial fitting period.

The eye will be expected to have excess discharge for three to five days as the tissues adapt to the "foreign body". Topical ointment is continued as needed. Medication can usually be discontinued after the first week.

e. Prosthesis retention - The eyelids will have contracted because of phthisis bulbi. This contraction limits the size of the prosthesis one can slip between the eyelids. Wearing the prosthesis will cause the eyelids to stretch and eventually return to near-normal size. As the eyelids stretch, the prosthesis becomes loose and may fall out. Therefore, the horse is kept in a confined area for about two weeks. When the prosthesis stays in place 7 to 10 days, this indicates an excellent fit and modifications will probably not be necessary for several months or more. Dental wax will be sent back with the prosthesis for "build up" if needed. If the prosthesis is too small or falls out, the dental wax is used to build up the edges until there is a snug eyelid fit. If the prosthesis has a tendency to rotate, dental wax can also be used to change the position of the pupil. The temporary prosthesis is returned to the ocularist with the wax in place for adjustment.

f. Coloring instructions for the final prosthesis - Color pictures or slides of the good eye are sent so the ocularist can match colors. If the iris is extremely dark, it is often desirable to omit the pupil. A pupil that is not horizontal with the eyelids is far more noticeable than the absence of a pupil in a dark eye. A pupil is recommended for eyes that have a light-colored iris.

g. Prosthesis care - The prosthesis will need to be removed every two to three weeks for cleaning. Animals with reduced tear production will require more frequent cleaning. Soap and water are excellent for cleaning the prosthesis. It is rinsed well and lubricated with ophthalmic ointment or artificial tear before replacing.

h. Prosthesis replacement - The client should check with the ocularist to see if they intend to save the final mold that was prepared to make the prosthesis. If not, the client should be advised to request the final mold so a replacement prosthesis can be made if the original is lost or damaged.

i. Comment - The author has a complete set of slides available for loan to anyone requesting additional information.

3. Severe phthisis bulbi - requires a large prosthesis which, because of its size, could be difficult to keep in the orbit. An alternate procedure would be to enucleate the eye, position a subconjunctival implant, and later fit with a corneoscleral prosthesis. This procedure is also indicated for animals with intraocular tumors.

A transconjunctival enucleation is performed with a limbal conjunctival incision. Tagging the conjunctival edges with clips or mosquito forceps during enucleation is suggested. After the eye has been removed, a silicone implant 2 to 4 mm greater than the horizontal diameter of the normal eye is positioned in the orbit and the conjunctival wound closed with 4-0 or 5-0 absorbable suture. Several interrupted sutures incorporating the conjunctiva and orbital fascia can be used to approximate edges over the implant. This is followed by a continuous suture pattern. A tarsorrhaphy or hood may be indicated for the next few days.

After 7 to 10 days, a temporary conformer is placed in the socket to maintain eyelid and conjunctival sac sizes. The conformer should remain four weeks or until healing is complete and the conjunctiva is smooth. Topical antibiotics should be continued during this period.

The socket is now ready to fit prosthesis in the same manner as previously described for a phthisical eye.

GLOBE PROPTOSIS

Globe proptosis (a prolapse displacement of the globe from the orbit sufficient to cause stretching or tearing of the extraocular muscles).

INCIDENCE - Common in dogs, seen less frequently in cats and rarely in animals with a complete bony orbit.

PREDISPOSING CAUSES

Brachycephalic dogs - with a shallow orbit. Occasionally dogs will proptose an eye from excess restraint of the head and the eye immediately returns to normal position with eyelid manipulation. The owner should be advised that nasal and/or temporal canthoplasty will prevent this from recurring.

Toy breeds - with relatively large eyes

ETIOLOGY - trauma to the head

Fighting - with other animals

Blunt trauma - to the head, especially automobile injuries

EVALUATION OF THE SERIOUSNESS OF THE INJURY (Table 17-1)

TABLE 17-1. Prognostic indicators for a prolapsed eye.

CLINICAL SIGNS	FAVORABLE	UNFAVORABLE
Duration	Short	Long
Damage to extraocular muscles	Muscle tension present	Muscle avulsion
Hyphema	None	Severe and masking pupil
Pupil size	Miosis	Dilated or flaccid
Pupillary light reflex	Positive direct	Absent indirect
Retrobulbar hemorrhage	Minimal	Severe
Intraocular pressure	Normal	Soft (ruptured globe)

Damage to the extrinsic muscles - Frequently one or two of the extrinsic muscles will be ruptured, allowing the eye to deviate. If only the medial rectus ruptures, the eye will deviate laterally. If the ventral rectus also ruptures, deviation is superior-temporal. If all of the extrinsic muscles are ruptured and the eye is hanging loosely from the orbit, there is no choice but to remove the eye.

Hyphema - Marked hyphema is an unfavorable sign because it generally is the result of severe damage to the ciliary body. In some cases, anterior luxation of the lens can also occur with ciliary damage. Severe ciliary damage may lead to permanent hypotension and subsequent phthisis of the eye.

Pupil size

1. Pinpoint pupil - the normal response to pain or injury is constriction of the pupil. A favorable sign.
2. Dilated pupil - this occurs when sympathetic innervation is undisturbed and there is severe damage to the oculomotor nerve or ciliary ganglion. The prognosis should be guarded to unfavorable if the pupil is dilated.

3. Near normal pupil - this occurs when both the sympathetic and parasympathetic innervation have been lost. The optic nerve is permanently injured in these cases.

Pupillary reflexes - the direct reflexes are not of much value in the injured eye but a consensual reflex in the uninjured eye when light is directed into the affected eye is a favorable sign. The absence of pupillary reflexes at the time of injury does not mean permanent loss of the optic nerve. If the pupillary reflexes are not returning in one week, sight loss will probably be permanent.

Retrobulbar hemorrhage - if minimal, replacement is simple and the recovery period after replacement is shorter.

Intraocular pressure

1. Normal if the globe is intact
2. Soft if the globe is ruptured. Digital pressure applied to the cornea will result in collapse of the anterior chamber.

TREATMENT (Figure 17-6)

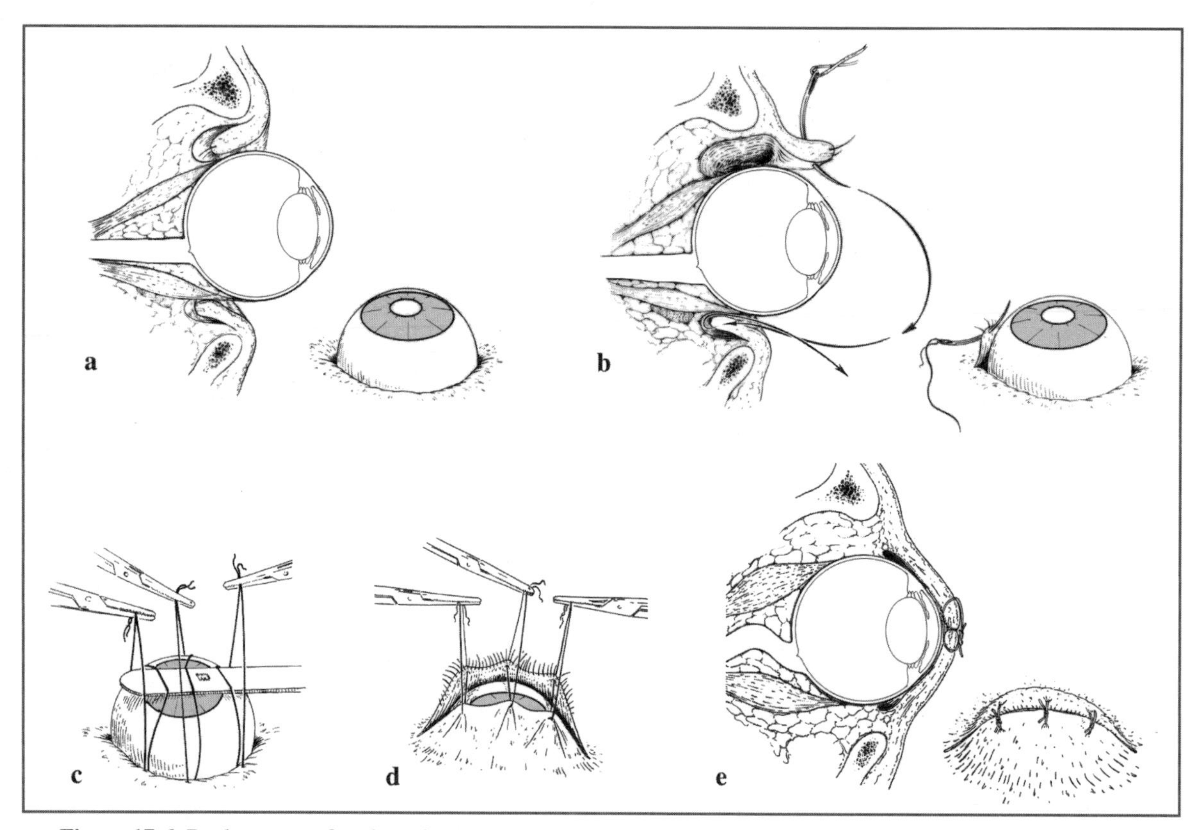

Figure 17-6. Replacement of prolapsed eye.

a. Cross-section and lateral view of prolapsed eye
b. Placing first suture in eyelid. The eyelid can be pulled away from the globe enough to place the suture. After the suture is placed the eyelid returns to the edge of the globe.
c. Three sutures have been placed. The globe is lubricated with ophthalmic ointment. A Bard-Parker handle is placed between the globe to the sutures. Tension on the sutures will simultaneously apply pressure to the globe and pull the eyelids around the eye.
d. The eye is replaced and the sutures are ready for tying
e. Sutures tied. Additional split thickness tarsorrhaphy sutures may be placed if needed.

A prolapsed eye is a true ophthalmic emergency in small animal practice. Correcting a prolapse within 15 to 30 minutes after it happens may save an eye or reduce the rehabilitation period by many days. Even if brought in immediately, some eyes will be beyond help. If the animal is in good health other than the prolapsed eye, immediate surgery should be recommended. If severe head or body injuries are present, one should wait until the patient is stable. Don't risk a patient's life to preserve a blind eye for cosmetic reasons. A prolapsed eye appears to result in minimal pain until the eye is manipulated. All prolapsed eyes should be replaced except those having ruptures of the fibrous tunic or those torn from nearly all supporting tissues. ***It is a less serious error to replace an eye that later has to be removed than to remove an eye that might have been saved for cosmetic purposes.***

Use general anesthesia

Preplace sutures - three or four simple interrupted sutures in the eyelid

Lubricate the eye - liberally with ophthalmic ointment

Pull all the preplaced sutures simultaneously - This will pull the eyelid forward and force the globe into the socket. In severe cases, sliding a scalpel handle between the eye and the sutures, contacting the eye, will facilitate reduction.

Tie the sutures - Split thickness mattress sutures can be placed between the first three sutures if there is excess tension on the eyelids. Orbital hemorrhage usually prevents the eye from returning to its original position. As the hemorrhage absorbs, the eye will become positioned normally in the orbit.

Retrobulbar injection of repository corticosteroids

AFTERCARE

Systemic antibiotics for 5 to 7 days

Medicate the eye - If the animal is easy to handle, the owner should medicate the eye at the nasal canthus with an antibiotic ointment two to three times daily. If the animal is not easy to medicate, ***do not prescribe topical medication.*** Excess manipulation to the eyelids and globe can do more harm than good.

Sutures should be left in the eyelids until there is minimal tension against the lids - usually one to three weeks, depending upon the cause. If the dog has lagophthalmos after removing the sutures, do not hesitate to suture the eyelids again and leave in place for another two or more weeks.

Corneal healing - A badly damaged cornea will regenerate from the limbus inward. Cortisone should not be used because it will delay this regeneration. A red ring of granulation will start at the limbus and progress to the center of the cornea. Clear cornea will be seen appearing at the limbus as the granulation moves centrally. When the granulation has served its purpose, topical corticosteroids can be started to hasten corneal clearing. Regeneration of badly injured corneas may require four to six weeks. Even if the eye is blind after a prolapse, its presence is more beneficial to the dog's appearance than absence of the eye.

Traumatic strabismus - will improve for six to eight weeks after injury. If it is still severe at that time, corrective surgery to straighten the eye out can be attempted but the author has been disappointed with the final result. The exposed nasal sclera often becomes pigmented, improving the appearance of the eye.

PROGNOSIS - Prognosis depends on the degree of ocular damage with the following possibilities.

Cosmetic eye - most traumatic proptosis cases will have a blind eye due to optic nerve damage. The cosmetic appearance is usually acceptable, with a dilated pupil and a slightly exophthalmic position. In some cases belpharoplastic surgery (nasal and/or temporal canthoplasty) to reduce the amount of exposed sclera will improve the appearance.

Noncosmetic eye or painful eye

1. Severe phthisis bulbi resulting in excessive discharge
2. Corneal vascularization and scarring from chronic exposure keratitis. If the eye ulcerates, healing is usually impaired and enucleation may be indicated.
3. Post-traumatic keratoconjunctivitis sicca

ENUCLEATION - EXENTERATION

TERMS

Enucleation - removal of the eye
Evisceration - surgical removal of intraocular contents
Exenteration - removal of the eye and all orbital tissues

SELECTING SURGICAL TECHNIQUE

Enucleation - is the preferred choice for eye removal when pathology is limited to the globe. Two basic techniques are most frequently used and modifications of these techniques have been described. The technique used is basically the surgeon's choice.

1. Transconjunctival approach
   a. Advantages - minimal hemorrhage until eye is removed, therefore easier for the less experienced surgeon
   b. Limitations
      1) Greater risk of contaminating the orbit if an infectious process is present
      2) Greater risk of leaving abnormal/diseased tissue in the orbit
2. Transpalpebral approach
   a. Advantage - allows better visualization of the globe and orbit, reducing risk of leaving diseased tissue behind
   b. Limitations
      1) Significantly more hemorrhage from the eyelids before starting surgery on the globe. This is especially true if the angularis oculi vein is severed.
      2) More difficult to access the sclera near the limbus for globe removal

TRANSCONJUNCTIVAL ENUCLEATION (Figure 17-7)

A lateral canthotomy is performed and the conjunctiva is grasped near the limbus with mosquito or fixation forceps to stabilize the globe. A 360° perilimbal incision is made and the conjunctiva undermined to expose the extraocular muscles. As the extraocular muscles are encountered, they are transected at their tendinous insertions to the globe. This dissection is continued until the optic nerve is encountered. The optic nerve is severed with scissors and ligated if desired. Ligation is not necessary. The third eyelid and gland are removed. Amputation of the margin of the eyelids is completed, using care to remove that portion containing the tarsal glands and caruncle. If residual conjunctiva remains, carefully remove the scissors. Conjunctiva will appear smooth and glistening. The conjunctival surface does not bleed because the mucosal layer is intact. On the other hand, subcutaneous and orbital connective tissue demonstrates capillary and small vessel hemorrhage.

If there is no danger of orbital infection or abnormal tissues (neoplasia), an orbital implant will result in a more cosmetic surgery (Fig 17-8).

A silicone sphere of the proper size is chosen so that the orbit is filled from dorsal to ventral rim. The anterior 1/4 of the prosthesis is trimmed away to give a flattened surface. The sphere is introduced into the orbit and several sutures are placed across the orbital opening from rim to rim in a star, horizontal or vertical direction, or as a simple continuous pattern. These sutures keep the sphere in position and prevent rotation or anterior displacement by the blood clot that will form in the orbit. Several horizontal mattress sutures or a simple continuous suture pattern are placed in the subcutaneous tissues to close dead space. The skin is closed with the surgeon's choice of an accepted skin closure suture pattern.

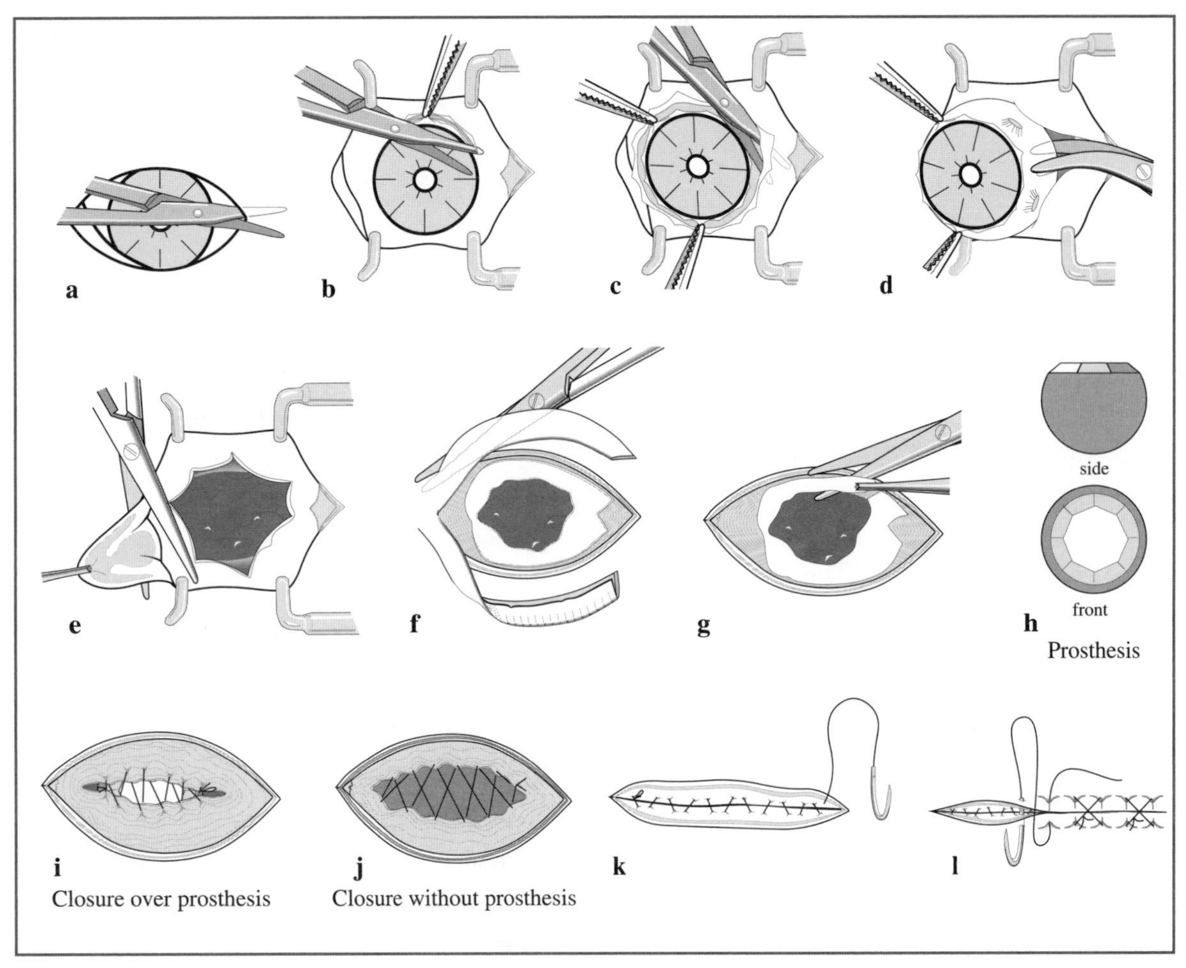

Figure 17-7. Transconjunctival enucleation. Modified from Slatter, Fundamentals of Veterinary Ophthalmology, 2nd ed, WB Saunders, 1990.

a. Canthotomy to gain exposure of the globe
b. Eyelids stabilized with eyelid speculum and globe stabilized with mosquito forceps. The conjunctiva is separated from the globe several millimeters from the limbus with blunt pointed scissors using blunt-sharp dissection.
c. Extrinsic ocular muscle insertions separated from the sclera with scissors
d. Globe moderately pulled from the orbit to cut optic nerve and retractor oculi muscle with enucleation or curved Mayo scissors
e. Third eyelid and gland removed with scissors
f. Margin of eyelids containing tarsal glands are removed with scissors
g. Remove remaining conjunction
h. Silicone rubber orbital implant trimmed for placement
i. Periorbital fascia and tissues closed over implant with absorbable sutures. Penicillin G injected behind implant (100,000 to 250,000 units)
j. If implant not available, fascia is closed as much as possible with nonabsorbable suture to reduce skin indentation after healing
k. Subcutaneous tissues closed and penicillin G injected in front of prosthesis
l. Skin closed with cruciate suture pattern

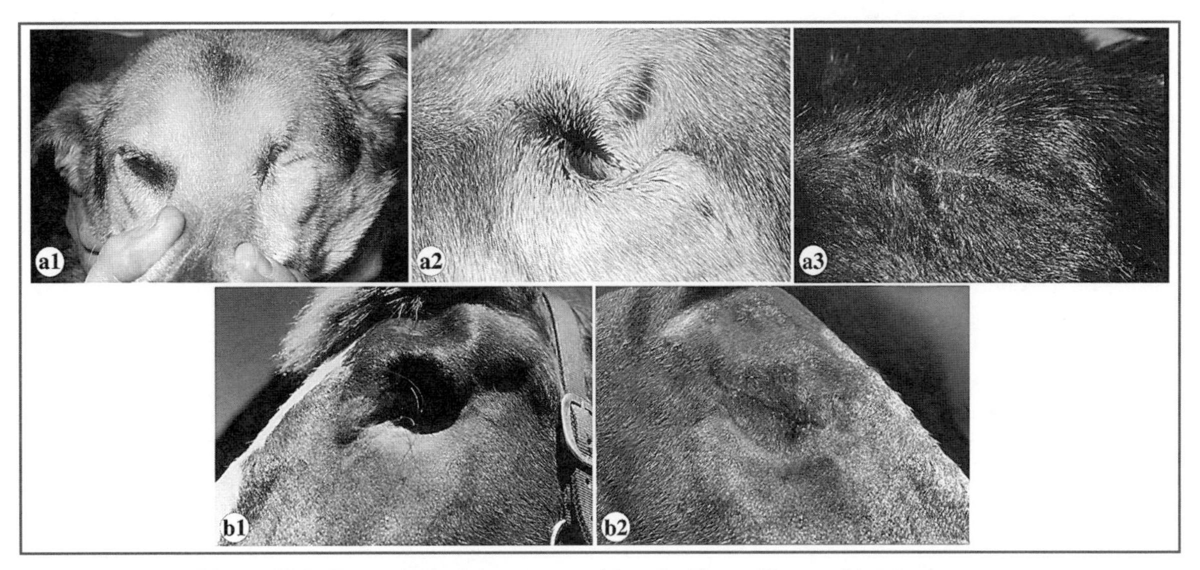

Figure 17-8. Comparison of appearance with and without silicone rubber implant.
a. Dogs
1) and 2). One year post surgery without implant. Front and lateral views.
3) One year post surgery with implant
b. Horses
1) Four months post surgery without implant
2) One year post surgery with implant

TRANSPALPEBRAL ENUCLEATION (Figure 17-9)

After standard surgical preparation of the eye and periocular region, the eyelids are sutured together, leaving the suture tails long enough to provide a handle for manipulation. Skin incisions are made parallel with the lid margins and far enough beyond the margins to avoid the tarsal glands. As the medial and lateral canthus regions are approached, the incisions are brought together forming an elliptical incision for smooth skin apposition. Dissection of the subcutaneous tissues is performed around the circumference of the incision. The lateral orbital ligament is transected with heavy scissors and the medial orbital ligament is severed with a scalpel blade. ***The angularis oculi vein should be avoided at the dorsomedial aspect of the orbital rim.*** If hemorrhage occurs from this vein, ligation should be performed.

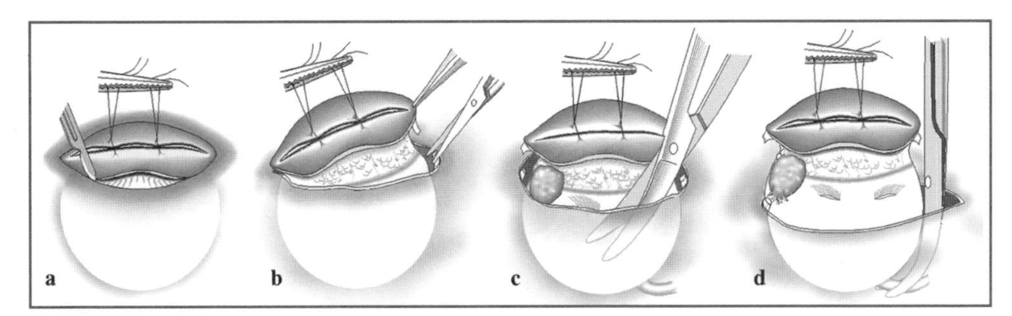

Figure 17-9. Transpalpebral enucleation. Modified from Slatter, Fundamentals of Veterinary Ophthalmology, 2nd ed, WB Saunders, 1990.
a. Eyelids sutured together and skin incised about 5 to 7 mm from palpebral border
b. Nasal and temporal attachments of eyelids severed. Blunt dissection with scissors continued to the conjunctival attachment at the limbus.
c. Extrinsic muscle insertions separated from the sclera with blunt scissors. Care should be taken to remove the gland of the third eyelid.
d. Carefully elevate the globe enough so the optic nerve and retractor oculi muscle can be severed with enucleation or curved Mayo scissors

Surgery is continued as illustrated by Figure 17-7, h to l.

Using scissors, a cut is made perpendicular to the surface of the globe, anterior to the equator. This form of dissection is continued until the sclera itself is visible. Once Tenon's capsule has been opened, one blade of the scissors can be introduced into Tenon's space. Without removing the scissor blade, a 360° cut is made around the globe, cutting the extrinsic ocular muscles at their insertions into the sclera. In the region of the nictitans, the scissors must be directed deeper into the orbit to assure complete removal of the nictitans gland. By cutting the muscles at the level of the tendons, most hemorrhage is avoided. Upward traction on the globe by means of the sutured eyelids will allow the optic nerve to be cut with scissors or a scalpel blade. Care should be used to avoid excessive tension on the globe after the muscles have been severed. This may cause tension on the optic nerve that could result in damage of the optic nerve fibers at the chiasm with blindness in the other eye. The globe is removed, a prosthesis is placed, and orbit and skin closed as in the transconjunctival approach.

EXENTERATION - is indicated when there is orbital pathology requiring removal of all orbital tissues. A transpalpebral approach is used. A cosmetic implant after surgery is usually contraindicated.

The healed surgery results in a deep cavity lined by skin, particularly in horses.

APPENDIX I

GLOSSARY

Abiatrophy: premature degeneration of a tissue after it has reached maturity

Accommodation: the adjustment of the eye for seeing different distances; produced by change in shape of lens, especially anterior surface.

Acorea: no pupil, solid iris

Adnexa: appendages of the eye (eyelids, conjunctiva, glands of the eye, and orbital contents)

Albinism: absence of pigment on a congenital basis

Amaurosis: blindness of unknown etiology without discoverable lesions

Amblyopia: reduced vision in an eye that appears normal at examination

Amblyopia ex anopsia: uncorrectable blurred vision due to disuse of the eye with no organic defect

Ametropia: imperfection in the refractive power of the eye so images are not brought into focus on the retina (hyperopia, myopia, or astigmatism)

Ancorea: no pupil, solid iris

Aniridia: absence of the iris

Anisocoria: difference in size of the pupils

Anisometropia: difference in refractive error of the eyes

Ankyloblepharon: adhesion between the ciliary edges of the eyelids (normal at birth in dog and cat)

Anophthalmos: absence of an eye

Anterior chamber: space in the eye filled with aqueous; bounded in front by the cornea, behind by the iris and lens, and peripherally by the filtration angle

Anterior segment: the anterior portion of the globe (cornea, iris and anterior sclera)

Aphakia: absence of lens

Aphakic crescent: a visible crescent between the iris and lens equator due to subluxation of the lens

Aqueous flare: Tyndall effect observed in the anterior chamber with a beam of light when excessive protein is present in the anterior aqueous

Aqueous humor: clear, watery fluid which fills the anterior and posterior chamber

Asteroid hyalosis: spherical and stellate calcium lipid opacities in normal vitreous; significance unknown

Astigmatism: refractive error which prevents the light rays from coming to a single focus on the retina because of different degrees of refraction in the various meridians of the cornea

Bergmeister's papilla: a remnant of the hyaloid artery in the center of the optic disc

Binocular vision: the ability to use the two eyes simultaneously to focus on the same object and to fuse the two images into a single image

Biomicroscope (slit lamp): an instrument providing magnification and well-focused illumination for examination of the anterior segment and hyaloid face

Blepharitis: inflammation of the eyelids

Blepharochalasis: redundancy of the upper lid skin

Blepharophimosis: narrowing of the slit between the eyes

Blepharoplasty: plastic surgery of the eyelids

Blepharospasm: spasm of the orbicularis oculi muscle

Blepharostenosis: inability to open eye to the normal extent

Blind spot: "blank" area in the visual field corresponding to the light rays that come to focus on the optic nerve

Blood-aqueous barrier: functional barrier between the vascular system and the aqueous

Bulbar conjunctiva: conjunctiva over the globe

Bullous keratitis: the formation of vesicles (bullae) on or in the cornea

Buphthalmos: enlargement of the eye due to glaucoma

Canal of Schlemm: a circular modified venous structure at the junction of the cornea and sclera, seen in primates

Canaliculus: small tear drainage tube in inner aspect of upper and lower lids leading from the puncta to the lacrimal sac

Canthoplasty: a plastic operation on the canthus

Canthorrhaphy: closing the palpebral fissure at either canthus

Canthotomy: incision of the canthus

Canthus: the angle at either end of the eyelid aperture, specified as outer or temporal and inner or nasal

Caruncle: a small piece of skin at the medial canthus from which hairs often protrude

Cataract: opacity of lens of eye, or its capsule, or both

Cataract, Morgagnian: a hypermature, partially liquefied cataract

Chalazion: chronic inflammatory granuloma or distention of a tarsal gland; sometimes called internal hordeolum

Chemosis: edema of the conjunctiva

China eye: a form of heterochromia; blue wall eye

Chorioretinitis: inflammation of the retina and choroid

Choroid: the vascular, intermediate coat which furnished nourishment of the retina and vitreous body

Ciliary body: that portion of the uveal tract between the iris and the choroid; it consists of ciliary processes and the ciliary muscle

Ciliary injection: hyperemia of the subconjunctival (ciliary) vessels

Cilium: eyelash (cilia pl.)

Cloquet's canal: potential space passing through the middle of the vitreous from the optic disc to the lens; the hyaloid canal

Collyrium: eye wash

Coloboma: a congenital fissure or cleft of any part of the eye or eyelid. Typical coloboma is due to incomplete closure of the fetal fissure. Atypical coloboma: any notch or defect not associated with the fetal fissure.

Cones and rods: two kinds of retinal receptor cells; cones are concerned with visual acuity and color discrimination; rods with peripheral vision and vision under decreased illumination

Conjunctiva: the mucous membrane lining the back of the lids (palpebral) and the front of the eye (bulbar), except for the cornea

Conjunctivitis: inflammation of the conjunctiva

Consensual reflex: indirect reflex; the response of the pupil of an eye when a light is directed into the other eye

Conus: a cone; in human ophthalmology, it refers to a myopic crescent around the optic nerve; the term has been applied to a hyperreflective ring around the optic disk of dogs and cats

Corectopia: displacement of the pupil from its normal position

Cornea: transparent portion of the outer coat of the eyeball forming the anterior wall of the aqueous chamber

Corneal graft (keratoplasty): operation to restore vision by replacing a section of opaque cornea with transparent cornea

Corpora nigra (granula iridica): irregular oval bodies on the dorsal and/or ventral pupillary edges of the iris

Cotton wool spots: a microinfarct causing acute edema of the nerve fiber layer of the retina (cytoid body)

Couching: an ancient surgical procedure of dislocating the lens from its optical axis

Cryotherapy: localized tissue destruction by freezing

Cul-de-sac: the area where the conjunctival layers covering the lower lid and the third eyelid meet

Cyclitic membrane: organized exudate seen as a transverse membrane covering the vitreous as a result of uveitis or following cataract surgery

Cyclitis: inflammation of the ciliary body

Cyclocryotherapy: localized destruction of parts of the ciliary body by freezing

Cyclodialysis: the establishment of communication between the anterior chamber and the suprachoroidal space in order to relieve intraocular pressure

Cycloplegia: paralysis of the ciliary muscle, resulting in loss of accommodation

Cycloplegic: a drug that temporarily puts the ciliary muscle at rest, paralyzes accommodation, and dilates the pupil

Dacryoadenitis: inflammation of the lacrimal gland

Dacryocystitis: inflammation of the lacrimal sac

Dacryostenosis: atresia of the lacrimal duct

Dark adaptation: the ability of the retina and pupil to adjust to decreased illumination

Decussation: referring to the crossing of nerve fibers or tracts from one side of the nervous system to the opposite side. The optic chiasm is the crossing of some fibers of the optic nerve to the opposite side of the brain.

Dellen: a slight corneal depression due to local drying

Dermoid: a congenital tumor (choristoma) consisting of skin and its dermal appendages

Descemetocele: protrusion of Descemet's membrane through the floor of an ulcer

Diopter: the unit in which the refracting strength of a lens is designed

Diplopia: seeing one object as two; double vision

Distichiasis: the presence of two separate rows of cilia on one lid; the aberrant row usually originates from the tarsal (meibomian) glands

Districhiasis: more than one cilia growing out of a follicle

Dyscoria: abnormally shaped pupil

Dysgenesis: defective development; malformation of an organ or structure

Dysplasia: defective development of a specific tissue within an organ

Dystrophy: defective or faulty nutrition

Ectasia: dilatation; distention

Ectropion: an eversion or turning out of the eyelid

Electroretinography: the recording of the changes in electric potential in the retina after light stimulation

Emmetropia: the refractive condition of the normal eye at rest so that the image of distant objects (parallel light rays) is brought to a focus on the retina

Enophthalmitis: inflammation of the inner structures of the eye

Enophthalmos: abnormal recession of the eye into the orbit

Entropion: a turning inward of the eyelid

Enucleation: removal of the eyeball after the eye muscles and optic nerve have been severed

Epilation: removal of hair (cilia)

Epiphora: pathologic overflow of tears

Episcleritis: localized inflammation of the superficial tissues of the sclera

Esophoria: a tendency of the eyes to turn inward

Esotropia: a manifest inward deviation of the eyes (crossed eyes)

Evisceration: removal of the contents of the eye with retention of the sclera and sometimes the cornea

Exenteration: removal of the eyeball and all soft tissues within the bony orbit including lids

Exophoria: a tendency of the eyes to turn outward

Exophthalmos: abnormal protrusion of the eyeball; proptosis

Exotropia: a manifest outward deviation of one or both eyes; divergent strabismus, walleye

Facet: a depression on the surface of the cornea lined with epithelium

Farsightedness: see hyperopia

Field of vision: the entire area which can be seen without shifting the gaze

Filtration angle: iridocorneal angle

Floaters: small particles in the vitreous

Fornix: the junction of the palpebral and bulbar conjunctivas

Fovea: small depression in the macula adapted for most acute vision in man

Fundus: the posterior layers of the eye which can be seen with an ophthalmoscope

Fusion: coordinating the images received by the two eyes into one image

Glands of Moll: sweat glands connected with the follicles of the eyelash

Glands of Zeis: modified sebaceous glands connected with the follicles of the eyelash

Glaucoma: increase in intraocular pressure

Gonioscopy: a technique of examining the iris-corneal angle utilizing a special contact lens, magnifying device, and light source

Haws: lay term for the third eyelid

Hemeralopia: day blindness

Hemianopia: loss of approximately one-half of the visual field

Heterochromia iridis: the irides or part of one iris has a different color

Heterophoria: a tendency of the eyes to deviate

Heterotropia: a manifest deviation of the eye in any direction in which binocular fixation is impossible; strabismus

Hippus: spontaneous rhythmic movements of the pupil independent of illumination; iridokinesia

Hordeolum, external (stye): infection of the glands of Moll or Zeis

Hordeolum, internal: tarsal gland infection

Horner's syndrome: sympathetic nerve paralysis with protrusion of the third eyelid, ptosis, miosis, and enophthalmus

Hyalitis: inflammation of the vitreous body

Hyaloid canal: potential space passing through the center of the vitreous from the optic disc to the lens; Cloquet's canal

Hydrophthalmus: marked enlargement of the eye from congenital glaucoma

Hyperopia, hypermetropia (farsightedness): a refractive error in which the focal point of light rays from a distant object is behind the retina

Hypertropia: elevation of one visual axis above the other

Hyphema: hemorrhage into the anterior chamber of the eye

Hypopyon: collection of pus in the anterior chamber

Hypotony: low intraocular tension

Injection: congestion of conjunctival blood vessels

Interstitial keratitis: deep keratitis, with involvement of all layers of the cornea

Intumescent lens: swollen or enlarged lens

Iridectomy: removal of a part of the iris

Iridencleisis: incarceration of a portion of the iris in a wound of the limbus, either accidentally or as an operative procedure to effect a displacement of the pupil, or as a filtering procedure for glaucoma

Iridocorneal angle: the angle between the iris and the cornea through which aqueous leaves the eye

Iridocyclitis: inflammation of the iris and ciliary body

Iridocyclitis, recurrent: moon blindness; equine periodic ophthalmia

Iridodialysis: separation of the base of the iris from the ciliary body

Iridodonesis: trembling of the iris with movement of the eye, indicating loss of lens support

Iris: colored, circular membrane, suspended behind the cornea and immediately ahead of the lens, the most anterior part of the uvea

Iris bombe´: a condition in which the iris is bowed forward by the collection of aqueous between the iris and lens in total posterior synechia

Keratectomy: excision of various parts of the cornea

Keratic precipitates (KPs): clumps of leukocytes adhering to the corneal epithelium. May have mutton fat or punctate appearance

Keratitis: corneal inflammation

Keratoconjunctivitis sicca: dry cornea as a result of lacrimal gland deficiency

Keratoconus: cone shaped cornea

Keratoglobus: globe shaped cornea

Keratomycosis: fungal infection of the cornea

Keratoplasty: plastic surgery of the cornea; corneal transplant

Lacrimal sac: the dilated area at the junction of the nasolacrimal duct and the canaliculi

Lacrimation: production of tears

Lagophthalmos: inadequate lid closure

Lens: transparent body suspended in the anterior portion of the eyeball between the aqueous and vitreous chambers

Lenticonus: conic bulging of the lens, either anterior or posterior

Lenticular intumescence: swollen lens

Leukokoria: a white pupil reflex due to changes behind the lens

Leukoma: a white opaque corneal opacity; adherent leukoma - iris adhered to corneal endothelium

Limbus: circular boundary between the cornea and sclera

Lysozyme: an antibacterial enzyme found in tears

Macula: a small spot or colored area; a moderate corneal scar; central area in human retina

Macula lutea: the small avascular area of the retina surrounding the fovea in man

Megalocornea: congenitally large cornea which may be confused with congenital glaucoma

Meibomian glands (tarsal glands): long sebaceous glands in the tarsal plate with openings on lid margin

Microphthalmos: an abnormally small eyeball

Miosis: constricted pupil

Miotic: a medication causing the pupil to become small

Mittendorf's dot: opacity of the posterior lens capsule marking the site of hyaloid artery attachment

Morgagnian cataract: a hypermature, cortically liquified cataract in which the nucleus falls ventrally

Mydriasis: dilated pupil

Mydriatic: a medication causing the pupil to become large

Myopia: a refractive error in which the point of focus for rays of light from distant objects is in front of the retina (nearsightedness)

Nanophthalmos: a congenital underdeveloped nonfunctional eye

Nebula: slight haziness in cornea; grayish opacity of the cornea

Nyctalopia: night blindness

Nystagmus: an involuntary, rapid movement of the eyeball, either horizontal, rotary or vertical

Occlusion (pupillary): closure of the pupil by an opaque membrane

Oculist: an old term for ophthalmologist

o.d.: oculus dexter, the right eye

Ophthalmologist: a doctor versed or expert in ophthalmology

Ophthalmoplegia: paralysis of the eye muscles; externa: paralysis of the extrinsic muscles; interna: paralysis of the intrinsic muscles; total (complete): paralysis of both extrinsic and intrinsic muscles of the eye

Optic disk: ophthalmoscopically visible portion of the optic nerve in the eyeball

Optic nerve: the nerve that carries visual impulses from the retina to the brain

Optometrist: a nonmedical person trained in the measurement of refraction of the eye

o.s.: oculus sinister, left eye

o.u.: oculi unitas, both eyes

Palpebral conjunctiva: conjunctiva on the inner surface of lids

Pannus: superficial vascularization of the cornea with infiltration of granulation tissue

Panophthalmitis: inflammation involving all coats of the eye

Papilla: a round-white disk in the fundus medial to the posterior pole of the eye; the optic disk

Papilledema: edema of the optic papilla (disk)

Papillitis: inflammation of the optic papilla (disk)

Persistent pupillary membrane: web-like strands stretching across the pupil

Photophobia: abnormal sensitivity to and discomfort from light

Photopic: pertaining to vision in bright light

Phthisis bulbi: shrunken, fibrotic globe resulting from injury or internal eye infection

Pigmentary keratitis: the deposition of pigment into the cornea as a response to an irritating factor

Plasmoid aqueous: fibrin in the anterior chamber

Polycoria: more than one pupil

Posterior chamber: space filled with aqueous between the back of the iris and the front of the lens

Posterior segment: behind the iris

Posterior scleral ectasia: underdevelopment of sclera

Posterior synechia: attachment of iris to lens capsule

Posterior uvea: choroid; posterior vascular tunic

Presbyopia: defect of vision in advancing age with loss of accommodation or recession of near point

Proptosis: forward displacement of the globe; exophthalmos

Pseudopterygium: a fold of bulbar conjunctiva attached to the cornea following a corneal ulcer

Pterygium: triangular thickening of bulbar conjunctiva on the cornea with apex toward pupil

Ptosis: drooping of the upper eyelid

Punctate keratitis: inflammation of the cornea characterized by small areas of homogenous opacity

Pupil: the round hole in the center of the iris which corresponds to the lens aperture in the camera

Pupillary cysts: black masses near the pupil that look much like the copra nigra in the horse

Refraction: 1) deviation in the course of rays of light in passing from one transparent medium into another of different density; 2) determination of refractive errors of the eye and correction by glasses

Refractive error (ametropia): a defect in the eye that prevents light rays from being brought to a single focus on the retina

Refractive media: the transparent parts of the eye having refractive power

Retina: innermost coat of the eye formed of light-sensitive nerve elements

Retina detachment: the separation of the sensory retina from the retina pigment epithelium

Retinal disinsertion: retinal dialysis at the ora ciliaris retinae in which the sensory retina is separated from the retinal pigment epithelium

Retinal dysplasia: abnormal differentiation of retinal layers

Retinitis pigmentosa: a hereditary degeneration and atrophy of the retina in man that is comparable to generalized progressive retinal atrophy in dogs

Retinoschisis: a congenital cleft of the retina; a cleavage of retinal layers

Retinoscope: a device for the objective determination of refractive error

Rheology: the gel-liquid state of the vitreous

Roots:

Blepharo - lid
Cor - pupil
Dacryo - tear
Hyal - vitreous
Hyp - anterior chamber
Irido - iris
Kerato - cornea
Ophthalmo - eye
Papilla - optic disk
Phaco/Phako - lens

Rubeosis irides: abnormal vascularization of the iris, usually associated with inflammation

Sclera: the white part of the eye; a tough covering which, with the cornea, comprises the connective tissue tunic of the eye

Schirmer tear test: a method of measuring tear production

Scotoma: a blind or partially blind area in the visual field

Scotopic: pertaining to vision in the dark (poor light)

Seclusion of the pupil: annular posterior synechia

Sicca: dry

Slit lamp: a combination light and microscope for examination of the eye, principally the anterior segment

Staphyloma: a bulging defect of cornea or sclera which is lined with uveal tissue

Strabismus (squint, heterotropia): a manifest deviation of the eye in which binocular fixation is impossible

Stye: infection of glands of Zies or Moll; external hordeolum

Subluxation of the lens: partial lens displacement

Sympathetic ophthalmia: inflammation in one eye following traumatic inflammation in the fellow eye occurring in man. Not observed in animals.

Symblepharon: adhesion of one or both eyelids to the eyeball

Synchysis: a fluid condition of the vitreous

Synchysis scintillans: flashes of reflected light from cholesterol crystals floating in the vitreous

Synechia: any adhesion of the iris
  a. Anterior synechia - adhesion of iris to cornea
  b. Posterior synechia - adhesion of iris to lens

Syneresis: the process of liquification of the vitreous

Tapetum: fluorescent layer in the choroid in the dorsal fundus

Tarsorrhaphy: suturing the lids together

Tenon's capsule: a connective tissue sheath encircling the eyeball posteriorly

Tonography: test to determine the amount of fluid forced from the eye by a constant pressure during a constant period

Tonometry: measurement of intraocular pressure in mm Hg

Trichiasis: the cilia follicle is normally placed but the direction of growth is toward the eye rather than away

Uvea: entire vascular coat of the eyeball; iris, ciliary body and choroid
  a. Anterior uveal tract; iris and ciliary body
  b. Posterior uveal tract; choroid

Uveitis: inflammation of the middle vascular coat of the eye

Vibrissae: stiff tactile hairs around the face of animals

Vitreous: transparent, colorless mass of soft, gelatinous material filling the eyeball behind the lens

Vitreous veils: faint, curtain-like opacities seen by focal light in the normal eye

Walleye: a parti-colored blue with yellow or brown iris; a form of heterochromia; lateral strabismus

Watch eye: a parti-colored blue with yellow or brown iris; a form of heterochromia

Xerophthalmia: conjunctivitis with atrophy and drying, predisposing to a dry and lusterless cornea

Zonules (Zonules of Zinn): the numerous fine tissue strands (ligaments) which stretch from the ciliary processes to the lens equator (360°) and hold the lens in place

Zonulolysis: lysis of the zonules, as with alpha-chymotrypsin, to facilitate removal of the lens in cataract surgery in man

APPENDIX II

MANUFACTURERS/DISTRIBUTORS INDEX

AO Reichert Scientific Instruments
PO Box 123
Buffalo, New York 14240
716-891-3000

Abbott Laboratories
100 Abbott Park Road
Abbott Park, IL 60064-3500
800-633-9110

Akorn, Inc
2500 Milbrook Dr.
Buffalo Grove, IL 60089
800-535-7155

Alcon Laboratories, Inc.
6201 South Freeway
Ft. Worth, TX 76134
817-551-8057
800-862-5266

Alcon Surgical
6201 South Freeway
Ft. Worth, TX 76134
800-862-5266

Aldrich Chemical Co.
PO Box 355
Milwaukee, WI 53201-9358
800-558-9160

Allergan Pharmaceuticals
2525 DuPont Drive
Irvine, CA 92715-9534
800-347-4500

Alza Corporation
950 Page Mill Road
Palo Alto, CA 94303-0802
650-496-5000

American Regent
Subsidiary, Luitpold Pharm. Inc.
1 Luitpold Dr
Shirley, NY 11967
516-924-4000

Arista Surgical Supply Co. Inc.
67 Lexington Ave
New York, NY 10010-1898
Orders: 800-223-1984
FAX: 212-696-9046

Astra Pharmaceutical Prod.
50 Otis
Westborough, MA 01581
508-366-1100

Bausch & Lomb Pharm.
8500 Hidden River Parkway
Tampa, FL 33637
813-975-7700

Bausch & Lomb
Personal Products Division
1400 No. Goodman St.
P O Box 450
Rochester, New York 14692-0450

Baxter Scientific
1118 Clay
N. Kansas City, MO 64116
800-444-7752

Bayer Corporation
36 Columbia Rd
Morristown, NJ 07962
800-331-4536

Becton Dickinson & Company
One Becton Drive
Franklin Lakes, NJ 07417-1881
201-847-6800

Bristol-Myers US Pharm.
Div. Bristol-Myers Squibb
2404 West Pennsylvania St
Evansville, IN 47721-0001
812-429-5000

Brymill Corporation
PO Box 2392
Vernon Industrial Place
Vernon, CT 06066
203-875-2460

Burroughs Wellcome Co.
See Glaxo Wellcome

Cabot Medical
2021 Cabot Blvd. West
Longhorne, PA 19047

Canada
The Orlo Division
I-MED Pharma Inc.
216 Brunswick Blvd.
Pointe-Claire
Quebec H9R 1A6
514-630-1818
Fax: 514-630-0016

Ciba Vision Ophthalmics
11460 Johns Creek Parkway
Duluth, GA 30136
770-418-4101

Concept Inc.
12707 US 19 South
Clearwater, FL 33516
800-237-0169

CooperVision Inc.
200 Willowbrook Office Park
Fairport, NY 14450
949-597-8130

The Cutting Edge Ltd.
870 North Circle Drive
Diamond Springs, CA 95619
530-621-2020
888-521-2020

Dallas Eye Prosthetics
William (Randy) Trownik
8226 Douglas Avenue, #415
Dallas, TX 75225
214-739-5355

Davis and Geck See
Kendall Health Care Products

Delmont Laboratories, Inc.
Biological Specialists
PO Box 269
Swarthmore, PA 19081-0269
610-543-3365

Denver Optic Co.
14 Inverness Drive East
D Suite 146
Englewood, CO 80112
303-649-9494

Deseret Health Medical
Al Gunther Associates
17485 Vancouver Street
Lakewood, CO 80228
303-986-3343
FAX: 303-985-9853

Dey Laboratories, Inc.
2751 Napa Valley Corporate Dr.
Napa, CA 94558
707-224-3200

Duffens Optical
2929 West 9th Ave
Denver, CO 80204
303-623-5301
800-358-9789

E. Fougera & Co.
60 Baylis Rd.
Melville, NY 11747
516-454-6996

Eagle Vision
6263 Poplar Ave., Suite 650
Memphis, TN 38119
901-683-9400
800-393-7584
FAX: 901-761-5736

Ellman International
Manufacturing Inc.
1135 Railroad Ave
Hewlett, NY 11557
516-569-1482

Ethicon
Route 22 West
Somerville, NJ 08876-0151
908-218-0707

Evsco Pharmaceuticals
PO Box 685
Harding Hwy
Buena, NJ 08310
800-225-0270
856-691-2411, ext. 265
Fax: 856-697-9711

Fisons Corp. - See
Medeva Pharmaceuticals

Fort Dodge Labs Inc.
PO Box 518
Fort Dodge, IA 50501
515-955-4600
FAX: 515-955-3730

Genentech, Inc.
1 DNA Way
South San Francisco, CA 94080
650-225-1000

Glaxo Wellcome
5 Moore Drive
Reasearch Triangle Pk, NC 27709
919-248-2100

Guardian Horse Mask Co.
PO Box 1811
La Quinta, CA 92253
619-564-5814

Henry Schein, Inc.
135 Duryea Rd.
Melville, NY 11747
800-472-4346

Immunovet Inc.
5810-G Breckenridge Parkway
Tampa, FL 33610-4253
813-621-9447
FAX: 813-621-0751

Interstate Drug Exchange - See
Henry Schein, Inc.

Iolab Pharmaceuticals - See
Ciba Vision Ophthalmics

Janssen Pharm. Inc.
1125 Trenton - Harbourton Rd.
P.O. Box 200
Titusville, NJ 08560-0200

Jardon Eye Prosthetics, Inc.
17100 West 12 Mile Road
Southfield, MI 48076
248-424-8560
FAX: 248-424-8196

Johnson & Johnson Medical
PO Box 130
Arlington, TX 76004-0130
800-433-5009

Jorgensen Labs
1450 N. VanBuren
Loveland, CO 80538
970-669-2500
FAX: 970-663-5042

Keeler Optical Products, Inc.
456 Parkway
Lawrence Park Industrial District
Broomall, PA 19008 or
31211 Floweridge Drive
Palos Verdes Peninsula, CA 90274

Kendall Health Care Products
15 Hampshire St.
Mansfield, MA 02048
800-962-9888

Lederle Laboratories
Div. of American Cyanamid Co.
North Middletown Road
Pearl River, NY 10965-1299
914-732-5000

Lehn & Fink Products - See
National Labs

Eli Lilly & Co.
Bldg. L1/3 Lilly Corp. Center
Indianapolis, IN 46285
317-276-2000

Luitpold Pharmaceuticals, Inc.
Animal Health Division
One Luitpold Dr.
Shirley, NY 11967
516-924-4000
800-458-0163
FAX: 516-924-1731

Lyphomed
3 Pkwy N.
Deerfield, IL 60015-2548
708-317-8800

MDS
Medical Diagnostic Services Inc
511 North Limon Road
Brandon, FL 33510
813-653-1800
FAX: 813-684-5953

MWI Veterinary Supply
PO Box 39888
Denver, Colorado 80239-0888
303-371-4437
800-525-4174

Mallinckrodt, Vet. Inc.
421 East Hawley St.
Mundelein, IL 60060
708-949-3300

Marion Scientific
Division of Marion Labs, Inc.
Kansas City, MO 64114

Mead Johnson
Div. of Bristol-Myers Squibb
2404 Pennsylvania Street
Evansville, IN 47721
812-426-6000

Medeva Pharmaceuticals
755 Jefferson Rd.
Rochester, NY 14623-0000
800-932-1950

Mentor O & O
300 Longwater Drive
Norwell, MA 02061-1672
617-871-6950
800-992-7557

Merck & Co.
P O Box 4
West Point, PA 19486
800-672-6372

Mila International
803 Nelson Rd.
Erlanger, KY 41018-2810
606-261-6637

Miles Inc.
1127 Myrtle Street
PO Box 340
Elkhart, IN 46515-0340
219-264-8111

Monarch Pharmaceuticals
335 Beecham St.
Bristol, TN 37620
800-776-3637

Muro Pharmaceutical, Inc.
890 East St.
Tewksbury, MA 01876-9987
978-851-5981

National Labs
225 Summit Avenue
Montvale, NJ 07645
800-388-1834

New World Medical Inc.
10574 Acacia St.
Suite D-1
Rancho Cucamonga, CA 91730-5448
714-466-4304
FAX: 714-466-4305

Novartis
59 Route 10
East Hanover, NJ 07936
908-277-5000

Norwich Eaton Pharm.
PO Box 191
Norwich, NY 13815
607-335-2111

Oasis Medical
514 South Vermont Avenue
Glendora, CA 91740
800-528-9786

Oculab
443 West Colorado St.
Glendale, CA 91204
818-247-4987
800-628-5227

Oculab Vet. Dist.
Dan Scott and Associates
235 Luke Court
Westerville, Ohio 43081
614-890-0370

Ortho Pharmaceutical Corp.
Route 202, PO Box 600
Raritan, NJ 08869-0600
908-218-6000

Otsuka America Pharmaceutical Inc
2440 Research Blvd
Rockville, MD 98101
301-990-0030

Parke-Davis
Div. of Warner-Lambert Co.
201 Tabor Road
Morris Plains, NJ 07950
973-540-2000

Parmed Pharmaceuticals, Inc.
4220 Hyde Park Blvd.
Niagara Falls, NY 14305
716-284-5666

Pasadena Research Labs See
Taylor Pharmaceuticals

Pfizer Animal Health
Whiteland Business Park
812 Springdale Dr.
Exton, PA 19341
800-438-1985

Pfizer Laboratories
235 E. 42nd St.
New York, NY 10017-5755
212-573-2422

Pharmics, Inc.
2350 So. Redwood Rd.
Salt Lake City, UT 84119
801-972-4138

Pharmacia & Upjohn
7000 Portage Road
Kalamazoo, MI 49001
616-833-4000

Purdue Frederick Co.
100 Connecticut Ave.
Norwalk, CT 06850-3590
203-853-0123

Ribi ImmunoChem Research
553 Old Corvallis Rd.
PO Box 1409
Hamilton, MT 59840
406-363-6214

Rhone Merierux
7101 College Blvd.
Overland Park, KS 66210
913-451-3434

Sandoz Pharmaceutical Corp. See
Novartis

Schering-Plough Corporation
Schering-Plough HealthCare
110 Allen Road
Liberty Corner, NJ 07938
908-604-1995

Schering-Plough Animal Health Corp.
1095 Morris Ave.
Union, NJ 07083
908-629-3490
800-648-2118

Schien Pharmaceuticals, Inc.
100 Campus Drive
Florham Park, NJ 07932
914-278-3724

Searle & Company
c/o Searle Pharmaceuticals
PO Box 5110
Chicago, IL 60680-5110
847-982-7000

Sherwood, Davis & Geck See
Kendall Health Care Products

Sigma Chemical Co.
PO Box 14508
St. Louis, MO 63178-9916
800-325-3010

SmithKline Beecham Pharm.
PO Box 7929
Philadelphia, PA 19101
215-751-4000

Solvay Veterinary Inc.
(Weck Instruments)
PO Box 7348
Princeton, NJ 08543
800-524-1645

Sontec Instruments
7248 South Tucson Way
Englewood, CO 80112
303-791-9411
800-821-7496

Steris Laboratories, Inc.
620 N. 51st Ave.
Phoenix, AZ 85043
602-278-1400

Storz Ophthalmics
Subs. American Cyanamid
3365 Tree Court Industrial
St. Louis, MO 63122-6694

Storz Instrument Co.
3365 Tree Court Industrial
St. Louis, MO 63122

Summit Hill Labs
PO Box 535
Novesink, NJ 07752
908-291-3600
FAX 908-872-1389

Sussex Drug Products Co.
PO Box 112
Edison, NJ 08818
800-255-7733

Taylor Pharmaceuticals
PO Box 5136
San Clemente, CA 92674-5136
714-492-4030

Thermotech
1 West Deer Valley Rd
Suite 300
Phoenix, AZ 85027-2128
602-780-9084

Topcon America Corporation
65 West Century Road
Paramus, NJ 07652-9990
Address inquiries to:
Medical Instrument Division
800-223-1130
201-261-9450
FAX 201-387-2710

The Upjohn Company See
Pharmacia & Upjohn

VETKO Inc.
4931 Northpark Drive
Colorado Springs, CO 80918-9986
800-525-9617
FAX: 719-598-6255

Vetrepharm Research Inc.
119 Rowe Road
Athens, GA 30601
706-549-4503
FAX: 404-548-0659

Vetroson - See
Summit Hill Laboratories

Edward Weck & Co. Inc.
Weck Division
PO Box 12600
Research Triangle Park, NC 27709
800-334-8511

Wedgewood Pharmacy
279-C EGG Harbor Road
Sewell, NJ 08080-3126
609-589-4200
800-331-8272
FAX: 800-589-4250

Welch Allyn Medical Division
State Street Road, Box 220
Skaneateles Falls, NY 13153-0020
315-685-4560
Fax 315-685-3361

Welch Allyn Intermountain Area
Phil Loftus, Sales Rep.
3102 Gamow Lane
Boulder, CO 80301
303-939-8761

Western Optical
Ophthalmic Instrument Division
1200 Mercer Street
Seattle, WA 98109
206-622-7627

Wyeth-Ayerst Laboratories
PO Box 8299
Philadelphia, PA 19101
610-688-4400

Zeneca Pharmaceuticals
Concord Pk. & New Murphy Rd.
Wilmington, DE 19897
302-886-3000

APPENDIX III

VETERINARY OPHTHALMOLOGY TEXTS

1. Animal Models of Ocular Diseases, Tabbara and Cello. Charles Thomas Publishers, 1984.
2. Feline Ophthalmology, Barnett and Crispin. WB Saunders Co, 1977.
3. Fundamentals of Veterinary Ophthalmology, Second Ed, Slatter. WB Saunders Co, 1990.
4. Handbook of Ophthalmic Surgery, Gelatt. Elsevier Science, Inc. (Pergamon Press), 1995. Volume 1 - Extrinsic Procedures; Volume 2 - Intraocular Procedures.
5. Inherited Eye Diseases of Purebred Dogs, Rubin. Williams and Wilkins, 1989.
6. Magrane's Canine Ophthalmology, Fourth Ed, Helper. Lea and Febiger, 1989.
7. Manual of Small Animal Ophthalmology, Pedersen-Jones and Crispin. BSVAA Books, 1993. Distributed USA by Iowa State Press.
8. Ocular Disorders Proven or Suspected to be Hereditary in Dogs, Second Ed, ACVO 1996.
9. Ophthalmic Pathology of Animals, Saunders and Rubin. S Kager, 1975.
10. Ophthalmology for the Veterinary Practitioner, Stades, Neumann, Boeve, and Wyman. Veterinary Practice Publishing Co, 1996.
11. Small Animal Ophthalmology - A Problem Oriented Approach, Second Ed, Peiffer and Peterson-Jones. WB Saunders Co, 1997.
12. Small Animal Ophthalmology, Self-assessment Picture Tests in Veterinary Medicine, Riis. Mosby-Wolfe, 1994.
13. The Eye in Veterinary Practice, Volume I, Blogg. WB Saunders Co, 1980.

    The Eye in Veterinary Practice, Volume II, (Eye examination of the performance horse), Blogg. Chilcote Publishing, Australia, 1985.

    The Eye in Veterinary Practice, Volume III, (Eye injuries), Blogg. Chilcote Publishing, Australia, 1987.
14. Veterinary Ophthalmology, Third Ed, Gelatt. Lippincott, Williams & Wilkins, 1999.
15. Veterinary Ophthalmology Notes, Martin. University of Georgia.
16. Veterinary Ophthalmology, Barnett. Mosby, 1997.

VETERINARY OPHTHALMOLOGY COLOR ATLASES

1. A Color Atlas of Veterinary Ophthalmology, Barnett. Wolfe Publishing Ltd, 1990.
2. Atlas of Breed-Related Canine Ocular Disorders, Ketring and Glaze. Veterinary Learning Systems, 1998.
3. Atlas of Feline Ophthalmology, Ketring and Glaze. Veterinary Learning Systems, 1994.

4. Color Atlas and Textbook, Equine Ophthalmology, Barnett, Crispin, Lavach & Mathews. Mosby-Wolfe, 1995.

5. The Retina, Ophthalmology Talking Manual, Volume I and II. AAHA.

VETERINARY OPHTHALMOLOGY BOOKS NO LONGER IN PRINT

1. Anatomy and Histology of the Eye and Orbit in Domestic Animals, Prince. CC Thomas, 1960.

2. Atlas of Ophthalmology in Dogs and Cats, Walde. BC Decker Inc, 1990.

3. Atlas of Veterinary Ophthalmic Surgery, Bistner, Aguirre and Batik. Saunders, 1977.

4. Atlas of Veterinary Ophthalmology, Rubin. Lea and Febiger, 1974.

5. Comparative Anatomy of the Eye, Prince. CC Thomas, 1956.

6. Diseases of the Canine Eye, Startup. Williams and Wilkins, 1969.

7. Large Animal Ophthalmology, Lavach. CV Mosby, 1990.

8. Manual of Small Animal Ophthalmology, Wyman. Churchill Livingstone, 1986.

9. The Fundus Oculi of Birds Especially as Viewed by the Ophthalmoscope, Case Albert Wood. The Lakeside Press, 1917.

10. Veterinary Ophthalmic Pharmacology and Therapeutics, Second Ed, Gelatt. VM Publishing Inc, 1978.

11. Veterinary Ophthalmology, Smythe. Bailliere Tindall and Cox, 1958.

GENERAL VETERINARY TEXTS WITH OPHTHALMOLOGY CHAPTERS

1. Current Technique in Small Animal Surgery, Bojrab. Lea and Febiger.

2. Current Therapy in Equine Medicine, Robinson. WB Saunders, 1992.

3. Current Veterinary Therapy in Food Animal Practice, Howard. WB Saunders Co, 1993.

4. Current Veterinary Therapy, Small Animal Practice, Kirk. WB Saunders and Co.

5. Equine Medicine and Surgery. American Vet Publications, Santa Barbara.

6. Handbook of Small Animal Practice, Morgan. Churchill Livingstone, Second edition, 1992.

7. Large Animal Internal Medicine, Smith. CV Mosby, 1990.

8. Manual of Small Animal Emergencies, Morgan. Churchill Livingstone, 1985.

9. Textbook of Small Animal Surgery, Second Edition, Slatter. WB Saunders Co, 1993.

10. Textbook of Veterinary Internal Medicine, Ettinger. WB Saunders.

11. Veterinary Clinics of North America, WB Saunders.

Small Animal Ophthalmology Issues:

Volume 3:3, 1973
Volume 10:2, 1980
Volume 20, 1990
Volume 27:5, 1997

Large Animal Ophthalmology Issues:

Volume 6:3, 1984
Volume 8:30, 1992

VETERINARY OPHTHALMOLOGY JOURNALS

1. Veterinary Ophthalmology. Published quarterly by American College of Veterinary Ophthalmologists. Blackwell Science Ltd, 1999.

HUMAN TEXTS USEFUL FOR COMPARATIVE OPHTHALMOLOGY

1. Adler's Physiology of the Eye, 9th Edition, Hart. CV Mosby, 1992.
2. An Atlas of Ophthalmic Surgery, Third Edition, King and Wadsworth. JB Lippincott, 1981.
3. General Ophthalmology, Vaughan and Asbury. Lange.
4. Havner's Ocular Pharmacology, 6th Edition. CV Mosby, 1994.
5. Histology of the Human Eye, Hogan. WB Saunders Co, 1971.
6. Ocular Pathology, Second Edition. Yanoff and Fine. Harper and Row Publisher, 1982.
7. Physiology of the Eye, 4th Edition, Davson. Academic Press, 1980.
8. Principles and Practice of Ophthalmology - 5 Volumes, Albert and Jakobiec. WB Saunders, 1994.
9. The Eye and Its Adaptive Radiation, Walls. Hafner Publishing Co, 1967.
10. The Eye, Volume 5, Comparative Physiology, Davson. Academic Press, 1974.
11. Wolf's Anatomy of the Eye and Orbit, 5th Edition, Last. WB Saunders Co, 1961.

APPENDIX IV

GUIDELINES USED BY THE ACVO GENETICS COMMITTEE FOR BREEDING RECOMMENDATIONS

Abstracted from *Ocular Disorders Proven or Suspected to be Hereditary in Dogs,* revised 1994

1. **NO** - Substantial evidence exists to support the heritability of this entity and/or the entity represents a potential compromise of vision or other ocular function (even a minor clinical form renders an animal unsuitable for breeding).

2. **BREEDER'S OPTION** - Entity is unknown or suspected to be inherited but does not represent potential compromise of vision or other ocular function.

3. **UNKNOWN** - Diseases under consideration with inadequate information available to give breeding advice.

The following disorders have the same recommendation against breeding for all dog breeds.

1. Progressive retinal atrophy (PRA) - Breeding is not advised for any animal demonstrating bilateral symmetrical retinal degeneration (considered to be PRA unless proven otherwise).
2. Cataract - Breeding is not recommended for any animal demonstrating partial or complete opacity of the lens or its capsule ***unless the examiner has also checked the space for "significance of above cataract is unknown".***
3. Retinal dysplasia - ***geographic or detached*** - breeding is not advised for any animal exhibiting a congenital retinal disorder consistent with retinal dysplasia.
4. Retinal detachment - Breeding is not recommended for any animal exhibiting retinal detachment.

KEY TO TABLE ABBREVIATIONS:

CEA - collie eye anomaly
CPRA - central progressive retinal atrophy
ON - optic nerve
PHPV - persistent hyperplastic primary vitreous
GT - gland of 3rd eyelid
NGE - nodular granulomatous episcleroconjunctivitis
PHA - persistent hyaloid artery
PK - pigmentary keraitis
PPM - persistent pupillary membrane
PRA - progressive retinal atrophy
Prolapse GT - prolapse gland of third eyelid
VKH - Vogt-Koyanagi-Harada-like syndrome, uveodermatologic syndrome

NO	OPTION	UNKNOWN
AFGHAN HOUND		
Cataract	Corneal dystrophy	Marg. corneal degeneration
AIREDALE TERRIER		
Corneal dystrophy	Distichiasis	Cataract
PRA	Entropion	Ret. dysplasia
	Pannus	Sclero-uveitis
AKITA		
Multi. defects	VKH	
PRA		
ALASKAN MALAMUTE		
Cataract		
Day blindness		
PRA		
Glaucoma		
AMERICAN STAFFORDSHIRE TERRIER		
Cataract	Entropion	
PHPV		
AMERICAN WATER SPANIEL		
Cataract	Ret. dysplasia -folds	
AUSTRALIAN CATTLE DOG		
PRA		Ret. dysplasia
Lens luxation		PHPV
Cataract		Vitreal degen.
		PPM
AUSTRALIAN KELPI		
PRA		Ret. dysplasia -folds
Cataract		Choroid. hypoplasia

NO	OPTION	UNKNOWN
AUSTRALIAN SHEPHERD		
Microphth./multi. defects	PPM	Corneal dystrophy
Coloboma/staphyloma		Ret. dysplasia -folds
Chorioret. hypoplplasia		
Cataract		
BASENJI		
PPM		Cataract
PRA		
ON coloboma		
BASSET GRIFFON VENDEEN, PETITE		
Ret. dysplasia -geographic	PPM	
	Ret. dysplasia -folds	
BASSET HOUND		
Glaucoma	Entropion	
	Ectropion	
BEAGLE		
Microphth./multi. defects	Prolapse GT	
	Tapetal degen.	
Glaucoma		
Cataract		
PRA		
BEARDED COLLIE		
Cataract	Ret. dysplasia -folds	
BEDLINGTON TERRIER		
Microphthalmia	Distichiasis	Lens luxation
Cataract	Imperf. puncta	
Ret. dysplasia -geog./detach.	Ret. dysplasia -folds	
BELGIAN MALINOIS		
PRA		
BELGIAN SHEEPDOG		
Retinopathy		PRA
Pannus		Micropapilla
Cataract		
BELGIAN TERVUREN		
Cataract	Micropapilla	ON hyploplasia
PRA		
Pannus		
BERNESE MOUNTAIN DOG		
PRA	Entropion	
Cataract		
BICHON FRISE		
Cataract	Entropion	
	Corneal dyst.	
BLOODHOUND		
Entropion	Ectropion	
	Prolapse GT	
BORDER COLLIE		
Lens luxation		Distichiasis
CPRA		Corneal dystrophy
PRA		Cataract
CEA		
BORDER TERRIER		
Cataract		
PRA		
BORZOI		
Microphthal./multi. defects		
Cataract		
PRA		
Ret. degen.		
BOSTON TERRIER		
Endoth. dystrophy		Iris cyst
Cataract		Vitreal degen.
BOUVIER DES FLANDRES		
Cataract	Entropion	
Glaucoma		
BOXER		
	Distichiasis	
	Prolapse GT	
	Corneal erosion	
	Nonpig.3rd lid	
BRIARD		
Cataract		
PRA		
CPRA		
Night blindness		

NO	OPTION	UNKNOWN
BRITTANY		
Cataract		Vitreal degen.
Lens luxation		Glaucoma
PRA		
BRUSSELS GRIFFON		
Cataract	Ectopic cilia	
PRA		
BULLDOG		
	Entropion	Ret. dysplasia
	Ectropion	-folds
	Exp. keratop.	
	Distichiasis	
	Dry eye	
	Ectop. cilia	
	Prolapse GT	
BULLMASTIFF		
Glaucoma	Entropion	
	Distichiasis	
	PPM	
	Ret. dysplasia	
BULL TERRIER		
	Entropion	
	Ectropion	
CAIRN TERRIER		
Cataract		
Glaucoma		
-pigmentary		
CAVALIER KING CHARLES SPANIEL		
Cataract	Entropion	
Microphth.	Corneal dystrophy	
Ret. dysplasia	Expos. keratop.	
-geog/detach.	Ret. dysplasia	
	-folds	
	Distichiasis	
CHESAPEAKE BAY RETRIEVER		
Cataract	Entropion	
PRA	Distichiasis	
Ret. dysplasia		
-folds/geographic		
CHIHUAHUA		
Endoth. dyst.		Lens luxation
PRA		

NO	OPTION	UNKNOWN
CHOW CHOW		
Glaucoma	Entropion	
PRA		
PPM		
CLUMBER SPANIEL		
	Ectropion	
	Entropion	
	Macrobleph.	
COCKER SPANIEL (AMERICAN)		
PRA	Ret. dysplasia	
Cataract (cortical)	-focal	
Glaucoma	Corneal dystrophy	
Ret. dysplasia	PPM	
-geog/detach.	Dry eye	
	Prolapse GT	
	Ectropion	
	Distichiasis	
	Imperf. puncta	
COLLIE		
Microph.	Distichiasis	Corneal dystrophy
CEA	Entropion	NGE
PRA	PPM	
Rod/cone dysp.	Ret. dysplasia	
Rod/cone degen.	-folds	
COONHOUND		
Entropion	Ectropion	
CURLY-COATED RETRIEVER		
Cataract	Entropion	
PRA	Ectropion	
DACHSHUND		
Dermoid		Punct. keratitis
Endo. dystrophy		
PK		
Cataract		
PRA		
Multi. defects		
DALMATIAN		
Glaucoma	Distichiasis	Pannus
	Entropion	PRA
	Dermoid	Microphthal./
		multi. defects
		PPM

NO	OPTION	UNKNOWN
DANDIE DINMONT TERRIER		
Cataract		
Glaucoma		
DOBERMAN PINSCHER		
Cataract	Entropion	
PHPV	Evert. cartilage 3rd lid	
PRA		
Microphth./multi. defects		
DOGO ARGENTINO		
Cataract		
ENGLISH COCKER SPANIEL		
Cataract	Ectropion	Glaucoma
PRA	Distichiasis	
	PPM	
	Ret. dysplasia -folds	
	Imperf. puncta	
ENGLISH SETTER		
Macroblepharon	Ectropion	
PRA		
ENGLISH SPRINGER SPANIEL		
Cataract	Entropion	
Ret. dysplasia		
PRA		
ENGLISH TOY SPANIEL		
Cataract	Entropion	
	Corneal dystrophy	
	Ret. dysplasia -folds	
FIELD SPANIEL		
Cataract	Ret. dysplasia -folds/geographic	
PRA		
FLAT-COATED RETRIEVER		
Cataract	Entropion	
PRA	Distichiasis	

NO	OPTION	UNKNOWN
FOX TERRIER		
Glaucoma		
Cataract		
Lens luxation		
FRENCH BULLDOG		
Cataract	Distichiasis	
	Entropion	
GERMAN SHEPHERD DOG		
Cataract (congen.)	Evert. cart. 3rd eyelid	Corneal dystrophy
Cataract (cortical)		Dermoid
PRA		
ON hypop./micropap		
Ret dysplasia -folds/geographic		
GERMAN SHORTHAIRED POINTER		
Cataract	Entropion	
PRA	Evert. cartilage 3rd lid	
GERMAN WIREHAIRED POINTER		
	Entropion	
GIANT SCHNAUZER		
Cataract	Ret. dysplasia -folds	Goniodysgenesis
PRA		PHPV
		Vitreal degeneration
GOLDEN RETRIEVER		
Cataract	Entropion	Glaucoma
PRA	Distichiasis	Ret. dysplasia
CPRA		Iris cysts
		Pigmentary uveitis
GORDON SETTER		
Cataract		
Dry eye		
Entropion/macroblepharon		
PRA		
GREAT DANE		
Cataract	Evert. cartilage 3rd lid	
Multi. defects/ albinism	Entropion	
PRA	Ectropion	
Glaucoma		

NO	OPTION	UNKNOWN
GREAT PYRENEES		
PRA	Entropion	
	Ectropion	
GREYHOUND		
Cataract	Pannus	
PRA		
HAVANESE		
Cataract		
PRA		
Ret. detach.		
IBIZAN HOUND		
Cataract		
IRISH SETTER		
Cataract	Entropion	Evert. cartilage 3rd lid
PRA		PPM
Rod-cone dysp.		PHPV
Late form PRA		Distichiasis
IRISH TERRIER		
PRA		
IRISH WATER SPANIEL		
Cataract		
PRA		
IRISH WOLFHOUND		
Cataract	Entropion	
	Evert. cartilage 3rd lid	
ITALIAN GREYHOUND		
Cataract	Vitreal degen.	
Glaucoma		
PRA		
JACK RUSSELL TERRIER		
Lens luxation		
JAPANESE CHIN		
Cataract	Distichiasis	
PRA		
KEESHOND		
Cataract		
CPRA		
PRA		
Glaucoma		

NO	OPTION	UNKNOWN
KERRY BLUE TERRIER		
Cataract	Entropion	
PRA		
KOMONDOR		
Entropion		Ectropion
Cataract		Distichiasis
		Prolapse GT
KUVASZ		
	Entropion	Ectropion
		Distichiasis
		Prolapse GT
		Cataract
		Evert. cartilage 3rd lid
LABRADOR RETRIEVER		
Cataract	Entropion	Corneal dyst.
PRA	Distichiasis	PHA
CPRA		PHPV
Ret. dysplasia		PTVL
Ret. dysplasia/ skeletal defects		
LHASA APSO		
Dry eye	Distichiasis	Ciliated caruncle
PRA	Entropion	
Cataract	Ectopic cilia	
Expos. keratop.	Prolapse GT	
LOWCHEN		
Cataract		
PRA		
MALTESE		
PRA	Distichiasis	Ciliated caruncle
MANCHESTER TERRIER (STANDARD)		
Cataract	Vitreal degeneration	
Lens luxation		
PRA		
MANCHESTER TERRIER (TOY)		
Cataract		
Lens luxation		
PRA		

NO	OPTION	UNKNOWN
MASTIFF		
PRA	PPM Ret. dysplasia -folds Entropion Ectropion Macrobleph.	Expos. keratopathy Distichiasis Prolapse GT Cataract Evert. cartilage 3rd lid Iris cysts
MINIATURE BULL TERRIER		
Lens luxation	Entropion PPM	
MINIATURE PINSCHER		
Corneal lipid dystrophy Cataract PRA		
MINIATURE SCHNAUZER		
Cataract Congen. catract/ microphthalmia PRA		Low amp. ERG
NEAPOLITAN MASTIFF		
Cataract PRA	Entropion Ectropion/ macrobleph. Dermoid Evert. cartilage 3rd lid Prolapse GT PPM	
NEWFOUNDLAND		
Cataract	Ectropion Macrobleph. Entropion Evert. cartilage 3rd lid	
NORBOTTENSPETS		
Cataract	PPM	
NORWEGIAN ELKHOUND		
Glaucoma Lens luxation PRA rod dysplasia early rod degen. Cataract	Entropion	

NO	OPTION	UNKNOWN
NOVA SCOTIA DUCK TOLLING RETRIEVER		
PRA Cataract		
OLD ENGLISH SHEEPDOG		
Cataract PRA Ret. detachment Microphth./multi. defects	Distichiasis Entropion	Corneal dystrophy Scleral uveitis
PAPILLON		
Cataract	Entropion Corneal dyst.	
PEKINGESE		
Expos. keratop. PRA Cataract Dry eye	Distichiasis Entropion Ciliated caruncle	
POINTER		
Cataract PRA	Entropion	Corneal dystrophy Pannus Chronic superficial keratitis
POMERANIAN		
Cataract PRA	Entropion	
POODLE (TOY, MINIATURE, STANDARD)		
PRA Microphthalmia Glaucoma Entropion Micropapilla Cataract	Imperf. punct. Distichiasis	Ectopic cilia
PORTUGUESE WATER DOG		
Cataract PRA Microphthal./multi. congen. defects	Distichiasis PPM	

NO	OPTION	UNKNOWN
PUG		
	Distichiasis	Cataract
	Entropion	
	Exposure keratopathy	
PULI		
Cataract	PPM	
PRA	Ret. dysplasia -folds	
REDBONE HOUND		
Entropion	Ectropion	
RHODESIAN RIDGEBACK		
Cataract	Entropion	
PRA		
ROTTWEILER		
Iris coloboma	Entropion	
PRA	Distichiasis	
Cataract	Ret. dysplasia	
SAINT BERNARD		
Entropion	Ectropion	
Cataract	Distichiasis	
Multi. defects	Dermoid	
SALUKI		
Cataract		
		Entropion
		Ectropion
		Distichiasis
		Prolapse GT
		Evert. cartilage 3rd lid
SAMOYED		
PRA	Distichiasis	VKH
Cataract	Corneal dystrophy	Vitreal degen.
Glaucoma		
Ret. dysplasia/ skeletal defects		
SCHIPPERKE		
PRA		
Cataract		

NO	OPTION	UNKNOWN
SCOTTISH TERRIER		
Cataract	PPM	
Lens luxation		
PRA		
SEALYHAM TERRIER		
Cataract	Imperf. puncta	
Lens luxation		
Retinal dysplasia		
PRA		
SHAR-PEI		
Entropion	Prolapse GT	Cataract
Glaucoma		
Lens luxation		
PRA		
SHETLAND SHEEPDOG		
PRA	Distichiasis	ON coloboma (without choroid. hypopl.)
Choroid hypoplasia	PPM	
Corneal dystrophy		
Cataract		
Coloboma/staphyloma		
SHIBA INU		
Cataract	Corneal dyst. epithilial/ stroma	
PRA	Distichiasis	
ON hypoplasia/ micropapilla	PPM	
	Ret. dysplasia -folds	
SHIH TZU		
Cataract	Distichiasis	Dry eye
PRA	Ectop. cilia	Ret. detachment
	Exposure keratopathy	Ciliated caruncle
		Lagophthalmos
		ON hypoplasia
SIBERIAN HUSKY		
PRA	Entropion	VKH
Cataract		Uveitis
Corneal dystrophy		
Glaucoma		
SILKY TERRIER		
Cataract		
PRA		

NO	OPTION	UNKNOWN
SOFT-COATED WHEATEN TERRIER		
Cataract	PPM	
PRA		
SPINONI ITALIANI		
	Ectropion	
STAFFORDSHIRE BULL TERRIER		
Cataract	Entropion	
PHPV		
STANDARD SCHNAUZER		
Cataract	Ret. dysplasia	Dry eye
	-folds	
SUSSEX SPANIEL		
Cataract	Entropion	
	Ret. dysplasia	
	-folds	
SWISS MOUNTAIN DOG, GREATER		
	Distichiasis	
	Ectropion	
	Entropion	
TIBETAN TERRIER		
Cataract	Ret. dysplasia	PHPV
Lens luxation	-folds	Vitreous degen.
PRA		
Ret. dysplasia		
-geographic		
VIZSLA		
Cataract		Corneal dystrophy
Entropion		
PRA		
WEIMARANER		
	Distichiasis	
	Entropion	
	Evert. cartilage	
	3rd lid	
WELSH CORGI, CARDIGAN		
PRA	PPM	
CPRA	Retinal dysplasia	
	-focal/multifocal	
WELSH CORGI, PEMBROKE		
Cataract	Ret. dysplasia	
PPM	-folds	
PRA		
Ret. dysplasia		
-geographic		
WELSH SPRINGER SPANIEL		
Cataract		
PRA		
Glaucoma		
WELSH TERRIER		
Lens luxation		
Glaucoma		
WEST HIGHLAND WHITE TERRIER		
Dry eye		
Cataract		
WHIPPET		
Cataract	Vitreal	Corneal dystrophy
PRA	degen.	
Lens luxation		
YORKSHIRE TERRIER		
Dry eye	Entropion	
Cataract		
PRA		

INDEX

INDEX

INDEX

INDEX

INDEX

NOTES

NOTES